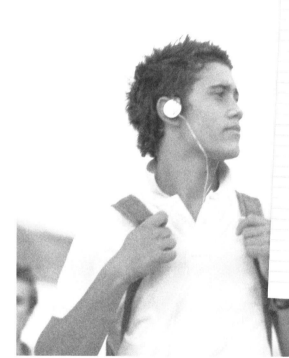

Pearson Nursing Reviews & Rationales

Pharmacology

Third Edition

SERIES EDITOR

MaryAnn Hogan, MSN, RN

Clinical Assistant Professor

School of Nursing

University of Massachusetts–Amherst

Amherst, Massachusetts

CONSULTING EDITORS

Sharon Burke, EdD, RN, CCRN, CEN

Assistant Professor

Thomas Jefferson University

Philadelphia, Pennsylvania

Margaret M. Gingrich, RN, MSN

Professor

Harrisburg Area Community College

Harrisburg, Pennsylvania

Traci Taylor, RN, MSN

Nursing Instructor

West Texas A&M University

Canyon, Texas

PEARSON

Boston   Columbus   Indianapolis   New York   San Francisco   Upper Saddle River
Amsterdam   Cape Town   Dubai   London   Madrid   Milan   Munich   Paris   Montréal   Toronto
Delhi   Mexico City   São Paulo   Sydney   Hong Kong   Seoul   Singapore   Taipei   Tokyo

Director of Readypoint™: Maura Connor
Executive Editor: Jennifer Farthing
Developmental Editor: Elisa Rogers
Editorial Assistant: Deirdre MacKnight
Director, Digital Product Development: Alex Marciante
Media Product Manager: Travis Moses-Westphal
Vice President, Director Sales & Marketing: David Gesell
Senior Marketing Manager: Phoenix Harvey
Marketing Coordinator: Michael Sirinides
Director of Media Production: Allyson Graesser

Media Project Manager: Rachel Collett
Managing Editor, Production: Patrick Walsh
Production Liaison: Maria Reyes
Production Editor: GEX Publishing Services
Manufacturing Manager: Ilene Sanford
Art Director/Cover Designer: Christopher Weigand
Cover Image: Blaj Gabriel/Shutterstock.com
Composition: GEX Publishing Services
Printer/Binder: Courier Kendallville
Cover Printer: Lehigh/Phoenix Color Hagerstown

Notice: Care has been taken to confirm the accuracy of the information presented in this book. The authors, editors, and the publisher, however, cannot accept any responsibility for errors or omissions or for the consequences for application of the information in this book and make no warranty, express or implied, with respect to its contents.

The authors and the publisher have exerted every effort to ensure that drug selections and dosages set forth in this text are in accord with current recommendations and practice at time of publication. However, in view of ongoing research, changes in government regulations, and the constant flow of information relating to drug therapy and drug reactions, the reader is urged to check the package inserts of all drugs for any change in indications of dosage and for added warnings and precautions. This is particularly important when the recommended agent is a new and/or infrequently employed drug.

The authors and publisher disclaim all responsibility for any liability, loss, injury, or damage incurred as a consequence, directly or indirectly, of the use and application of any of the contents of this volume.

Library of Congress Cataloging-in-Publication Data

Hogan, Mary Ann, MSN
  Pharmacology / MaryAnn Hogan; consulting editors, Sharon Burke, Margaret M.
Gingrich, Traci Taylor. -- 3rd ed.
      p. ; cm. -- (Pearson nursing reviews & rationales)
  Rev. ed. of: Pharmacology, c2008.
  Includes bibliographical references and index.
  ISBN-13: 978-0-13-304599-4 (pbk.)
  ISBN-10: 0-13-304599-4 (pbk.)
  I. Burke, Sharon Ogden. II. Gingrich, Margaret M. III. Taylor, Traci. IV. Title. V. Series:
Pearson nursing reviews & rationales series.
  [DNLM: 1. Pharmaceutical Preparations--Examination Questions. 2. Pharmaceutical
Preparations--Nurses' Instruction. 3. Pharmaceutical Preparations--Outlines. QV 18.2]
  LC Classification not assigned
  615.1'9--dc23
                              2012019904

10 9 8 7 6 5 4 3 2

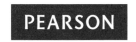

ISBN 10: 0-13-304599-4
ISBN 13: 978-0-13-304599-4

Contents

Welcome to the Pearson Nursing Reviews & Rationales Series!

This series has been specifically designed to provide a clear and concentrated review of important nursing knowledge in the following content areas:

- Anatomy & Physiology
- Nursing Fundamentals
- Nutrition & Diet Therapy
- Fluids, Electrolytes, & Acid–Base Balance
- Medical-Surgical Nursing
- Pathophysiology
- Pharmacology
- Maternal-Newborn Nursing
- Child Health Nursing
- Mental Health Nursing
- Health & Physical Assessment
- Leadership & Management

The books in this series are designed for use either by current nursing students as a study aid for nursing course work, for NCLEX-RN® exam preparation, or by practicing nurses seeking a comprehensive yet concise review of a nursing specialty or subject area.

This series is truly unique. One of its most special features is that it has been developed and reviewed by a large team of nurse educators from across the United States and Canada to ensure that each chapter is edited by a nurse expert in the content area under study. The series editor, MaryAnn Hogan, designed the overall series in collaboration with a core Pearson Education team to take full advantage of Pearson Education's cutting-edge technology. The consulting editors for each book, also experts in that specialty area, then reviewed all chapters and test questions submitted for comprehensiveness and accuracy. Finally, MaryAnn Hogan reviewed the chapters in each book for consistency, accuracy, and applicability to the NCLEX-RN® Test Plan.

All books in the series are identical in their overall design for your convenience. As an added value, each book comes with a comprehensive support package, including access to additional questions online, complete eText, and a tear-out *NursingNotes* card for clinical reference and quick review.

Study Tips

Use of this book should help simplify your review. To make the most of your valuable study time, also follow these simple but important suggestions:

1. Use a weekly calendar to schedule study sessions.
   - Outline the timeframes for all of your activities (home, school, appointments, etc.) on a weekly calendar.
   - Find the "holes" in your calendar, which are the times in which you can plan to study. Add study sessions to the calendar at times when you can expect to be mentally alert and follow your plan!
2. Create the optimal study environment.
   - Eliminate external sources of distraction, such as television, telephone, etc.
   - Eliminate internal sources of distraction, such as hunger, thirst, or dwelling on items or problems that cannot be worked on at the moment.
   - Take a break for 10 minutes or so after each hour of concentrated study both as a reward and an incentive to keep studying.
3. Use prereading strategies to increase comprehension of chapter material.
   - Skim read the headings in the chapter (because they identify chapter content).
   - Read the definitions of key terms, which will help you learn new words to comprehend chapter information.
   - Review all graphic aids (figures, tables, boxes) because they are often used to explain important points in the chapter.

4. Read the chapter thoroughly but at a reasonable speed.
   - Comprehension and retention are actually enhanced by not reading too slowly.
   - Do take the time to reread any section that is unclear to you.
5. Summarize what you have learned.
   - Use the accompanying online resource, NursingReviewsandRationales.com, to test yourself with hundreds of NCLEX-RN®-style practice questions.
   - Review again any sections that correspond to questions you answered incorrectly or incompletely.

Test-Taking Strategies

Test-taking strategies accompany the rationales for every question in the series. These strategies will assist you to select the correct answer by breaking down the question, even if you don't know the correct response. Use the following strategies to increase your success on nursing tests or examinations:

- Get sufficient sleep and have something to eat before taking a test. Avoid eating concentrated sweets, though, to prevent rapid upward and then downward surges in your blood glucose. Avoid also high-fat foods that will make you sleepy.
- Take deep breaths during the test as needed. Remember, the brain requires oxygen and glucose as fuel.
- Read the question carefully, identifying the stem, the 4 options, and any key words or phrases in either the stem or options.
  - Key words in the stem such as "most important" indicate the need to set priorities, since more than one option is likely to contain a statement that is technically correct.
  - Remember that the presence of absolute words such as "never" or "only" in an answer option is more likely to make that option incorrect.
- Determine who is the client in the question; often this is the person with the health problem, but it may also be a significant other, relative, friend, or another nurse.
- Decide whether the stem is a true response stem or a false response stem. With a true response stem, the correct answer will be a true statement, and vice-versa.

- Determine what the question is really asking, sometimes referred to as the issue of the question. Evaluate all answer options in relation to this issue, and not strictly to the "correctness" of the statement in each individual option.
- Eliminate options that are obviously incorrect, then go back and reread the stem. Evaluate the remaining options against the stem once more to make a final selection.
- If two answers seem similar and correct, try to decide whether one of them is more global or comprehensive. If the global option includes the alternative option within it, it is likely that the more global response is the correct answer.

The NCLEX-RN® Licensing Examination

Upon graduation from a nursing program, successful completion of the NCLEX-RN® licensing examination is required to begin professional nursing practice. The NCLEX-RN® licensing examination is a Computer Adaptive Test (CAT) that ranges in length from 75 to 265 individual (stand-alone) test items, depending on your performance during the examination. The blueprint for the exam is reviewed and revised every three years by the National Council of State Boards of Nursing using the results of a job analysis study of new graduate nurses practicing within the first six months after graduation. Each question on the exam is coded to a *Client Need Category* and an *Integrated Process*.

Client Need Categories There are four categories of client needs, and each exam will contain a minimum and maximum percent of questions from each category. Each major category has subcategories within it. The *Client Needs* categories according to the NCLEX-RN® Test Plan effective April 2010 are as follows:

- Safe, Effective Care Environment
  - Management of Care (16–22%)
  - Safety and Infection Control (8–14%)
- Health Promotion and Maintenance (6–12%)
- Psychosocial Integrity (6–12%)
- Physiological Integrity
  - Basic Care and Comfort (6–12%)
  - Pharmacological and Parenteral Therapies (13–19%)
  - Reduction of Risk Potential (10–16%)
  - Physiological Adaptation (11–17%)

Integrated Processes   The integrated processes identified on the NCLEX-RN® Test Plan effective April 2010, with condensed definitions, are as follows:

- Nursing Process: a scientific problem-solving approach used in nursing practice; consisting of assessment, analysis, planning, implementation, and evaluation.
- Caring: client–nurse interaction(s) characterized by mutual respect and trust and that are directed toward achieving desired client outcomes.
- Communication and Documentation: verbal and/or nonverbal interactions between nurse and others (client, family, health care team); a written or electronic recording of activities or events that occur during client care.
- Teaching/Learning: facilitating client's acquisition of knowledge, skills, and attitudes that lead to behavior change.

More detailed information about this examination may be obtained by visiting the National Council of State Boards of Nursing website at http://www.ncsbn.org and viewing the *2010 NCLEX-RN® Detailed Test Plan.*[1]

[1]Reference: National Council of State Boards of Nursing, Inc. *2010 NCLEX Test Plan.* Effective April, 2010. Retrieved from http://www.ncsbn.org/2010_NCLEX_RN_TestPlan.pdf.

HOW TO GET THE MOST OUT OF THIS BOOK

Each chapter has the following elements to guide you during review and study:

Chapter Objectives describe what you will be able to know or do after learning the material covered in the chapter.

Objectives

➤ Describe general goals of therapy when administering gastrointestinal system medications.
➤ Describe the use and side effects of antacids.
➤ Identify the actions of various forms of laxatives.
➤ Discuss the effects of H_2-receptor antagonists, proton pump inhibitors, and mucosal protectants on the gastrointestinal tract.
➤ Describe nursing considerations related to administration of antiemetics.

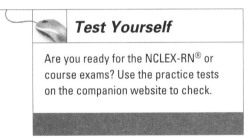

Test Yourself

Are you ready for the NCLEX-RN® or course exams? Use the practice tests on the companion website to check.

Review at a Glance contains a glossary of key terms used in the chapter, with definitions provided up-front and available at your fingertips, to help you stay focused and make the best use of your study time.

Review at a Glance

antacid agent that reduces or neutralizes acidity

anticholinergic antagonist to parasympathetic action or other cholinergic receptors

antispasmodic agent that prevents or relieves spasms

cathartic agent with purgative action

H_2 antagonist antagonist agent against histamine that decreases gastrin secretion

Helicobacter pylori bacteria found in gastric mucosa that produces urease and is associated commonly with gastric and duodenal ulcers

laxative agent used to cause a bowel movement or loosening of the bowels

surfactant a surface-active agent also known as a wetting agent, tension depressant, detergent, and emulsifier

Pretest provides a 10-question quiz as a sample overview of the material covered in the chapter and helps you decide in what areas you need the most—or the least—review.

PRETEST

1 After a 2-year-old ingested a full bottle of children's aspirin, the parent gives the child 2 doses of ipecac syrup found hidden at the back of the medicine cabinet and then rushes the child to the urgent care clinic. It has been over 40 minutes and the child has not vomited. What should the nurse be prepared to do at this time?

1. Call poison control center.
2. Administer activated charcoal.
3. Offer milk or carbonated soda.
4. Explain that ipecac is no longer sold over the counter.

Practice to Pass questions are open ended, stimulate critical thinking, and reinforce mastery of the chapter information.

Practice to Pass

What GI drug has been withdrawn by the Food and Drug Administration because of adverse effects of QT prolongation?

NCLEX® Alert identifies concepts that are likely to be tested on the NCLEX-RN® examination. Be sure to learn the information highlighted wherever you see this icon.

Case Study, found at the end of the chapter, provides an opportunity for you to use your critical thinking and clinical reasoning skills to "put it all together." It describes a true-to-life client case situation and asks you open-ended questions about how you would provide care for that client and/or family.

Case Study

A 45-year-old male client comes to the nurse practitioner stating he wakes often at night with coughing and burning he describes as heartburn. He drinks 1–2 alcoholic beverages per evening, usually with distilled liquor, and then wine with dinner. He eats heavy dinners with dessert. He prefers mint ice cream and coffee for dessert. The nurse practitioner prescribes a regimen with omeprazole (Prilosec) every morning and Maalox 30 mL qid.

1. How will you instruct the client about gastroesophageal reflux disease and its relationship to symptoms?
2. What will you instruct the client about his diet, particularly the evening meal?
3. What medication will be prescribed if the client is diagnosed with *H. pylori*?
4. How will you instruct the client about his medications?

For suggested responses, see page 543.

Posttest provides an additional 10-question quiz at the end of the chapter. It provides you with feedback about mastery of the chapter material following review and study. All pretest and posttest questions contain comprehensive rationales for the correct and incorrect answers, and are coded according to cognitive level of difficulty, NCLEX-RN® Test Plan category of client need, and integrated process.

POSTTEST

1 When the nurse teaches a client about the side effects of anticholinergic medications, what signs or symptoms should be included?

1. Urinary retention, constipation, or dilated pupils
2. Pupillary constriction, bronchoconstriction, or bradycardia
3. Inability to obtain an erection, irregular heart rhythm
4. Increased salivation, dysphagia, confusion, restlessness

NCLEX-RN® Test Prep: NursingReviewsandRationales.com

For those who want to prepare for the NCLEX-RN®, practicing online will help you become more familiar with the computer-based testing experience, especially for new alternate item formats such as audio, media-enhanced, hot spot, and exhibit questions. With this new edition, use the code printed inside the front cover of the book to access Nursing Reviews & Rationales, which offers 800 practice questions using all NCLEX®-style formats. This includes the practice questions found in all chapters of the book as well as 30 additional questions per chapter. Nursing Reviews & Rationales allows you to choose the two ways to prepare for the NCLEX-RN®. Both approaches personalize your practice experience according to what stage you are at in your NCLEX® preparation.

Nursing Reviews & Rationales includes the eText version of *Pearson Nursing Pharmacology,* Third Edition. This eText is fully searchable and includes features like note-taking, highlighting, and more. The eText allows you to take your review with you anywhere you have an internet connection to NursingReviewsandRationales.com.

Pearson NursingNotes Card

This tear-out card provides a reference for frequently used facts and information related to the subject matter of the book. This is designed to be useful in the clinical setting, when quick and easy access to information is so important!

About the Pharmacology Book

Chapters in this book cover "need-to-know" information about medications that belong to a wide variety of drug classes and associated nursing management. The first chapter reviews general principles of pharmacology with an emphasis on safety. Chapters 2 through 15 explore drug classes used to treat health problems that affect specific body systems. The final chapter explores the use of herbal agents as supplements and phytomedicines. Mastery of the information in this book and effective use of the test-taking strategies described will help you be confident and successful in testing situations, including the NCLEX-RN®, and in actual clinical practice.

Pharmacology is an ever-evolving field because drug therapy changes over time as new research evidence becomes available. Care has been taken to ensure that drug information in this book is accurate and current; however, this is a condensed review book, not a full pharmacology textbook or official drug reference. Before administering any medication, check the manufacturer's product literature to verify recommended dose, route, duration of therapy, and any contraindications. Neither the publisher nor the author assumes liability for any injury or damage arising from information contained in this condensed review book.

Acknowledgments

This book is a monumental effort of collaboration. Without the contributions of many individuals, this edition of *Pharmacology: Reviews and Rationales* would not have been possible. Thank you to all the contributors and reviewers who devoted their time and talents to the third edition. The contributors for this edition are Sharon Burke, EdD, RN, CCRN, CEN, Thomas Jefferson University, Philadelphia, Pennsylvania; Margaret M. Gingrich, RN, MSN, Harrisburg Area Community College, Harrisburg, Pennsylvania; Traci Taylor, RN, MSN, Nursing Instructor, West Texas A&M University, Canyon, Texas. The reviewers for this edition are Nathaniel M. Apatoy, MHS, MSN, PhD, CRNA, University of Miami, Coral Gables, Florida; Ilene Borze, MS, RN, Gateway Community College, Phoenix, Arizona.

Thanks also to the contributors and reviewers who assisted with the previous editions of this book: Julie A. Adkins, RN, MSN, FNP, Private Practice, West Frankfort, Illinois; Carolyn M. Burger, MSN, RN, C, OCN, Miami University, Middletown, Ohio; Janet Courtney, RN, MSN, Holyoke Community College, Holyoke, Massachusetts; Joseann Helmes DeWitt, MSN, RN, C, CLNC, Alcorn State University, Natchez, Mississippi; Suzanne Kay Marnocha, PhD, RN, MSN, CCRN, University of Wisconsin, Oshkosh, Wisconsin; Caron Martin, MSN, RN, Northern Kentucky University, Highland Heights, Kentucky; Lee Murray, MSN, RN, CS, CADAC, Holyoke Community College, Holyoke, Massachusetts; Lynn Wemett Nicholls, PhD, RN, St. John Fisher College, Rochester, New York; Donna Polverini, RN, MS, America International College, Springfield, Massachusetts; Roni Ruhlandt, MSN, RN, CCRN, CNRN, University of Phoenix, Grand Rapids, Michigan; Susan K. Steele, MN, RN, AOCN, Clinical Nurse Specialist General Health System, Clinical Instructor, Southeastern Louisiana University College of Nursing, Hammond, Louisiana; Bethany Hawes Sykes, EdD, RN, CEN, Salve Regina University, Newport, Rhode Island; Geralyn M. Frandsen, EdD, MSN, RN, Maryville University, St. Louis, Missouri; Daryle Wane, MS, APRN, BC, Pasco-Hernando Community College, New Port Richey, Florida; Skip Davis, PhD, MSN, BSN, San Francisco State University, San Francisco, California; Pattie Garrett Clark, RN, MSN, Abraham Baldwin College, Tifton, Georgia; Janice Hausauer, MSN, BSN, ANCC-FNP, Montana State University, Bozeman, Montana; Mercy Popoola, RN, CND, PhD, Georgia Southern University, Statesboro, Georgia; Anita K. Reed, BSN, MSN, St. Joseph College, Rensselaer, Indiana. Their work will surely assist both students and practicing nurses alike to extend their knowledge in the area of pharmacology.

I owe a special debt of gratitude to the wonderful team at Pearson Nursing for their enthusiasm for this project, as well as their good humor, expertise, and encouragement as the series developed. Maura Connor, Director of Readypoint™, was unending in her creativity, support, encouragement, and belief in the need for this series. Jennifer Farthing, Executive Editor, Readypoint™, coordinated this revision with insight, talent, and zeal, and fostered a culture of true collaboration and teamwork. Elisa Rogers, Developmental Editor, devoted many long hours to coordinating different facets of this project. Her high standards and attention to detail contributed greatly to the final "look" of the book. Editorial Assistant, Deirdre MacKnight, helped to keep the project moving forward on a day-to-day basis, and I am grateful for her efforts as well. A very special thank you goes to the designers of the book and the production team, led by Patrick Walsh, Managing Editor, who brought the ideas and manuscript into final form.

Thank you to the team at GEX Publishing Services, led by Project Coordinator Kelly Morrison, for the detail-oriented work of creating this book. I greatly appreciate their hard work, attention to detail, and spirit of collaboration.

Finally, I would like to acknowledge and gratefully thank my children, Michael Jr., Kathryn, Kristen, and William, who sacrificed precious hours of family time so this book could be revised. I would also like to thank my students, past and present, for continuing to inspire me with their quest for knowledge and passion for nursing. You are the future!

–MaryAnn Hogan

Basic Principles and Safety in Pharmacology

1

Chapter Outline

Pharmacology and the
  Nursing Process
Legal Regulation
Prescription and
  Nonprescription Medications

Medication Classification
  Systems
Terminology Related to
  Pharmacology

Issues Related to
  Medication Administration

Objectives

➤ Describe legal regulatory issues related to medication
  administration.
➤ Identify the difference between generic and trade names.
➤ Identify differences between prescription and over-the-counter
  medications.
➤ Define terms commonly used in pharmacology.
➤ Describe differences between a side effect and an adverse or toxic
  effect of a medication.
➤ Describe factors that affect medication absorption and response.
➤ List the rights of safe medication administration.
➤ Calculate medication dosages accurately.
➤ Explain nurses' roles and responsibilities related to client education
  regarding medication therapy.
➤ Describe cultural considerations related to medication therapy and
  associated client education.

NCLEX-RN® Test Prep

Use the accompanying online resource,
NursingReviewsandRationales, to test
yourself with hundreds of NCLEX®-style
practice questions.

Review at a Glance

absorption what happens to a drug
from the time it is introduced into the
body until it reaches the circulating fluids
and tissues
biotransformation enzymatic
alteration of drug structure; often takes
place in liver; also called drug
metabolism
critical concentration amount
of a drug needed to cause a therapeutic
effect
distribution movement of a drug to
body tissues following absorption

drug chemical that is introduced into
body to cause some sort of change; used
interchangeably with the term *medication*
drug abuse use of a drug in a
fashion inconsistent with medical or
social norms
drug metabolism enzymatic
alteration of drug structure; most drug
metabolism takes place in liver; also
called biotransformation
excretion removal of a drug from
body, such as via skin, saliva, lungs, bile,
kidneys, or feces

first-pass effect a phenomenon
that occurs following ingestion of an oral
drug in which a large percentage of drug
is destroyed in the gastrointestinal
system and never reaches tissues
half-life the time it takes for the amount
of drug in the body to decrease to one-half
of the peak level it previously achieved
negligence failure to provide care
that a reasonable person would provide
in a similar circumstance
pharmacodynamics process of
how a drug affects the body

pharmacogenetics area of pharmacology that examines how heredity affects one's response to drug therapy

pharmacokinetics process of how the body acts on a drug

pharmacology study of drugs and their interactions with living systems

pharmacotherapeutics branch of pharmacology that involves the use of drugs to treat, prevent, or diagnose

disease; also known as clinical pharmacology

selective toxicity ability of a drug, such as penicillin, to attack only those systems found in foreign cells

PRETEST

1 When administering medication to a hospitalized client who is awake and carrying on a conversation with visitors, what would be the most accurate way for the nurse to check this client's identity?

1. Ask the client, "Are you Dale Jones?"
2. Ask the client, "Can you tell me your name and date of birth?"
3. Check the client's room number and bed assignment.
4. Match the medication with the client's diagnosis.

2 The mother of the pediatric client asks the nurse, "What is the difference between Advil and ibuprofen? I can buy ibuprofen at a cheaper price, but the instructions from the clinic say to use Children's Advil Liquid." What would be the nurse's best response?

1. "Similarities do exist, but the liquid medication is a different formulation designed for children."
2. "There is no difference between Advil and ibuprofen."
3. "Advil and ibuprofen are 2 different drugs with similar effects."
4. "You need to talk to the health care provider that prescribed the drug."

3 A pregnant client tells the clinic nurse at the first prenatal visit that she heard it is good to take an over-the-counter (OTC) iron preparation during pregnancy. Which statement by the nurse would be the best response?

1. "You should not take any OTC products during pregnancy."
2. "Most prenatal vitamins contain iron."
3. "It is safe to take iron during pregnancy, but tell your health care provider you are using it; many prenatal vitamins also contain iron."
4. "There may be staining of your baby's first teeth if you take this medication during pregnancy."

4 A client taking diltiazem hydrochloride (Cardizem) 30 mg by mouth 4 times per day is experiencing symptoms of toxicity. Which intervention by the nurse should take highest priority?

1. Assess for elevation of body temperature.
2. Evaluate rate, depth, and regularity of respirations.
3. Assess for weight loss by obtaining a daily weight.
4. Evaluate client's intake of grapefruit juice.

5 The nurse is caring for a 78-year-old client who has multiple medications ordered to treat various health problems. The nurse considers that which common age-related physical changes are most likely to require a reduction in medication dosage for this client?

1. Increased rate of drug retention
2. Decreased total body fluid proportionate to body mass
3. Decreased efficiency in drug distribution
4. Decreased rate of drug metabolism by the liver
5. Significant weight gain

6 A 3-year-old client weighing 33 pounds is to receive liquid ibuprofen (Advil) 150 mg PO q6h prn for temperature above 101°F. The nurse should administer how many mL to the client from a bottle labeled 100 mg/5 mL? Provide a numeric answer.

_____ mL

7 A client receiving nadolol (Corgard) for hypertension tells the nurse, "I get dizzy when I stand up." What is the most appropriate response by the nurse?

1. "This is an expected side effect of the drug, and you should use caution and move slowly when standing up."
2. "You may be experiencing a toxic effect of the drug, and I will notify the physician."
3. "Dizziness is not related to the drug, but I will need to ask you a few more questions."
4. "Episodes of dizziness when moving are common symptoms of elevated blood pressure."

8 An older adult client is given a prescription for celecoxib (Celebrex) to treat pain and stiffness from osteoarthritis of the hips and back. The nurse should take which action first?

1. Complete a thorough medication assessment to see what other drugs the client is taking.
2. Provide client with a printed pamphlet describing the drug and its uses.
3. Inform client where a medication organizer can be purchased.
4. Give short, simple, verbal explanation about drug and its side effects.

9 The medication administration record shows that a client is to receive lisinopril (Zestril) 10 mg PO at 9:00 a.m. On hand are tablets labeled fosinopril (Monopril) 20 mg. What action should the nurse take next?

1. Give 1 tablet of Monopril from the drug supply.
2. Give one-half tablet of Monopril from drug supply.
3. Ask client if the 20 mg tablet looks familiar.
4. Read original physician order to verify the drug order.

10 The nurse plans to administer oral medication for hypertension to a client. To safely administer the medications, in which order should the nurse complete the following interventions?

1. Review client's medication history and drug allergies.
2. Record drug administration in medication administration record.
3. Identify the client and explain the intended action of the medications.
4. Administer medication after verifying proper drug, route, time, and dose.
5. Obtain medication and compare the drug label against the healthcare provider's order.

➤ *See pages 19–21 for Answers and Rationales.*

I. PHARMACOLOGY AND THE NURSING PROCESS

A. Assessment of client

1. Client's current condition, health history, and presence of factors that are relative or absolute contraindications for some drugs (i.e., pregnancy, lactation, liver or renal disease)
2. Client's history of allergies
3. Drug history, including prescription and over-the-counter (OTC) medications, herbal therapies, home remedies, and recreational drugs
4. Lifestyle factors that could affect medications, including caffeine intake and nicotine use, alcohol consumption, and dietary patterns (number of meals per day and food restrictions)
5. Client's ability to swallow oral medications
6. Client's understanding of purpose of medication(s), how to self-administer, adverse effects to report, and routine follow-up care

B. Assessment of drug
  1. Medication prescription
  2. Need for conversion when preparing drug dose

C. Analysis/nursing diagnosis
  1. Risk for Injury
     a. Can occur if client takes a medication to which he or she is hypersensitive (allergic)
     b. Can occur if medication is taken incorrectly
        1) An insufficient dose will lead to development of signs and symptoms of original disorder
        2) An excessive dose can lead to signs and symptoms of toxicity or other adverse effects
  2. Deficient Knowledge
     a. Is often pertinent when a client is given a prescription for a new medication
     b. Should also be assessed with each client encounter to ensure ongoing knowledge
     c. Insufficient knowledge of medication therapy may lead to suboptimal results of therapy or other complications

D. Planning/goal setting
  1. Client will remain free of injury
  2. Client will verbalize purpose of medication, how to take it, expected effects, side effects and adverse effects, and proper storage of medication
  3. Client will respond appropriately to medication

E. Implementation
  1. Review medication prescription for completeness and accuracy
  2. Determine client history of allergies
  3. Review client's condition for which medication is ordered
  4. Measure client's vital signs if indicated
  5. Determine need for conversion when calculating correct dose of medication
  6. Prepare and administer medication dose correctly
  7. Determine client's understanding of the prescribed medication
  8. Teach client about medication, including name, dose, route, frequency, purpose, any follow-up lab work, side/adverse effects including when to notify prescriber, and how to store medication properly
  9. Document medication administration
  10. Assess and document client's response to medication

F. Evaluation
  1. Client receives correct medication and dosage
  2. Client's vital signs remain within normal limits
  3. Client responds appropriately to medication
  4. Client does not experience adverse effects of medication

II. LEGAL REGULATION

A. Food and Drug Administration (FDA)
  1. An agency of the United States Department of Health and Human Services (USDHHS) that regulates development and sale of **drugs** (chemicals that exert an effect on body) to assure safety and efficacy
  2. Drug legislation in Canada includes the Canadian Food and Drugs Act and the Canadian Controlled Drugs and Substances Act
  3. Controls the process of scientific testing to evaluate therapeutic and toxic effects of a chemical that may potentially become a drug/medication

Box 1-1	
Phases of Drug Development	***Investigational Drug Studies:*** New drugs must be tested *in vitro* and using animal studies prior to testing in humans; allows for determination of presumed effects on living tissue and also adverse effects. ***Phase 1 Clinical Trials:*** A tightly controlled study is conducted that involves the use of healthy human volunteers to test the drug. ***Phase 2 Clinical Trials:*** The drug is administered to clients who have the disease that the drug was intended to treat. ***Phase 3 Clinical Trials:*** The drug is used in the clinical setting to determine any unanticipated effects or lack of effectiveness. ***Food and Drug Administration (FDA) Approval:*** Drugs that complete Phase 3 are evaluated by the FDA after submission of a New Drug Application (NDA), and if FDA approval is received, the drug may be marketed. ***Phase 4 Post-Marketing Surveillance:*** A phase that involves continual evaluation of the drug following approval for marketing.

4. Phases of drug development
   a. A drug must pass through several stages of development before receiving final FDA approval to be marketed to public
   b. Stages of development include preclinical research, Phase I clinical trials, Phase II clinical trials, Phase III clinical trials, FDA approval, and post-marketing surveillance (Phase IV) (Box 1-1)
5. Generic formulations of currently marketed drugs may be approved using an expedited process known as an Abbreviated New Drug Application
6. In 2002, the USDHHS reauthorized the Prescription Drug User Fee Act of 1992 and provided resources to review drug applications in an expedited fashion

B. **Controlled substances**
   1. Are substances that are considered to have potential for **drug abuse**, use of the substance in a manner inconsistent with medical or social norms
   2. The Comprehensive Drug Abuse Prevention and Control Act (also known as the Controlled Substance Act) of 1970 regulates the manufacturing, distribution, and dispensing of drugs that are known to have abuse potential
   3. The FDA studies a drug and determines its abuse potential
   4. The Drug Enforcement Agency (DEA), a part of the Department of Justice, enforces the control of a drug
   5. The DEA monitors the prescription, distribution, storage, and use of a controlled substance in an attempt to decrease substance abuse of prescribed medications
   6. Controlled substances are assigned to one of 5 DEA schedules based on their potential for abuse and physical and psychological dependence (Box 1-2 and Box 1-3)

C. **Pregnancy categories (Box 1-4)**
   1. Are guidelines for use of a particular drug during pregnancy
   2. Indicate a drug's potential or actual teratogenic or adverse effects on the fetus
   3. FDA requires that each new drug be assigned a pregnancy category
   4. FDA recommends that no drug be administered during pregnancy regardless of pregnancy category, unless the drug's benefit clearly outweighs the risks of use

Box 1-2	
DEA Schedules of Controlled Substances	***Schedule I:*** High abuse potential and no accepted medical use ***Schedule II:*** High abuse potential with severe dependence liability ***Schedule III:*** Less abuse potential than Schedule II drugs and moderate dependence liability ***Schedule IV:*** Less abuse potential than Schedule III drugs and limited dependence liability ***Schedule V:*** Limited abuse potential

Box 1-3	**Schedule I:** Heroine, marijuana, cocaine
Examples of Controlled Substances by DEA Schedule	**Schedule II:** Opioids, amphetamines, barbiturates
	Schedule III: Nonbarbiturate sedatives, nonamphetamine stimulants, limited amounts of certain opioids
	Schedule IV: Some sedatives, nonopioid analgesics, antianxiety agents
	Schedule V: Drugs that may contain small amounts of opioids such as codeine, used as antitussives or antidiarrheals

D. Investigational medications and informed consent

1. *Informed consent*: an autonomous decision made by a specific individual based on the nature of the condition, treatment options, and risks involved
2. The client must be competent to give consent for procedures and treatment
3. Informed consent should be in writing; it should include explanation of procedure, medication, or treatment; description of benefits and harmful results; and an opportunity for client to ask questions
4. Information should be written in language understandable to the client
5. Consent must be obtained by the medical practitioner ordering the medication, treatment, or procedure
6. The nurse administering a medication explains the drug's purpose and answers questions the client may have
7. A client has the right to decline information and waive the informed consent and undergo treatment; this decision must be documented in the medical record
8. During urgent medical or surgical intervention, such as severe bleeding, fractured skull, or gunshot or stab wounds, an informed consent can be waived
9. When the client is a minor, unconscious, or incompetent, consent must be obtained from a responsible family member or legal guardian
10. When a nurse is involved in the informed consent process, in most states the nurse is only responsible for witnessing the client's signature on the informed consent form
11. The most common concern in the use of investigational drugs is that all adverse effects have not been identified; the client is not able to be fully informed about these; therefore, the decision-making process is not ideal
12. A placebo-controlled study implements the use of placebos on certain clients; neither the research staff nor the client know whether the client receives a placebo or an actual drug

Practice to Pass

A pregnant client experiences occasional headaches and backaches. She asks you what over-the-counter (OTC) medication she can take to relieve these discomforts. How will you respond?

Box 1-4	**Category A:** Controlled human studies in pregnant women fail to demonstrate a risk to the fetus in the first trimester of pregnancy, and there is no evidence of risk in later trimesters.
Pregnancy Categories	**Category B:** Animal studies have not demonstrated a risk to the fetus but there are no adequate studies in pregnant women. Or, animal studies have shown an adverse effect, but adequate studies in pregnant women have not demonstrated a risk to the fetus during the first trimester of pregnancy, and there is no evidence of risk in later trimesters.
	Category C: Animal studies have shown an adverse effect on the fetus but there are no adequate studies in humans; the benefit from the use of the drug in pregnancy may be acceptable despite its potential risks. Or, there are no animal reproduction studies and no adequate studies in humans.
	Category D: There is evidence of human fetal risk, but the potential benefits from the use of the drug in pregnant women may be acceptable despite its potential risks.
	Category X: Studies in animals or humans demonstrate fetal abnormalities or adverse reactions and reports indicate evidence of fetal risk. The risk of use in a pregnant woman clearly outweighs any possible benefits.

E. Regulation of nursing practice related to medication therapy
1. Nurse Practice Act
    a. A series of statutes enacted by each state legislature to regulate the practice of nurses in that state
    b. The Nurse Practice Act describes the role of the nurse in relation to medication administration
    c. Advanced practice nurses may have prescriptive privileges; check individual state statute to determine laws governing prescriptive authority in that state
2. Standards of care
    a. Some standards of care are global guidelines by which the nurse should practice, without a specific focus on medication therapy
    b. Other standards of care may be based on research of specific health problems and include recommendations for care including medication therapy
    c. An example is the "stepped-care" approach to treating hypertension; medication therapy is recommended in specific sequences based on client response
3. *Professional misconduct*: a violation of the Nurse Practice Act that can result in disciplinary action against a nurse; examples of professional misconduct are failing to wear an identification badge or sharing client's personal information with others without the client's consent; medication therapy as part of the plan of care can be construed to be personal information
4. *Disciplinary action*: denying or suspending any license to practice by boards of nursing because of unprofessional conduct; nurses who are involved in drug diversion are subject to disciplinary action
5. *Malpractice*: a form of **negligence** or professional misconduct; includes actions that are poor, wrong, or injudicious in the professional care of a client that result in injury, unnecessary suffering, or death to the client (such as a serious medication error); this may also occur through omission of a necessary act, such as failure to give a prescribed medication

F. Legal liability
1. Administration of medications by the nurse includes several aspects of legal liability
2. A legal prescription from a health care provider with prescription-writing authority, such as a physician or nurse practitioner, begins the process of medication delivery to a client; see Box 1-5 for a list of elements of a complete drug prescription
3. Nurses are responsible for their actions even when there is a written medication prescription
    a. If a drug prescription is incorrect (inaccurate dose or the drug prescribed is not indicated for the client's health condition), the nurse who administers the drug is liable for the error along with the prescriber
    b. The nurse must question any prescription that appears inappropriate and can refuse to give the drug until the prescription is clarified

---

Box 1-5	**The following points should be included in a complete drug prescription:**
Elements of a Drug Prescription	• Full name of the client • Date and time the drug prescription is written • Name of the drug to be given to the client • Dosage of the drug • Frequency of drug administration • Route of drug administration • Signature of person writing the prescription

4. Nurses, along with physicians and pharmacists, participate in the system used in an agency to maintain medication safety

    a. One important feature of such a system is the recording of allergy to medications that a client reports

    b. The nurse is the "last stop" in the system and has a crucial role in ensuring accuracy in medication administration

    c. The use of, storage, dispensing of, and documentation for drugs that are controlled substances is a highly regulated part of the medication administration system in a health care agency

    d. The nurse participates in a process of system analysis that addresses the entire system of medication administration, which includes the prescription and method of dispensing, as well as preparation, administration, and documentation

5. The nurse ensures that the *right client* receives the *right medication* in the *right dose* via the *right route* at the *right time*; the nurse then completes the *right documentation* (time of medication administration and client responses to medication)

    a. Included in the process noted above is ensuring that the dosage is appropriate for the client's size and age

    b. It is critical to verify the client's identity prior to medication administration by using 2 unique identifiers, such as checking identification band and asking client to state his or her name and date of birth

6. The nurse is responsible for assessing the client's condition as it relates to the ordered medication, the client's response to the medication (including expected or unexpected responses)

7. The nurse must have knowledge of the effects and potential effects of every drug that is given to a client

8. The nurse takes measures to protect the client from any safety hazards that may be expected from a medication's effects; an example is taking measures to protect the client from falling if a medication has a sedative effect

9. Professional liability insurance: nurses need their own liability insurance for protection against malpractice lawsuits, including those involving medication errors

III. PRESCRIPTION AND NONPRESCRIPTION MEDICATIONS

A. Generic, chemical, and trade names

1. *Generic name*: original designation that is given to a drug when the drug company applies for the approval process; each drug has only 1 generic name such as acetaminophen

2. *Chemical name*: name that reflects chemical structure of a drug; is often long and complex; is of use to pharmacists and researchers

3. *Trade name*: also known as brand name; a name given to an approved drug by the pharmaceutical company that developed it; the number of trade names that a drug can have is large; for instance, acetaminophen has 31 trade names, including Tylenol

B. Nonprescription or over-the-counter (OTC) medications

1. Are products that are available without a prescription for self-treatment of a variety of minor problems

2. The regulation and evaluation of OTC drugs is under FDA supervision

3. OTC medications may have been previously approved as prescription medications, usually at a higher strength

4. Advantages of using OTC medications include reduced health care costs, less time lost from work, less travel, and fewer side effects

5. Potential problems with OTC drug use include improper use, lack of counseling, labeling concerns, and possible delay in obtaining needed treatment

IV. MEDICATION CLASSIFICATION SYSTEMS

A. Two possible approaches

1. Medications with similar characteristics might be classified together based on clinical indication; an example is analgesic medications, which relieve pain
2. Medications can also be grouped together by the body system upon which they act; an example is central nervous system medications

B. Benefits of a classification system

1. Knowledge of a drug's classification helps the nurse to understand intended effects and common side effects of a drug being administered
2. It also assists the nurse to organize knowledge of thousands of drugs that are used for a wide variety of therapeutic indications

V. TERMINOLOGY RELATED TO PHARMACOLOGY

A. **Critical concentration:** the amount of a drug needed to cause a therapeutic effect

B. **Distribution:** the transport of a drug in body fluids from the bloodstream to various tissues of the body and then to its site of action

C. **Drug:** any substance used in the diagnosis, treatment, or prevention of a disease or condition; this term is used interchangeably with the word *medication*

D. **Drug–enzyme interactions:** drugs can cause interference with enzyme systems

E. **First-pass effect:** a phenomenon that occurs following ingestion of an oral drug, in which a large percentage of the drug is inactivated in the liver after being absorbed from the GI tract as the drug is carried from the GI circulation through the hepatic portal circulation; this explains why oral medication doses need to be larger than parenteral doses

F. **Half-life:** the time required to reduce to one half that amount of unchanged drug that is in the body at the time equilibrium is established

G. **Orphan drugs:** drugs that are not profitable financially, but may be useful in treating rare diseases

H. **Pharmacodynamics:** what drugs do to the body and how drugs interact with body tissues

I. **Pharmacokinetics:** what the body does to a drug or how a drug is altered as it travels through the body

J. **Pharmacology:** the study of drugs and their interactions with living systems

K. **Pharmacotherapeutics:** also known as clinical pharmacology; the branch of pharmacology that involves using drugs to treat, prevent, or diagnose disease

L. **Selective toxicity:** ability of a drug, such as penicillin, to attack only those systems found in foreign cells

VI. ISSUES RELATED TO MEDICATION ADMINISTRATION

A. **The "rights" of safe medication administration:** right medication, right dose, right client, right route, right time, and right documentation; additional "rights" may include right assessment, right to refuse, right response, and right education

B. **Factors affecting absorption and response**

1. **Absorption:** movement of a drug from its site of administration into the blood
2. Physiological factors affecting drug absorption
   a. Weight: the recommended dosage of a drug is based on drug evaluation studies and is targeted at a 70-kg (150-lb) person
   b. Volume of distribution (Vd): may be used along with client weight to calculate a loading dose of a drug needed by a client
   c. Age: a factor to be considered primarily in children and older adults
   d. Gender: because males have more vascular muscles than females, the effects of an intramuscular (IM) injection are noted sooner in a male than in a female; females have more fat cells than males; therefore, drugs that deposit in fat may be slowly released in a female and cause effects for a longer period of time than in a male

   3. Chemical and physical factors affecting drug absorption
      a. Lipid solubility: highly soluble drugs are absorbed more rapidly than drugs whose lipid solubility is low
      b. pH partitioning: the difference between the pH of plasma and the pH at the site of administration is such that drug molecules will have a greater tendency to be ionized in plasma
      c. Range of dissolution: the faster the dissolution of medication, the more rapid the onset of drug absorption will be
      d. Blood flow: medications are absorbed most rapidly from sites where blood flow is high
      e. Routes of administration: the barriers to absorption associated with each route are different, so the patterns of absorption differ between routes

C. Unintended responses to drugs
   1. Side effect: unavoidable secondary drug effect produced at therapeutic doses (e.g., gastric irritation caused by aspirin)
   2. Adverse drug reaction: undesired response to a drug; may range from mild to life-threatening
      a. Toxicity: an adverse drug reaction caused by excessive dosing (e.g., coma from morphine overdose); some drugs have a narrow therapeutic index, that is, the dose required to produce a therapeutic effect is close to the toxic dose
      b. Allergic reaction: an adverse physiological reaction of immunologic origin; in order for an allergic reaction to occur, there should be prior sensitization of the immune system; the drug dosage has no effect on the intensity of allergic reactions
      c. Idiosyncratic effect: an adverse drug reaction based on a client's genetic predisposition
   3. Iatrogenic disease: a drug- or health care provider-induced disease
   4. Teratogenic effect: a drug-induced birth defect
   5. Carcinogenic effect: ability of a drug to cause cancer

D. Medications and children
   1. Children metabolize drugs differently than adults in that they metabolize medications faster than adults
   2. Children have immature body systems for handling drugs
      a. Drug responses may be unusually intense and prolonged
      b. Absorption of intramuscular (IM) medications in neonates is slower than in adults; Figure 1-1 shows the vastus lateralis site for IM injection for a newborn and children up to 3 years of age

Figure 1-1

The vastus lateralis muscle is used for IM injections in newborns, infants, and children up to 3 years of age

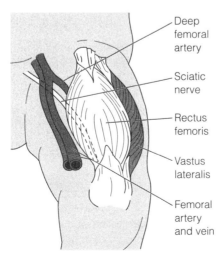

Deep femoral artery

Sciatic nerve

Rectus femoris

Vastus lateralis

Femoral artery and vein

c. Absorption of IM medications in infants is more rapid than in adults

d. Neonates are more sensitive to medications that affect the central nervous system (CNS) because the blood–brain barrier is not fully developed

e. The medication-metabolizing capacity of neonates is low

f. Renal **excretion** (a process whereby drugs and pharmacologically active or inactive metabolites are eliminated from body) of medications is low in neonates

g. Most pharmacokinetic parameters in children 1 year and older are similar to those in adults

E. Medications and older adults

1. Older adults undergo physical changes as part of the aging process that affect the response to a drug that is administered

2. Altered response may be due to less effective absorption, less efficient **distribution** (transport of a drug in body fluids from bloodstream to various body tissues and then to its site of action), less efficient perfusion, altered metabolism, and less efficient excretion

3. The rate of drug absorption may be slowed in older adults

4. Concentrations of water-soluble drugs may be high, and concentrations of lipid-soluble drugs may be low in older adults

5. Reduced liver and/or renal function may prolong medication effects; this is because with reduced metabolism and/or excretion of a drug, the drug may work for a prolonged amount of time or toxic effects may become apparent

6. Adverse drug reactions are more common in older adults than in younger adults

7. Nonadherence is more common among older adults; the factors contributing to nonadherence include low income, forgetfulness, complex regimens, side effects, failure to follow instructions, and inability to obtain medications

F. Calculating medication dosages

1. Calculation of medication dosage by body weight
   a. 1 kg = 2.2 lb
   b. To convert from pounds to kilograms, divide by 2.2
      1) Example: a client weighs 154 pounds: 154 ÷ 2.2 = the client weighs 70 kg
   c. To convert from kilograms to pounds, multiply by 2.2
      1) Example: a client weighs 20 kg: 20 × 2.2 = the client weighs 44 lb

2. Calculating daily dosages
   a. Dosages are expressed in terms of mg/kg/day, or mg/lb/day
      1) Example: the drug vancomycin (Vancocin) can be given to a pediatric client with pseudomembranous colitis in doses up to 40 mg/kg/day
      2) The pediatric client above, who weighs 20 kg (44 lb), can receive 40 mg × 20 kg/day; 40 mg × 20 kg = 800 mg/day in 3 to 4 divided doses
   b. The total daily dosage is usually administered in divided doses per day
      1) Example: from above drug prescription for vancomycin: 800 mg ÷ 4 = 200 mg each dose; this dose is within the recommended range for this client
   c. The nurse is responsible for verifying that a drug prescription is within the recommended dosage range; if not, the prescription should be questioned and clarified

3. Intravenous fluid calculations
   a. First step: determine how many milliliters per hour (volume) needs to be given; this may be part of the original prescription or it may need to be calculated when the total volume and hours are given
      1) Example: the provider prescribes 1,000 mL IV solution to be given over 8 hours
      2) 1,000 ÷ 8 = 125 mL per hour (mL/hr)

Practice to Pass

The physician orders morphine sulfate 15 mg subQ for a client with pain. The medication is supplied as morphine sulfate 25 mg/mL. What volume of the drug will the nurse prepare to administer the right dose?

  b. Second step: calculate the drops per minute (gtts/min); when the mL/hr is given, calculate the gtts/min
    1) Example: the client's IV set delivers 10 gtt/mL
    2) 1.25 mL 3 10 gtts/mL ÷ 60 minutes = 20.83 gtts/min
    3) Since a fractional drop cannot be counted, the nurse will set the IV drip rate at 21 gtts/min after rounding the decimal up or down appropriately
  c. The drop factor is the number of drops in 1 mL; drop factors of 10, 15, and 60 are the most common (the drop factor is determined by the manufacturer and is found on the IV tubing box)

G. Routes of medication administration
  1. See Table 1-1 for a detailed description of very commonly used routes for administering medications
  2. Enteral (via GI tract): including oral administration as well as administration via a GI feeding tube; classic routes include
    a. PO: typical oral administration
    b. SL: sublingual, under the tongue
    c. Buccal: between the cheek and gum
    d. Via feeding tube
  3. Parenteral
    a. Intravenous (IV): through an IV catheter into a vein; is the fastest-acting route
    b. Subcutaneous (subQ): Figure 1-2 illustrates the angle of insertion for subQ injections; typical volume is 0.5 to 1 mL per injection but should not exceed 1.5 mL; needle gauge is 25 to 29 and a 3/8- to 5/8-in. needle should be used
    c. Intramuscular (IM): Figure 1-3 illustrates the angle of insertion for IM injections using the Z-track method; total volume varies by age and injection site, commonly 1 to 2 mL in adults and 0.5 to 1 mL in children; needle size varies by age, commonly 21- to 23-gauge and 1 to 1.5 in. long

Table 1-1   **Commonly Used Routes of Administration**

Routes	Barriers to Absorption	Absorption Pattern	Advantages	Disadvantages
Intravenous	No barriers	Instantaneous and complete	Rapid onset Control over levels of drug in the blood Use of large fluid volumes Use of chemically irritant drugs such as anticancer	High cost Difficulty and inconvenience Irreversibility Fluid overload Infection Embolism
Intramuscular and subcutaneous	Capillary wall	Rapidly or slowly; depends on the water solubility of the drug and blood flow to the site of the injection Intramuscular absorption faster than subcutaneous because of better blood flow to muscle tissue	Poorly soluble drugs in water Depot preparations (preparations from which medication is absorbed gradually over an extended time)	Discomfort and inconvenience Possible nerve damage
Oral	a. The layer of epithelial cells b. The capillary wall	Varies according to: a. Solubility and stability of the drug b. Gastric and intestinal pH c. Gastric emptying time d. Food in the gut e. Co-administration of other drugs f. Special coatings on the preparation	Easy and convenient Inactivation Inexpensive Safer than parenteral injection	Variability of absorption Client requirements (i.e., cooperation, local irritation)

Figure 1-2

Inserting a needle for subQ injection

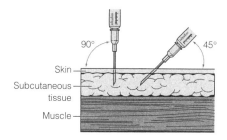

Figure 1-3

Inserting a needle using *Z*-track method for IM injections

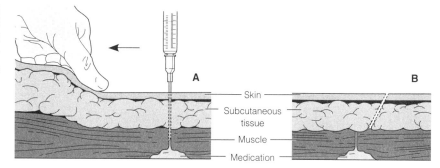

    d. Intradermal (ID): used for diagnostic testing, such as allergens or tuberculosis screening; uses a tuberculin syringe, usual dose is 0.01 mL to 0.1 mL using 25- to 27-gauge, ¼- to ½-in. needle

  4. Topical

    a. Transcutaneous: some medications may be given as a paste (e.g., nitroglycerin) or as a patch (e.g., nitroglycerin or scopolamine) to the skin, so medication is absorbed continually over time

    b. Instillations or irrigations: medications may be administered to various body orifices or cavities, such as ophthalmic (eye), otic (ear), intranasal (nose), vaginal, rectal, or into joints or urinary bladder

    c. Inhalations: some medications may be inhaled into respiratory tract using an inhaler, nebulizer, or positive pressure breathing machine

  5. Intrathecal (less common): some drugs, such as chemotherapy, are administered into spinal fluid in the subarachnoid space, using a device such as an Ommaya reservoir implanted in a ventricle in the brain

H. Medication interactions

  1. *Drug–food interaction* is important because it can result in toxicity or therapeutic failure

    a. Impact of food on drug absorption: food may increase or decrease a drug's absorption rate and consequently affect the extent of absorption; for example, if tetracyclines are administered with milk products or calcium supplements, absorption is reduced and antibacterial effects may be lost

    b. Impact of food on drug metabolism: food may change the metabolism of certain medications; grapefruit juice produces a 406% increase in blood levels of some calcium channel blockers used for hypertension

    c. Impact of food on drug toxicity: interaction between monoamine oxidase (MAO) inhibitors and foods rich in tyramine (including yeasts extracts, aged cheese) can raise blood pressure to a life-threatening level and cause other symptoms such as headache, nausea and vomiting, tachycardia, sweating, and rarely brain hemorrhage

    d. Impact of food on drug action: food may have direct impact on drug action, such as foods rich in vitamin K (e.g., broccoli, cabbage), which can reduce the effects of sodium warfarin (Coumadin)

      e. Timing of drug administration with respect to meals: may result in significant increase or decrease in drug absorption

2. *Drug–drug interaction* can occur whenever a client takes 2 or more medications; some interactions are intended and desired, but others are unintended

    a. Mechanisms of drug–drug interaction

      1) *Direct chemical or physical interaction*: when drugs are combined in IV solutions and cause formation of a precipitate; the nurse carefully inspects any solution that has been mixed with a drug to detect crystals or cloudiness

      2) *Pharmacokinetic interaction*: may alter absorption, distribution, metabolism, and excretion; for example, heparin cannot cross the GI tract membrane, so absorption via oral route is not possible; the drug must be given via parenteral route

      3) *Pharmacodynamic interaction*: includes interactions at the same receptors or interactions at separate sites; for example, naloxone (Narcan) is a drug that blocks access of opiate drugs to receptor sites, so it is used to reverse the action of opiates in the event of opiate overdose

    b. Consequences of drug–drug interactions

      1) Increased/decreased therapeutic effects

      2) Increased/decreased adverse effects

      3) Creation of a unique response

3. Incompatibility: occurs when the mixture of one medication with another results in an undesirable reaction

    a. These reactions could include chemical alteration, destruction, or pharmacologic effect

    b. An example is that diluting phenytoin (Dilantin) in 5% dextrose in water will result in precipitation of solution, which can be fatal if administered to a client

I. Client education

1. Process of client education

    a. Assessment of need to learn

    b. Assessment of motivation

    c. Formulation of a nursing diagnostic statement and setting objective goals with client

    d. Teaching–learning activities aimed at client's preferred learning style and general ability and educational level

    e. Evaluation and reteaching if necessary, depending on achievement of learning objectives

2. Nursing roles and responsibilities

    a. Applying the nursing process to client teaching

      1) Assessment: assess for client's readiness for education; organize, analyze, and summarize the collected data

      2) Nursing diagnosis: formulate nursing diagnoses to address learning needs

      3) Planning and goals: assign priority to nursing diagnoses; identify teaching strategies appropriate for goal; establish expected outcome

      4) Implementation: put the teaching plan into action; encourage client to participate in learning

      5) Evaluation: evaluate the collected objective data; identify alterations that need to be made in the teaching plan; make referrals to appropriate sources

    b. Establish a good teacher–learner rapport

    c. Plan the best time for teaching and reduce noise and distractions in the teaching environment

    d. Match teaching methods to client's primary learning style, such as visual, auditory, and/or tactile, for optimum effectiveness

    e. Use teaching tools appropriate to client's primary learning style, such as lecture or verbal teaching, demonstration, written materials, videotapes or visual materials or physical models

---

Practice to Pass

For a client with severe pain, which route of analgesic drug administration would provide the most rapid effect? Explain your answer.

    f. Identify barriers to learning, such as disabilities, cultural or socioeconomic factors, communication, and excessive volume of learning materials

3. Client adherence

    a. A goal of client education is that clients adhere to the therapeutic regimen

    b. Direct the teaching program toward stimulating client motivation to adhere to therapy

    c. Perform ongoing assessment of variables that affect client's ability to accept specific behaviors; examples are age, gender, socioeconomic status, education, severity of illness, complexity of regimen, religious or cultural beliefs, and costs associated with a prescribed regimen

    d. Identify potential nonadherence to therapeutic regimens and plan counteractive strategies

    e. Establish comprehensive adherence-enhancing interventions (see Box 1-6)

4. Cultural considerations: cultural competence refers to a complex integration of attitudes, knowledge, and skills that direct the nurse to provide care in a culturally sensitive manner (Table 1-2)

    a. Recognize special dietary needs for clients from selected cultural groups; sometimes foods that clients prefer may be those that interact with prescribed medications

    b. Review drug information to be aware of variations in individual response to medications based on ethnic and racial differences; some clients may require lower doses and some may have faster clearance rates of selected drugs based on cultural background

    c. Create an environment in which the traditional healing practices of clients are respected; recognize that some clients may not value drug therapy as a primary mode of treatment for a health problem

    d. Establish effective communication by overcoming language barriers (see Box 1-7)

    e. Establish flexible regulations pertaining to visitors, such as length of visits

    f. View each client as an individual and avoid stereotyping

    g. Be aware of cultural preferences the client has in regards to space and distance, eye contact, time, touch, observance of holidays, and diet

    h. Maintain a broad and open attitude; expect the unexpected

    i. Try to understand the reasons for any behavior that you do not understand; ask for clarification

    j. Use any words you know in the client's language

Practice to Pass

The client, who does not speak English, is being discharged with 3 prescriptions for medications. What strategies will the nurse use to meet responsibilities for client teaching in this situation?

Box 1-6	**Consider using the following interventions to promote client adherence to treatment plan:**
Enhancing Adherence to Treatment Plan	**1.** Provide verbal instruction in small amounts, specific to activity
	2. Dispense optimal amounts of printed instructions
	3. Use material at client's comprehension level
	4. Dispense materials over time
	5. Assess level of client's understanding
	6. Encourage questions
	7. Augment verbal instructions with demonstrations
	8. Refer to community resources for additional skill development
	9. Goal setting: make goals attainable and very specific
	10. Reinforcement: provide feedback and praise for attempt
	11. Problem solving: identify problems and potential solutions for adherence
	12. Habit building: such as placing bedtime medication by clock radio
	13. Cueing: set up system of reminders to take medications, such as calendars or medication box
	14. Social support: involve others in behavior change plan

Table 1-2 Comparative Characteristics of Culturally Diverse Clients

Cultures	Communication	Social Roles	Health Risks	Implementation
African Americans	Direct eye contact is viewed as being rude, nonverbal communication is very important	Large extended family networks are important	Hypertension Coronary heart disease Sickle cell anemia Cancer	Be flexible and avoid rigidity in scheduling care Encourage involvement with family An herbalist may be consulted before an individual seeks medical care
Asian Americans	Silence is valued, eye contact considered rude, the word "no" considered disrespectful	Large extended family networks, devoted to tradition, education is highly valued	Hypertension Cancer Lactose intolerance Thalassemia	Limit eye contact Avoid gesturing with hands A healer may be consulted prior to medical treatment
European Americans	Eye contact is considered as trustworthiness	The nuclear family is the basic unit, the man is the dominant figure	Breast cancer Thalassemia Diabetes	Eye contact is acceptable
Hispanic Americans	Eye contact indicates disrespect	The nuclear family is the basic unit, men are the decision makers, the extended family is highly valued	Diabetes Parasites Lactose intolerance	Protect privacy Offer to call priest or other clergy
Native Americans	Silence is valued, eye contact is avoided	Family oriented, elders are honored	Diabetes Tuberculosis Alcohol abuse Heart disease Gallbladder disease Accidents	Be attentive Clarify communication Obtain input from members of extended family May consult a medicine man

Box 1-7

Enhancing Communication to Overcome Language Barriers

Consider using the following interventions to assist in overcoming a language barrier:

1. Greet client using the last or complete name
2. Smile
3. Pay attention to any effort by the client to communicate
4. Avoid talking loudly
5. Use short and simple sentences
6. Summarize and repeat frequently
7. Use a qualified interpreter to ensure appropriate communication about plan of care and prescribed medications; family members may not be the best choices for this task, depending on a number of variables, including age and sensitivity of information
8. Identify cues that may signal a lack of effective communication, including absence of questions, efforts to change the subject, inappropriate laughter, and nonverbal cues

5. Health care beliefs
   a. Values are beliefs and attitudes that may influence behavior and the process of decision making; they evolve from personal experiences
   b. Decisions about whether or not to use drugs as therapy for health problems are often influenced by a client's overall health care beliefs

    c. Ethical principles are codes that direct a person's actions
       1) They include the ability to make choices without external constraints, the need to maintain a balance between benefits and harms, and the obligation to tell the truth
       2) These are some areas in which ethical concerns arise for nurses and for clients related to treatment with drugs
    d. Ethical codes: provide broad principles for determining and evaluating client care
    e. American Nurses Association (ANA) Code of Ethics: an ideal framework for nurses to use in ethical decision making
    f. Ethical dilemma: occurs when there is a conflict between 2 or more ethical principles, including confidentiality, use of restraint, trust issues (not lying to the client, communicating to family and physician), refusing treatment or care, and end-of-life issues; drug therapy may play a role from time to time when issues arise in any of these areas; the nurse's role is to maintain ethical behavior in the course of administering drug therapy

Case Study

The nurse is visiting a 75-year-old client in the home. The client has type 1 diabetes mellitus, hypertension, and osteoarthritis in both knees. The client's sight is moderately impaired despite the use of eyeglasses. The client's medication regimen includes Humulin insulin 70/30 (combination insulins) 35 units subcutaneously in the morning, lisinopril (Zestril) 5 mg by mouth daily, and nabumetone (Relafen) 500 mg by mouth twice daily.

1. What are 2 important medication administration safety issues that the nurse will assess in the client?

2. What data will the nurse gather to evaluate the effects of the ordered medications?

For suggested responses, see pages 539–540.

3. What measures can the nurse suggest to the client to ensure accuracy and compliance with the medication regimen?

4. The client reports feeling "dizzy" at times. How will the nurse evaluate this concern?

5. What criteria will the nurse use to select printed educational materials for this client's use?

POSTTEST

POSTTEST

1 The nurse is administering tetracycline hydrochloride (Tetracyn) 500 mg PO 4 times daily to a client with gonorrhea. The nurse should plan to take which action to enhance absorption of this medication?

1. Administer drug with meals.
2. Give drug with a full glass of milk to prevent gastric irritation.
3. Give drug on an empty stomach with a full glass of water.
4. Give drug with a glass of orange juice or other source of vitamin C.

2 After observing the client taking phenelzine sulfate (Nardil) after eating a lunch of yogurt, sliced bananas, and chocolate milk, the nurse should take which action?

1. Monitor client's body temperature for elevated temperature.
2. Observe client for dyspnea.
3. Test urine specimen for glucose and ketones.
4. Monitor client for elevated blood pressure.

POSTTEST

3 A client who is taking several prescribed oral medications for the treatment of chronic heart failure tells the nurse, "I usually take all of my medications with my breakfast." The nurse's best response includes which statements? Select all that apply.

1. "It might be a good idea to review each drug to determine the best times and conditions for taking it."
2. "That depends on what you eat at breakfast."
3. "Has the swelling in your lower legs decreased?"
4. "What time do you usually have breakfast?"
5. "That's a great idea."

4 The client received isophane (NPH) insulin 30 units subcutaneously at 7:30 a.m. What time is the nurse most likely to observe signs and symptoms of hypoglycemia?

1. 9:30 to 10:30 a.m.
2. 11:30 a.m. to 2:30 p.m.
3. 11:30 a.m. to 7:30 p.m.
4. 3:30 p.m. to 7:30 p.m.

5 The client taking theophylline (TheoDur) 16 mg/kg PO for asthma has a serum theophylline level of 22 mcg/mL. Because the client is experiencing nausea and vomiting and headache, which action should the nurse take?

1. Seek an order for an antiemetic from the prescriber.
2. Withhold the next scheduled dose and notify the prescriber.
3. Ask if client expectorated any mucus after the last respiratory therapy treatment.
4. Stop prescribed doses of theophylline for 24 hours.

6 Morphine sulfate 10 mg PO is prescribed for a first-day postoperative client with a large abdominal wound. The nurse would do which of the following as the most appropriate nursing action?

1. Request a prescription that changes the route from oral to parenteral.
2. Administer drug with food.
3. Dissolve tablet in a small amount of warm liquid.
4. Encourage coughing and deep breathing 2 hours after ingestion.

7 A pregnant client is at the clinic for a routine evaluation and asks the nurse about continuing to take her routine medications. The nurse provides a response based on which principles established by the Food and Drug Administration (FDA)? Select all that apply.

1. No drug should be administered during pregnancy unless the benefits outweigh the risks.
2. The Pregnancy Categories were established in order to indicate the potential for a drug to cause birth defects.
3. A Pregnancy Category A designation indicates that studies demonstrate abnormalities or adverse reactions in the fetus and that the risk of use outweighs any benefit.
4. The Pregnancy Category guidelines were developed in order to rank the abuse potential of various drugs in pregnancy.
5. Schedule V medications have limited abuse potential and are generally safe for pregnancy.

8 A health care provider prescribed a prochlorperazine (Compazine) 12.5 mg suppository for a client with severe nausea. The nurse has on hand a 25 mg suppository. What is the next step that the nurse should take?

1. Cut suppository in half and insert the rounded edge.
2. Administer drug orally.
3. Contact pharmacist if unable to locate the correct dosage.
4. Clear rectal vault of the contents before administering half of the suppository.

9 A health care provider prescribes 1,000 mL 5% dextrose in 0.9% sodium chloride over 6 hours. The nurse calculates the flow rate for this infusion to be how many mL per hour? Provide a numerical response rounded to a whole number.

_____ mL

10 The home health nurse plans to provide additional education after hearing an older adult client taking glyburide (Micronase) 1.25 mg PO daily make which statement?

1. "I take the tablet with breakfast every day."
2. "If I forget the dose on one day, I will take 2 tablets the next day."
3. "I will avoid drinking alcohol while taking this drug."
4. "I will keep appointments to have my HBA_{1c} checked every 4 months."

➤ *See pages 21–22 for Answers and Rationales.*

ANSWERS & RATIONALES

Pretest

1 **Answer: 2** **Rationale:** Asking the client to state his or her name is an accurate way to identify a client, provided the client is alert. A second unique identifier, such as date of birth or medical record number, should also be used. This information may be found on the client's identification bracelet, although the client may be asked to state date of birth. Asking the client his name is incorrect because hospitalized or ill clients are often anxious, medicated, or confused and could respond incorrectly to this question. Because clients' bed assignments are sometimes changed to meet unit needs, simply checking the client's room number and bed assignment poses a risk for incorrect client identification. Because the same diagnosis with the same medication may be appropriate for more than one client, matching the medication to the diagnosis or need will place the client at risk. **Cognitive Level:** Applying **Client Need:** Pharmacological and Parenteral Therapies **Integrated Process:** Communication and Documentation **Content Area:** Pharmacology **Strategy:** Analyze each option and select the option that minimizes the risk for obtaining incorrect information. Recall that having the client provide information directly is generally a preferred option as long as the client is alert. **Reference:** Adams, M., Holland, L., & Bostwick, P. (2011). *Pharmacology for nurses: A pathophysiologic approach* (3rd ed.). Upper Saddle River, NJ: Pearson Education, p. 19.

2 **Answer: 1** **Rationale:** Stating that similarities exist but that instructions were specific to the child answers the question and reaffirms the health care provider's instructions. Changing from brand-name drugs to generic drugs should be done by the health care provider. Advil, an enteric-coated tablet, is a brand name of ibuprofen. Not all ibuprofen is enteric-coated, although the active ingredient is the same—ibuprofen (which is also the generic name). Answering that Advil and ibuprofen are 2 different drugs with similar effects is inaccurate. It is inappropriate to make a referral when the nurse is capable of meeting the need of the client. **Cognitive Level:** Applying **Client Need:** Pharmacological and Parenteral Therapies

Integrated Process: Communication and Documentation **Content Area:** Pharmacology **Strategy:** Select the option that is most accurate and that places the client at the least amount of risk. **Reference:** Wilson, B. A., Shannon, M., & Shields, K. (2011). *Pearson nurse's drug guide 2011.* Upper Saddle River, NJ: Pearson Education, pp. 768–770.

3 **Answer: 3** **Rationale:** Iron is a Pregnancy Category A drug, and this category is assigned to drugs that have not been shown to have adverse effects on fetal development. Therefore, it is safe to ingest the drug during pregnancy. The statement that no OTC products should be taken during pregnancy is inaccurate because of the word *any*. An example of a safe product to use during pregnancy is a multivitamin. Answering that "most prenatal vitamins contain iron" is accurate; however, it does not answer the client's question directly. Staining of the teeth is a side effect of the tetracyclines. **Cognitive Level:** Analyzing **Client Need:** Pharmacological and Parenteral Therapies **Integrated Process:** Teaching and Learning **Content Area:** Pharmacology **Strategy:** To answer this question correctly, recall the Pregnancy Category of iron and use knowledge of the safety of Pregnancy Category A drugs to select the option that most closely correlates with that category. **Reference:** Wilson, B. A., Shannon, M., & Shields, K. (2011). *Pearson nurse's drug guide 2011.* Upper Saddle River, NJ: Pearson Education, pp. 639–641.

4 **Answer: 4** **Rationale:** Grapefruit juice changes the metabolism of the calcium channel blocker drugs and leads to increase in serum drug levels. This can lead to toxicity manifested by dysrhythmias (heart block, bradycardia), angina, heart failure, and hypotension. Assessment of respiratory pattern may be important because of the toxicity, but does not address the primary problem directly; assessment should focus on the cause. There is no direct relationship between elevated body temperature and toxic levels of this drug. Weight gain (not loss) is an adverse effect of this drug. The highest priority is assisting the client to ingest this drug safely. Identification of the cause of the toxicity takes the highest priority. **Cognitive Level:** Analyzing **Client Need:** Pharmacological and Parenteral Therapies **Integrated Process:** Nursing Process: Assessment **Content Area:** Pharmacology **Strategy:** The core issue of the question is knowledge of factors that increase the risk of toxicity with use of calcium channel blockers. Recall that grapefruit juice interferes with drug biotransformation to help you choose correctly. **Reference:** Wilson, B. A., Shannon, M., & Shields, K. (2011). *Pearson nurse's drug guide 2011.* Upper Saddle River, NJ: Pearson Education, pp. 477–478. Adams, M., Holland, L., & Bostwick, P. (2011). *Pharmacology for nurses: A pathophysiologic approach* (3rd ed.). Upper Saddle River, NJ: Pearson Education, pp. 308, 366.

5 **Answer: 1, 2, 4** **Rationale:** Since older adult clients experience a decreased rate of drug excretion, a reduction in dosage would be appropriate. The decreased total body fluid proportion that accompanies physical aging increases the concentration of water-soluble drugs and requires lower dosing in older adults. Decreased efficiency in drug distribution would not correlate with a need to lower the dosage. Older adult clients experience a decreased rate of drug metabolism. Many older adults tend to lose weight with lean muscle mass loss. **Cognitive Level:** Analyzing **Client Need:** Pharmacological and Parenteral Therapies **Integrated Process:** Nursing Process: Diagnosis **Content Area:** Pharmacology **Strategy:** The core issue is the effect of age-related changes on drug metabolism. Select the options that would place the client at greatest risk and that correlate closest to the information in the stem. **Reference:** Adams, M., Holland, L., & Bostwick, P. (2011). *Pharmacology for nurses: A pathophysiologic approach* (3rd ed.). Upper Saddle River, NJ: Pearson Education, pp. 73–74.

6 **Answer: 7.5** **Rationale:** Use the following formula as one way to calculate the dose: 100 mg/5 mL = 150 mg/x mL $100x = 750$; $x = 7.5$ mL **Cognitive Level:** Analyzing **Client Need:** Pharmacological and Parenteral Therapies **Integrated Process:** Nursing Process: Implementation **Content Area:** Pharmacology **Strategy:** Use the "solving for x" equation or any other pharmacological dosage calculation formula to determine the correct amount. **Reference:** Olsen, J., Giangrasso, A., Shrimpton, D., & Dillon, P. (2012). *Medical dosage calculations: A dimensional analysis approach* (10th ed.). Upper Saddle River, NJ: Pearson Education, pp. 144–151.

7 **Answer: 1** **Rationale:** Feeling dizzy when moving from lying or sitting to standing position is referred to as orthostatic hypotension and is a common side effect of beta-blocker drugs such as nadolol. The client should be instructed to change positions slowly. Signs and symptoms should diminish after a few weeks of treatment. Dizziness is not a sign of toxicity, but is related to the body's adjustment to reduced decreased cardiac output and reduced central circulating volume. Dizziness can be a sign or symptom of hypertension. Since the client is ingesting an antihypertensive drug, postural hypotension related to decreased central circulating volume should be suspected. **Cognitive Level:** Analyzing **Client Need:** Pharmacological and Parenteral Therapies **Integrated Process:** Teaching and Learning **Content Area:** Pharmacology

Strategy: The core issue of the question is the ability to recognize a drug side effect and provide appropriate teaching to protect the client from falls and possible harm. With this in mind, select the option that provides the greatest safety to the client, which is to ask the client to use caution and move slowly when standing up. **Reference:** Wilson, B. A., Shannon, M., & Shields, K. (2011). *Pearson nurse's drug guide 2011.* Upper Saddle River, NJ: Pearson Education, pp. 1049–1050.

8 **Answer: 1** **Rationale:** Older clients often take other prescribed drugs, herbs, or other alternative remedies, and client may be ingesting an over-the-counter (OTC) remedy for arthritis. Because there is a potentially high risk for drug–drug or drug–herb interaction, getting a thorough picture of the client's current drug regimen is the first step in planning for client education when a new drug is ordered. Providing written materials is appropriate as a supplement after the nurse has taught the client about the medication. Because of cognitive changes, the client may need a strategy to help in maintaining the drug schedule, but it should not be the first action. First action is based on the potential risk to the client. Teaching about the drug is very relevant to the management of the client's health needs, but assessing the risk to the client should occur before implementation. **Cognitive Level:** Analyzing **Client Need:** Pharmacological and Parenteral Therapies **Integrated Process:** Nursing Process: Assessment **Content Area:** Pharmacology **Strategy:** The critical term in the question is *older adult.* Correlate knowledge associated with older adult clients and drug therapy. Assessment is the first step in managing client needs. **Reference:** Adams, M., Holland, L., & Bostwick, P. (2011). *Pharmacology for nurses: A pathophysiologic approach* (3rd ed.). Upper Saddle River, NJ: Pearson Education, pp. 467–470.

9 **Answer: 4** **Rationale:** This is an example of 2 different drugs in the same subcategory with very similar names. The question of which drug should be administered to the client is answered by checking the original prescriber order and giving that drug. The actions of giving medications that are not ordered are dangerous because they do not involve rechecking the original prescriber order against the medication administration record (MAR) and could lead to a medication error (wrong drug) if the MAR is written correctly. Asking the client if the pill looks familiar violates using the appropriate sources to validate the accuracy of a transcribed order. **Cognitive Level:** Analyzing **Client Need:** Pharmacological and Parenteral Therapies **Integrated Process:** Nursing Process: Planning **Content Area:** Pharmacology **Strategy:** The core issue of the question involves application of the principles of the *rights* of medication administration. Use the process of elimination and select the option that best ensures delivery of the *right drug.* **Reference:** Adams, M., Holland, L., & Bostwick, P. (2011). *Pharmacology for nurses: A pathophysiologic approach* (3rd ed.). Upper Saddle River, NJ: Pearson Education, p. 19.

10 **Answer: 1, 5, 3, 4, 2** **Rationale:** First, review the client's medication history and drug allergies as part of the assessment phase of medication administration. The client's medical history can influence a drug's effect; knowledge of client history and allergies can prevent inadvertent administration of a medication that could cause harm to the client. Second, obtain the medication, compare the drug label against the health care provider's order, and prepare the medication. Third, identify the client and explain the intended action of the medications before administration, to prevent errors. Fourth, verify proper drug route, time, and dose, and then administer the medication. Fifth, record the drug administration at bedside in the medication administration record. **Cognitive Level:** Applying **Client Need:** Pharmacological and Parenteral Therapies **Integrated Process:** Nursing Process: Implementation **Content Area:** Pharmacology **Strategy:** Visualize correct and safe sequence of events; apply knowledge of appropriate drug administration techniques. **Reference:** Berman, A., Snyder, S., & McKinney, D. (2011). *Nursing basics for clinical practice*. Upper Saddle River, NJ: Pearson Education, pp. 662–665. Karch, A. (2011). *Focus on nursing pharmacology* (5th ed.). Philadelphia, PA: Lippincott Williams & Wilkins, pp. 42–53.

Posttest

1 **Answer: 3** **Rationale:** The drug tetracycline is absorbed best when given to the client on an empty stomach with a glass of water. Intake of food or juices, dairy products, iron, and antacids decrease the absorption of this drug. **Cognitive Level:** Applying **Client Need:** Pharmacological and Parenteral Therapies **Integrated Process:** Nursing Process: Planning **Content Area:** Pharmacology **Strategy:** Remember that oral administration of this drug with any type of food or other medication poses a risk to appropriate drug absorption. **Reference:** Wilson, B. A., Shannon, M., & Shields, K. (2011). *Pearson nurse's drug guide 2011.* Upper Saddle River, NJ: Pearson Education, pp. 1487–1490.

2 **Answer: 4** **Rationale:** Ingesting foods that are high in tyramine (such as those in the question) can result in a hypertensive crisis in the client who is also taking a monoamine oxidase inhibitor (MAOI) such as phenelzine. The central nervous system side effects involve mental alterations such as confusion and anxiety rather than physical changes such as temperature elevation. Respiratory depression is more likely to occur than dyspnea. Diabetes mellitus or hyperglycemia is not associated with the drug. **Cognitive Level:** Applying **Client Need:** Pharmacological and Parenteral Therapies **Integrated Process:** Nursing Process: Assessment **Content Area:** Pharmacology **Strategy:** The core issue of the question is recognizing that the phenelzine is an MAOI and then associating this drug class with a risk for hypertension when taken with foods high in tyramine. Memorize this information if the question was difficult, because of its importance to client safety. **Reference:** Wilson, B. A., Shannon, M., & Shields, K. (2011).

Pearson nurse's drug guide 2011. Upper Saddle River, NJ: Pearson Education, pp. 1212–1214.

3 **Answer: 1, 3** **Rationale:** Drug interactions, drug side effects, drug actions, and drug absorption should be examined before ingesting multiple prescriptions. Reaching the goals of the drug therapy such as a decrease in peripheral edema would indicate that this approach is appropriate. Stating "that depends on what you eat at breakfast" contains a correct statement, but is not comprehensive. Time is only one of the elements of concern. The nurse needs to be sure there are no significant risks to the timing of the drugs rather than just affirming the client's plan. **Cognitive Level:** Analyzing **Client Need:** Pharmacological and Parenteral Therapies **Integrated Process:** Nursing Process: Planning **Content Area:** Pharmacology **Strategy:** Select option providing most effective approach to the drug therapy. **Reference:** Adams, M., Holland, L., & Bostwick, P. (2011). *Pharmacology for nurses: A pathophysiologic approach* (3rd ed.). Upper Saddle River, NJ: Pearson Education, pp. 324–330.

4 **Answer: 3** **Rationale:** Four to twelve hours is the peak time period for NPH. Two to three hours is the peak time period for regular insulin. Four to seven hours is the peak time period for Semilente. Eight to twelve hours is the peak time period for Lente. **Cognitive Level:** Applying **Client Need:** Pharmacological and Parenteral Therapies **Integrated Process:** Nursing Process: Planning **Content Area:** Pharmacology **Strategy:** Associate this drug with an intermediate range and then select a time frame that is not the shortest range available but also not the longest. **Reference:** Wilson, B. A., Shannon, M., & Shields, K. (2011). *Pearson nurse's drug guide 2011.* Upper Saddle River, NJ: Pearson Education, pp. 805–806.

5 **Answer: 2** **Rationale:** Since the drug has a narrow therapeutic range, toxicity can develop quickly. The normal therapeutic dose level is 10–20 mcg/mL. Hence, the signs and symptoms are indicative of toxicity. The nurse should suspend the order until the prescriber is contacted. Procuring and administering antiemetic would reduce the signs and symptoms but would not resolve the problem. The lab test validates that toxicity exists. The nurse should suspend the order until the dosage can be changed. The drug's duration is 4–8 hours. Holding it for 24 hours could create the opposite problem. **Cognitive Level:** Analyzing **Client Need:** Pharmacological and Parenteral Therapies **Integrated Process:** Nursing Process: Planning **Content Area:** Pharmacology **Strategy:** Recall that this drug has profound effects on GI tract and cardiac function. Then consider that toxicity is likely to have an effect on the 2 systems. **Reference:** Wilson, B. A., Shannon, M., & Shields, K. (2011). *Pearson nurse's drug guide 2011.* Upper Saddle River, NJ: Pearson Education, pp. 1492–1495.

6 **Answer: 1** **Rationale:** Because a parenteral route (IM or IV) is a more efficient route, the drug is likely to be effective more rapidly. Food will delay absorption. The capsule may prevent the delay caused by food, but the oral route is not the most appropriate route for this client).

Peak time period is 1 hour. **Cognitive Level:** Applying **Client Need:** Pharmacological and Parenteral Therapies **Integrated Process:** Nursing Process: Implementation **Content Area:** Pharmacology **Strategy:** Associate the route with the magnitude of the client's needs. **Reference:** Wilson, B. A., Shannon, M., & Shields, K. (2011). *Pearson nurse's drug guide 2011.* Upper Saddle River, NJ: Pearson Education, pp. 1037–1040.

7 **Answer: 1, 2** **Rationale:** Regardless of the FDA's designated Pregnancy Category, the recommendations include to not administer any drug unless necessary. Differentiation between the categories depends on adequate and reliable documentation and the risk-benefit ratio. The categories are intended to indicate birth defect potential. The FDA developed the Schedules of Controlled Substance to regulate drugs known to have abuse potential; these are not specific for pregnancy. Client education of medications would be based on the FDA's Pregnancy Categories, not the controlled substance schedules. The Schedules for Controlled Substances do not address pregnancy specifically, and routine medication that the pregnant woman receives should be based on the Pregnancy Categories. **Cognitive Level:** Analyzing **Client Need:** Pharmacological and Parenteral Therapies **Integrated Process:** Teaching and Learning **Content Area:** Pharmacology **Strategy:** Base knowledge of safe medication administration considerations and FDA recommendations to the education of a maternal client **Reference:** Karch, A. (2011). *Focus on nursing pharmacology* (5th ed.). Philadelphia, PA: Lippincott Williams & Wilkins, pp. 10–12.

8 **Answer: 3** **Rationale:** The nurse should consult with the pharmacist before contacting the prescriber. Drug companies do not guarantee that the medication is equally distributed throughout the medium. The dosage is not stable across routes. Nurses may not change prescriptions. After the dosage problem is resolved, the rectal vault should be cleared adequately to guarantee maximum absorption.

Cognitive Level: Analyzing **Client Need:** Pharmacological and Parenteral Therapies **Integrated Process:** Nursing Process: Planning **Content Area:** Pharmacology **Strategy:** Recall that the active drug in a suppository may not be evenly distributed and use the process of elimination to make a selection. **Reference:** Wilson, B. A., Shannon, M., & Shields, K. (2011). *Pearson nurse's drug guide 2011.* Upper Saddle River, NJ: Pearson Education, pp. 277–287.

9 **Answer: 167** **Rationale:** The rate for administration is calculated by dividing 1,000 mL by 6 hours: 1,000 / 6 = 166.66 mL/hr, which rounds to 167 mL/hr. **Cognitive Level:** Applying **Client Need:** Pharmacological and Parenteral Therapies **Integrated Process:** Nursing Process: Planning **Content Area:** Pharmacology **Strategy:** Note that this is a simple calculation. Divide the total volume in mL by the number of hours calculate the number of mL/hr. **Reference:** Olsen, J., Giangrasso, A., Shrimpton, D., & Dillon, P. (2012). *Medical dosage calculations: A dimensional analysis approach* (10th ed.). Upper Saddle River, NJ: Pearson Education, pp. 277–287.

10 **Answer: 2** **Rationale:** Because of the drug's action (hypoglycemic), duration (24 hrs) and the half-life (10 hrs), the client could be at significant risk if the dose is doubled. The common dosage is once daily before or with breakfast. Ingestion of alcohol with the drug can result in a disulfiram reaction or excessive sympathomimetic reaction. HBA_{1c} provides information regarding the glucose level over a 4-month period. **Cognitive Level:** Applying **Client Need:** Pharmacological and Parenteral Therapies **Integrated Process:** Teaching and Learning **Content Area:** Pharmacology **Strategy:** Determine the client's health maintenance ability based on the content of the statement. The incorrect statement is the correct answer based on the wording of the question. **Reference:** Wilson, B. A., Shannon, M., & Shields, K. (2011). *Pearson nurse's drug guide 2011.* Upper Saddle River, NJ: Pearson Education, pp. 713–715.

References

Abrams, A. (2009). *Clinical drug therapy: Rationales for nursing practice* (9th ed.). Philadelphia: Lippincott Williams & Wilkins.

Adams, M., Holland, L., & Bostwick, P. (2011). *Pharmacology for nurses: A pathophysiologic approach* (3rd ed.). Upper Saddle River, NJ: Pearson Education.

Adams, M., & Koch, R. (2010). *Pharmacology: Connections to nursing practice.* Upper Saddle River, NJ: Pearson Education.

Agency for Health Care Policy and Research, http://www.ahcpr.gov.

Aschenbrenner, D., & Venable, S. (2012). *Drug therapy in nursing* (4th ed.). Philadelphia: Lippincott Williams & Wilkins.

Berman, A., & Snyder, S. (2012). *Kozier & Erb's fundamentals of nursing: Concepts, process, and practice* (9th ed.). Upper Saddle River, NJ: Pearson Education.

Food and Drug Administration, http://www.fda.gov.

Karch, A. (2009). *Focus on nursing pharmacology* (5th ed.). Philadelphia: Lippincott Williams & Wilkins.

Kee, J. (2009). *Laboratory and diagnostic tests and nursing implications* (8th ed.). Upper Saddle River, NJ: Prentice Hall.

Lehne, R. (2010). *Pharmacology for nursing care* (7th ed.). St. Louis, MO: Mosby.

NANDA International (2012). *NANDA-I Nursing diagnoses: Definitions and classification 2012–2014.* Des Moines, IA: Wiley-Blackwell.

National Institutes of Safety and Health, http://www.cdc.gov/niosh.

Olsen, J., Giangrasso, A., Shrimpton, D., & Dillon, P. (2012). *Medical dosage calculations: A dimensional analysis approach* (10th ed.). Upper Saddle River, NJ: Pearson Education.

Smeltzer, S., Bare, B., Hinkle, J., & Cheever, K. (2010). *Brunner & Suddarth's textbook of medical-surgical nursing* (12th ed.). Philadelphia: Lippincott Williams & Wilkins.

ANSWERS & RATIONALES

Anti-Infective Medications

2

Chapter Outline

Antibiotics
Antimycobacterials

Antivirals
Antifungals

Antiprotozoals
Antihelminthics

Objectives

➤ Describe general goals of therapy when administering anti-infective medications.
➤ Explain why antibiotics should not be discontinued until the prescribed therapy is complete.
➤ Identify actions and common side effects of various anti-infective medications.
➤ Describe most common adverse reactions to anti-infective medications.
➤ Explain nursing considerations related to anti-infective medications prescribed to treat human immunodeficiency virus and acquired immunodeficiency syndrome.
➤ Describe why medication combinations are commonly used to treat tuberculosis and leprosy.
➤ Identify significant client education points related to the use of anti-infective medications.

NCLEX-RN® Test Prep

Use the accompanying online resource, NursingReviewsandRationales, to test yourself with hundreds of NCLEX®-style practice questions.

Review at a Glance

amebiasis infection of large intestine by a protozoan parasite called *Entamoeba histolytica*; transmitted via fecal to oral route from contaminated food or water or from person to person contact; found throughout the world

bactericidal term for an agent that *destroys* a bacterial microorganism

bacteriostatic agent that *inhibits* growth of bacteria and depends on host's immune system to destroy bacteria

candidiasis a fungal infection caused by *Candida albicans* transmitted by direct contact or as a superinfection; occurs in mucous membranes in warm, dark, moist areas such as oral cavity (thrush), vagina, intestine, and cutaneously beneath breasts and in diaper areas of infants

cross-sensitivity a condition in which one class of drugs is chemically

very similar to another; allergy to one class may suggest allergy to another class of drugs; cross-sensitivity occurrence between penicillins and cephalosporins has been reported to be 1 to 18%

cytomegalovirus (CMV) a common virus that resides in salivary glands; may cause CMV pneumonia (potentially fatal) and CMV retinitis (with potential blindness) in immunosuppressed clients; newborns are also at higher risk if mother is infected; requires use of standard precautions

disulfiram-like reaction also called antabuse effect; a reaction when certain medications are taken with even small amounts of alcohol; causes abdominal cramping, facial and upper body flushing, pulsating headache, weakness, uneasiness, vertigo, hypotension, palpitations, shortness of breath, sweating,

pruritic macular rash, tachycardia, nausea and vomiting; may occur within 10–30 minutes of alcohol ingestion and last 30 minutes to several hours

empiric therapy drug therapy initiated based on clinical manifestations of a pathologic or infectious process rather than diagnosis by culture and sensitivity (C&S); selection of agent is based on most common known cause of infection and may be adjusted if needed after C&S results are known

giardiasis most common protozoan intestinal (usually duodenal) infection transmitted by contaminated food or water or stool of infected clients; causes diarrhea, abdominal distention, and malodorous stools

helminths disease-producing parasites such as *Nematoda* (roundworms) and *Platyhelminthes* (flatworms) that include *Cestodes* (tapeworms), and *trematodes* (flukes), which may be isolated in stool, urine, blood, sputum, or host tissues

herpes simplex a viral infection classified as Type 1 (of facial areas including cold sore or fever blister) or Type 2 (genital herpes)

herpes varicella virus that causes chickenpox

herpes zoster virus of chickenpox that has lain dormant in nerves; eruptions of infection occur along nerve routes, especially of trunk; may be activated by immunosuppressed states or stress of disease

peak drug level serum blood level of antibiotic drawn 15–30 minutes after IV infusion is complete to determine that peak level is not at a toxic level

pneumocystis (carinii) jiroveci pneumonia very serious protozoan

infection of lungs occurring only in immunosuppressed clients

pseudomembranous colitis a type of superinfection that occurs when an antibiotic decreases or completely eliminates normal flora needed to maintain normal function in GI tract; permits overgrowth of other bacteria or fungi or yeasts (not susceptible to antibiotic) that cause infection

Stevens-Johnson syndrome an adverse skin reaction that resembles appearance of partial thickness burns with erythema multiforme, fever, and bullae (blister) lesions of mucous membranes of oropharynx, conjunctiva, vagina, and anus

superinfection a condition in which an antibiotic decreases or eliminates normal bacterial flora that consists of certain bacteria and fungi or yeasts needed to maintain normal function in various organs;

permits overgrowth of other bacteria or fungi or yeasts (not susceptible to the antibiotic) that cause infection (e.g., vaginal yeast infection, pseudomembranous colitis, candidiasis)

tinea fungal infections, called ringworm, caused by dermatophytes on foot (tinea pedis or "athlete's foot"), on scalp (tinea capitis), on body (tinea corporis), and in the groin (tinea cruris or "jock itch")

toxoplasmosis protozoan systemic infection transmitted by contact with oocysts in feces of domesticated animals, primarily in feline species

trough drug level blood specimen drawn just prior to next scheduled IV dose of antibiotic to determine that therapeutic level has been maintained between drug doses; it is also measured to ensure that adequate renal clearance of drug has occurred to avoid toxicity

PRETEST

1 When overseeing drug therapy for a client taking isoniazid (INH), the nurse should assess for which of the following? Select all that apply.

1. Elevated aspartate aminotransferase (AST)
2. Clinical manifestations of hypercalcemia
3. Concurrent self-administration of aluminum antacids
4. Compliance with ingestion of pyridoxine vitamin B_6 supplements
5. Excessive bruising on the skin

2 A client receiving an intravenous infusion of a cephalosporin medication reports pain and irritation at the infusion site. Which action would be most appropriate for the nurse to take when thrombophlebitis of the site is observed?

1. Slow the infusion and apply a cold compress to the site.
2. Dilute the infusion by running it concurrently with a normal saline infusion.
3. Stop the infusion and notify the primary care provider.
4. Select an alternate infusion site and administer the medication slowly.

3 A client with benign prostatic hyperplasia (BPH) is receiving amantadine (Symmetrel) for *influenza A*. The nurse should monitor for which side effect?

1. Urinary retention
2. Hypermotility of bowel
3. Excessive urination
4. Nephrotoxicity

4 Which intervention is of highest priority for the nurse working with a client who has *herpes zoster* (shingles) and who recently began drug therapy with acyclovir (Zovirax)?

1. Monitor for jaundice and elevated liver enzymes.
2. Teach client to avoid sexual intercourse during therapy.
3. Administer the dose early in the day, as it may cause insomnia.
4. Encourage fluid intake of 2,500 to 3,000 mL daily if not contraindicated.

5 The nurse concludes that a client with an upper respiratory infection understands principles of self-administration of a prescribed oral antibiotic after the client makes which statement?

1. "I will continue to take the antibiotic as it is ordered, even though I no longer have a cough with yellow sputum."
2. "When I missed a dose of my antibiotic this morning, I made up by taking 2 doses when it was time to take the next dose."
3. "I am careful to take the antibiotic every day at breakfast, lunch, and dinner."
4. "Even though the doctor prescribed an amoxicillin (Amoxil) chewable tablet, I have no problem swallowing it whole."

6 After ingesting amoxicillin (Amoxil) for 10 days, the client has developed diarrhea, with approximately 8 watery stools per day. The nurse should anticipate the need for which priority interventions? Select all that apply.

1. Monitor for clinical manifestations of metabolic acidosis.
2. Administer an antiperistaltic agent such as dicyclomine hydrochloride (Bentyl).
3. Administer an antidiarrheal agent such as kaolin and pectin (Kaopectolin).
4. Collect stool specimen for a cytotoxin assay to detect *Clostridium difficile*.
5. Instruct client to increase intake of fruit juices.

7 When assessing a client for toxicities associated with aminoglycoside therapy, the nurse should include evaluation of which of the following? Select all that apply.

1. Hand strength
2. Creatinine levels
3. Alanine aminotransferase (ALT) levels
4. Amylase levels
5. Hearing acuity

8 Which client statement indicates a need for more teaching from the nurse regarding the use of the macrolide erythromycin (EES)? Select all that apply.

1. "I will always take this medication with fruit juices."
2. "If I experience abdominal pain and fullness I will contact my provider."
3. "I know I should not crush the pills."
4. "I understand it is common to have some hearing loss while taking this medication."
5. "I will let my provider know if I begin to have a lot of diarrhea."

9 The prescriber has just ordered cefdinir (Omnicef), a third-generation cephalosporin, for a client with a staphylococcal infection. The nurse collaborates with the prescriber about which data related to the client?

1. Blood urea nitrogen (BUN) 14 mg/dL
2. Elevated granulocyte count
3. Culture and sensitivity (C&S) results not yet available
4. History of Type I hypersensitivity to penicillin

10 When a client's white blood cell count (WBC) differential shows a "shift to the left," the nurse should assess the client for signs of what type of infection?

1. Bacterial
2. Acute viral
3. Parasitic
4. Chlamydia *trachomatis*

➤ *See pages 81–83 for Answers and Rationales.*

I. ANTIBIOTICS

A. Aminoglycosides

1. Action and use
   a. **Bactericidal**: aminoglycosides kill bacteria cells by interfering with protein synthesis
   b. Effective against aerobic gram-negative infections; used in combination with another antibiotic to treat gram-positive infections
   c. Used to remove enterococcal bacteria prior to bowel surgery
   d. Used to destroy urease-producing bacteria in bowel to prevent absorption of ammonia in hepatic encephalopathy (Neomycin)
   e. Toxicity limits the drug's use to serious gram-negative infections and specific conditions involving gram-positive cocci
   f. Used in infections caused by *Acinetobacter, Citrobacter, E. coli, Klebsiella pneumoniae, proteus, pseudomonas, Providencia, Salmonella, Serratia,* and *staphylococcus* organisms; also active against protozoal infections

2. Common medications (Table 2-1)

3. Administration considerations
   a. Intravenous (IV) route preferred for optimal distribution to tissues
    b. May be used intramuscularly (IM) as well
   c. Oral route: poorly absorbed so effective orally only to cleanse bowel prior to abdominal surgery or to prevent absorption of ammonia in hepatic encephalopathy
   d. Intrathecal or intraventricular injection: these routes may be used because of poor penetration of cerebrospinal fluid (CSF) by other routes
   e. Periocular instillations: because of poor penetration of eye fluids, direct instillations may be used
    f. Topical route: neomycin combined with other antibiotics provides broad spectrum coverage in a cream or ointment

4. Contraindications
   a. Allergy to aminoglycosides
   b. Preexisting renal disease
   c. Concurrent order for renal toxic agents such as amphotericin B (Fungizone), vancomycin (Vancocin), or loop diuretics as furosemide (Lasix)
   d. In myasthenia gravis
   e. Should be used cautiously in pregnancy and lactation
   f. Should be used cautiously in neonates and preterm infants due to immaturity of renal system

Table 2-1	Aminoglycosides
Generic (Trade) Name	**Route**
Amikacin sulfate (Amikin)	IM, IV
Gentamicin sulfate (Garamycin)	IM, IV, topical
Kanamycin sulfate (Kantrex)	PO, IM, IV, irrigation, intraperitoneal, inhalation
Neomycin sulfate (Mycifradin)	PO, IM
Paromomycin sulfate (Humatin)	PO
Streptomycin sulfate (Streptomycin)	IM
Tobramycin sulfate (Nebcin)	IM, IV, topical

5. Significant drug interactions

    a. Aminoglycosides may be microbiologically inactivated with concurrently high concentration of penicillins greater than 200 mcg/mL

    b. Do not mix other medications in the same IV fluid

    c. With oral anticoagulant therapy, bleeding may increase because aminoglycosides decrease vitamin K synthesis in intestinal tract

    d. Concurrent administration of dimenhydrinate (Dramamine) may mask signs of toxicity

6. Significant food interactions: none reported

7. Significant laboratory studies

    a. Peak drug level: blood specimen drawn 15–30 minutes after completion of IV infusion of aminoglycoside to determine that toxic level does not occur; dose may need to be decreased if peak too high; peak levels may not be drawn with once daily dosing since dose is short-lived

    b. Trough drug level: blood specimen drawn immediately prior to administering next IV dose of aminoglycoside to assure that therapeutic levels of drug are maintained between doses and also to ensure adequate renal clearance of drug has occurred; if a therapeutic level is not sustained, an increase in dose and/or dosing frequency may be needed; if trough levels are too high, dosage will need to be decreased

    c. White blood count (WBC) to monitor effectiveness of drug therapy

        1) Neutrophils and immature neutrophils, called stabs or bands, are increased in acute bacterial infections

        2) Neutrophils and lymphocytes make up 75 to 90% of leukocytes; when one part of the differential increases, as in response to an acute infection, another part has to decrease; a "shift to the left" signifies an increase in neutrophils and, therefore, an acute bacterial infection

        3) This knowledge facilitates selection of an appropriate type of anti-infective drug by health care provider

    d. Serum creatinine and blood urea nitrogen (BUN) to monitor renal function; expected BUN to creatinine ratio is 20:1 or 15:1 depending on criteria of laboratory; creatinine is most specific test for renal function; if creatinine level rises 3 to 4 days into treatment, it indicates renal damage has occurred

8. Side effects: headache, paresthesia, skin rash, fever

9. Adverse effects/toxicity

    a. Nephrotoxicity and ototoxicity are 2 common toxicities associated with therapy with aminoglycosides

    b. Occur when trough levels are elevated

    c. Nephrotoxicity: risk factors include infancy or advanced age (with associated immature or declining renal function), hypotension, dehydration, preexisting renal disease, and coadministration of other nephrotoxic drugs

    d. Ototoxicity: may be irreversible

        1) Auditory impairment and vestibular damage

        2) Possible damage to 8th cranial nerve

        3) Risk increased with nephrotoxic drugs, prolonged treatment with aminoglycosides, impaired renal function, and other ototoxic drugs, such as furosemide (Lasix), vancomycin (Vancocin), amphotericin B, and certain antineoplastic agents

    e. Neuromuscular blockade: secondary to inhibition of acetylcholine release; may be seen in clients with myasthenia gravis or clients receiving neuromuscular blocking agents such as pancuronium bromide (Pavulon) or succinylcholine (Anectine); use calcium salts to reverse blockade

     f. Hypersensitivity reactions include purpura, rash, urticaria, and exfoliative dermatitis

     g. Superinfection: a secondary infection caused by eradication of normal flora

         1) Candidiasis: secondary infection usually of skin and mucous membranes caused by *Candida albicans*

           a) Often associated with immunosuppression

           b) Occurs on mucous membranes of oropharynx (thrush), bronchi, vagina, and anus

           c) Appears as discrete white plaques; red, scaly, papular skin rash can occur in warm, moist, dark areas, such as in breast folds, axilla, and/or groin

         2) Pseudomembranous colitis: secondary infection of bowel usually caused by *Clostridium difficile*

           a) Manifested by 4 to 6 watery stools/day with blood and/or mucus, abdominal pain, and fever

           b) Antibiotic is discontinued and vancomycin (Vancocin) orally (PO) or metronidazole (Flagyl) IV or PO is prescribed

10. Nursing considerations

     a. Collect appropriate specimen for culture and sensitivity (C&S) prior to initiating anti-infective therapy to ensure appropriate drug is prescribed; **empiric therapy** (based on probable offending organism) is usually begun before test results become available because of seriousness of infection

     b. Assess for other current medications that could cause drug–drug interaction

     c. Ensure client takes complete course of antibiotic for full beneficial effects, even if clinical manifestations of infection resolved; premature discontinuation can result in regrowth of microorganisms as well as development of drug resistance

     d. Monitor peak and trough aminoglycoside levels

     e. Monitor for nephrotoxicity

         1) Monitor serum creatinine (normal 0.8 to 1.6 mg/dL), BUN (normal 8–22 mg/dL), urine creatinine clearance and urinalysis results; client may exhibit azotemia

         2) Nephrotoxicity manifestations include urinary casts and proteinuria

         3) Make certain the client is not taking other nephrotoxic drugs

         4) Keep accurate record of intake and output (I & O)

     f. Monitor for ototoxicity

         1) Assess baseline hearing and existing hearing impairments (may be noted by presence of hearing aids) and monitor for hearing loss once therapy begins; may include audiometry testing; determine if client already wears hearing aids

         2) Clinical signs of ototoxicity include dizziness, light-headedness, tinnitus, fullness in ears, and hearing loss

         3) Monitor vestibular integrity: perform Romberg's test, if possible; have client stand alone with hands at sides and eyes open, then have client close eyes; minimum swaying of body is expected, but if unable to maintain standing position or balance, Romberg's test is positive indicating problem with balance

     g. Question prescriber about dosage adjustment or medication change if indicated by results of above tests or assessments

     h. Maintain hydration to protect kidneys; fluid intake should be 2,500 to 3,000 mL/day unless contraindicated by other conditions

     i. Observe for evidence that infection is resolving within 48–72 hours of therapy (fever and local manifestations)

     j. Observe an IM injection site regularly for irritation, if used

     k. Provide small, frequent, nutritious meals with high-quality proteins; drugs that may be taken with food may be associated with decreased gastrointestinal (GI) upset

     l. Assess for adverse reactions

     m. Evaluate effectiveness of teaching plan

11. Client education
    a. See universal teaching points for anti-infectives (Box 2-1)
    b. Keep premixed drug refrigerated as recommended
    c. Take safety precautions according to side effects that occur
    d. Take oral gentamicin on an empty stomach, 1–2 hours before any meal or other drugs
    e. Eat small, frequent meals with at least 6–8 glasses of fluid daily
    f. Report sore throat, watery stools greater than 4–6 per day, and severe nausea or vomiting, which indicate possible superinfection
    g. Instruct on signs and symptoms of ototoxicity: headache, nausea, unsteady balance or gait, tinnitus, vertigo, high-frequency hearing loss, and dizziness

B. Carbapenems
1. Action and use
    a. Are among the broadest spectrums of antibiotics; inhibit cell wall synthesis and are bactericidal; they are effective against many gram-positive organisms and most gram-negative cocci and bacilli and anaerobic bacteria
    b. Are usually reserved for complicated body cavity and connective tissue infections in hospitalized clients
    c. Imipenem (Primaxin) is rapidly inactivated in kidneys by renal dehydropeptidase 1 and is always combined with cilastatin, a drug that inhibits this renal enzyme; Primaxin (cilastatin-imipenem) has a high resistance to bacterial enzymes, making it a very useful antibiotic
    d. May be used in serious infections of urinary tract, lower respiratory tract, bones, joints, skin–skin structures, intra-abdominal, gynecologic, and mixed infections
    e. Used in bacterial septicemia and endocarditis
    f. Meropenem (Merrem) used in bacterial meningitis because of its ability to enter CSF, especially if inflammation present
2. Common medications (Table 2-2)
3. Administration considerations
    a. Carbapenems have been associated with drug-induced seizure activity in a small percentage of clients; they are contraindicated in anyone with a history of hypersensitivity to any of their ingredients
    b. Reduced doses are indicated in the presence of renal insufficiency
    c. Preparations are specific to IM or IV use; do not interchange
    d. If administering IM, inject deep into gluteal muscle

Box 2-1	
Universal Client Teaching Points for Anti-Infective Therapy	• Know drug name, dose, route, administration schedule, and whether to take with or without food • Take at evenly spaced intervals around the clock as much as possible (but without interrupting sleep) in order to maintain therapeutic levels between doses • Take full course of therapy as prescribed to prevent repeat infection or development of drug resistance • Do not double the next dose if a dose is skipped or missed • Discard any outdated or unused drug; self-administration or use of drugs with decreased potency could adversely affect future treatment and increase risk of development of drug resistance • Do not use drug if expiration date has passed • Before taking any over-the-counter (OTC) drugs, check efficacy and possible adverse reactions with health care provider • Teach client to monitor for and report signs of superinfection (candidiasis or pseudomembranous colitis)

Table 2-2	Carbapenems
Generic (Trade) Name	**Route**
Imipenem and cilastin (Primaxin)	IV
Doripenem (Doribax)	IV
Ertapenem (Invanz)	IV, IM
Meropenem (Merrem)	IV, IM

4. Contraindications
   a. A small risk of allergenicity exists in clients with penicillin allergies; clients who experience anaphylactic-type reactions to penicillin should not receive carbapenem
   b. Ertapenem is not approved for use in children
   c. Use caution in clients with (central nervous system) CNS disorders, renal dysfunction, asthma, or in pregnancy or lactation
   d. IV use is not recommended in children due to risk of seizures
   e. Imipenem and cilastin are stable in dextrose-containing solutions for only 4 hours; are incompatible in Lactated Ringers solution
5. Significant drug interactions
   a. CNS effects may be additive when given with cyclosporine, ganciclovir, and theophylline
   b. Meropenem may interact with valproic acid; monitor levels of valproic acid to ensure they are therapeutic
   c. Concurrent use of imipenem or cilastin with cyclosporine, tramadol, theophylline, or ganciclovir may increase risk of seizures and other CNS effects
   d. Concurrent administration with penicillin, cephalosporins may antagonize antimicrobial effects with Primaxin and Azactam
6. Significant food interactions: this drug class is only given IV or IM
7. Significant laboratory studies
   a. Monitor renal function; reduced doses of Primaxin may be needed for clients with renal insufficiency since this drug is substantially excreted by kidneys
   b. Monitor liver function tests (LFTs), electrolytes, BUN, creatinine, and complete blood count (CBC) with differential
8. Side effects
   a. Nausea or vomiting (N/V), anorexia, dizziness, diarrhea, rash, pruritus, headache
   b. Drug fever
   c. Hyperkalemia, hyponatremia, polyuria, oliguria, weakness, arthralgias
9. Adverse effects/toxicity
   a. Superinfections with bacteria or fungi may occur
   b. Pseudomembranous colitis and blood dyscrasias may occur
   c. CNS effects such as seizures, especially in older adults with compromised renal function, or when concurrently taking ganciclovir
   d. Transient hearing loss
   e. Hypersensitivity reactions with fever, chills, dyspnea, chest discomfort, hyperventilation, pruritus
10. Nursing considerations
    a. Clients allergic to other beta-lactam antibiotics may be cross-allergic to imipenem
    b. These drugs are not absorbed by GI tract and must be given IV or IM
    c. Monitor renal function studies and electrolyte levels closely
    d. Monitor for neurotoxicity, nephrotoxicity, hepatotoxicity, transient hearing loss

      e. Provide measures for seizures and other CNS alterations when appropriate; call prescriber to discontinue drug if seizures occur

      f. Monitor client for signs of superinfections such as candidiasis

      g. Monitor injection site closely for phlebitis

      h. Imipenem and cilastin (Primaxin) are a pregnancy category C drugs; ertapenem and meropenem are category B

      i. Do not interchange IM and IV solutions

  11. Client education

      a. See Box 2-1 for universal teaching points for anti-infective therapy

      b. Determine whether or not client is pregnant before starting imipenem

      c. Instruct client to inform nurse if IV site is burning or painful

      d. Instruct client to report severe or persistent diarrhea, intense itching, difficulty breathing, confusion, or seizures

      e. Do not breastfeed or become pregnant while taking imipenem or cilastin

      f. Report excessive diarrhea (a sign of pseudomembranous colitis) or secondary infection (sore mouth, vaginal irritation)

C. Cephalosporins

  1. Action and use

      a. Structurally and chemically related to penicillins; practically identical to penicillin in mechanism of action, drug effects, therapeutic effects, side effects, adverse effects, and drug interactions; also considered to be beta-lactam antibiotics; **cross-sensitivity** may occur between penicillins and cephalosporins, meaning that allergy to one class may indicate hypersensitivity to the other in some clients

      b. Four generations of cephalosporins

         1) First through third generations: increased activity against gram-negative organisms and anaerobes; less activity against gram-positive organisms; first generation does not enter CSF and has limited activity against aerobic gram-negative organisms such as *E. coli*, *P. mirabilis*, *Klebsiella pneumoniae*

         2) Fourth generation: increased activity against gram-positive cocci and gram-negative bacilli

         3) Fifth generation: effective against gram-positive and -negative organisms; are being used to treat community-acquired bacterial pneumonias (CABP), resistant strains of methicillin-resistant *Staphylococcus aureus*, and soft tissue and skin infections

      c. Usually bactericidal; differences between generations include activity against gram-negative bacteria, resistance to beta-lactam drugs, and distribution in CSF

      d. Sexually transmitted infections (STIs)

         1) Third generation for cervicitis, urethritis, pharyngitis, and proctitis caused by *Neisseria gonorrhea*

         2) Chlamydia is commonly associated with gonorrhea so client may be given azithromycin (Zithromax) as a single dose or doxycycline (Vibramycin) concurrently

         3) Ceftriaxone (Rocephin): treats chancroid, syphilis; doxycycline may be added to treat pelvic inflammatory disease (PID), epididymitis, or orchitis

      e. Used to treat respiratory infections such as bronchitis, pharyngitis, otitis media, sinusitis, and pneumonia

      f. Used to treat urinary tract infections (UTI), skin and tissue infections, Lyme disease

      g. Used prophylactically and therapeutically in orthopedic disorders; cefazolin (Ancef) is drug of choice to prevent or treat bone infections associated with orthopedic surgery

     h. Used for endocarditis prophylaxis prior to surgery for clients with history of rheumatic heart disease

     i. Important to reserve use for appropriate clinical infections because bacterial resistance increasing

     j. Most cephalosporins are excreted through urine except cefoperazone (Cefobid) and ceftriaxone (Rocephin), which are excreted in bile

2. Common medications (Table 2-3)

3. Administration considerations

     a. Collect specimen for C&S from site of infection, whenever possible, prior to initiation of antibiotic; empiric therapy may be started if results not available to enhance effectiveness with early antibiotic administration

     b. Well absorbed from GI tract

         1) Absorption delayed with food but amount absorbed not affected

         2) Absorption not delayed with cefadroxil and cefprozil

Table 2-3 Cephalosporins

Generic (Trade) Name	Route
First generation	
Cefadroxil (Duricef)	PO
Cefazolin (Ancef, Kefzol)	IM, IV
Cephalexin (Keflex)	PO
Cephapirin (ToDAY)	PO, IM, IV
Cephradine (Velosef)	PO, IM, IV
Second generation	
Cefaclor (Ceclor)	PO
Cefotetan (Cefotan)	IM, IV
Cefoxitin (Mefoxin)	IM, IV
Cefprozil (Cefzil)	PO
Cefuroxime (Ceftin, Zinacef)	PO, IM, IV
Third generation	
Cefdinir (Omnicef)	PO
Cefditoren (Spectracef)	PO
Cefixime (Suprax)	PO
Cefoperazone sodium (Cefobid)	IM, IV
Cefotaxime (Claforan)	IM, IV
Cefpodoxime proxetil (Vantin)	PO
Ceftazidime (Fortaz)	IM, IV
Ceftibuten (Cedax)	PO
Ceftizoxime (Cefizox)	IM, IV
Ceftriaxone (Rocephin)	IM, IV
Fourth generation	
Cefepime (Maxipime)	IM, IV
Fifth generation	
Ceftraroline (Teflaro)	IV

    c. Do not readily enter CSF except for cefuroxime; third-generation drugs readily enter CSF in presence of meningeal inflammation

    d. Check renal function before and during therapy to allow for appropriate dosage adjustment; renal impairment significantly extends drug half-life

    e. Crosses placenta

    f. Separate oral administration of antacids, histamine H2-receptor blockers, iron supplements and foods fortified with iron by 2 hours before and after oral administration of cephalosporins

    g. Separate oral administration of cefdinir from iron supplements and foods fortified with iron by 2 hours

    h. Intramuscular administration is painful and irritating; administer deep IM into large muscle; avoid repeated IM injections; IV is the preferred parenteral route; addition of prescribed 1% xylocaine solution can help to reduce pain with IM injections

    i. Shake suspensions to disperse or dissolve particles of drug immediately before measurement

    j. Continue drug administration for at least 10 days to decrease risk of rheumatic fever in beta-hemolytic streptococcal infections such as "strep throat"; also acute glomerulonephritis can become a sequela of this infection if treatment is inadequate

  4. Contraindications

    a. Cross-sensitivity with penicillins; not recommended for those who have had a Type I (anaphylactic) reaction to penicillin

    b. Use extreme caution if creatinine clearance is less than 50 mL/minute

    c. Hepatotoxicity with cefoperazone and ceftriaxone

    d. Should be used cautiously in pregnancy and lactation

  5. Significant drug interactions

    a. Probenecid (Benemid): increases and prolongs half-life of cephalosporins

    b. Loop diuretics and aminoglycosides increase risk of nephrotoxicity

    c. Anticoagulants increase the risk of bleeding

    d. Use of ethanol with some cephalosporins such as cefoperazone and cefotetan can cause **disulfiram-like reaction** (weakness, pulsating headache, and abdominal cramps) during therapy and up to 72 hours after drug discontinued; can occur within 30 minutes of alcohol ingestion

    e. Antacids: concurrent use interferes with absorption of cefaclor, cefdinir, cefpodoxime

    f. Histamine H2-receptor antagonists: decrease plasma concentration of cephalosporins

  6. Significant food interactions

    a. Iron supplements and iron-fortified foods decrease absorption of cefdinir

    b. May take with food or milk if drug causes gastric irritation except ceftibuten, which is taken 1 hour before and 2 hours after meals

    c. Drug absorption enhanced with food with cefuroxime and cefpodoxime

  7. Significant laboratory studies

    a. With parenteral use and/or prolonged therapy, check urinalysis, BUN, and serum creatinine to monitor renal function

    b. Monitor liver function tests when giving cefoperazone and ceftriaxone

    c. Monitor baseline and periodic prothrombin time (PT) and international normalized ratio (INR) if taking oral anticoagulants, and assess for increased bleeding, such as bleeding gums and easy bruising

      1) With long-term therapy of parenteral cefamandole, cefoperazone, cefotetan, or moxalactam (Moxam)

      2) If PT prolonged, give exogenous vitamin K (Phytonadione) as prescribed

8. Side effects
   a. Central nervous system (CNS): lethargy, hallucinations, anxiety, depression, twitching, seizures, coma
   b. GI: N/V, mild diarrhea, abdominal cramps or distress, increased LFTs such as aspartate aminotransferase (AST) and alanine aminotransferase (ALT), abdominal pain, colitis
   c. Hematologic: anemia, increased bleeding time, bone marrow depression, granulocytopenia
   d. Metabolic: hyperkalemia, hypokalemia, alkalosis
   e. Phlebitis can occur with IV administration of cephalosporins
   f. Abscess formation can occur with IM injection
   g. Other: taste alteration, sore mouth; dark, discolored or sore tongue; hives, pruritis, rash, edema

9. Adverse effects/toxicity
   a. Hypersensitivity occurs in 5–16% of clients
   b. Cross-sensitivity with penicillins
   c. Serum sickness–like illness
      1) Erythema multiforme and other skin rashes, arthralgia, and fever
      2) Usually follows second course of treatment and may be delayed at least 10 days after initiation of drug
      3) Treated with antihistamines and corticosteroids
   d. Seizure activity
      1) Especially in renal impairment or in intraventricular administration
      2) Discontinue the cephalosporin to resolve activity
   e. In renal impairment, cancer, impaired vitamin K synthesis, malnutrition, or low vitamin K stores, there is increased risk for the following:
      1) Coagulation disturbances with parenteral use or concurrent anticoagulant use
      2) Disulfiram-like reaction in those who consume, or less frequently, inhale or absorb alcohol as in perfume, aftershave, alcohol swabs
   f. Immune hemolytic anemia: rare
   g. Pseudomembranous colitis: treated by stopping cephalosporin and giving oral vancomycin (Vancocin) or metronidazole (Flagyl)
   h. Accumulation of biliary sludge or pseudolithiasis with ceftriaxone; clears after drug is discontinued

10. Nursing considerations
   a. Monitor clinical therapeutic response
      1) Heat, redness, swelling, tenderness, or discharge abate after 48–72 hours
      2) Fever and malaise improve; WBC count decreases
      3) Pulmonary infiltrates resolve and pulse oximetry normalizes in pneumonia
   b. Monitor site of infection throughout course of treatment; re-culture site if improvement is not observed in 48 hours
   c. Monitor injection sites for induration and tenderness; provide warm compresses and gentle massage to injection sites if painful or swollen; if phlebitis or redness at IV site develops, remove IV device and restart IV
   d. Monitor for renal toxicity: check serum creatinine, BUN, and urine creatinine clearance, and keep accurate I & O
   e. Monitor for unusual lethargy beginning after drug started; provide safety measures, including adequate lighting, use of side rails, and assistance with ambulation to protect client if CNS effects occur
   f. For client with diabetes mellitus, use blood glucose monitoring; although urine glucose testing is generally an outdated therapy, false-positive urine glucose can occur with copper sulfate technique (Clinitest)

    g. Offer small, frequent meals with quality protein as tolerated

    h. Provide frequent oral care; offer ice chips or sugarless candy if stomatitis and sore mouth occur

    i. Monitor for superinfections

       1) Often subtle and nonspecific with clinical manifestations of oral or pharyngeal discomfort with oral candidiasis or perineal itching or discharge with vaginal candidiasis

       2) Differentiate antibiotic diarrhea from pseudomembranous colitis; the latter is characterized by fever, abdominal cramping, at least 4 to 6 watery stools/day, stools with blood and/or mucus; send stool specimen culture for *Clostridium difficile*

    j. Monitor for increased bleeding if taking anticoagulants

       1) Assess for easy bruising or bleeding

       2) If PT or INR prolonged, give exogenous vitamin K as ordered

    k. Monitor for hemolytic anemia (rare): check RBCs with indices, tiredness or weakness, yellow skin or eyes; check the hard palate to observe for icterus in dark-skinned clients

    l. Monitor effectiveness of teaching plan with regard to adherence and comfort and safety measures

  11. Client education

    a. See again Box 2–1 for universal teaching points for anti-infectives

    b. Take safety precautions including changing position slowly and avoiding driving and hazardous tasks if CNS effects occur

    c. Drink fluids and maintain nutrition, especially protein, to ensure adequate protein for drug binding and efficacy of action

    d. Shake suspensions well to dispense or dissolve particles of drug immediately before measurement: to ensure dosage accuracy, use a measuring device for suspension or other liquid and not a kitchen teaspoon (may vary from 2 to 10 mL/teaspoon)

    e. Report manifestations of hypersensitivity or superinfection to health care provider

       1) Hypersensitivity: difficulty breathing, severe rash, hives, severe headache, dizziness or weakness, aching joints

       2) Severe diarrhea: call health care provider; do not take antiperistaltic agent that would promote retention of toxins, such as *C. difficile* in pseudomembranous colitis; mild diarrhea: may take absorbent antidiarrheal agent

       3) Vaginal itching or discharge, sore mouth or throat, white patches on oral mucous membranes

    f. Report side effects to the health care provider: anorexia, epigastric pain, nausea or vomiting indicating biliary sludge or pseudolithiasis if on ceftriaxone; discontinue drug and manifestations will resolve

    g. Refrain from alcohol use during therapy and for 72 hours after drug discontinued to avoid disulfiram-like reaction

D. Fluoroquinolones

  1. Action and use

    a. Are broad-spectrum bactericidal antibiotics that interfere with enzyme DNA gyrase

    b. Used against gram-negative and selected gram-positive organisms; used in various bacterial infections depending on bacteria and site: lower respiratory tract infections, sinusitis, bone and joint infections, infectious diarrhea, skin and soft tissue infections, intra-abdominal infections, STIs, and UTIs

    c. Many of the oral formulations are as effective as the parenteral forms

    d. Postexposure prophylaxis to anthrax

2. Common medications (Table 2-4)
3. Administration considerations
   a. Administer evenly spaced around the clock and do not interrupt sleep, if possible, to maintain therapeutic blood level
   b. Oral drug is tolerated better with food
4. Contraindications
   a. Known hypersensitivity to fluoroquinolones
   b. Use cautiously in clients with renal dysfunction including those with advanced age, children, pregnant or lactating women, those with history of seizures
5. Significant drug interactions
   a. Oral antacids, iron, zinc preparations, and sucralfate reduce absorption
   b. Probenecid (Benemid) prolongs half-life of fluoroquinolones
   c. Beta-agonist effects of theophylline (TheoDur) may be increased; monitor clients with hypertension, ischemic heart disease, coronary insufficiency, congestive heart failure (CHF), or history of cerebrovascular accident (CVA or stroke)
   d. Class IA or Class III antidysrhythmics may enhance adverse cardiovascular (CV) effects
   e. Cimetidine (Tagamet) may prolong half-life
   f. Cyclosporine (Sandimmune) increases risk of nephrotoxicity
   g. Glucocorticosteroids may increase risk for rupture of tendon, especially in older adults
   h. Caffeine elimination with ciprofloxacin (Cipro) and norfloxacin (Noroxin) is decreased
   i. Use of ciprofloxacin with phenytoin (Dilantin) may lower levels of phenytoin
   j. Nitrofurantoin (Furadantin) may reduce the efficacy of norfloxacin
   k. Use of nonsteroidal anti-inflammatory drugs (NSAIDs) with levofloxacin (Levaquin) increases CNS stimulation including seizures; levofloxacin may also increase or decrease blood glucose in conjunction with oral antidiabetic agents
   l. Risk of significant CV side effects may occur with use of certain CV agents and sparfloxacin (Zagam) or moxifloxacin (Avelox)
   m. Increased bleeding risk may occur with oral anticoagulants because antibiotic alters intestinal flora and interferes with vitamin K synthesis
6. Significant food interactions
   a. Limit alkaline foods that can alter pH of stomach and absorption
   b. Alkaline foods include dairy products, vegetables, and legumes
7. Significant laboratory studies
   a. Monitor ALT (SGPT), AST (SGOT), alkaline phosphatase, and bilirubin for elevation in liver toxicity
   b. Monitor for normalization of WBC and other appropriate laboratory findings, such as cultures of infectious site, to evaluate therapy effectiveness
   c. Monitor PT and INR if on warfarin (Coumadin)

Table 2-4 Fluoroquinolones

Generic (Trade) Name	Route
Ciprofloxacin (Cipro)	PO, IV, Ophthalmic
Gatifloxacin (Tequin)	PO, IV
Levofloxacin (Levaquin)	PO, IV
Lomefloxacin (Maxaquin)	PO
Moxifloxacin (Avelox)	PO
Norfloxacin (Noroxin)	PO, Ophthalmic
Ofloxacin (Floxin)	PO, IV, Otic, Ophthalmic

    8. Side effects

        a. Headache, dizziness, fatigue, lethargy, insomnia, depression, restlessness, confusion, and seizures

        b. N/V, diarrhea, constipation, flatulence, epigastric distress, oral candidiasis, dysphagia, pseudomembranous colitis; and elevated liver function tests, such as ALT, AST, bilirubin, and alkaline phosphatase

        c. Rash, pruritus, urticaria, photosensitivity, flushing

        d. Fever, chills, piloerection, blurred vision, tinnitus

    9. Adverse effects/toxicity

        a. Superinfections: more common in prolonged therapy

        b. Hypersensitivity reaction

        c. Quinolones contain an FDA black box warning because of an increased risk of tendonitis and tendon rupture with use of these drugs; this effect is seen more commonly in older adults and clients with renal failure or receiving a glucocorticoid; they are not approved for use under age 18

    10. Nursing considerations

        a. Assure appropriate specimens have been sent for C&S prior to beginning antibiotic therapy

        b. Check current medications for possible drug interactions

        c. Separate drug from oral antacids, iron and zinc salts, or sucralfate by 2 hours

        d. Monitor PT, INR, and manifestations of increased bleeding or bruising if also on oral anticoagulants

        e. Monitor renal function

        f. Provide more frequent meals with complete or complementary proteins to better ensure adequate albumin levels for drug efficacy

        g. Monitor for increased CNS irritability if client has history of epilepsy, ethanol abuse, or is concurrently taking theophylline

        h. Maintain hydration with 3 liters of fluid/day, if not contraindicated

    11. Client education

        a. Refer to Box 2-1 again for universal teaching points for anti-infectives therapy

        b. Take safety precautions including changing position slowly and avoiding driving and hazardous tasks if CNS effects occur

        c. Drink fluids and maintain nutrition, especially protein, to provide adequate protein for drug-binding and drug efficacy

        d. Report difficulty breathing, severe headache, dizziness, or weakness to health care provider

        e. May obtain baseline electrocardiogram with sparfloxacin or moxifloxacin

        f. Teach to wear sunglasses, long-sleeved and long-legged garments, and hat to protect from direct sunlight; sunscreen or sunblock may not prevent photosensitivity reaction; avoid ultraviolet lights, tanning beds, and direct sunlight

        g. Report unexplained joint or muscle pain

E. Macrolides and lincosamides

    1. Action and use

        a. Bacteriostatic (inhibiting growth of bacteria) but can be bactericidal in high doses with some bacteria; often considered when person is allergic to penicillins

        b. Is highly protein-bound

        c. Inhibit bacterial protein synthesis by binding to the 50S ribosomal subunit; they do not bind to human ribosome, thus providing selective toxicity

        d. Used in upper and lower respiratory tract infections, skin and soft tissue infections caused by *Streptococcus* or *Haemophilus* organisms

        e. Used to treat syphilis, gonorrhea, chlamydia, Lyme disease, and *mycoplasma*, *listeria*, and *corynebacterium* infections

     f. Clarithromycin (Biaxin) is used with omeprazole (Prilosec) to treat *Helicobacter pylori* associated with peptic ulcers

     g. Lincosamides may be bactericidal and bacteriostatic; used to treat chronic bone infections, genitourinary (GU) infections, intra-abdominal infections, pneumonia, and streptococcal or staphylococcal septicemia

2. Common medications (Table 2-5)

3. Administration considerations

     a. If erythromycin form has bitter taste, give with juice or applesauce

     b. Give clindamycin (Cleocin) and lincomycin (Lincocin) with at least 8 ounces of fluid or on an empty stomach

     c. If clindamycin (Cleocin) is given IV, do not give by intravenous push (IVP) method; instead give by IV infusion

     d. Azithromycin has longer half-life with less frequent dosing, shorter term of therapy and has fewer or less intense GI side effects than others (may contribute to better compliance)

     e. Give azithromycin suspension on an empty stomach, as food can significantly inhibit absorption

4. Contraindications

     a. Hypersensitivity

     b. Use caution with liver or renal dysfunction, GI disorders, in older adults and pregnant or lactating women

     c. Lincosamides are also contraindicated in ulcerative colitis or enteritis and children less than 1 year of age

5. Significant drug interactions

     a. Clindamycin and lincomycin: many drugs may be antagonistic, such as muscle relaxants, chloramphenicol (Chloromycetin), erythromycin, theophylline, antihistamines, penicillins, and oral anticoagulants

     b. Many drug interactions can occur when taken concurrently with the macrolides: carbamazepine (Tegretol), cyclosporine (Sandimmune), warfarin, and theophylline result in increased effects of these drugs

     c. Erythromycin (E-mycin) may increase risk of bleeding with warfarin (Coumadin)

     d. Erythromycin (E-mycin) and clarithromycin (Zithromax) increase risk of myopathy and rhabdomyolysis with lovastatin or simvastatin

6. Significant food interactions: grapefruit juice may increase bioavailability of erythromycin

7. Significant laboratory studies

     a. Monitor WBC with differential to monitor therapeutic response

     b. Monitor for hepatotoxicity (e.g., ALT, AST, alkaline phosphatase, bilirubin elevations)

     c. Monitor for nephrotoxicity (e.g., adverse changes in serum creatinine, BUN, creatinine clearance, urinalysis)

Table 2-5   **Macrolides and Lincosamides**

Generic (Trade) Name	Route
Azithromycin (Zithromax, Z-Pak, AzaSite)	PO, IV Ophthalmic solution
Clarithromycin (Biaxin)	PO
Erythromycin (E-Mycin, Erythrocin)	PO, topical
Clindamycin (Cleocin)	PO, IM, IV, topical
Lincomycin (Lincocin)	PO, IM, IV

8. Side effects

    a. Diarrhea from stimulation of smooth muscle and GI motility (may be used thera-peutically as a GI stimulant to facilitate passage of intestinal tube or to prevent gastroesophageal reflux and diabetic gastroparesis)

    b. Palpitations and chest pain

    c. Headache, dizziness, vertigo, lethargy, somnolence, confusion, hearing loss usually preceded by tinnitus

    d. Stomatitis, flatulence, epigastric distress, anorexia, nausea, vomiting; abnormal taste (clarithromycin [Biaxin])

    e. Jaundice, rash, pruritis, urticaria

    f. Thrombophlebitis at peripheral IV site

9. Adverse effects/toxicity

    a. Hepatotoxicity

    b. Nephrotoxicity

    c. Ototoxicity: erythromycin (Erythrocin)

    d. Superinfections (e.g., pseudomembranous colitis, candidiasis)

    e. High doses of erythromycin (E-mycin) may be cardiotoxic, increasing risk for a torsades de pointes dysrhythmia

10. Nursing considerations

    a. Collect data such as age, hypersensitivity to drugs, hepatic and renal function; also check cardiac status if appropriate for drug ordered

    b. Ensure client takes complete course of antibiotic for full beneficial effects, even if clinical manifestations resolved

    c. Collect specimen from infection site for C&S before initiating therapy, if possible

    d. Assess GI function and elimination pattern

    e. Observe for bleeding if taking oral anticoagulants

    f. Observe for superinfections

    g. Review OTC and prescribed client medications for drug–drug interactions

    h. Monitor ALT, AST, bilirubin, and alkaline phosphatase as indicated for hepatic dysfunction prior to and during therapy

    i. Monitor serum creatinine, BUN, creatinine clearance, I & O as appropriate for development of renal dysfunction

    j. Assess baseline hearing and monitor for hearing loss; arrange for discontinuation of drug if occurs

    k. Hydrate with at least 2,000 to 2,400 mL/day if not contraindicated

11. Client education

    a. See again Box 2-1 for universal teaching points for anti-infective therapy

    b. Report signs and symptoms of increasing infection such as fever, pain, redness, drainage, edema, lethargy, or exacerbation of presenting manifestations

    c. Include protein in diet since these drugs are highly protein-bound and need protein for therapeutic efficacy

    d. Report signs of ototoxicity including dizziness, vertigo, nausea, tinnitus, roaring noises, or hearing impairment

F. Penicillins (beta-lactams) and penicillinase-resistants

    1. Action and use

        a. Beta-lactams are chemical structure of penicillins

        b. Derived from fungus or mold evidenced on bread or fruit

        c. There is similarity among penicillins, cephalosporins, monobactams, carbapenems, and beta-lactamase inhibitors; they share many of the same actions and uses; cross-sensitivity is possible

        d. Penicillin is least toxic of these drugs; usually is antibiotic of choice because of low toxicity potential in nonallergic client

     e. Bactericidal; bacteriostatic effect with adequate dosing or blood levels

     f. Increased efficacy during replication of bacterial cells; prevent bacteria from biosynthesizing, which results in swelling and bursting of bacterial cells

     g. Only cross blood–brain barrier if meningeal inflammation present

     h. Most effective against gram-positive organisms; less effective against gram-negative organisms

     i. Used to treat infections caused by meningococci, pneumococci, streptococci, *treponema pallidum*, staphylococci as in upper respiratory infections, pneumonia, STIs such as syphilis but not gonorrhea, wound infections, and UTIs

     j. Used prophylactically against endocarditis for oral, GI, pulmonary procedures when bacteria may enter circulation; usually amoxicillin (Amoxil) or ampicillin (Omnipen) are used

     k. Used in beta-hemolytic streptococci Group A infections that can be associated with rheumatic fever or acute glomerulonephritis, such as pharyngitis; penicillin V (V-Cillin) PO route is preferred

     l. Because of history of possible overuse by prescribers, increasing resistance is developing, especially in facility-acquired infections; a C&S should be obtained prior to use

     m. Gonorrhea is mostly resistant to penicillins

     n. *Streptococcus pneumoniae* is most frequent microorganism in otitis media and sinusitis; has increased resistance to penicillins, tetracyclines, macrolides, and sulfonamides

2. Common medications (Table 2-6)

3. Administration considerations

     a. Oral dosing needs to be 3 to 4 times the parenteral dose because of hepatic first-pass effect and instability of penicillin in acidic environment of stomach

     b. For serious systemic infections, parenteral route is recommended

     c. Absorption erratic from IM route; limit due to irritability of tissue; IM injection should be slow and steady over 12–15 seconds to minimize discomfort and prevent obstructing the needle, especially with thick preparations

4. Contraindications

     a. Not for use in hypersensitivity reaction and anaphylaxis, serum sickness, exfoliative dermatitis, blood dyscrasias

     b. Penicillin G procaine or benzathine not to be given IV: lethal

     c. Is most likely drug category to cause allergic reactions

     d. Use caution in anemia, thrombocytopenia, bone marrow depression, and concurrently with anticoagulants because some penicillins cause increased bleeding

5. Significant drug interactions

     a. Loop and thiazide diuretics may exacerbate hypokalemia and rash

     b. Potassium-sparing diuretics may contribute to hyperkalemia

Table 2-6   **Penicillins (Beta-lactams) and Penicillinase-Resistants**

Generic (Trade) Name	Route
Amoxicillin (Amoxil)	PO
Ampicillin (Omnipen)	PO, IM, IV
Piperacillin (Pipracil)	IM, IV
Ticarcillin (Ticar)	IM, IV
Carbenicillin (Geopen)	PO
Oxacillin (Bactocil)	PO, IM, IV
Penicillin G (Pentids)	PO, IM, IV
Penicillin V (V-Cillin)	PO

c. Leads to decreased efficacy of oral contraceptives
   d. Probenecid (Benemid) delays excretions and increases serum levels
   e. Avoid coadministration with tetracycline because it may interfere with effectiveness of penicillins and increases risks of adverse effects
   f. Atenolol (Tenormin) levels may be decreased when given with ampicillin (Omnipen); increased risk for anaphylaxis
   g. Allopurinol (Zyloprim) increases risk for rash
   h. Piperacillin (Pipracil) may alter elimination of lithium
   i. Aspirin, phenylbutazone (ibuprofen-like), sulfonamides, furosemide, thiazide diuretics, and indomethacin prolong half-life of penicillin-G (Pentids)
   j. When penicillin is administered concurrently with aminoglycosides and both are given parenterally, the aminoglycoside may be inactivated
   6. Significant food interactions
   a. Take on empty stomach
   b. Amoxicillin not affected by food
   7. Significant laboratory studies
   a. CBC with WBC and differential
   b. PT and INR if on oral anticoagulants; activated partial thromboplastin time (aPPT) if receiving heparin
   c. ALT, AST, bilirubin, alkaline phosphatase
   d. Electrolytes, especially potassium and sodium
   8. Side effects
   a. Most common allergic responses are skin rash, urticaria, pruritis, angioedema; a maculopapular, pruritic rash that is like measles with ampicillin or amoxicillin is not a true allergic reaction, but develops after 7–10 days of therapy and may last a few days after drug discontinuation; is not a contraindication to give drug in future
   b. Most common side effects are GI, such as N/V, diarrhea, epigastric distress, abdominal pain, colitis, elevated liver enzymes; also taste alteration, sore mouth, or dark, discolored, sore tongue
   c. Hypokalemia or hyperkalemia, metabolic alkalosis
   9. Adverse effects/toxicity
   a. Type I hypersensitivity often fatal immediately if untreated within 2 to 30 minutes
      1) Urticaria, pruritis
      2) Severe dyspnea, stridor, tachycardia, hypotension
      3) Diaphoresis, vertigo, loss of consciousness and circulatory collapse
   b. Serum sickness–like reaction: skin rash, arthralgia, fever
   c. Exfoliative dermatitis: red, scaly skin
   d. Blood dyscrasias: hemolytic anemia, neutropenia, leukopenia
   e. Lethargy, anxiety, depression, hallucinations, twitching, seizures, coma
   f. Superinfections with broader-spectrum penicillins, especially with prolonged therapy; pseudomembranous colitis possible up to several weeks after drug discontinued; treated with anti-infectives such as metronidazole (Flagyl) PO or IV or vancomycin (Vancocin) PO
10. Nursing considerations
   a. Assess for allergies and hypersensitivity history
   b. Assess all medications taken to avoid drug–drug interactions
   c. Collect appropriate specimen for C&S, if possible, prior to initiating antibiotic therapy to ensure appropriate drug employed; empiric therapy is usually begun before test results available because of seriousness of infection
   d. Ensure client takes complete course of antibiotic for full beneficial effects, even if clinical manifestations of infection resolve; premature discontinuation can result in both regrowth of organisms and development of drug resistance

e. Do not administer with fruit juices, milk, or carbonated beverages because of poor absorption

f. Monitor renal studies, liver enzymes, and electrolytes; many penicillins contain sodium salts that can result in hypokalemia

g. Arrange for dose or drug adjustment as indicated by lab results

h. Monitor for evidence of clinical improvement of infection

i. Monitor for adverse effects; may not be necessary to discontinue drug if mild diarrhea develops; give yogurt or buttermilk to restore normal flora; use absorbent antidiarrheal agents (kaolin and pectin or Kao-tin); avoid antiperistaltic agents that delay or prevent elimination of intestinal toxins

j. Provide good nutrition and hydration

k. Some penicillins cause false-positive results on urine glucose testing; use Clinistix, or Testape for glucose urine testing or use blood glucose monitoring

l. Evaluate effectiveness of teaching plan

11. Client education

a. See Box 2-1 for universal teaching points for anti-infectives

b. Take oral drug on empty stomach; take 1 hour before meals or 2 hours after meals, except amoxicillin (which is not affected by food); take dose with a full glass of water

c. Chewable tablets must be crushed or chewed in order for penicillin to be effectively absorbed

d. Shake suspensions to disperse particles prior to measurement; use a calibrated device to measure liquid since kitchen teaspoons may vary by 2 to 10 mL; most suspensions maintain potency for 14 days if refrigerated

Practice to Pass

The client taking an antibiotic develops diarrhea. What assessments and interventions would you perform?

e. Ensure antibiotic drops used for correct route (i.e., oral, eye, ear)

f. Report rash, urticaria, pruritis, difficulty breathing

g. Report sore throat, watery stools equal to or greater than 4–6 stools/day or stools with blood/mucus, severe N/V, unusual bleeding or bruising

h. Take small frequent meals with high-quality protein and drink equal to or greater than 6–8 glasses of water per day, if not contraindicated by other conditions

G. Sulfonamides

1. Action and use

a. First effective group of antibiotics (1935)

b. Bacteriostatic, inhibit folic acid synthesis to prevent cell growth

c. Used to treat UTIs (especially caused by *Escherichia coli*, the most common cause), *Chlamydia trachomatis* causing blindness, pneumonia, brain abscesses, mild to moderate ulcerative colitis, active Crohn disease, and rheumatoid arthritis; with pyrimethamine as only effective drug treatment for toxoplasmosis; drugs of choice for treatment of nocardiosis

d. Sulfacetamide (silver sulfadiazine) to prevent bacterial growth in burns and wounds

e. Cross-sensitivity possible with penicillins and cephalosporins

2. Common medications (Table 2-7)

Table 2-7 Sulfonamides

Generic (Trade) Name	Route
Sulfisoxazole (Gantrisin)	PO, vaginal
Sulfadiazine (Microsulfon)	PO
Sulfamethoxazole–Trimethoprim (Bactrim)	PO, IM, IV
Sulfasalazine (Azulfidine)	PO

3. Administration considerations

    a. Fluid intake should be 3,000–4,000 mL/day if tolerated to promote urinary output at least 1,500 mL/day to prevent crystalluria/stone formation; if not possible, may administer antacids or sodium bicarbonate to alkalinize urine; alkaline ash diet may be helpful, which includes fruit (except plums, prunes, and cranberries), vegetables, and milk

    b. Store in light-resistant, tightly closed container at room temperature

4. Contraindications

    a. History of hypersensitivity to sulfonamides, salicylates, penicillins, or cephalosporins

    b. During pregnancy because of risk of birth defects or kernicterus; use cautiously

    c. During lactation and in children younger than 2 months unless used to treat congenital toxoplasmosis

    d. In porphyria, advanced or severe renal or hepatic dysfunction, or with intestinal and urinary blockage; use with caution in impaired renal or hepatic function, asthma, blood dyscrasias, or glucose-6-phosphate dehydrogenase (G6PD) deficiency

5. Significant drug interactions

    a. Increased risk for bleeding with oral anticoagulants

    b. More significant drop in blood glucose with oral antidiabetic agents (such as tolbutamide, tolazamide, glyburide, glipizide, acetohexamide, or chlorpropamide)

    c. Increased risk for phenytoin toxicity with phenytoin (Dilantin)

    d. Trimethoprim and sulfamethoxazole (Bactrim): combines sulfonamide with folic acid antagonist; increases synergistic effect

    e. Iron and some antibiotics may interfere with absorption of sulfonamide, such as sulfasalazine (Azulfidine)

6. Significant food interactions

    a. Some drugs, such as sulfamethoxazole (Gantanol), may be crushed and taken with liquids of choice

    b. Some, such as sulfasalazine, are best taken after meals to prolong time in intestine

7. Significant laboratory studies

    a. Creatinine, BUN, creatinine clearance, urinalysis to monitor renal function

    b. ALT, AST, bilirubin, alkaline phosphatase to monitor hepatic function

    c. CBC to monitor for blood dyscrasias and response to therapy

8. Side effects

    a. Rash common; most are urticaria and maculopapular

    b. N/V, diarrhea, abdominal pain, jaundice, stomatitis

    c. Headache, insomnia, drowsiness, depression, psychosis

    d. Photosensitivity

    e. Crystalluria

9. Adverse effects/toxicity

    a. Peripheral neuritis and neuropathy

    b. Tinnitus, hearing loss, vertigo

    c. Ataxia, seizures

    d. Hepatitis, pancreatitis

    e. Anemia, agranulocytosis, thrombocytopenia, leucopenia, eosinophilia, hypothrombinemia

    f. Exfoliative dermatitis, **Stevens–Johnson syndrome** (an adverse reaction of skin that resembles appearance of partial-thickness burns)

    g. Serum sickness, drug fever

10. Nursing considerations

    a. Collect appropriate specimen for C&S, if possible, prior to beginning therapy to ensure appropriate drug employed; empiric treatment is usually begun before test results are available because of seriousness of infection

    b. Assess for allergies and history of hypersensitivity; assess for allergy to thiazide diuretics

    c. Assess drugs being taken to avoid drug–drug interaction

    d. Assess baseline laboratory findings for liver function and renal function (creatinine) and monitor during therapy; a baseline skin assessment will provide a basis for detecting hypersensitivity reaction later if it occurs

    e. Provide hydration to assure daily urinary output of equal or greater than 1,500 mL to prevent stone and crystal formations; alkalinize urine as indicated; keep accurate I & O record

    f. Consult prescriber for dose adjustment or discontinuation of drug if toxicities develop

    g. Provide for safety if neurotoxicities develop, such as ataxia or seizures

    h. Provide small, frequent, nutritious meals with high quality proteins; drugs that may be taken with food may decrease GI upset

    i. Ensure client takes complete course of sulfonamides for full beneficial effects, even if clinical manifestations of infection resolve; premature discontinuation can result in regrowth of organisms and/or development of drug resistance

    j. Assess for clinical improvement, adverse effects, and effectiveness of client education

11. Client education

    a. See Box 2-1 for universal teaching points for anti-infectives

    b. Take safety precautions if client experiences vertigo, ataxia, seizures

    c. Avoid driving or performing hazardous tasks if drowsiness occurs

    d. Take with food, if not contraindicated, to minimize GI upset

    e. Eat small, frequent meals with at least 2,500–3,000 mL fluid intake a day

    f. Empty bladder frequently, at least every 2 hours while awake

    g. Report flank or suprapubic pain, increased dysuria, disruption of skin integrity to health care provider

H. Urinary tract antiseptics

    1. Action and use

        a. These drugs act against bacteria in urine but have little or no systemic antibacterial effects

        b. Used for UTIs only; destruction of bacteria based on acidification of urine

    2. Common medications (Table 2-8)

    3. Administration considerations: shake suspensions well just prior to measuring with a calibrated device (household teaspoons may vary by 2 to 10 mL)

    4. Contraindications

        a. Methenamine hippurate (Hiprex): avoid concurrent use of drugs that could alkalinize urine and interfere with effectiveness (e.g., antacids, carbonic anhydrase inhibitors, citrates, sodium bicarbonate, thiazide diuretics)

        b. Sulfamethizole (Thiosulfil Forte): increased risk for crystalluria

Table 2-8	**Urinary Tract Antiseptics**
Generic (Trade) Name	**Route**
Cinoxacin (Cinobac)	PO
Fosfomycin (Monurol)	PO
Methenamine (Hiprex)	PO
Methylene blue (Urolene blue)	PO
Nalidixic acid (NegGram)	PO
Nitrofurantoin (Furadantin)	PO
Norfloxacin (Noroxin)	PO

   c. Caution with nitrofurantoin (Furadantin): can increase neurotoxicity in clients with neurologic disorders such as peripheral neuropathy and seizures, and can cause pulmonary reaction in clients with pulmonary conditions

   d. Use caution in clients with impaired renal and/or hepatic function

   e. Use caution during lactation and pregnancy

5. Significant drug interactions
   a. See contraindications listed earlier
   b. Probenecid (Benemid): may increase risk for toxicity with sulfinpyrazone; decreased urinary tract effectiveness may occur with nitrofurantoin

6. Significant food interactions
   a. Controversial if pH of urine has any effect on UTI (may inhibit adherence of bacteria to bladder wall)
   b. Alkaline ash diet may interfere with required acidity of urine for antiseptic action; alkaline ash foods include fruits (except cranberries, prunes, plums), milk, vegetables
   c. Acid ash foods that may or may not increase urine acidity; include meat, cheese, eggs, whole grains, as well as cranberries, prunes, and plums
   d. Fluids that may acidify the urine and potentially facilitate the action of the drugs include cranberry or prune juice

7. Significant laboratory studies
   a. Urinalysis and urine C&S: baseline and repeated regularly
   b. CBC with WBC and differential
   c. Baseline ALT, AST, alkaline phosphatase, and bilirubin; repeat as necessary
   d. Baseline creatinine, BUN, creatinine clearance; repeat as needed
   e. Pulmonary tests with nitrofurantoin

8. Side effects: (do not commonly occur)
   a. N/V, anorexia, diarrhea, epigastric distress
   b. Rash, pruritus, photosensitivity, photophobia, tinnitus, insomnia, headache, dizziness, drowsiness
   c. Low back pain, dysuria
   d. Nitrofurantoin: urine may become brown

9. Adverse effects/toxicity: see contraindications and significant drug interactions sections earlier

10. Nursing considerations
   a. Review client history for allergies, previous renal or liver dysfunction
   b. Assess current drugs being taken to avoid drug interactions
   c. Ensure client takes full course of treatment for optimal benefit and to deter risk for development of drug resistance
   d. Discard any unused or outdated drug to ensure drug not taken with decreased potency or self-treatment will not occur in future infections
   e. Monitor for evidence of drug effectiveness
      1) Upper UTI or pyelonephritis: resolution of pain in lower back, flank, or epigastric area; fever, diaphoresis, piloerection, N/V, headache, generalized weakness are resolved
      2) Lower UTI or cystitis: resolution of urinary urgency, burning, frequency and of suprapubic discomfort; improvement in increasing the amounts of urine on voiding; resolution of incontinence if occurs
      3) Resolution of hematuria and pyuria
      4) No red or white blood cells, no casts, protein, crystals, or bacteria in urine
      5) Normalization of CBC with WBC differential
   f. Monitor for clinical manifestations of adverse effects

     g. Encourage at least 3,000 mL/day fluids, including cranberry juice if not contraindicated by fluid restriction, diabetes mellitus, or other conditions

     h. Monitor urine pH at bedside with test strip as indicated

     i. Give medication with or after food to limit GI adverse effects

11. Client education

     a. See Box 2-1 for universal teaching points for anti-infectives

     b. Take with or after food to minimize GI distress

      c. Drink at least 3 liters of fluid a day including cranberry and prune juice unless contraindicated by other conditions

      d. Include acid ash foods in diet, such as cranberries or cranberry juice, prunes, plums, cheese, eggs, meat, whole grains; limit or avoid alkaline ash foods, such as citrus fruits and juices, vegetables

     e. Do not take other medications unless approved by prescriber; avoid drugs that may alkalinize urine, such as antacids, Alka-Seltzer, sodium bicarbonate (baking soda); ascorbic acid (vitamin C) acidifies urine

     f. Report to health care provider if improvement not noted in 2–3 days or if severe adverse effects occur

     g. Nalidixic acid (NegGram) can cause photophobia, and client should avoid bright sunlight, wear sunglasses, and report any visual disturbances; photosensitivity can also occur several weeks after drug is discontinued so client should avoid direct sunlight or ultraviolet light

     h. Nitrofurantoin may cause urine to be brown; may stain

     i. Do not drive or perform hazardous tasks if drowsiness or dizziness occurs

     j. If diabetic, urine testing for glucose with Clinitest can yield a false-positive result; test blood glucose instead

     k. Instruct client on urinary hygiene measures and perineal care, including a cotton liner in underwear, avoiding hot tubs and bubble baths, wiping from front to back, and voiding after intercourse

I. Tetracyclines

  1. Action and use

     a. Broad spectrum; bacteriostatic (by inhibiting protein synthesis); can be bactericidal in high concentrations

     b. Effective against most chlamydia, mycoplasmas, rickettsiae, cholera, and certain protozoa

      c. Suppress *Proprionibacteriium acnes* in treating acne; topical application may be as effective as oral preparation for acne; both forms may be used for severe acne

     d. Used prophylactically for traveler's diarrhea

     e. Drug of choice for Rocky Mountain Spotted Fever, **amebiasis** (a protozoan infection), brucellosis, shigellosis, cholera, tetanus, chronic bronchitis, Lyme disease

     f. Used to treat syphilis and gonorrhea in client with penicillin allergy

     g. Used as a sclerosing agent for pleural and pericardial effusion, such as in metastasis of cancer; causes inflammation resulting in fibrosis, leaving scar tissue that does not allow fluid to accumulate

     h. Used in *Helicobacter pylori* peptic ulcer disease, Q fever, Rickettsia pox, typhus, Mycoplasma pneumonia, epididymo-orchitis, pelvic inflammatory disease (PID)

     i. Used with quinine for treatment of malaria

     j. Anti-infective prophylaxis for rape victims

     k. Treat syndrome of inappropriate antidiuretic hormone (SIADH) with demeclocycline (Declomycin) by inhibiting antidiuretic hormone (ADH)

     l. Topical application of Atridox and oral tablets of Periostat are used to treat chronic peridontitis in adults

     m. Inflammatory rosacea is treated with Oracea, which contains immediate and delayed release beads

  2. Common medications (generic name ends in "-cycline"; Table 2-9)

Table 2-9	Tetracyclines
Generic (Trade) Name	**Route**
Demeclocycline (Declomycin)	PO
Tetracycline (Achromycin)	PO, IM, topical
Doxycycline (Vibramycin)	PO, IV
Minocycline (Minocin)	PO, IV
Tigecycline (Tygacil)	IV

3. Administration considerations
    a. Avoid administering outdated drug: Fanconi-like syndrome with polyuria, poly-dipsia, nausea and vomiting, glycosuria, proteinuria; acidosis can occur; renal tubular dysfunction and lupus-erythematosus–like syndrome have occurred and are attributed to preparations used beyond expiration date
    b. Oral: give with full glass of water on empty stomach at least 1 hour before or 2 hours after meals; food, milk, and milk products decrease absorption by one half
    c. Shake oral suspension well to distribute particles
    d. Use calibrated measuring device (kitchen teaspoon can vary by 2 to 10 mL)
    e. IM injection contains procaine so assess for allergies to local anesthetics ending with *-caine*
    f. Administer deep IM into large muscle as the gluteus; alternate sites
    g. If topical, clean area with soap and water, rinse and dry well prior to application
    h. Not to be administered IV
4. Contraindications
    a. Hypersensitivity to tetracyclines
    b. Severe renal or hepatic dysfunction
    c. Contraindicated during last half of pregnancy when tooth development occurs, from birth to 8 years of age, and in lactating women; tetracyclines bind to calcium, preventing normal bone growth and causing tooth hypoplasia in developing fetus or child younger than 8 years old; this produces discoloration of the teeth
    d. Use caution with history of renal or liver dysfunction, allergy, asthma, hay fever, urticaria, or in myasthenia gravis
    e. Use caution with concurrent use of oral anticoagulants
    f. Tetracyclines may antagonize other antibiotics; see product literature
    g. Oracea, Tygacil, and Minocin are Pregnancy Category D drugs
5. Significant drug interactions
    a. Antacids and antidiarrheal agents with kaolin and pectin decrease absorption
    b. Oral anticoagulants potentiate hypoprothrombinemia
    c. Decreased effectiveness of oral contraceptives
    d. Increased effect against brain abscess with sulfonamide
    e. Decreased effect of penicillin
    f. Increased or decreased level of digoxin (Lanoxin) depending on specific tetracycline
    g. Can cause fatal nephrotoxicity with methoxyflurane, an anesthetic
6. Significant food interactions
    a. Milk and dairy products and iron supplements interfere with absorption
    b. Take on empty stomach
7. Significant laboratory studies
    a. Obtain C&S of infection site prior to initiating drug therapy; obtain follow-up culture from gonoccocal infection site 3–7 days post-treatment to ensure elimination of infection, or culture from other sites if improvement not observed

    b. Baseline and periodic renal function tests: serum creatinine, BUN, creatinine clearance, urinalysis

    c. Baseline and periodic hepatic function tests: ALT, AST, alkaline phosphatase, bilirubin

!   **d.** CBC including WBC with differential to monitor response to therapy (decreased WBC), to check for thrombocytopenia, and for hemolytic anemia

8. Side effects

    a. N/V, diarrhea, epigastric distress, abdominal discomfort, flatulence, dry mouth, dysphagia, bulky or loose stools, steatorrhea

    b. Headache, photosensitivity, increased intracranial pressure (rare)

!   **c.** Maculopapular rash, urticaria, exfoliative dermatitis, angioedema

    d. Stinging or burning with topical application

!   **e.** Discoloration of developing teeth

    f. Pigmentation of conjunctiva related to drug deposits

    g. Discoloration and loosening of nails

    h. Retrosternal pain

9. Adverse effects/toxicity

    a. Elevated liver function tests and decreased cholesterol level

    b. Drug fever, serum sickness, and anaphylaxis

    c. Hepatotoxicity, pancreatitis, nephrotoxicity

    d. Blood dyscrasias such as thrombocytopenia, hemolytic anemia

    e. Superinfections: increased risk for candidiasis in clients taking oral contraceptives, with diabetes mellitus, leukemia, systemic lupus erythematosus (SLE); possible stomatitis, glossitis, black, hairy tongue (lingua nigra), and pseudomembranous colitis

    f. Fatty degeneration of liver results in jaundice, azotemia, increased nitrogen retention, hyperphosphatemia, and metabolic acidosis

    g. Tetracycline topical application can cause itching, wheezing, and anaphylaxis in client with asthma allergies

10. Nursing considerations

!   **a.** Collect C&S specimen from infection site prior to initiation of drug therapy, if possible; recheck C&S 3–7 days after therapy completed for gonococcal infection to assure infection eradicated or culture other infected sites if improvement not observed

    b. Assess for history of renal or liver problems and related laboratory results

    c. Assess history of immunosuppression

    d. Check CBC including WBC with differential, RBC indices, and platelet count

    e. Assess other medications being taken to avoid drug–drug interactions

    f. Collaborate with prescriber regarding dosage or drug change if indicated by adverse effects

    g. Observe for superinfections such as candidiasis and pseudomembranous colitis; consult prescriber for discontinuation of drug if they occur

    h. Monitor I & O

    i. Check IM injection sites every day for induration, redness, edema

11. Client education

    a. See Box 2-1 for universal teaching points for anti-infectives

!   **b.** Unstable with age and light exposure; store in tightly covered container in dry area, protected from light at room temperature

    c. Report side effects, particularly severe diarrhea

    d. Practice good oral care and hygiene

!   **e.** Avoid exposure to direct sunlight or ultraviolet light or tanning beds; wear hat, long sleeves, long-legged pants, and sunglasses outside during and for a few days after treatment; sunscreen or sunblock may not prevent erythema

    f. If on long-term treatment, report onset of severe headache or visual disturbances that may indicate increased intracranial pressure (rare); requires discontinuation of tetracycline to prevent irreversible vision loss

---

Practice to Pass

Tetracycline capsules have been prescribed for an 18-year-old female client to treat acne. What specific teaching would you include on the client education plan?

g. Take oral doses with full glass of water on empty stomach (1 hour before or 2 hours after meal or dairy product) to promote absorption and decrease risk of esophagitis; report sudden dysphagia to health care provider

h. Topical form may stain clothing

i. Topical application can cause affected skin to reflect yellow or green fluorescence under an ultraviolet or "black" light

J. Miscellaneous antibiotics (Table 2-10)

1. Aztreonam (Azactam)

   a. Action and use: a monobactam that has bactericidal against gram-negative rods; has similar activity as beta-lactam antibiotic (penicillins) and cephalosporins; used for infections with gram negative aerobes, such as *pseudomonas aeruginosa*

   b. Administration considerations: given IM; no cross-sensitivity to penicillins or cephalosporins

   c. Contraindications: known hypersensitivity to aztreonam

   d. Significant drug interactions: cefoxitin, imipenem; incompatible with nafcillin sodium, cephradine, vancomycin, or metronidazole; yields false positive results with cupric sulfate-type urine glucose testing products

   e. Significant food interactions: none significant

   f. Significant laboratory studies

     1) Monitor ALT, AST, bilirubin, and alkaline phosphatase for hepatotoxicity

     2) Monitor creatinine, creatinine clearance, and BUN for nephrotoxicity

     3) Monitor WBC with differential to monitor therapeutic effectiveness; note linezolid may decrease WBC count, neutrophils, and platelet count

   g. Side effects

     1) N/V, diarrhea

     2) Superinfections such as candidiasis

     3) Local pain at injection site

   h. Adverse effects/toxicity (rare): anaphylaxis, pseudomembranous colitis

   i. Nursing considerations

     1) Collect appropriate specimen for C&S, if possible, prior to initiating antibiotic to ensure appropriate drug employed; empiric therapy is usually begun before test results are available because of seriousness of infection

     2) Ensure client takes complete course of drug for full beneficial effects, even if clinical manifestations of infection resolved; premature discontinuation can result in regrowth of organisms as well as development of drug resistance

     3) Assess for allergies, adverse reactions, and effectiveness of client teaching

   j. Client education: same as for penicillins and cephalosporins

Table 2-10 Miscellaneous Antibiotics

Classification	Generic (Trade) Name	Route
Monobactam	Aztreonam (Azactam)	IM, IV
Streptogramins	Quinupristin/dalfopristin (Synercid)	IV
None (unique cell wall inhibitor)	Vancomycin (Vancocin)	IV, off-label PO use
Ketolide (similar to Macrolide)	Telithromycin (Ketek)	PO
Oxazolidinones	Linezolid (Zyvox)	PO, IV
Cyclic lipopeptide	Daptomycin (Cubicin)	IV
Macrolide for C. Diff-associated diarrhea	Fidaxomicin (Dificid)	PO
None (antibacterial and antiparasitic)	Metronidazole (Flagyl)	PO, IV

2. Quinupristin and dalfopristin (Synercid)

    a. Action and use

        1) Two streptogramin antibacterials work synergistically; it is in a new class of antibiotics called *streptogramins* that work by binding the 50S ribosome, similar to the action of macrolides

        2) Used to treat bacteremia and life-threatening infections caused by *Enterococcus faecium* (VREF); also complicated skin and skin structure infections caused by *Staphylococcus aureus*, including vancomycin-resistant strains and *Streptococcus pyogenes*

    b. Administration considerations

        1) For IV use only, preferably via central line

        2) Incompatible with normal saline or heparin; flush line with D^5W before and after each dose and to reconstitute drug

        3) Infuse using an infusion pump

    c. Contraindications: known hypersensitivity to Synercid, pristinamycin or virginiamycin

    d. Significant drug interactions

        1) Do not mix with other drugs; use cautiously with cephalosporins

        2) Close monitoring of cyclosporine levels should be done if client taking this drug, as increased levels may occur

    e. Significant food interactions: none reported

    f. Significant laboratory studies

        1) Monitor CBC with WBC and differential to monitor therapeutic effectiveness

        2) Baseline, and as needed, liver and renal serum tests

    g. Side effects: arthralgias, myalgias (possibly severe)

    h. Adverse effects/toxicity: with peripheral IV administration, frequently pain, inflammation, edema, and thrombophlebitis

     i. Nursing considerations: same as with other antibiotics; avoid infusion into peripheral sites; it is associated with high incidence of phlebitis

    j. Client education: same as with other antibiotics

3. Vancomycin (Vancocin)

    a. Action and use

        1) Bactericidal

        2) Bacteria mainly killed through inhibition of bacterial cell wall synthesis, but it also interferes with plasma membrane and RNA synthesis

        3) Antibiotic of choice for methicillin-resistant *Staphylococcus aureus* (MRSA) and other gram-positive bacteria, yeast, fungi

        4) Oral: for antibiotic-induced pseudomembranous colitis caused by *Clostridium difficile* and for staphylococcal enterocolitis

        5) IV: for bone and joint infections or septicemia caused by staphylococcal organisms

    b. Administration considerations

        1) Poorly absorbed from GI tract so oral therapy for treatment of local, surface infected areas of GI tract

        2) IV administration should be through a central venous access device because of high risk for phlebitis; can cause necrosis if it extravasates

        3) Increasing reports of resistance to enterococcus strains; concern about MRSA resistance developing; quinupristin and dalfopristin (Synercid) used in place of vancomycin sometimes to limit evolution of resistance to vancomycin

        4) Incidence of "red man syndrome" can be minimized by infusing over at least 60 minutes

    c. Contraindications

        1) Known hypersensitivity

        2) Use cautiously in renal dysfunction, prior hearing loss, in pregnancy and lactation, in older adults and neonates

        3) Do not give IM

    d. Significant drug interactions

        1) Do not mix intravenously with other drugs

        2) Increased risk of ototoxicity and nephrotoxicity when used with other drugs having potential for these toxicities

    e. Significant food interactions: none reported

    f. Significant laboratory studies

        1) Serum creatinine, BUN, creatinine clearance, urinalysis (for casts in urine)

        2) Peak and trough drug levels

        3) ALT, AST, bilirubin, alkaline phosphatase

        4) CBC with WBC and differential

        5) Audiometry testing

    g. Side effects

        1) Nausea, hypotension, flushing

        2) Pain and thrombophlebitis at injection site

        3) "Red man syndrome": too rapid IV infusion results in profound hypotension, erythematous rash on face, neck, upper chest, and arms

        4) Too rapid infusion can cause increased sense of warmth, nausea, and generalized tingling and paresthesia

    h. Adverse reactions/toxicity

        1) Ototoxicity of auditory branch of 8th cranial nerve; possible irreversible hearing loss; hearing loss may continue after drug is discontinued

        2) Nephrotoxicity with possible uremia

        3) Hypersensitivity: anaphylaxis

        4) Superinfections

        5) Leukopenia and eosinophilia: temporary

    i. Nursing considerations

        1) Monitor baseline and regular lab results for early detection of toxicities

        2) Ensure central venous access available

        3) Assess baseline hearing; assess regularly for early detection of hearing loss, tinnitus, and loss of hearing high-pitched tones that may precede deafness

        4) Record accurate I & O

        5) Assess for improvement in clinical manifestations of infection

        6) Give over 60 to 90 minutes to avoid too rapid administration

        7) Monitor for hypotension and tachycardia during infusion; if red man syndrome occurs, stop infusion and report to health care provider

        8) Collect appropriate specimen for C&S, if possible, prior to institution of vancomycin therapy to ensure appropriate drug employed

        9) Ensure client takes complete course of drug for full beneficial effects

        10) Consult with prescriber for dose adjustment or drug discontinuation if toxicities develop

        11) Ensure adequate nutrition and hydration

        12) Evaluate effectiveness of teaching plan

    j. Client education

        1) Refer to Box 2-1 for universal teaching points for anti-infectives

        2) Keep appointments for laboratory testing, drug administrations at home when indicated, and follow-up visits with health care provider

        3) If to receive IV therapy in home, ensure appropriate person's knowledge and ability to perform procedures correctly, including monitoring blood pressure (BP) and heart rate

        4) Report ringing in ears or change in hearing

Practice to Pass

The client states, "I don't know why the doctor wants me to have the vancomycin every 6 hours now instead of every 8 hours as I had been getting it. It seems as though I am so tied down." How do you respond?

    5) Report sore throat, watery stools more than 4 to 6 per day or if blood or mucus in stools, severe N/V, change in color or consistency of urine, which may indicate superinfection or toxicity

    6) Maintain adequate fluid intake (2–3 liters/day)

4. Telithromycin (Ketek)

  a. Actions and uses

    1) Blocks protein synthesis of bacteria, similar to macrolides; approved for use in community acquired pneumonias, bronchitis, and sinusitis; is sole drug in a new class of antibiotics called *ketolides*

    2) Is indicated in treatment of acute bacterial exacerbation of chronic bronchitis due to *Streptococcus pneumoniae*, *Haemophilus influenzae*, or *Moraxella catarrhalis*; acute bacterial sinusitis due to *Streptococcus pneumoniae*, *Haemophilus influenzae*, *Moraxella catarrhalis*, or *Staphylococcus aureus*, and community-acquired pneumonia due to *Streptococcus pneumoniae*

    3) Derived from erythromycin A, it is similar to macrolides; recently associated with severe liver damage and so use is very limited

  b. Administration considerations: it is only available in oral tablets

  c. Contraindications

    1) It may cause hepatotoxicity and should be used cautiously in those with impaired liver function

    2) Contraindicated in myasthenia gravis

    3) May cause prolonged QT intervals; avoid use in clients with a history of torsade de pointes

  d. Significant drug interactions

    1) Avoid concurrent administration with simvastatin, lovastatin, atorvastatin; may cause increased drug levels of "statins"

    2) Administration with Class IA or III antiarrhythmics may lead to life-threatening dysrhythmias

  e. Significant food interactions

    1) Greater than 1 quart/day of grapefruit juice may increase drug levels and side effects

  f. Significant laboratory studies: elevated liver enzymes, BUN, creatinine, potassium

  g. Side effects

    1) Diarrhea, nausea, headache, dizziness, vomiting, loose stools, dysgeusia

    2) May cause blurred or double vision and difficulty focusing, which may necessitate discontinuation of drug

  h. Adverse reactions/toxicity: increased risk for ventricular dysrhythmias in clients with history of prolonged QT interval

  i. Nursing considerations

    1) Assess liver and renal function prior to administration

    2) Pregnancy Risk Category C

  j. Client education

    1) Stop taking drug and notify provider if dizziness or fainting occurs

    2) Report signs of jaundice, unexplained fatigue, loss of appetite, nausea, dark urine, or clay-colored stools

    3) If visual changes occur, avoid quick changes in viewing between close and distant objects

5. Linezolid (Zyvox)

  a. Actions and uses

    1) Inhibits bacterial protein synthesis; is the first antibacterial drug in a class known as oxazolidinones

    2) Bactericidal against gram-positive, gram-negative, and anaerobic bacteria; bacteriostatic against enterococci and staphylococci

          3) Developed to treat infections associated with vancomycin-resistant *Enterococcus faecium*, or VRE

          4) Used to treat hospital- and community-acquired pneumonias, complicated and uncomplicated skin and skin structure infections

   b. Administration considerations: has excellent oral absorption

   c. Contraindications

          1) Known hypersensitivity to linezolid

          2) Concurrent use with monoamine oxidase inhibitors (MAOIs)

   d. Significant drug interactions

          1) May increase effect of vasopressor drugs, such as dopamine

          2) May lead to serotonin syndrome when given with other serotonergic drugs, such as selective serotonin reuptake inhibitor (SSRIs) and MAOIs

   e. Significant food interactions: tyramine-containing foods, such as soy sauce, aged cheeses, wines, smoked foods, and fish, can raise blood pressure

   f. Significant laboratory studies: monitor electrolytes, liver and renal functions, WBC with differential, and CBC

   g. Side effects

          1) Headache, N/V, diarrhea

          2) Thrombocytopenia, leukopenia

   h. Adverse reactions/toxicity

          1) Serotonin syndrome may occur if given with serotonin reuptake inhibitors, tricyclic antidepressants, serotonin 5ht1-receptor agonists, meperidine, or buspirone

          2) Myelosuppression, including anemia, leukopenia, pancytopenia, and thrombocytopenia (long-term use)

   i. Nursing considerations

          1) Monitor client for signs of low platelets, such as easy bruising, prolonged bleeding

          2) Monitor for signs of pseudomembranous colitis

   j. Client education

          1) Report diarrhea, easy bruising, or bleeding to prescriber

          2) Avoid foods and beverages high in tyramine, such as aged, fermented, pickled, or smoked foods

          3) Avoid use of OTC cold remedies or decongestants containing pseudoephedrine

6. Daptomycin (Cubicin)

   a. Actions and uses

          1) Is a drug in the new class known as *lipopeptides*

          2) Binds to gram-positive cells in a calcium-dependent process, which causes rapid depolarization of cell membrane potential, leading to inhibition of protein, DNA, and RNA synthesis

          3) Used for complicated skin and soft tissue infections caused by gram-positive bacteria, including MRSA and VRE

   b. Administration considerations

          1) It is only available IV

          2) Safe use in infants and children less than 18 years is not known

          3) Use cautiously in presence of renal or hepatic impairment, peripheral neuropathy, history of rhabdomyolysis

   c. Contraindications: pseudomembranous colitis, myopathy, allergy to daptomycin

   d. Significant drug interactions: potential increased risk for myopathy if given with HMG-COa reductase inhibitors ("statins")

   e. Significant food interactions: none identified

    f. Significant laboratory studies
        1) Liver function tests; renal function
        2) Baseline C&S before treatment is initiated
        3) PT/INR during first few days of therapy if client taking warfarin (Coumadin)
        4) Weekly creatine phosphokinase (CPK) levels
        5) Daily blood glucose in clients with diabetes mellitus
        6) Serum electrolytes if signs of hypokalemia or hypomagnesemia appear
    g. Side effects
        1) Hypotension and hypertension
        2) Headache, dizziness, rash, GI discomfort
        3) Dyspnea
        4) Thrombocytopenia, anemia, fever
    h. Adverse reactions/toxicity: elevated liver enzymes, renal failure, fungal infection
    i. Nursing considerations
        1) Monitor LFTs and for signs of impaired liver function such as anorexia, abdominal pain, dark urine
        2) Withhold drug if signs of myopathy appear (muscle pain or weakness) or CPK is elevated greater than 1,000 units
        3) Monitor serum electrolytes; monitor blood glucose in clients with diabetes mellitus
    j. Client education: report muscle pain, weakness, unusual tiredness; numbness or tingling; difficulty breathing or shortness of breath; severe diarrhea or vomiting; skin rash or itching

7. Fidaxomicin (Dificid)
    a. Actions and uses
        1) Is an oral macrolide antibiotic approved in 2011 for treatment of *Clostridium difficile* associated diarrhea
        2) Is bactericidal against *C. difficile*, inhibiting RNA synthesis by RNA polymerases
        3) Is mainly confined to GI tract following oral administration and excreted in feces
    b. Administration considerations
        1) Should be taken twice a day for 10 days
        2) Is indicated for use in adults (greater than 18 years of age)
        3) Should only be used to treat infections that are proven or strongly suspected to be caused by *C. difficile*
        4) Pregnancy risk is Category B, but safety in lactation not determined
    c. Contraindications: none indicated
    d. Significant drug interactions
        1) Levels of cyclosporine and Dificid may both be elevated if given concurrently, but levels of either drug are not toxic
    e. Significant food interactions: none reported
    f. Significant laboratory studies: none indicated
    g. Side effects: nausea, headache, abdominal pain, diarrhea
    h. Adverse reactions/toxicity: none reported
    i. Nursing considerations: may be given with or without food
    j. Client education
        1) Instruct on importance of completing entire 10 days of treatment
        2) Do not treat diarrhea with OTC antidiarrheal agents

8. Metronidazole (Flagyl)
    a. Action and use
        1) Is the protype antiprotozoal medication for amebiasis, giardiasis (off label), and trichomoniasis
        2) Has both antiprotozoal and anti-infective properties
        3) Is frequently used to treat pseudomembranous colitis, Crohn disease, and colitis (off-label uses)

           4) In combination with bismuth and tetracycline (Helidac), it is FDA-approved to treat *Helicobacter pylori* infection

           5) Used to treat intraabdominal and gynecological infections caused by anaerobes *Eubacterium spp.*, *Bacteroides spp.*, and *Clostridium spp.*

           6) Topical drug form is used to treat rosacea

           7) Binds to DNA and RNA of intracellular proteins, causing cell death

      b. Administration considerations

           1) Available in PO, IV, topical skin and vaginal creams

           2) In 2011, Pregnancy Risk Category was changed from a C to a D for high dose (400–800 mg daily); long-term administration during first trimester may be associated with birth defects

      c. Contraindications

           1) Allergy to metronidazole

           2) Blood dyscrasias; may cause bone marrow depression

      d. Significant drug interactions

           1) May cause disulfiram-like reaction if taken with alcohol

           2) May increase toxicity of lithium, benzodiazepines, cyclosporine, calcium channel blockers, warfarin, and antidepressants

           3) Phenytoin and phenobarbital may reduce effects of metronidazole

      e. Significant food interactions: none reported

      f. Significant laboratory studies: monitor liver function in clients with alcoholism or hepatic impairment

      g. Side effects

           1) Dizziness, headache, nasal congestion

           2) GI discomfort, anorexia, N/V, diarrhea

           3) Reversible neutropenia, thrombocytopenia

           4) Dry mouth, unpleasant metallic taste

      h. Adverse reactions/toxicity

           1) Bone suppression may occur in presence of blood dyscrasias

           2) Dosage adjustment needed if client on warfarin or has hepatic impairment

      i. Nursing considerations

           1) Discontinue therapy if client develops seizures or peripheral neuropathy

           2) Monitor total and differential WBC counts before, during, and after therapy

           3) Monitor for lithium toxicity if client is taking lithium

      j. Client education

           1) Instruct client to avoid alcohol consumption 24 hours before beginning therapy and for 36 hours after cessation of therapy

           2) Avoid use of OTC products containing alcohol, such as cold and cough remedies

           3) Refrain from sexual intercourse during therapy when treatment is for trichomoniasis; sexual partner should also be treated

           4) Report symptoms of candidiasis, including vaginitis, milky vaginal discharge, proctitis, furry tongue, glossitis, or stomatitis

           5) Do not breastfeed without permission of health care provider

II. ANTIMYCOBACTERIALS

    A. Antituberculins

      1. Action and use

         a. Inhibit cell wall synthesis or mycocolic acid coat of bacteria (INH); protein synthesis, DNA or RNA synthesis (rifampin and rifapentine), or cell wall division (ethionamide)

         b. Effects limited primarily to *Mycobacterium tuberculosis* and then certain other mycobacterium strains

   c. Prophylaxis or treatment of pulmonary tuberculosis (TB)
   d. Extrapulmonary TB in adults and children
   e. Often used in combination with other antituberculin agents
   f. Used to prevent or delay onset of *Mycobacterium avium* bacteremia in clients with advanced HIV, in combination with other antituberculin antibiotics
   g. Rifampin eradicates meningococci from nasopharynx of asymptomatic *Neisseria meningitides* carriers when there is increased risk for infection outbreaks among a community
   h. Rifampin is used prophylactically with exposure to *Haemophilus influenzae* Type B (hib) infection
   i. Antituberculins are used in combination to treat leprosy
   j. Used to treat endocarditis with methicillin-resistant staphylococci, chronic prostatitis with staphylococcal organisms, and anti-infective-resistant pneumococci
   k. Used as combination treatment for mycobacterial infections including TB
      1) Effective treatment requires compliance and therapy over months to years
      2) Common medications (Table 2-11)
3. Administration considerations
   a. Effectiveness depends on correct drug, correct combination therapy, adequate dosing, adequate duration of therapy, and compliance
   b. Empiric treatment is initiated with isoniazid, rifampin, pyrazinamide, and ethambutol or streptomycin
   c. TB medications are classified as first- or second-line drugs (See Table 2-11); first-line drugs are safer and more effective agents; second-line drugs exhibit greater toxicity, are less effective, and prescribed when resistance develops to first-line drugs
   d. Multicombination drug therapy decreases risk or rate of developing resistance to any single drug
   e. Give isoniazid 1 hour before meals on empty stomach
   f. Give clofazimine (Lamprene) with meals

Table 2-11 Antituberculins

Generic (Trade) Name	Route
First-Line Antituberculins	
Isoniazid (INH)	PO, IM
Ethambutol HCL (Myambutol)	PO
Pyrazinamide (Tebrazid)	PO
Rifampin (Rifadin)	PO, IV
Rifapentine (Priftin)	PO
Rifabutin (Mycobutin)	PO
Second-Line Antituberculins	
Aminosalicylic acid (Paser)	PO
Capreomycin (Capostat sulfate)	IM
Clofazimine (Lamprene)	PO
Cycloserine (Seromycin)	PO
Ethionamide (Trecator-SC)	PO
Kanamycin (Kantrex) (also an aminoglycoside)	PO, IM, IV
Streptomycin (Streptomycin) (also an aminoglycoside)	IM

4. Contraindications
   a. Hypersensitivity to drug
   b. Hepatic or renal damage
   c. Variable by specified drug: caution in pregnancy unless risk is significant
   d. Caution in renal or liver dysfunction, history of seizures, ethanol abuse, or CNS dysfunction
   e. Caution in older clients, children, diabetics, those with gout or blood dyscrasias, and optic neuritis or defects
5. Significant drug interactions
   a. Increased effect of antituberculin agent with antigout agents such as probenecid (Benebid) and sulfinpyrazone (Antazone), glucocorticosteroids such as methylprednisolone (Medrol) and prednisolone (Pred-Forte), nonsteroidal anti-inflammatory drugs (NSAIDs), aminoglycosides, and testosterone agents
   b. Decreased effect of antituberculin drug with quinidine (Quinidex), metoprolol (Lopressor), propranolol (Inderal), oral anticoagulants, oral contraceptives, phenytoin (Dilantin), methadone, verapamil (Isoptin), cyclosporine (Neoral), and ketoconazole (Nizoral)
   c. Increased toxicity
      1) Salicylates, other antitubercular agents, nephrotoxic and hepatotoxic drugs, alcohol
      2) Increased neurotoxicity: cycloserine (Seromycin), isoniazid (INH), ethionamide (Trecator-C), and phenytoin (Dilantin)
   d. Hyperkalemia with potassium-sparing diuretics and angiotensin converting enzyme (ACE) inhibitors
   e. Crystalluria with ascorbic acid (vitamin C)
   f. Decreased efficacy of oral contraceptives
6. Significant food interactions: decreased rate or extent of absorption of isoniazid (INH) when taken with food (take 1 hour before meals)
7. Significant laboratory studies

   a. Monitor for hepatic dysfunction with ALT, AST, alkaline phosphatase, bilirubin

   b. Purified protein derivative (PPD) tuberculin skin test to check for positive reaction indicating prior exposure to *M. tuberculosis* and T-lymphocyte production; cellular response to tubercle bacillus occurs 3–10 weeks after infection and does not diagnose active infection; chest x-rays and sputum tests for tubercle bacillus are done to clarify actual status
   c. Chest x-ray if PPD positive
   d. Sputum smear culture to confirm diagnosis if chest x-ray positive
   e. Drug levels if suspected toxicity, such as with phenytoin
8. Side effects
   a. Fairly well tolerated
   b. N/V, anorexia, constipation, diarrhea, dyspepsia
   c. Headache, dizziness, malaise, fever, chills, arthralgia, flulike symptoms, weakness
   d. Skin rash, dry skin, peripheral paresis, photophobia, photosensitivity, vision changes
   e. Dysrhythmias
   f. Urinary retention (in males)
   g. Change in color to orange-red of excretions or secretions as urine, tears, feces, perspiration (with rifampin and rifabutin)
   h. Electrolyte imbalances
   i. Metallic taste with ethionamide (Trecator-SC)
   j. Disulfiram-like effect with alcohol ingestion
9. Adverse effects/toxicity
   a. Nephrotoxicity, hepatotoxicity, or ototoxicity (tinnitus, hearing loss)
   b. Hematologic disorders: agranulocytosis, thrombocytopenia, eosinophilia, anemia
   c. Seizure, depression, confusion, ataxia, paresis, paresthesias, drowsiness

10. Nursing considerations

a. Assess baseline laboratory findings and monitor during therapy the client's liver and renal function, C&S results, CBC with WBC differential, RBC indices, platelet count

b. Assess for hypersensitivity reactions

c. Assess concurrent medications being taken to avoid adverse drug–drug interactions

d. Assess for shortness of breath, numbness, tingling, or hallucinations

e. Assess for pregnancy; instruct female clients of ineffectiveness of oral contraceptives

f. Evaluate drug effectiveness by resolution of fever and other signs and symptoms of infection

g. Coadminister pyridoxine (vitamin B_6) and/or cyanocobalamin (vitamin B_{12})

h. Encourage food high in B-complex vitamins, (especially pyridoxine) such as meat (chicken, beef, and pork), liver, soybeans, baked potato with skin, raw avocado

i. Evaluate client compliance; ensure full course of therapy is completed to lessen risk of reinfection or development of drug resistance

j. Encourage good hydration and good nutrition with high-quality protein

11. Client education

a. See Box 2-1 for universal teaching points for anti-infectives

b. Take isoniazid (INH) 1 hour before meals

c. Report adverse reactions

d. Rifampin (Rifadin): may discolor urine, tears, saliva, and stain contact lens and undergarments

e. Keep follow-up appointments with health care provider and for tests

f. Use infection control measures to protect self and others

g. Avoid alcohol because of increased risk for hepatitis or disulfiram-like effect

h. Use alternative contraception during therapy and for at least 1 month after therapy is discontinued if using oral contraceptives

i. For dry skin, use emollients or oils

j. Explain pharmacotherapy noncompliance is most common cause of treatment failure; explain need to treat close contacts prophylactically due to infectiousness of tuberculosis

B. Leprostatics

1. Action and use

a. Treat leprosy and *pneumocystis carinii*, an AIDS-related opportunistic infection

b. Bacteriostatic against *Mycobacterium leprae*, *Pneumocystis carinii*, *Plasmodium*, *Mycobacterium tuberculosis*: dapsone (DDS)

c. Bactericidal against *Mycobacterium leprae* and *Mycobacterium avium*: clofazimine (Lamprene)

d. Clofazimine (Lamprene) and dapsone (DDS) are used in combination to prevent development of resistant strains

2. Common medications (Table 2-12)

3. Administration considerations: give clofazimine with food

4. Contraindications

a. Hypersensitivity to DDS and possible sulfonamides

Table 2-12 **Leprostatics**

Generic (Trade) Name	Route
Dapsone (DDS)	PO
Clofazimine (Lamprene)	PO
Thalidomide (Thalomid)	PO

      b. Use cautiously in clients with hepatic disease or glucose-6-phosphate dehydrogenase (G6PD) deficiency (an inherited hemolytic anemia associated with stress or certain drug interactions)

      c. Not established for safe use in pregnant and lactating clients

  5. Significant drug interactions

      a. Rifampin decreases levels of dapsone by 7- to 10-fold

      b. Trimethoprim (Proloprim, Trimpex), a urinary tract anti-infective, and pyrimethamine (Daraprim), an anti-infective and antimalarial; each increases levels and risk for adverse effects

  6. Significant food interactions: none reported

  7. Significant laboratory studies: monitor CBC for hemoglobin decline and reticulocyte count increase

  8. Side effects

      a. Skin pigmentation changes, as pink to brownish-black color; may resolve in weeks to months

      b. Dry skin

      c. N/V, diarrhea, abdominal pain

      d. Headache, insomnia, malaise, paresthesias, nervousness, tinnitus, vertigo, vision changes, neuritis

  9. Adverse effects/toxicity

      a. Agranulocytosis

      b. Hepatotoxicity

      c. Dose-related hemolysis (increased in G6PD deficiency)

      d. Methemoglobinemia may occur resulting in rhinitis, fatigue, difficulty breathing, cyanosis

      e. Phototoxicity

      f. Male infertility with DDS

  10. Nursing considerations

      a. Ensure pregnancy test is negative

      b. Give clofazimine with food

      c. Monitor laboratory tests for hemoglobin and reticulocyte count

      d. Assess concurrent medication regimen to avoid or minimize drug–drug interactions, such as with rifampin and trimethoprim

      e. Evaluate for drug effectiveness with resolution of infection; ensure client takes complete course of therapy

  11. Client education

      a. See Box 2-1 for universal teaching points for anti-infectives

      b. Take clofazimine with meals; skin discoloration may be pink to brownish-black; resolves in months to years after drug is discontinued

      c. Keep follow-up appointments with health care provider and for tests

      d. Ensure infection control measures are used

      e. Encourage hydration and good nutrition with complete or complementary proteins for tissue healing

III. ANTIVIRALS

A. Medications to treat herpes and cytomegalovirus

  1. Action and use

      a. Virustatic; prevents viral replication by inhibiting DNA replication

      b. Drug has little effect on host cells; effective only during acute phase of infection, not during latent phase; virus must be in living cell to survive and replicate

      c. Used to treat broad spectrum of diseases including cold sores, viral encephalitis, shingles, and genital infection

d. Viruses include **herpes simplex** virus-1 (HSV-1) in oral herpes or herpes labialis, herpes simplex virus-2 (HSV-2) in genital herpes, **herpes zoster** in shingles, **herpes varicella** zoster virus (VZV) in chickenpox, and some Epstein-Barr viruses

e. Acyclovir (Zovirax) is most frequently used to treat genital herpes and the drug of choice in herpes simplex encephalitis; used prophylactically with immunosuppressed seropositive clients before bone marrow transplantation and after other organ transplants; not found to be beneficial in treating those who have normal immune status, although it may help prevent shedding of virus

f. Ganciclovir (DHPG) is approved to treat only cytomegalic retinitis (caused by **cytomegalovirus** or **CMV**) in immunosuppressed clients; has good intraocular penetration; foscarnet (Foscavir) is used to treat ganciclovir-resistant CMV retinitis; cidofir (Vistide) is also given by IV administration for CMV-induced retinitis

g. Famciclovir (Famvir) is used to treat acute herpes zoster (shingles)

h. Trifluridine is a topical treatment for keratoconjunctivitis caused by herpes simplex

i. Valacyclovir (Valtrex) is the drug of choice for genital herpes; it is an improved oral form of acyclovir

j. Penciclovir (Denavir) is used to treat herpes infections; topical only; it is negligibly absorbed so is well tolerated and shortens pain or healing by one-half day

k. Cidofir (Vistide) IV to treat CMV retinitis in client with AIDS

2. Common medications (Table 2-13)

3. Administration considerations

a. Hydrate client to decrease risk or extent of nephrotoxicity

b. Administer as soon as possible to improve effectiveness

c. Wear gloves for topical application to limit exposure to drug or lesions

d. Preferred central venous access when given IV

e. Foscarnet: precipitates with many drugs when given IV; use with D_5W or NaCl solutions

Table 2-13 Antivirals: Medications to Treat Herpes Virus and Cytomegalovirus (CMV)

Generic (Trade) Name	Route	Uses
Acyclovir (Zovirax)	PO, IV	Herpes zoster, varicella zoster, CMV, varicella pneumonia, Herpes simplex infection, disseminated primary eczema herpeticum
Cidofovir (Vistide)	IV	Cytomegalovirus retinitis clients with HIV
Docosanol (Abreva)	topical	Herpes simplex cold sores and fever blisters
Ganciclovir (DHPG, Cytovene)	PO, IV	CMV retinitis, prevention of CMV disease in transplant recipients or immunocompromised clients
Famciclovir (Famvir)	PO	Acute herpes zoster, recurrent orolabial or genital herpes simplex infections in HIV-infected clients
Foscarnet (Foscavir)	IV	CMV retinitis in clients with HIV; monocutaneous acyclovir-resistant herpes simplex virus infections; varicella zoster
Penciclovir (Denavir)	Topical	Herpes labialis on lips and face
Trifluridine (Viroptic)	Ophthalmic	Herpes simplex 1 and 2; primary keratoconjunctivitis; recurrent epithelial keratitis
Valacyclovir (Valtrex)	PO	Herpes zoster, recurrent genital herpes
Valganciclovir (Valcyte)	PO	CMV retinitis, prevention of CMV disease in immunocompromised clients
Vidarabine (Ara-A)	Ophthalmic, IV	Acute keratoconjunctivitis; recurrent epithelial keratitis

4. Contraindications
   a. Hypersensitivity to drug
   b. Use caution in preexisting hepatic or renal dysfunction or concurrent use of nephrotoxic drugs
   c. Use caution in pregnant and lactating women
5. Significant drug interactions
   a. Increased drowsiness with zidovudine (AZT)
   b. Nephrotoxic drugs potentiate renal effects
   c. Probenecid (Benemid) can prolong effects of antiviral agent
6. Significant food interactions: none reported
7. Significant laboratory studies
   a. CBC including WBC with differential, T-cell count, and platelet count
   b. Serum and urine creatinine, BUN, and creatinine clearance
   c. ALT, AST, alkaline phosphatase, and bilirubin
8. Side effects
   a. Anemia, headache, mood changes, depression, seizures
   b. N/V, diarrhea
   c. Local irritation including phlebitis at IV site; inflammation with topical application
   d. Neutropenia; often dose-dependent because of bone marrow suppression
   e. Fever, hypocalcemia, hypomagnesemia, hypokalemia, metabolic acidosis, dysrhythmias
   f. Increased risk for CNS disturbances and fluid overload in clients with impaired hepatic or renal function
   g. Ocular hypotony
9. Adverse effects/toxicity
   a. Additive neutropenia with zidovudine
   b. Carcinogenic, embryotoxic, and teratogenic in experimental animals
   c. Infertility in males and females: ganciclovir
   d. Nephrotoxicity or hepatotoxicity
   e. Thrombocytopenic purpura
   f. Pancreatitis
10. Nursing considerations
    a. Check allergies, including allergy to antiviral agents
    b. Use protective gloves to administer topical antivirals
    c. Assess for neutropenic infection if immunosuppressed
    d. Assess renal function: creatinine, BUN, creatinine clearance, I & O
    e. Check hepatic function: ALT, AST, alkaline phosphatase, bilirubin
    f. Collaborate with prescriber if dosage needs adjustment for hepatic or renal dysfunction
    g. Analyze findings of CBC with differential, CD4 count, platelet count to monitor bone marrow activity and for effectiveness of drug therapy
    h. Preexisting CNS disturbances may be exacerbated; assess orientation and reflexes; implement safety measures to protect against injury if CNS disturbances exist
    i. Assess skin and lesions regularly
    j. Hydrate to decrease risk of nephrotoxicity (e.g., 2,000–3,000 mL/fluids per day if not contraindicated by other conditions)
    k. Monitor relief of infection and of pain
    l. Monitor platelets and evidence of petechiae or increased risk of bleeding
    m. Monitor electrolytes and fluid balance
    n. Monitor nutritional status, especially if GI side effects occur; ensure adequate protein intake

      11. Client education

         a. See Box 2-1 for universal client teaching points

         b. Self-administration techniques if indicated; wear gloves for topical applications

         c. Clinical manifestations to report: severe side effects; evidence of increased bleeding, edema, fatigue; severe rash, especially if accompanied by blisters, fever, and other indications of infection to avert serious complications

         d. Avoid sexual intercourse if genital herpes being treated

         e. Avoid tactile contact of lesions by self and others to avoid spreading infection to new sites

         f. Avoid hazardous tasks and driving if drowsiness, dizziness, seizure activity occurs

         g. Ensure client follows up with labs and appointments with health care provider

         h. Offer frequent, small, high-protein meals

         i. Encourage 2,000–3,000 mL/day intake

         j. Female clients should have annual Papanicolaou smear since there is increased risk of cervical cancer with genital herpes infection

         k. Antiviral agents do not cure herpes and CMV infections

         l. Notify health care provider if lesions do not heal or recur

   B. Medications for HIV, AIDS, and hepatitis

      1. Antiretroviral protease inhibitors

         a. Action and use

            1) Most potent of antiviral agents; inhibit cell protein synthesis that interferes with viral replication; block protease activity in HIV

            2) Is not curative but slows progression of disease and prolongs life

            3) Used prophylactically because viral replication peaks before clinical manifestations emerge and antiviral efficacy is then more limited; virus relies on using resources within live host cell and there is increased risk for toxicity to host cell

            4) Used in AIDS, AIDS-related complex (ARC), and hepatitis B and C to decrease viral load and opportunistic infections

            5) Used in combination to decrease viral load, increase CD4 counts, and decrease incidence or rate of development of drug resistance

            6) Is rapidly absorbed from GI tract

            7) Treatment of chronic hepatitis B may include use of interferon alfa and antivirals lamivudine, adefovir, and entecavir

            8) Treatment of chronic hepatitis C includes use of interferon and ribavirin, as well as the new drug boceprevir

         b. Common medications (Table 2-14)

         c. Administration considerations

            1) Saquinavir (Invirase): take with high-fat meals or within 2 hours of full meal

            2) Ritonavir (Norvir): unpalatable; take with chocolate milk, nutritional supplement, or food

            3) Indinavir (Crixivan) requires an acidic gastric environment for absorption; take 1 hour before or 2 hours after a light, low-fat snack; drink greater than 1.5 liters of fluid daily

         d. Contraindications

            1) Not recommended for pregnant or lactating women, or children

            2) Hypersensitivity

         e. Significant drug interactions

            1) To decrease risk of resistance, drug may be combined with reverse transcriptase agents

            2) Rifampin and rifabutin lower blood levels of protease inhibitors; mycobacterium prophylaxis may be changed to clarithromycin

         f. Significant food interactions (see section on administration considerations)

Table 2-14	**Antiviral Medications for HIV and AIDS: Protease Inhibitors**
Generic (Trade) Name	**Route**
Amprenavir (Agenerase)	PO
Atazanivir (Reyataz)	PO
Boceprevir (Victrelis)	PO
Darunavir (Prezista)	PO
Fosamprenavir (Lexiva)	PO
Indinavir (Crixivan)	PO
Lopinavir (Kaletra)	PO
Nelfinavir (Viracept)	PO
Ritonavir (Norvir)	PO
Saquinavir (Fortovase)	PO
Tipranavir (Aptivus)	PO

g. Significant laboratory studies
  1) Aminotransferase and triglyceride levels may be elevated with ritonavir
  2) ALT, AST, alkaline phosphatase, bilirubin
  3) CBC
  4) Creatinine, BUN, creatinine clearance
h. Side effects
  1) Headache, fatigue, N/V, diarrhea, abdominal discomfort, anemia, taste perversion, asthenia, circumoral paresthesia with ritonavir
  2) Reversible hyperbilirubinemia and nephrolithiasis with indinavir (Crixivan): greater than 1.5 liters fluid daily are needed to prevent nephrolithiasis
i. Adverse effects/toxicity: hepatotoxicity; reduce dose in liver dysfunction
j. Nursing considerations
  1) Assess current medications to avoid drug interactions
  2) Assess allergies
  3) Monitor for hepatotoxicity: ALT, AST, alkaline phosphatase, bilirubin; observe for N/V, jaundice, upper right abdominal quadrant enlargement and tenderness
  4) Monitor for nephrotoxicity: creatinine, BUN, creatinine clearance, urinalysis; keep accurate I & O
  5) Monitor CBC for blood dyscrasias such as neutropenia, thrombocytopenia, or anemia, and for improvement as evidenced by increased T-cell count
  6) Monitor for side effects; if neutropenic, observe for occult signs of infection (e.g., low back, flank, or suprapubic pain, normal temperature or low-grade fever related to UTI)
  7) Collaborate with prescriber if dosage change indicated by analysis of data collected to determine adverse effects
  8) Saquinavir (Invirase): take with high-fat foods or within 2 hours of full meal
  9) Ritonavir (Norvir): take with chocolate milk, nutritional supplement, or food to counteract unpleasant taste
  10) Indinavir (Crixivan): take 1 hour before or 2 hours after light, low-fat snack; drink more than 1,500 mL/day of fluids
  11) Provide neutropenic care as appropriate
k. Client education
  1) See Box 2-1 for universal teaching points for anti-infectives
  2) Ensure fluid intake of at least 1,500 mL/day

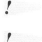

3) Take with food: saquinavir (Invirase) (high-fat foods recommended) and ritonavir (unpalatable taste)

4) Take 1 hour before or 2 hours after light, low-fat snack: indinavir

5) Eat small, frequent meals with complete or complementary proteins

6) Keep appointments for follow-up examinations and laboratory testing

7) Use neutropenic precautions

2. Reverse transcriptase inhibitors

   a. Action and use

      1) Block viral reverse transcriptase; stop replication and growth

      2) Are used for all symptomatic, HIV clients with a CD4 count less than 500/mm^3 and some with higher counts

      3) Penetrate blood–brain barrier

      4) Possible prophylaxis for known occupational HIV exposure

      5) Effectiveness diminishes over time

      6) AZT is used to prevent maternal transmission of HIV

      7) A major advantage of nonnucleoside reverse transcriptase inhibitors is that they do not adversely affect development of blood cells

      8) There is no cross-resistance between nucleoside and nonnucleoside reverse transcriptase inhibitors

      9) Are used in combination because resistant strains rapidly evolve if used as single agent therapy

   b. Common medications (Table 2-15)

   c. Administration considerations

      1) Crush or chew buffered tablets that are chewable because drug has acid lability

      2) Food may slow absorption but does not affect total absorption

      3) May administer at bedtime for better tolerance of CNS adverse effects

   d. Contraindications

      1) Concurrent use of drugs that cause peripheral neuropathy, such as choramphenicol (Chloromycetin), vinca alkaloids (vincristine [Oncovin], vinblastine

Table 2-15 Antiviral Medications for HIV and AIDS: Reverse Transcriptase Inhibitors

Generic (Trade) Name	Route
Nucleoside Reverse Transcriptase Inhibitors	
Abacavir (Ziagen)	PO
Abacavir/amivudine (Epzicom)	PO
Didanosine (Videx, DDI)	PO
Emitricitabine (Emtriva)	PO
Lamivudine (Epivir, 3TC)	PO
Stavudine (Zerit)	PO
Tenofovir disoproxil fumarate (Viread)	PO
Tenovir/emtricitabine (Truvada)	PO
Zalcitabine (Hivid, DDC)	PO
Zidovudine (Retrovir, AZT)	PO, N
Nonnucleoside Reverse Transcriptase Inhibitors	
Nevirapine (Viramune)	PO
Delavirdine (Rescriptor)	PO
Efavirenz (Sustiva)	PO
Etravine (Intelence)	PO

[Velban], etoposide [VP 16], cisplatin [Platinol]), dapsone (DDS), hydralazine (Apresoline), isoniazid (INH), metronidazole (Flagyl), nitrofurantoin, phenytoin (Dilantin), and ribavirin

2) Avoid or use with caution drugs that can increase toxicity, such as probenecid (Benemid), acetaminophen (Tylenol), lorazepam (Ativan), indomethacin (Indocin), and cimetidine (Tagamet)

3) If neurotoxic signs occur, discontinue drug until signs are resolved

4) Abacavir must be stopped if flulike symptoms occur and is contraindicated with anticoagulants

5) Not contraindicated in clients with AIDS dementia

e. Significant drug interactions

1) Many drug class interactions; see individual product literature

2) Antivirals will decrease effect of oral contraceptives

3) Tenofovir can increase serum level of didanosine

4) May be given with other drugs to enhance antiviral effect: acyclovir, interferon (Intron-A), didanosine (Videx), granulocyte colony-stimulating factor (GCSF) such as epoetin alfa (Procrit)

f. Significant food interactions: decreased absorption of didanosine when taken with food

g. Significant laboratory studies

1) Amylase, cholesterol, liver function tests (ALT, AST, alkaline phosphatase, bilirubin)

2) CBC including WBC with differential, platelet count, and CD4 count

3) Electrolytes

4) Serum creatinine, BUN, creatinine clearance

h. Side effects

1) Neurologic side effects of insomnia, confusion, peripheral neuropathies, and seizures

2) Diarrhea

3) Hypermagnesemia

4) Discolored fingernails, rash

5) Myalgias, numbness and tingling of extremities, altered taste sensations, dizziness, anxiety, tremors

6) Cough

i. Adverse effects/toxicity

1) Pancreatitis

2) Anemia, leukopenia, thrombocytopenia with nucleosides

3) Nevirapine (Viramune): severe hepatotoxicity and dermatologic effects such as Stevens–Johnson syndrome

j. Nursing considerations

1) Assess for hypersensitivity

2) Assess current drug therapies for drug interactions

3) Assess baseline renal and liver tests and monitor at intervals

4) Ensure client takes complete course and all drugs included in regimen to improve effectiveness and retard risk for resistant strains emerging

5) Administer around the clock as needed to maintain therapeutic levels

6) Stop administration if severe rash or other hypersensitivity reaction occurs

7) Assess client for complications of HIV infection (e.g., opportunistic infections, cancer, neurologic disease)

8) Monitor level of consciousness (LOC), strength, appropriateness of activity, short-term memory, ability to follow complex commands, reasoning and calculation abilities, and peripheral sensation

!

        9) Assess for compromised respiratory or cardiovascular status
      10) Provide safety measures to protect from injury if CNS adverse effects occur
      11) Assess nutritional intake and tolerance
      12) Monitor skin and mucous membranes frequently
      13) Monitor renal function with labs, I & O, daily weight
      14) Monitor for alleviation of clinical manifestations of AIDS or ARC and for increase in CD4 count

    k. Client education
        1) See Box 2-1 for universal teaching points for anti-infectives
        2) Caution about risks of dizziness or altered mentation; do not drive or perform hazardous tasks
        3) Avoid crowds and persons with infections
        4) Hair loss possible with zidovudine (AZT)
        5) Drug does not cure but helps manage infection; it reduces viral load, decreases risk for complications, and extends survival
        6) Practice good hygiene and safe-sex practices
        7) Explain use of combination of drugs that work by different mechanisms; improves client's survival by reducing viral resistance to drug therapy

!

Practice to Pass

The client with HIV states, "I quit taking the acyclovir. I don't have any symptoms. I don't want to take it now and risk becoming resistant to it when I may really need it." How do you respond?

3. Enfurvitide (Fuzeon) is sole drug in a class called *fusion inhibitors*, which bind to viral envelope and limit ability of virus to attach to CD4 cells administered subcutaneously bid; indicated in clients resistant to other antiretroviral classes; injection site reactions may include erythema, severe pain, pruritis, cysts, abscesses, and cellulitis; clients should be monitored for pneumonia secondary to increased risk of lung infections; no significant drug interactions

4. Maraviroc (Selzentry) is a *chemokine coreceptor 5 antagonist* (CCR5 antagonist), which reversibly binds to chemokine coreceptor located on CD4 cells; used in treatment-experienced clients with resistant strains of HIV; FDA-approved guide required prior to administration; drug interactions may occur with azole antifungals, clarithromycin, doxycycline, quinidine, telithromycin, verapamil, phenytoin, carbamazepine, naficillin, and rifanmpin; it may cause hepatotoxicity and caution should be used in clients with preexisting cardiac disease due to risk for cardiac ischemia or infarction

5. Raltefravir (Isentress) is an *integrase inhibitor* that inhibits activity of integrase enzyme, needed by HIV to insert viral DNA into human chromosome; it is indicated in combination treatments with clients who are treatment experienced and drug resistant; myopathy and rhabdomyolysis have been reported; no significant drug interactions; headache, diarrhea, and nausea are most common side effects

6. Combination drugs (See Table 2-16)

Table 2-16   **Other Antiretroviral Medications**

Classification	Generic (Trade) name	Route
Fusion Inhibitor	Enfuritide (Fuzeon)	subQ
CCR5 Coreceptor Antagonist	Maraviroc (Selzentry)	PO
Integrase Inhibitor	Raltegravir (Isentress)	PO
Combination Products	Efavirenz/emtritabine/tenofovir (Atripla) Abacavir/lamivudine/zidovudine (Trizivir) Lamivudine/zidovudine (Combivir) Lopinavir/ritonavir (Kaletra) Ripivirine/ tenofovir/emtricitabine (Complera)	PO for all

C. Medications for influenza and respiratory viruses
 1. Action and use
  a. Virustatic
  b. Most viral replication has occurred before clinical evidence appears; bacterial replication occurs as clinical manifestations of infection emerge so antibacterial agents are more effective against bacterial infections than antiviral agents are against viral infections, since drug therapy relies on viral replication for effectiveness
  c. Ribavirin (Virazole)
   1) Aerosolized administration for respiratory syncytial virus (RSV) or severe infections of the respiratory tract secondary to RSV
   2) Virustatic
   3) May decrease length of disease
   4) Efficacy demonstrated in influenza A and B and in hepatitis A
  d. Amantadine (Symmetrel) and rimantadine (Flumadine)
   1) Used prophylactically for influenza A; increased efficacy if initiated at time of exposure or at least within 48 hours
   2) Adjunctive therapy for temporary immunization of influenza A
   3) May limit severity of clinical manifestations of influenza and/or decrease length or duration
 2. Common medications (Table 2-17)
  a. Amantadine (Symmetrel): prophylactically and therapeutically used for respiratory viral infections such as influenza; also used to treat Parkinson disease; recommendations for use of amantadine change yearly based on type of influenza that is prevalent; refer to Centers for Disease Control website for the most current information
  b. Ribavirin (Virazole): treat influenza A, RSV, and herpes infections
  c. Rimantadine (Flumadine): used prophylactically against influenza A
 3. Administration considerations
  a. Initiate drug therapy as soon as possible to enhance effectiveness and to deter complications of infection
  b. Administer before flu season for prophylactic purpose as indicated, but do not use as substitute for influenza vaccination
  c. If given within 48 hours of onset of symptoms, the neuraminidase inhibitors, oseltamivir (Tamiflu), and zanamivir (Relenza), will shorten the normal 7-day duration of symptoms
 4. Contraindications
  a. Known hypersensitivity
  b. Ribavirin (Virazole) contraindicated in pregnancy (teratogenic); use cautiously in lactating clients and children

Table 2-17 **Medications for Influenza and Respiratory Viruses**

Generic (Trade) Name	Route	Uses
Amantadine (Symmetrel)	PO	Respiratory viral infections Decrease Parkinson-related symptoms
Oseltamivir (Tamiflu)	PO	Uncomplicated influenza
Ribavirin (Virazole)	PO	Chronic hepatitis C in clients who relapse after interferon alpha therapy; treatment of influenza A, respiratory syncytial virus, and herpes virus infections
Rimantadine (Flumadine)	PO	Prevention and treatment of influenza A
Zanamivir (Relenza)	Inhalation	Treatment of uncomplicated influenza

    c. Caution in clients with renal or liver dysfunction

    d. Caution in clients with psychotic disorders or seizures

5. Significant drug interactions

    a. Alcohol increases CNS effects

    b. Anticholinergics increase atropine-like effects

    c. Ribavirin with digoxin increases risk for digitalis toxicity

6. Significant food interactions: none reported

7. Significant laboratory studies

    a. CBC with WBC differential

    b. Possible C&S of pharynx or of sputum

    c. ALT, AST, alkaline phosphatase, bilirubin to evaluate liver function

    d. Creatinine, BUN, creatinine clearance to evaluate renal function

8. Side effects

    a. Most are transient and resolve quickly after drug is discontinued

    b. Dizziness, light-headedness, headache, palpitations, mood and mental changes, drowsiness, insomnia, irritability, nightmares

    c. Dyspnea, rash, peripheral edema

    d. Orthostatic hypotension, N/V, mouth dryness, urinary retention

9. Adverse effects/toxicity

    a. Slurred speech, ataxia, seizures

    b. Leukopenia

    c. Possible digitalis toxicity with concurrent digoxin therapy

    d. Possible teratogenic

10. Nursing considerations

    a. Assess for allergies

    b. Assess hepatic and renal dysfunction

    c. Assess baseline neurological status (e.g., orientation, affect, coordination, reflexes)

    d. Assess drugs currently taking to avoid drug interactions

    e. Maintain hydration with 2,000–3,000 mL fluids/day if not contraindicated by other conditions

    f. Initiate drug therapy as soon as possible after exposure

    g. Ensure complete course of therapy taken to enhance drug effectiveness

    h. Evaluate for resolution of signs or symptoms, such as fever, lethargy, respiratory difficulty

    i. Monitor for adverse effects; monitor for respiratory deterioration in infants; assess for adventitious breath sounds in all clients

    j. Provide safety precautions if CNS adverse effects develop

    k. Keep accurate I & O; monitor for urinary retention (have client void before dose administration)

    l. Avoid commercial mouthwashes that may potentiate dryness of mouth; provide oral care with water or saline rinses

11. Client education

    a. See Box 2-1 for universal teaching points for anti-infectives

    b. Initiate therapy as soon as possible when prescribed

    c. Change position slowly to minimize risks of orthostatic hypotension

    d. Report increased respiratory distress or severe adverse effects to health care provider

    e. If drowsiness, dizziness, light-headedness, confusion, ataxia, or blurred vision occurs, do not drive or perform hazardous tasks

    f. If improvement is not noted within 2–3 days, notify health care provider

    g. If dry mouth develops, rinse mouth as needed with warm water or glass of warm water with 1 teaspoon of salt; commercial mouth rinses with alcohol and hydrogen peroxide may dry mouth further; hard sugarless candy may stimulate salivation

!

!

Practice to Pass

The client taking amantadine (Symmetrel) reports symptoms of xerostomia. What is this complaint? What intervention or teaching would you provide?

!

h. Drink at least 6–8 glasses of fluids a day

i. Keep appointments with health care provider and for tests

j. Obtain influenza A vaccine before flu season begins

D. Locally active antiviral agents

    1. Action and use: not absorbed systemically; interfere with viral replication and metabolic processes

    2. Common medications (Table 2-18)

    3. Administration considerations

        a. Wash hands well before applying medication

        b. Wear gloves and may use cotton-tip applicator to apply to skin lesions, being cautious not to contaminate drug or other sites on skin

        c. Ensure proper administration technique

        d. Stop drug if severe local adverse effect or open lesions develop

    4. Contraindications: caution if known hypersensitivity, pregnancy, lactation; fomivirsen should not be used if treated with cidofovir in last 2–4 weeks

    5. Significant drug interactions: do not apply other topical agents to same lesions

    6. Significant food interactions: none reported

    7. Significant laboratory studies: none reported

    8. Side effects

        a. Local burning, stinging, discomfort may occur at time of application but usually resolve without intervention

        b. Temporary visual impairment possible with optic application

    9. Adverse effects/toxicity: skin eruptions; hypersensitivity

    10. Nursing considerations

        a. See previous administration considerations

        b. Assess for allergies

        c. Assess site prior to administration to evaluate effectiveness of previous dose(s)

        d. Monitor for therapeutic response and adverse effects, and for client comfort, safety, and compliance

    11. Client education

        a. See Box 2-1 for universal teaching points for anti-infectives

        b. Use proper administration technique

        c. Does not cure but alleviates pain and discomfort and prevents extended damage to uninvolved tissue

        d. Report severe local discomfort or reaction to health care provider

Table 2-18   Locally Active Antiviral Agents

Generic (Trade Name)	Route	Uses
Docosanol (Abreva)	Topical	Herpes simplex cold sores and fever blisters
Fomivirsen (Vitravene)	Injected into affected eye	CMV retinitis
Ganciclovir (Vitrasert)	Implanted into eye	CMV retinitis
Idoxuridine (Herplex)	Topical	Herpes simplex keratitis
Imiquimod (Aldara)	Topical	Genital and perianal warts
Penciclovir (Denavir)	Topical	Herpes labialis
Trifluridine (Viroptic)	Ophthalmic	Herpes simplex of eye
Vidarabine (Vira-A)	Ophthalmic	Herpes simplex of eye that does not respond to idoxuridine

IV. ANTIFUNGALS

    A. Systemic

        1. Action and use

            a. Are fungistatic or fungicidal depending on therapeutic serum levels and sensitivity to fungi

            b. Treat candida infections, cryptococcus, blastomycosis, histoplasmosis, and aspergillus fumigates, **tinea** infections (a fungal infection caused by ringworm)

            c. Increased permeability of cell membranes better enables other drugs to enter fungus cell

        2. Common medications (Table 2-19)

        3. Administration considerations

            a. Administer carefully as ordered, especially IV dosages

            b. Combination of antifungal agents may deter or retard drug resistance

            c. Amphotericin B

                1) May premedicate with an antipyretic such as acetaminophen (Tylenol), an antihistamine such as diphenhydramine (Benadryl), an antiemetic, and meperidine (Demerol) to reduce severity of fever or chills response; heparin or hydrocortisone (Cortaid) added to the IV solutions may reduce risk for thrombophlebitis at IV site

                2) Give with heparin or hydrocortisone and over 4–6 hours to avert clinical manifestations of hypersensitivity or drug toxicity

                3) Hydrate with IV fluids usually 2 hours before and 2 hours after drug administration to decrease risk for nephrotoxicity

                4) To test for hypersensitivity prior to administration, deliver 1 mg/20 mL D_5W IV over 10–30 minutes; if hypersensitivity response occurs, a lipid preparation such as amphotericin B liposomal complex (Ambisome) may minimize severe fever, shaking, and chills; premedicate as discussed earlier

                5) Mix in D_5W only; precipitates form in any solution containing sodium chloride

                6) Abelcet (another name for Amphotericin B Liposomal Complex): shake gently to distribute drug particles; use 5-micrometer filter needle to inject agent into container of D_5W and thoroughly disperse drug throughout solution; redisperse drug in solution every 2 hours if infusion time extends beyond 2 hours; no in-line filter used

Table 2-19   **Systemic Antifungal Medications**

Generic (Trade) Name	Route
Amphotericin B preparations (Fungizone, Abelcet, others)	IV
Anidulafungin (Eraxin)	IV
Caspofungin acetate (Cancidas)	IV
Fluconazole (Diflucan)	PO, IV
Flucytosine (Ancobon)	PO
Griseofulvin (Fulvicin, Grifulvin V, Grisactin, Gris-PEG)	PO
Itraconazole (Sporanox)	PO
Ketoconazole (Nizoral)	PO, topical
Micafungin (Mycamine)	IV
Nystatin (Mycostatin, Nilstat, Nystex)	PO, topical
Terbinafine (Lamisil)	PO
Voriconazole (Vfend)	PO, IV

4. Contraindications
  a. Hypersensitivity
  b. If IV test dose of amphotericin B elicits hypersensitivity response, lipid preparations (which are much more expensive) may be given to avoid the severe response of fever, shaking, chills
  c. Avoid H_2-histamine antagonists unless scheduled so not to interfere with absorption of antifungals
  d. Use caution with IV administration of miconazole (Monistat) because of risk of cardiotoxicity
  e. Use caution in pregnant and lactating clients
  f. Use caution with amphotericin B agents in renal impairment and/or severe bone marrow depression
5. Significant drug interactions
  a. Increased risk for bleeding with concurrent administration of anticoagulants or corticosteroids
  b. Increased risk for nephrotoxicity if given concurrently with other nephrotoxic drugs, such as aminoglycosides, cisplatinum (Platinol) and other antineoplastic agents, furosemide (Lasix), vancomycin (Vancocin), fluconazole (Diflucan), and cyclosporine (Sandimmune)
  c. Antidiabetic agents given concurrently with miconazole, fluconazole, and itraconazole may exaggerate hypoglycemia effect
  d. Ketoconazole and itraconazole depend on acid environment; give antifungal agent 1 hour before or 2 hours after administration of antacid
  e. Ketoconazole and fluconazole prolong effect of cyclosporine (Sandimmune)
  f. Ketoconazole: rifampin decreases effect of the antifungal
  g. Fluconazole: increases phenytoin (Dilantin) level and decreases serum levels of fluconazole with administration of rifampin (Rifadin); interacts with benzodiazepines, anticoagulants, and oral contraceptives; should use aspirin instead of acetaminophen for pain relief
  h. Amphotericin B (Fungizone): synergistic effect with tetracyclines, rifampin, or 5-flucytosine (Ancobon); do not administer with any other nephrotoxic drugs or with conticosteroids, digoxin, or thiazide diuretics
  i. Griseofulvin (Grifulvin V)
    1) Flushing and tachycardia with alcohol
    2) Decreased antifungal effect with barbiturates
    3) Increased risk of bleeding with anticoagulants
    4) Decreased efficacy of oral contraceptives and risk for breakthrough bleeding
6. Significant food interactions
  a. Itraconazole (Sporanox): take with food to enhance absorption
  b. Ketoconazole (Nizoral): take with food to decrease nausea and vomiting
7. Significant laboratory studies
  a. Creatinine, BUN, creatinine clearance as baseline and at intervals to evaluate renal function
  b. ALT, AST, alkaline phosphatase, bilirubin as baseline and at intervals to evaluate liver function
  c. PT and INR if taking oral anticoagulants
  d. Electrolytes, especially potassium, magnesium, and sodium
  e. Monitor metabolic acidosis development during amphotericin B therapy
  f. Monitor CBC with hemoglobin and hematocrit, RBC indices, and platelet count
8. Side effects
  a. Thrombophlebitis with administration through peripheral vein
  b. Fever, chills, shaking, headache

    c. Anorexia, N/V during or after administration, heartburn, diarrhea, flatulence

    d. Myalgia, arthralgia, weakness, hypotension

    e. Insomnia, vertigo, confusion

    f. Taste acuity diminished or causes unpleasant taste

    g. Photosensitivity

    h. Rash, pruritus, dry skin, urticaria

    i. Hypokalemia, hypomagnesemia: especially with concurrent use of glucocorticosteroids or diuretics

    j. Furry tongue with griseofulvin (Grifulvin V)

    k. Ketoconazole (Nizoral): sexual impotency, hair loss, and gynecomastia

9. Adverse reactions/toxicity

    a. Bone marrow depression resulting in neutropenia, thrombocytopenia, anemia

    b. Ototoxicity and nephrotoxicity with amphotericin B preparations

    c. Superinfections

    d. Drug toxicity or hypersensitivity: fever, chills, shaking, piloerection, headache, anorexia, nausea and vomiting

    e. Stevens–Johnson syndrome

    f. Renal dysfunction with amphotericin B may result in severe hypokalemia

    g. Cardiovascular collapse with too rapid infusion

    h. Hepatic necrosis: rare

10. Nursing considerations

    a. Assess concurrent medications to avoid drug interactions; check for incompatibility of solutions as there are many

    b. Ensure C&S specimen of infection site is collected before starting agent

    c. Assess for pregnancy, lactation, liver or renal dysfunction; monitor liver and renal laboratory studies throughout therapy

    d. Monitor serum levels of antifungal agents

    e. Monitor WBC for improvement and for early detection of developing neutropenia, thrombocytopenia, anemia

    f. Ensure complete course of medication taken for full benefit of therapy and to minimize risk of regrowth of fungus or development of drug resistance

    g. Evaluate for resolution of clinical signs of infection, such as fever

    h. Give potassium supplements if hypokalemia occurs

    i. Amphotericin B (IV)

        1) Use in-line filter with pores greater than 1 micron

        2) Premedicate with acetaminophen, diphenhydramine, an antiemetic, corticosteroids, and opioid analgesics as indicated

        3) Assess vital signs and for adverse reactions every 15 minutes twice, then every 30 minutes for 4 hours with initial administration and thereafter as indicated; administer IV over 2–6 hours

        4) Hydrate with 2,000–3,000 mL/day unless contraindicated by other conditions; keep accurate I & O

        5) Use strict aseptic technique since there is no preservative in solution and client may be compromised

        6) Use in life-threatening infections

        7) Protect drug solution from light with foil covering

        8) Closely monitor for hypokalemia and hypomagnesemia and impaired renal function

11. Client education

    a. See Box 2-1 for universal teaching points for anti-infectives

    b. Amphotericin B may be given over weeks or months

    c. Explain administration procedure

Practice to Pass

The client with AIDS is to be given a first dose of amphotericin B intravenously after a central line is inserted. The client states, "I'm scared to get this stuff. The doctor told me all the bad things that can happen." How would you respond?

    d. Report adverse effects such as burning at IV site, increased bleeding or bruising, or evidence of superinfection

    e. Febrile reaction may decrease over time

    f. Maintain fluid intake of 2,000–3,000 mL/day if not contraindicated by other conditions

    g. Eat small, frequent meals with high-quality protein

    h. Take oral agents with food to minimize GI distress

b. Topical antifungals

    1. Action and use

      a. Local infections of skin and mucous membranes of oropharnyx, vagina, or intestines caused by *Candida* species; infections of tinea pedis (athlete's foot), tinea cruris (in scrotal, crural, anal, and genital areas, called "jock itch"), tinea corporis (skin), tinea unguium or onychomycosis (nail fungus), tinea manus, tinea versicolor (infection of skin with yellow or beige-colored brawny patches)

      b. Use vaginal tablets up to 6 weeks prior to delivery to prevent newborn thrush

    2. Common medications (Table 2-20)

    3. Administration considerations

      a. Oral tablets or lozenges or troches are not to be chewed or swallowed whole; swallow saliva as lozenge or troche dissolves slowly over 5–30 minutes; avoid food or drink during and for 30 minutes after dose

      b. For oral infections in client with dentures, remove dentures at bedtime; with oral suspension, remove dentures before each rinse or before each oral lozenge or troche

Table 2-20 **Topical Antifungal Medications**

Generic (Trade) Name	Route
Azole Type	
Butaconazole (Femstat-3)	Topical
Clotrimazole (Mycelex, Lotrimin)	PO, lozenges, topical, vaginal
Econazole (Spectazole)	Topical
Ketoconazole (Nizoral)	PO, topical, shampoo, vaginal
Miconazole (Monistat)	Topical, vaginal suppository and cream, spray, shampoo, IV rarely due to high risk fo cardiotoxicities
Oxiconazole (Oxistat)	Topical
Sertaconazole (Ertaczo)	Topical
Sulconazole (Exelderm)	Topical
Terconazole (Terazol)	Topical
Tioconazole (Vagistat, Monistat 1-Day, Tioconastat-1)	Topical
Others	
Amphotericin B (Fungizone, Abelcet, others)	Topical, IV
Butenafine (Mentax)	Topical
Ciclopirox cream, gel shampoo (Loprox) or nail lacquer (Penlac)	Topical
Griseofulvin (Fulvicin)	Topical
Naftifine (Naftin)	Topical cream
Nystatin (Mycostatin)	PO tablet and suspension, troches, vaginal, topical
Terbinafine (Lamisil)	Topical
Tolnaftate (Aftate, Tinactin)	Topical
Undecylenic acid (Fungi-Nail, Gordochom	Topical

    c. For application to skin: wear latex gloves, cleanse area with tepid water (soap if prescribed), dry thoroughly (without application of heat), and apply to infected area sparingly; do not cover with an occlusive dressing or tight clothing; wash hands well after gloves removed

    d. For treatment of tinea pedis (athlete's foot), apply antifungal powder such as nystatin (Mycostatin) to inside of shoes and stockings

    e. For vulvovaginal use: insert one applicator full or one vaginal tablet into vagina at bedtime as instructed; continue therapy during menstruation

    f. Avoid contact of antifungal with eyes; with certain agents, avoid contact with mucous membranes

    g. Do not apply occlusive dressing unless prescribed; client to avoid restrictive clothing in areas of infection

    h. Store creams, vaginal application, and topical preparation at room temperature; if specified for vaginal tablets and troches, refrigerate but do not freeze

4. Contraindications: hypersensitivity (skin blistering, burning)

5. Significant drug interactions: do not apply other preparations on same surface area

6. Significant food interactions: none reported

7. Significant laboratory studies: liver enzymes in hepatic impairment

8. Side effects

    a. Topical: stinging, burning, erythema, edema, dry skin, vesication, pruritus, urticaria, desquamation, skin fissures

    b. Vaginal: slight burning, lower abdominal discomfort, bloating, erythema, itching, vaginal soreness during intercourse

    c. Oral troches or swish and swallow: nausea and vomiting

9. Adverse effects/toxicity: possible hepatotoxicity in client with liver impairment

10. Nursing considerations

    a. Ensure complete course of therapy taken on consecutive days

    b. Observe for clinical signs of improvement

    c. Observe for clinical evidence of liver dysfunction, such as upper right quadrant tenderness, abdominal discomfort or bloating, lethargy, mentation changes, icterus, enlarged liver, elevated liver enzymes (ALT, AST, alkaline phosphatase, bilirubin)

    d. Stop application if severe burning or exacerbation of lesions occur and collaborate with prescriber

11. Client education

    a. See Box 2-1 for universal teaching points for anti-infectives

    b. Explain how to apply or instill dose

    c. Observe for resolution of signs or symptoms within first week of therapy; some infections require 2–4 weeks of treatment; notify prescriber if condition worsens or no improvement is noted in 1–2 weeks

    d. Store in tightly covered container at room temperature; if vaginal tablet or suppository, store as recommended, usually in refrigerator or above 59°F; avoid freezing or excess heat of all products

    e. If taken vaginally, refrain from sexual intercourse or have partner wear condom to avoid burning or irritation of penis or urethra

    f. Wash clothing and linens in contact with infectious sites with soap and water after each treatment; ointments may be removed from fabric with commercial cleaning products

    g. If severe burning, stinging, or eruptions occur, discontinue use and notify prescriber

V. ANTIPROTOZOALS

A. Antimalarials (schizonticides)

1. Action and use
   a. Therapeutic use to treat acute episodes or prophylaxis to prevent malarial infection and/or relapse
   b. Chloroquine treatment for **giardiasis** (a protozoan intestinal infection) and amebiasis outside the GI tract, as well as rheumatoid arthritis and discoid lupus erythematosus
   c. Quinacrine (Atabrine): treat dwarf tapeworm giardiasis and cestodiosis (infestation with tapeworms); pleural sclerosing agent to prevent recurrence of pneumothorax
2. Common medications (Table 2-21)
3. Administration considerations
   a. Separate drug from antacid administration by 4 hours (before or after)
   b. Take quinine sulfate with food to decrease gastric distress and mask bitter taste; do not crush capsule
   c. Quinacrine HCL (Atabrine): take after food with full glass of water, tea, or juice
   d. Chloroquine (Aralen), hydroxychloroquine sulfate (Plaquenil Sulfate), and pyrimethamine (Daraprim): take with food to minimize gastric distress
   e. For prophylaxis, take as prescribed, such as same day every week when entering high-risk area and for 10 weeks after departing
   f. Mefloquine (Lariam): take with at least 8 ounces water; separate by at least 8 hours from dose of quinine or quinidine, an antiarrhythmic
4. Contraindications
   a. Quinine sulfate: tinnitus, optic neuritis, myasthenia gravis, G6PD deficiency, pregnancy; use caution with dysrhythmias and cardiac disorders
   b. Pyrimethamine (Daraprim): caution with antiseizure agents
   c. Mefloquine (Lariam): hypersensitivity; with calcium channel blockers; in dysrhythmias, psychotic or seizure disorders; in pregnancy and in infants
   d. Chloroquine: renal disease; caution in hepatic dysfunction, ethanol abuse, eczema, G6PD deficiency, children, blood dyscrasias, GI and neurological disorders; and psoriasis or porphyria (may precipitate attacks)
   e. Primaquine: administer cautiously to clients of Eastern Mediterranean or African origins (pharmacogenetics) and clients with preexisting hematologic conditions

Table 2-21 Antiprotozoal Medications

Generic (Trade) Name	Route	Uses
Chloroquine (Aralen)	PO	*Plasmodium* malaria; extraintestinal amebiasis
Atovaquone/proguanil (Malarone)	PO	*Plasmodium* malaria
Hydroxychloroquine sulfate (Plaquenil Sulfate)	PO	*Plasmodium* malaria
Mefloquine (Lariam)	PO	*Plasmodium* malaria
Primaquine (generic)	PO	Toxoplasmosis; prevent relapses of *Plasmodium* malaria in combination with other agents to suppress transmission
Pyrimethamine (Daraprim)	PO	Toxoplasmosis; prevent relapses of *Plasmodium* malaria in combination with other agents to suppress transmission
Pyrimethamine and sulfadiazine (Fansidar)	PO	Toxoplasmosis
Quinine (Quinamm)	PO	Chloroquine-resistant *Plasmodium* infections
Tinidazole (Tindamax)	PO	Amebiasis, giardiasis, trichomonas infection

5. Significant drug interactions
   a. Quinine sulfate: may increase digoxin levels; increased vagolytic effects with anti-cholinergics; decreased effectiveness if concurrent use of rifampin, antiseizure agents, or barbiturates; increased risk for toxicity with systemic and oral antacids; increased anticoagulant effects with oral anticoagulants; decreased mefloquine HCL levels; increased risk for seizures from possible lowered levels of valproic acid
   b. Disulfiram-like effects with alcohol and some antimalarials
   c. Pyrimethamine: decreased effectiveness against **toxoplasmosis** (protozoan systemic infection transmitted by contact with oocysts in feces of domesticated animals) with concurrent use of folic acid or para-aminobenzoic acid (PABA)
   d. Chloroquine: interacts with cimetidine, digoxin, penicillamine, and rabies vaccine; has decreased absorption if taken with kaolin or magnesium-containing antacids
   e. Mefloquine: beta blockers, calcium blockers, and digoxin can prolong cardiac conduction
   f. Decreased absorption with antacids or laxatives containing aluminum or magnesium
   g. May interfere with rabies vaccine
6. Significant food interactions: none reported
7. Significant laboratory studies
   a. ALT, AST, alkaline phosphatase, bilirubin
   b. CBC with differential, reticulocyte count, red blood cell indices, hemoglobin, hematocrit, platelet count
   c. Evaluate electrolytes affected by GI side effects
   d. Prior to therapy, test for G6PD deficiency in African Americans and clients of Mediterranean descent
8. Side effects
   a. Dizziness, vertigo, headache, visual impairment, angina
   b. N/V, diarrhea, gastric distress, abdominal cramps
   c. Confusion, apprehension, insomnia, nightmares, syncope, delirium
   d. Cutaneous flushing, pruritus, rash, paresthesia, dyspnea, weight loss, fatigue
   e. Quinacrine: may cause reversible yellowing of skin or gray-blue hue to ears, nasal cartilage, and nail beds (not jaundice or cyanosis)
   f. Chloroquine and hydroxychloroquine sulfate: alopecia, bleaching of scalp or hair (including eyebrows and body hair) and freckles; bluish-black hue of skin or mucous membranes, rash, pruritis; photophobia
9. Adverse effects/toxicity
   a. Tinnitus, hearing loss
   b. Cardiotoxicity in clients with atrial fibrillation
   c. Leukopenia, thrombocytopenia, agranulocytosis, hypoprothrombinemia, hemolytic anemia
   d. Hypotension, tachypnea, tachycardia, hypothermia
   e. Seizures, coma, cardiovascular collapse, blackwater fever (extensive intravascular hemolysis with renal failure), death
   f. Visual halos, blurring, inability to focus
10. Nursing considerations
   a. Ensure complete course of medication is taken for full benefit
   b. Assess drugs being taken to avoid drug interactions
   c. Assess hepatic and cardiac function at intervals
   d. Assess for electrolyte disturbances, blood disorders as anemia, thrombocytopenia
   e. If taking antiepileptics, monitor drug levels of these agents
   f. Ensure regular ophthalmic exams, electrocardiograms, and lab tests as ordered
   g. Assess for G6PD deficiency as indicated

    h. Assess for muscle weakness and depressed deep tendon reflexes periodically

    i. Assess for CNS side effects; collaborate with prescriber regarding discontinuation of agent

  11. Client education

    a. See Box 2-1 for universal teaching points for anti-infectives

    b. If weekly, take on same day every week

    c. Do not drive or perform hazardous tasks if drowsiness, dizziness, vertigo, or visual disturbances occur

    d. Report fever, sore throat, myalgias, visual disturbances, anxiety, mental changes, hallucinations

    e. Chloroquine: sunglasses may decrease risk of photophobia or ocular changes; urine may become rusty yellow or brown; do not take OTC antacids or laxatives containing magnesium

B. Other antiprotozoals

  1. Action and use

    a. Amebic dysentery, hepatic amebiasis, or abscess

    b. Some are bactericidal as well as amebicidal, especially in GI tract

    c. Destroy intestinal bacteria that forms nitrogen to decrease ammonia in hepatic disease and coma

    d. Pentamidine isoethionate (Pentem 300): treat **pneumocystis (carinii) jiroveci pneumonia**, an opportunistic infection in client with AIDS

    e. Kills insects and parasites and their ova as in head lice, body lice, and scabies

  2. Common medications: paromomycin (Humatin), pentamidine isoethionate (Pentam 300), lindane (Kwell), atovaquone (Mepron)

  3. Administration considerations

    a. Pentamidine isoethionate: decreased doses in renal dysfunction

    b. Rotate IM injection sites

    c. Administer atovaquone with high-fat meal greater than 23 grams to increase absorption

  4. Contraindications

    a. Caution in pregnancy and lactation

    b. Hypersensitivity to drug or to iodine, iodoquinol (Dioquinol), or primaquin

  5. Significant drug interactions: none reported

  6. Significant food interactions: none reported

  7. Significant laboratory studies

    a. Electrolytes including potassium, magnesium, and calcium if GI problems

    b. CBC with WBC and differential: check for infection and blood disorders such as leukopenia, anemia, neutropenia, thrombocytopenia if indicated

    c. Blood glucose for hypoglycemia if pancreatitis develops

  8. Side effects

    a. Hypotension, tachycardia, dizziness, headache, syncope

    b. Flushing, pruritis, dyspnea

    c. Abdominal cramps, diarrhea, N/V, epigastric distress, unpleasant taste

    d. Myalgia, precordial stiffness

    e. Tremors, restlessness

  9. Adverse effects/toxicity

    a. Nephrotoxicity: mild and reversible

    b. Leukopenia, neutropenia, anemia, thrombocytopenia

    c. Dysrhythmias

    d. Hypoglycemia related to pancreatitis

    e. Large doses can cause abscess, cellulitis, or lesion in muscle in the GI tract, heart, liver, and kidneys

f. Pain at injection site

g. Lindane (Kwell) topical shampoo can cause CNS problems such as seizures or eczematous eruptions

10. Nursing considerations

a. Ensure complete course of therapy is taken for full benefit

b. Assess other drugs being taken to avoid drug interactions

c. Assess skin for scabies, tracking, lesions, nits

d. For scabies: warm (not hot) shower and apply topical Kwell, then rinse off after 24 hours

e. For lice: massage Kwell into head or area infected; leave on for 5 minutes and shampoo out; do not get agent into eyes or on face; do not repeat in less than 1 week

11. Client education

a. See Box 2-1 for universal teaching points for anti-infectives

b. Report side or adverse effects to health care provider

c. Wash clothes and linens after treatment to prevent reinfection

d. Know clinical manifestations of infections to recognize and report

VI. ANTIHELMINTHICS

A. Action and use

1. *Ascaris lumbricoides* (intestinal worm infestation)
2. *Enterobius vermicularis* (pinworm)
3. *Ancytostoma duodenale* (hookworm)
4. *Necator americanus* (hookworm)
5. *Trichostrongylus* (intestinal worm infestation)
6. Most antihelminthics work by inhibiting glucose transport and uncoupling metabolism in the parasite's mitochondria

B. Common medications (Table 2-22)

C. Administration considerations

1. Mebendazole: may be chewed, swallowed whole, crushed, mixed with food
2. Pyrantel: may take with food
3. Thiabendazole: take after meals

D. Contraindications

1. Known hypersensitivity
2. Piperazine citrate: in renal or hepatic impairment, seizure disorders
3. Mebendazole: use cautiously in inflammatory bowel disease; contraindicated with liver disease or during pregnancy
4. Use cautiously with other anthelmintics in clients with hepatic or renal dysfunction
5. Safety not established in pregnancy and lactation

E. Significant drug interactions

1. Piperazine citrate: may decrease pyrantel pamoate (Antiminth) levels
2. Phenothiazines: may increase extrapyramidal effects or risk for seizures

Table 2-22 Antihelminthics for Worm Infestations

Generic (Trade) Name	Route
Mebendazole (Vermox)	PO
Albendazole (Albenza)	PO
Ivermectin (Stromectol)	PO
Pyrantel (Antiminth, Pin-X)	PO
Thiabendazole (Mintezol)	PO
Praziquantel (Biltricide)	PO

F. Significant food interactions: none reported

G. Significant laboratory studies

1. ALT, AST, alkaline phosphatase, bilirubin for liver assessment
2. Creatinine, BUN, creatinine clearance for renal assessment
3. Stool for ova and parasites (O & P) for accurate diagnosis of **helminths** (disease-producing parasites)

H. Side effects

1. N/V, diarrhea, abdominal cramps, anorexia
2. Rash, urticaria, erythema multiforme, photosensitivity, purpura, lacrimation, rhinorrhea
3. Dizziness, drowsiness
4. Fever, productive cough, anemia
5. Vision changes
6. Thiabendazole: urinary odor

I. Adverse effects/toxicity

1. Low toxicity; adverse effects usually with large doses
2. Neurotoxicity: headache, vertigo, ataxia, tremors, jerking movements, muscle weakness, paresthesia, depressed reflexes, mental changes abnormal ECG, seizures
3. Dose-related neutropenia; reversed with discontinuation of drug

J. Nursing considerations

1. Assess other drugs being taken to avoid drug interactions
2. Assess laboratory findings for hepatic, renal, or blood disorders and to verify diagnosis
3. Assess allergies
4. Ensure complete regimen taken to optimize therapeutic benefit
5. Collect stool specimen for ova and parasites (O & P) for baseline and follow-up to verify eradication of infectious agents

K. Client education

1. See Box 2-1 for universal teaching points for anti-infectives
2. Recognize and report evidence of effectiveness as well as adverse effects that may require discontinuation of drug
3. Agents may be taken with or after food to minimize gastric disturbances
4. Store drug at room temperature protected from light and heat
5. Do not repeat drug therapy for continued infection until 1 week after initial treatment
6. Practice personal hygiene to prevent transmission
7. Urine odor may occur with thiabendazole
8. Mebendazole may be chewed, swallowed whole, crushed, or mixed with food
9. Do not drive or operate machinery after dose of praziquantel

Case Study

A 25-year-old married female client has tested positive for group A streptococcus of the oropharyngeal area. The sensitivity report is not yet available. Amoxicillin (Amoxil) PO is to be initiated as empiric treatment.

1. What baseline assessment, including laboratory findings, is indicated prior to administering the first dose of amoxicillin?

2. How would you evaluate drug effectiveness?

3. If the client developed diarrhea, how would you differentiate the diarrhea from pseudomembranous colitis? What interventions would you implement to manage the diarrhea? For what fluid and electrolyte imbalance would you monitor?

4. Why is it important to ensure completion of the antibiotic therapy? What two infectious sequela may occur with inadequate therapy against group A streptococcus?

5. What client education would be appropriate?

For suggested responses, see pages 540–541.

POSTTEST

1 While teaching the client about taking a new prescription of oral metronidazole (Flagyl), which information would be most important for the nurse to include?

1. Avoid intake of alcoholic beverages.
2. Headache may accompany ingesting the drug.
3. Drug may cause constipation.
4. Drug may cause vaginal dryness.

2 Which of the following statements best indicates that an immunocompromised client understands self-application of the topical drug acyclovir (Zovirax)?

1. "I need to wash my hands for at least 10 seconds before and after applying the drug."
2. "I need to apply several thin layers of the medication on the lesions."
3. "I need to avoid touching the lesions and the opening of the container with the same finger cot."
4. "I should not allow anyone else to use this drug."

3 A nurse returning to work after 10 days off is assigned to a client who has received amphotericin B (Fungilin) 0.3 mg/kg/day IV for 5 days. The nurse should place priority on reviewing the client's record for which of the following?

1. Alanine aminotransferase (ALT) and aspartate aminotransferase (AST) levels
2. Sodium level and serum protein
3. Blood urea nitrogen (BUN) and creatinine
4. Number and consistency of stools in the past 24 hours

4 A client has prescriptions for an antipyretic, antihistamine, and an antiemetic to decrease the risk of infusion-related reactions to anti-infective therapy. The nurse anticipates the client may have orders for which intravenous (IV) anti-infectives? Select all that apply.

1. Amphotericin B (Fungizone)
2. Acyclovir (Zovirax)
3. Gentamicin (Garamycin)
4. Amoxicillin (Sumox)
5. Cefixime (Suprax)

5 The nurse is teaching a group of clients who are infected with the HIV about the various drug groups available to treat the disease. Which point of information would be important for the nurse to explain during the discussion using appropriate terminology?

1. Fusion inhibitors enhance release of reverse transcriptase.
2. Protease inhibitors are the most potent anti-HIV drugs.
3. Nonnucleoside reverse transcriptase inhibitors (NNRTIs) prevent replication of HIV.
4. Nucleoside transcriptase inhibitors (NRTIs) suppress production of reverse transcriptase.

6 The nurse should include which information when instructing a client who has been started on mebendazole (Vermox) for the treatment of pinworms?

1. Do not chew or crush the tablets.
2. Take the mediation with food.
3. Use sunscreen when going outdoors.
4. The drug may cause constipation.

7 A client is scheduled to receive a dose of clarithromycin (Biaxin) 100 mg suspension by mouth. If the reconstituted dosage concentration is 250 mg/5mL, the nurse should prepare a dose of how many mL?

_____ mL

8 When hanging an intravenous dose of vancomycin (Vancocin), the nurse administers the drug over 90 minutes to prevent which speed-related adverse drug effect?

1. Hypertension
2. Projectile vomiting
3. Flushing of face, neck, and chest
4. Pseudomembranous colitis

9 After liquid tetracycline (Sumycin) is ordered for a 2-year-old child, the nurse provides which most important instruction to the licensed practical or vocational nurse (LPN/LVN) who is administering the medication?

1. "Have the client drink the dose through a straw."
2. "Withhold the dose until I telephone the prescriber."
3. "Monitor the client for diarrhea."
4. "Administer with 6 to 8 ounces of milk."

10 A client has been prescribed to take both a tetracycline and a sulfonamide drug. When providing client teaching, what priority information should the nurse give the client related to adverse drug effects?

1. "Avoid exposure to upper respiratory infections."
2. "Use protective measures when exposed to the sun."
3. "Report problems with constipation to your provider."
4. "Change position slowly to avoid orthostatic hypotension."

➤ *See pages 83–84 for Answers and Rationales.*

ANSWERS & RATIONALES

Pretest

1 Answer: 1, 3, 4, 5 Rationale: Isoniazid (INH) can be hepatotoxic and aspartate aminotransferase (AST) levels reflect liver inflammation or damage. The client should be monitored for elevated levels. Antacids interfere with absorption of INH when taken within 1 to 2 hours of the INH, so the nurse should ensure that ingestion of the antacid dose is separated from the INH dose by 2 hours. Vitamin B_6 should be administered with INH therapy to reduce the incidence of peripheral neuritis. Thrombocytopenia is an adverse effect of INH, which can lead to the potential for bleeding and excessive bruising. INH can cause hypocalcemia, not hypercalcemia. **Cognitive Level:** Applying **Client Need:** Pharmacological and Parenteral Therapies **Integrated Process:** Nursing Process: Assessment **Content Area:** Pharmacology **Strategy:** Correlate drug major side effects with the client's signs and symptoms and also consider drug interactions (antacids and vitamin B$_6$). **Reference:** Wilson, B. A., Shannon, M., & Shields, K. (2012). *Pearson nurse's drug guide 2012*. Upper Saddle River, NJ: Pearson Education, pp. 814–816.

2 **Answer: 4** **Rationale:** Selecting an alternate infusion site and administering the medication slowly is correct. The infusion must be stopped to prevent further vein trauma and another site selected. Thrombophlebitis indicates that the infusion should be discontinued altogether, not slowed or diluted. A cold compress may ease the discomfort. It is not necessary to notify the primary care provider; the nurse can take responsibility for obtaining another site. **Cognitive Level:** Applying **Client Need:** Pharmacological and Parenteral Therapies **Integrated Process:** Nursing Process: Implementation **Content Area:** Pharmacology **Strategy:** Note the question is asking for what the most appropriate action would be, indicating that all answers may be correct, but one will be a better choice. Recall the dangers of thrombophlebitis to be directed to the correct option. **Reference:** Adams, M. P., & Koch, R. W. (2010). *Pharmacology: Connections to nursing practice*. Upper Saddle River, NJ: Pearson Education, pp. 795–800.

3 **Answer: 1** **Rationale:** Amantadine can cause anticholinergic effects such as bladder relaxation and detrusor muscle contraction. Urinary retention is more likely to occur in a client with benign prostatic hyperplasia (BPH). The anticholinergic effects can also contribute to constipation. There is no evidence that amantadine is nephrotoxic. **Cognitive Level:** Applying **Client Need:** Pharmacological and Parenteral Therapies **Integrated Process:** Nursing Process: Assessment **Content Area:** Pharmacology **Strategy:** Specific knowledge of drug side effects is needed to answer the question. Note that a critical term in the question is *benign prostatic hyperplasia (BPH)*, which should guide you to look for an option that relates to genitourinary symptoms. **Reference:** Wilson, B. A., Shannon, M., & Shields, K. (2012). *Pearson nurse's drug guide 2012*. Upper Saddle River, NJ: Pearson Education, pp. 58–60.

4 **Answer: 4** **Rationale:** Acyclovir (Zovirax) can be nephrotoxic and so it is important to ensure high fluid intake to keep the client well hydrated and perfuse the kidneys. Acyclovir is not hepatotoxic. It would not be necessary to avoid sexual intercourse while taking this medication. This drug may cause headaches, nausea, and vomiting, but not insomnia. **Cognitive Level:** Applying **Client Need:** Pharmacological and Parenteral Therapies **Integrated Process:** Nursing Process: Implementation **Content Area:** Pharmacology **Strategy:** To answer this question correctly, it is necessary to know specific information about this drug. Determine nursing interventions according to knowledge of drug characteristics. **Reference:** Wilson, B. A., Shannon, M., & Shields, K. (2012). *Pearson nurse's drug guide 2012*. Upper Saddle River, NJ: Pearson Education, pp. 18–21.

5 **Answer: 1** **Rationale:** A full course of antibiotic therapy must be taken in order to decrease the risk of resistance to the antibiotic or reoccurrence of the infection. Clients often discontinue drug therapy when the signs or symptoms subside. Missed doses should be taken as soon as they are remembered and the dose should not be doubled. Antibiotic doses are to be taken at regular intervals spaced throughout the 24 hours, without interrupting sleep when possible, to maintain effective therapeutic blood level of the antibiotic. Chewable tablets must be crushed or chewed, or the drug may not absorb adequately. Attempting to swallow chewable tablets could put the client at risk for airway obstruction. **Cognitive Level:** Analyzing **Client Need:** Pharmacological and Parenteral Therapies **Integrated Process:** Nursing Process: Evaluation **Content Area:** Pharmacology **Strategy:** The core issue of the question is knowledge that antibiotic therapy needs to be taken for the full course of therapy to effectively eradicate infection and prevent development of drug resistance. Apply knowledge of client compliance issues and potential outcomes. **Reference:** Adams, M. P., & Koch, R. W. (2010). *Pharmacology: Connections to nursing practice*. Upper Saddle River, NJ: Pearson Education, pp. 775–785.

6 **Answer: 1, 4** **Rationale:** The client is at risk for developing metabolic acidosis because of increased loss of bowel contents that consist primary of alkaline fluids. Excessive watery stools or stools that contain blood may indicate pseudomembranous colitis, caused by the toxins released by *C. difficile*. A stool specimen should be collected as a priority measure. If the cause of the diarrhea is *C. difficile*, the toxin needs to be eliminated. Antiperistaltic agents such as Bentyl or antidiarrheal agents such as Kapectolin can promote retention of toxins and should not be given. Some fruit juices could further exacerbate diarrhea and would not be encouraged. **Cognitive Level:** Applying **Client Need:** Pharmacological and Parenteral Therapies **Integrated Process:** Nursing Process: Implementation **Content Area:** Pharmacology **Strategy:** Correlate the most life-threatening side effects exhibited by gastrointestinal (GI) alterations with the specific drug and the specific microorganism. This will allow you to systematically select the options that should be anticipated by the nurse. **Reference:** Adams, M. P., & Koch, R. W. (2010). *Pharmacology: Connections to nursing practice*. Upper Saddle River, NJ: Pearson Education, pp. 794–798.

7 **Answer: 2, 5** **Rationale:** Aminoglycosides, such as tobramycin, can cause ototoxicity and nephrotoxicity. Hearing abilities and renal function should be monitored when clients are receiving any aminoglycoside. **Cognitive Level:** Applying **Client Need:** Pharmacological and Parenteral Therapies **Integrated Process:** Nursing Process: Evaluation **Content Area:** Pharmacology **Strategy:** Recall that aminoglycosides tend to be cause ototoxicity and nephrotoxicity. Evaluate each option in relation to these toxicities to select the correct options. **Reference:** Adams, M. P., & Koch, R. W. (2010). *Pharmacology: Connections to nursing practice.* Upper Saddle River, NJ: Pearson Education, pp. 816–820.

8 **Answer: 2, 3, 5** **Rationale:** Erythromycin (EES) is a macrolide that should be taken with a full glass of water for best absorption. Fruit juices and some carbonated beverages can interfere with complete absorption and so should be avoided. EES can cause severe diarrhea with life-threatening pseudomembranous colitis, liver impairment, and ototoxicity. **Cognitive Level:** Applying **Client Need:** Pharmacological and Parenteral Therapies **Integrated Process:** Nursing Process: Evaluation **Content Area:** Pharmacology **Strategy:** Recall the toxicities and drug interactions that could occur with erythromycin (EES) to choose the correct options. **Reference:** Adams, M. P., & Koch, R. W. (2010). *Pharmacology: connections to nursing practice*. Upper Saddle River, NJ: Pearson Education, pp. 814–815.

9 **Answer: 4** **Rationale:** A cross-allergenicity with penicillin may exist. If a history of a penicillin allergy exists, the prescriber may choose a drug from another category. The BUN is within normal limits and it is expected that granulocytosis (such as elevated neutrophils) would occur in response to a bacterial infection. It is common practice to collect the specimen for culture and sensitivity (C&S), then begin therapy with a broad-spectrum antibiotic that can be changed if the C&S reveals that a different drug would be more appropriate. **Cognitive Level:** Analyzing **Client Need:** Pharmacological and Parenteral Therapies **Integrated Process:** Nursing Process: Planning **Content Area:** Pharmacology **Strategy:** Identify common, life-threatening side effects of antibiotics, such as hypersensitivity. Next associate this risk with the appropriate nursing action. **Reference:** Wilson, B. A., Shannon, M., & Shields, K. (2012). *Pearson nurse's drug guide 2012*. Upper Saddle River, NJ: Pearson Education, pp. 284–285.

10 **Answer: 1** **Rationale:** A "shift to the left" refers to an increase in the production of immature neutrophils called bands or stab cells. Production of these white blood cells is stimulated by an acute bacterial infection. Lymphocytes, T cells, and B cells are increased primarily in viral infections. There is no evidence that parasites cause increased production of immature neutrophils. Chlamydia is an intracellular parasite. **Cognitive Level:** Analyzing **Client Need:** Pharmacological and Parenteral Therapies **Integrated Process:** Nursing Process: Planning **Content Area:** Pharmacology **Strategy:** Use knowledge of responses to infections related to types of microorganisms. The words *shift to the left* constitute a critical phrase. Viral infections are not likely to result in increased WBCs. **Reference:** Pagana, K., & Pagana, T. (2010). *Mosby's manual of diagnostic and laboratory tests* (4th ed.). St. Louis, MO: Elsevier Mosby, pp. 478–479.

Posttest

1 **Answer: 1** **Rationale:** Ingesting alcoholic beverages with Flagyl can result in a *disulfiram-reaction*, including exaggerated sympathomimetic signs/symptoms. Headache, constipation, and vaginal dryness may occur and can be easily managed, but are not as significant as tachycardia and flushing. **Cognitive Level:** Analyzing **Client Need:** Pharmacological and Parenteral Therapies **Integrated Process:** Teaching and Learning **Content Area:** Pharmacology **Strategy:** Note the critical words *most important* in the question. Evaluate each option and select the one that will likely have the greatest negative effect on the client. **Reference:** Wilson, B. A., Shannon, M., & Shields, K. (2012). *Pearson nurse's drug guide 2012*. Upper Saddle River, NJ: Pearson Education, Inc., pp. 988–991.

2 **Answer: 3** **Rationale:** A different gloved finger or a different finger cot should be used to apply acyclovir to each lesion not only to prevent spread on client's own body, but also to prevent spread of the virus. Hand hygiene is a standard precaution associated with infection control for all clients. One thin layer of medication is sufficient. Not sharing medication with others is a universal principle associated with drug therapy. **Cognitive Level:** Applying **Client Need:** Pharmacological and Parenteral Therapies **Integrated Process:** Nursing Process: Evaluation **Content Area:** Pharmacology **Strategy:** Correlate the characteristics of the target microorganism with the client's needs. **Reference:** Wilson, B. A., Shannon, M., & Shields, K. (2012). *Pearson nurse's drug guide 2012*. Upper Saddle River, NJ: Pearson Education, Inc., pp. 19–21.

3 **Answer: 3** **Rationale:** Since this drug can be nephrotoxic, it would be most important to check BUN and creatinine as indicators of renal function. Alanine aminotransferase (ALT) and aspartate aminotransferase (AST) reflect liver function and damage and would be assessed prior to beginning drug therapy as a general routine measure. Serum sodium levels could indirectly reflect renal function, but are not as important as checking direct indicators of kidney function. Diarrhea can be a side effect but the priority assessment is the client's renal function. **Cognitive Level:** Applying **Client Need:** Pharmacological and Parenteral Therapies **Integrated Process:** Nursing Process: Assessment **Content Area:** Pharmacology **Strategy:** Associate the drug with nephrotoxicity. From this point, determine which option *best* reflects kidney function. **Reference:** Wilson, B. A., Shannon, M., & Shields, K. (2012). *Pearson nurse's drug guide 2012*. Upper Saddle River, NJ: Pearson Education, Inc., pp. 89–93.

4 **Answer: 1, 4, 5** **Rationale:** Since most all clients receiving Amphotericin B (Fungizone) experience fever, chills, nausea, and itching, they are premedicated with antipyretics, antihistamine, and antiemetics. Penicillins have a propensity for causing allergic reactions so the client may need to be premedicated with an antihistamine. Cephalosporins may lead to allergic reaction, which may require use of an antihistamine. Premedication with these types of drugs would not be indicated prior to administration of acyclovir (Zovirax) or gentamicin (Garamycin). **Cognitive Level:** Analyzing **Client Need:** Pharmacological and Parenteral Therapies **Integrated Process:** Nursing Process: Diagnosis **Content Area:** Pharmacology **Strategy:** Note first that the premedication drugs are used to decrease the risk of allergic or hypersensitivity reactions. Associate penicillins, amphotericin B, and cephalosporin drugs with a higher risk of allergic reaction to choose correctly. **Reference:** Wilson, B. A., Shannon, M., & Shields, K. (2012). *Pearson nurse's drug guide 2012*. Upper Saddle River, NJ: Pearson Education, Inc., pp. 19–21, 84–86, 89–93, 291–292, 755–758.

5 **Answer: 4** **Rationale:** NRTIs suppress production of reverse transcriptase, which prevents conversion of viral RNA to DNA similar to human DNA. Fusion inhibitors work by blocking the attachment of the HIV virus to the host cell. Protease inhibitors block protease (which is needed for cell replication) and are used in conjunction with other drugs to reduce the viral load in HIV. NNRTIs drugs work by reducing the synthesis of reverse transcriptor A. **Cognitive Level:** Applying **Client Need:** Pharmacological and Parenteral Therapies **Integrated Process:** Teaching and Learning **Content Area:** Pharmacology **Strategy:** Compare and contrast the major elements existing among the drug categories. Associate the conclusions with the disease process. **Reference:** Adams, M. P., & Koch, R. W. (2010). *Pharmacology: Connections to nursing practice.* Upper Saddle River, NJ: Pearson Education, pp. 927–940.

6 **Answer: 2** **Rationale:** Taking mebendazole with food will help to reduce gastric irritation. The tablets may be chewed, swallowed whole, crushed, or mixed with food. Mebendazole does not cause photosensitivity so sunscreen is not necessary because of this drug. It may cause abdominal cramping and diarrhea. **Cognitive Level:** Applying **Client Need:** Pharmacological and Parenteral Therapies **Integrated Process:** Teaching and Learning **Content Area:** Pharmacology **Strategy:** Recall that mebendazole is an antihelminthic and recall specific information about this medication. **Reference:** Wilson, B. A., Shannon, M., & Shields, K. (2012). *Pearson nurse's drug guide 2012*. Upper Saddle River, NJ: Pearson Education, Inc., pp. 922–923.

7 **Answer: 2** **Rationale:** Use the formula "Desired dose divided by dose on hand multiplied by the quantity = *x*"

$$\frac{100}{250} \times 5 = x$$ Multiple 100 by 5 to yield 500 and divide that by 250 to calculate that *x* = 2 **Cognitive Level:** Applying **Client Need:** Pharmacological and Parenteral Therapies **Integrated Process:** Nursing Process: Implementation **Content Area:** Pharmacology **Strategy:** First recognize the ordered drug dose is less than the available dose. Recall the prescribed dose (desired) over dose on hand (have) times quantity to calculate your answer. **Reference:**

Olsen, J., Giangrasso, A., Shrimpton, D., & Dillon, P. (2012). *Medical dosage calculations* (10th ed.). Upper Saddle River, NJ: Pearson Education, Inc., pp. 133–135.

8 **Answer: 3** **Rationale:** Flushing of the face, neck, and chest, which is known as "red man syndrome" or "red neck syndrome," is associated with too rapid administration of vancomycin (Vancocin). Hypotension, not hypertension, is associated with vancomycin (Vancocin) administration. Vancomycin (Vancocin) may cause nausea, but not projectile vomiting. Vancomycin (Vancocin) is often used to treat *Clostridium difficile*, associated with pseudomembranous colitis. This complication is not associated with speed of the transfusion. **Cognitive Level:** Applying **Client Need:** Pharmacological and Parenteral Therapies **Integrated Process:** Nursing Process: Assessment **Content Area:** Pharmacology **Strategy:** Recall that "red neck syndrome" or "red man syndrome," occurs with rapid infusion and use this to choose from the available options. **Reference:** Wilson, B. A., Shannon, M., & Shields, K. (2012). *Pearson nurse's drug guide 2012*. Upper Saddle River, NJ: Pearson Education, Inc., pp. 1567–1568.

9 **Answer: 2** **Rationale:** Tetracycline is contraindicated in children less than 8 years of age because it causes permanent tooth discoloration. The order should be questioned by the nurse. Drinking through a straw is necessary when administering liquid iron preparations, but not tetracycline. Tooth discoloration is caused by systemic absorption, not direct contact. The drug may cause diarrhea, but this is not the most important consideration. Milk and other dairy products will decrease the absorption of tetracycline. **Cognitive Level:** Applying **Client Need:** Pharmacological and Parenteral Therapies **Integrated Process:** Nursing Process: Planning **Content Area:** Pharmacology **Strategy:** Associate this drug with staining of teeth in children less than 8 years old and use this information to eliminate the incorrect options. **Reference:** Wilson, B. A., Shannon, M., & Shields, K. (2012). *Pearson nurse's drug guide 2012*. Upper Saddle River, NJ: Pearson Education, Inc., pp. 1470–1473.

10 **Answer: 2** **Rationale:** Photosensitivity is a side effect of both classes of antibiotics. The client should avoid sun exposure and tanning beds. These drugs would not increase the client's risk for upper respiratory infections. Orthostatic hypotension and constipation are not side effects of either drug. **Cognitive Level:** Applying **Client Need:** Pharmacological and Parenteral Therapies **Integrated Process:** Teaching and Learning **Content Area:** Pharmacology **Strategy:** Look for the option that illustrates teaching associated with an adverse drug effect that occurs with both drugs. In this case, the correct option relates to photosensitivity. **Reference:** Adams, M. P., & Koch, R. W. (2010). *Pharmacology: Connections to nursing practice.* Upper Saddle River, NJ: Pearson Education, pp. 810–813, 840–844.

References

Abrams, A. (2009). *Clinical drug therapy: Rationales for nursing practice* (9th ed.). Philadelphia, PA: Lippincott Williams & Wilkins.

Adams, M., Holland, L., & Bostwick, P. (2011). *Pharmacology for nurses: A pathophysiologic approach* (3rd ed.). Upper Saddle River, NJ: Pearson Education.

Adams, M. P., & Koch, R.W. (2010). *Pharmacology: Connections to nursing practice.* Upper Saddle River, NJ: Pearson Education.

Aschenbrenner, D., & Venable, S. (2012). *Drug therapy in nursing* (4th ed.). Philadelphia, PA: Lippincott Williams & Wilkins.

Drug Facts & Comparisons® (Updated monthly). St. Louis, MO: A. Wolters Kluwer.

Ignatavicius, D. D., & Workman, M. L. (2010). *Medical-surgical nursing: Critical thinking for collaborative care* (6th ed.). Philadelphia, PA: W. B. Saunders.

Karch, A. M. (2010). *Focus on nursing pharmacology* (5th ed.). Philadelphia: Lippincott Williams & Wilkins.

Kee, J. (2009). *Laboratory and diagnostic tests and nursing implications* (8th ed.). Upper Saddle River, NJ: Pearson Education.

Lehne, R. (2010). *Pharmacology for nursing care* (7th ed.). St. Louis, MO: Mosby, Inc.

LeMone, P., Burke, K. M., & Bauldoff, G. (2011). *Medical-surgical nursing: Critical thinking in patient care* (5th ed.). Upper Saddle River, NJ: Pearson Education.

Lilley, L. L., Collins, S. R., et al. (2011). *Pharmacology and the nursing practice* (6th ed.). St. Louis, MO: Mosby, Inc.

Tucker, S., & Dauffenbach, V. (2011). *Nutrition and diet therapy for nurses.* Upper Saddle River, NJ: Pearson Education.

Wilson, B. A., Shannon, M. T., & Shields, K. M. (2012). *Pearson nurse's drug guide 2012.* Upper Saddle River, NJ: Pearson Education.

3 Antineoplastic Medications

Chapter Outline

Alkylating Agents
Antimetabolites
Antitumor Antibiotics
Plant-Based Antineoplastic
  Agents

Hormones and Hormone
  Modulators
Other Antineoplastics
Safe Handling of
  Chemotherapeutic Agents

Nursing Management of
  Treatment Side Effects

NCLEX-RN® Test Prep

Use the accompanying online resource,
NursingReviewsandRationales, to test
yourself with hundreds of NCLEX®-style
practice questions.

Objectives

➤ Describe the general goals of antineoplastic therapy.
➤ Describe the common side effects of antineoplastic medications.
➤ Identify primary toxic effects associated with antineoplastic therapy.
➤ Identify nursing interventions for the client with depressed white
  blood cell production, bleeding tendencies, or stomatitis.
➤ List the significant client education points related to antineoplastic
  medications.

Review at a Glance

acral erythema red palms
alopecia partial or complete hair loss
anticipatory nausea conditioned
response resulting from repeated
association of chemotherapy-induced
nausea and vomiting and a stimulus
from the environment
cell cycle specific chemotherapy
agent that exhibits its cytotoxic effect at
a certain stage of cell division

cell cycle nonspecific
chemotherapy agent that exhibits its
cytotoxic effect regardless of the stage
of cell division
hemorrhagic cystitis chemical
irritation of bladder that causes bleeding
and hematuria
irritant a chemotherapy agent that
causes redness and irritation of skin upon
extravasation, but without sloughing

nadir lowest point to which blood counts
will drop after chemotherapy administration
myelosuppression decrease
in blood counts usually related to
chemotherapy
vesicant medication that causes
severe skin and tissue necrosis if it
extravasates from the vein

PRETEST

1 A client with cancer is receiving vincristine (Oncovin). The nurse would assess for which of the following as an early indicator of neurotoxicity from vincristine?

1. Confusion
2. Short-term memory loss
3. Depression of the Achilles reflex
4. Decreased hand-grasp strength

2 The nurse would focus on which of the following nursing interventions that are most likely to prevent cardiotoxicity in a client receiving doxorubicin (Adriamycin)?

1. Exercise and smoking cessation
2. Smoking cessation and oxygen (O_2) administration
3. Exercise and administration of dexrazoxane (Zinecard)
4. O_2 administration and a low-fat diet

3 A client is experiencing signs and symptoms of pulmonary toxicity related to administration of chemotherapy. In order to maximize the client's pulmonary potential, the nurse teaches the client to do which of the following? Select all that apply.

1. Elevate head of the bed.
2. Exhale through pursed lips.
3. Perform shallow, slow breathing during activity.
4. Exhale using accessory muscles.
5. Plan rest and exercise periods.

4 The nurse should include management of pulmonary toxicity in the plan of care for clients receiving which of the following antineoplastic agents?

1. 5-fluorouracil (5-FU)
2. Bleomycin (Blenoxane)
3. Etoposide (Vepesid)
4. Paclitaxel (Taxol)

5 The nurse explains to a client receiving chemotherapy that taking action to reduce the risk of mucositis will have which of the following as the most important benefit?

1. Increased comfort
2. Decreased risk of infection
3. Prevention of changes in self-image
4. Reduced risk of cancer recurrence

6 Several clients have received chemotherapy in an outpatient clinic. Which client will the nurse expect to have increased episodes of nausea and vomiting?

1. Mother of 2 who experienced severe morning sickness during both of her pregnancies
2. Navy pilot who experienced motion sickness as a child
3. 38-year-old male who has alcoholism
4. Young woman with no significant history of emesis

7 The nurse would plan to include which nursing intervention in the care of a client experiencing neutropenia?

1. Insert an indwelling urinary catheter to maintain accurate intake and output.
2. Leave all wounds open to the air for better healing.
3. Encourage regular oral care and perianal care after each stool.
4. Flush all lumens of the long-term intravenous catheter with heparinized saline every 8 hours.

8 A client with cancer has the nursing diagnosis of impaired oral mucous membranes related to side effects of fluorouracil (5-FU), an antimetabolite. The nurse would plan which of the following as an optimal nursing intervention?

1. Schedule oral hygiene every 2 hours during the day with warm saline rinses.
2. Rinse mouth every 2 hours during the day and every 4 hours at night with a baking soda and peroxide rinse.
3. Schedule oral care every 2 to 4 hours with a soft toothbrush and fluorinated toothpaste, followed by a dilute baking soda rinse.
4. Continue oral hygiene twice daily with baking soda and rinse with commercial mouthwash.

9 A client receiving vincristine (Oncovin) is at risk for developing constipation. In order to reduce this risk, the nurse should help the client to make which of the following lifestyle changes? Select all that apply.

1. Increase physical activity.
2. Add fiber to the diet.
3. Use laxative of choice.
4. Increase fluid intake.
5. Ingest antiflatulent of choice.

10 During a seminar the nurse explains to a group of clients that an important advantage of combination chemotherapy over single-drug regimens includes which the following?

1. Reduce potential for nausea and vomiting.
2. Reduce potential for tumor resistance.
3. Spare normal cells from severe toxicity.
4. Decrease likelihood of drug-induced gonadal sterility.

➤ *See pages 115–116 for Answers and Rationales.*

I. ALKYLATING AGENTS

A. Action and use

1. Interfere with DNA replication through cross-linking of DNA strands, DNA strand breaking, and abnormal base pairing proteins
2. Most agents are **cell cycle nonspecific**, which means that they exhibit a cytotoxic effect in multiple phases of cell cycle; most effective in the G_0 phase
3. Major toxicities occur in hematopoietic, gastrointestinal (GI), and reproductive systems
4. There are 3 major types of alkylating agents:
   a. Nitrogen mustards: commonly cyclophosphamide, ifosfamide
   b. Platinum compounds: commonly cisplatin, carboplatin
   c. Nitrosoureas: commonly carmustine, streptozocin

B. Common medications (Table 3-1)

C. Administration considerations

1. Nitrogen mustards
   a. Hydrate with oral or intravenous (IV) fluids before administering dose
   b. Administer PO on an empty stomach; if nausea and vomiting are severe it may be taken with food; antiemetic agent should be given before the drug is administered
   c. Administer IV piggyback (IVPB) dose over 60 to 90 minutes
2. Mechlorethamine (Mustargen)
   a. Potent **vesicant** (causes severe skin and tissue necrosis if medication extravasates from vein)
   b. Should be administered through side-arm portal of a freely running IV to avoid extravasation
   c. If drug should extravasate, subcutaneous and intradermal injection with isotonic sodium thiosulfate and application of ice compresses may reduce local irritation
   d. Short **nadir** period (6–8 days), which is the lowest point to which blood counts will drop after chemotherapy administration
   e. Wear surgical gloves during preparation and avoid inhalation of powder and vapors
3. Platinum compounds
   a. General information
      1) Plan to administer a parenteral antiemetic agent before therapy is instituted and give it on a scheduled basis throughout day and night as long as necessary
      2) Needles or IV sets containing aluminum should not be used
   b. Cisplatin (Platinol)
      1) Does not cause significant myelosuppression, unlike other alkylating agents
      2) Provide hydration with 1 to 2 liters of IV fluid before and after administration
      3) Obtain baseline electrocardiogram (ECG) and cardiac monitoring during therapy

Table 3-1 Common Alkylating Agents

Generic (Trade) Name	Route
Nitrogen mustards	
Bendamustine (Treanda)	IV
Chlorambucil (Leukeran)	PO
Cyclophosphamide (Cytoxan)	PO, IV
Estramustine (Emcyt)	PO
Ifosfamide (Ifex)	IV
Mechlorethamine (Mustargen)	IV, IT, T
Melphalan (Alkeran)	PO, IV
Nitrosoureas	
Carmustine (BiCNU)	IV
Lomustine (CeeNU)	PO
Streptozocin (Zanosar)	IV
Platinum compounds	
Carboplatin (Paraplatin)	IV
Cisplatin (Platinol)	IV
Oxaliplatin (Eloxatine)	IV
Miscellaneous alkylating agents	
Busulfan (Myleran)	PO, IV
Dacarbazine (DTIC-Dome)	IV
Procarbazine (Matulane)	PO
Temozolomide (Temodar)	PO, IV
Thiotepa	PO, IC

Legend: PO, oral; IV, intravenous; IT, intrathecal; IC, intracavitary; T, topical

    c. Carboplatin (Paraplatin)
      1) First-line palliative treatment of advanced ovarian cancer, less toxic than cisplatin
      2) Do not repeat dosage until neutrophil count is at least $2,000/mm^3$
      3) Monitor closely for anaphylaxis during first 15 minutes of infusion
    d. Nitrosourea: carmustine (BiCNU)
      1) One of the few drugs that can penetrate blood–brain barrier, is used for brain tumors
      2) Administer over 1 to 2 hours by slow IV infusion with constant monitoring if given peripherally
      3) Vesicant: if possible, avoid starting IV in dorsum of hand, wrist, or antecubital veins, since extravasation may cause damage to underlying tissues
D. Contraindications
   1. Nitrogen mustards
    a. Cyclophosphamide (Cytoxan)
      1) Use with extreme caution in men and women of childbearing years because of effects on reproductive system
      2) Serious infections including chicken pox and herpes zoster
      3) Immunosuppression
      4) Pregnancy (Risk Category D) and nursing mothers

  b. Ifosfamide (Ifex)
   1) Severe bone marrow suppression or known hypersensitivity to ifosfamide
   2) Cautious use in clients with impaired renal function, prior radiation therapy, or prior cytotoxic agents
   3) Cautious use in pregnancy (Category D) and nursing mothers
  c. Mechlorethamine (Mustargen)
   1) **Myelosuppression**: a decrease in blood counts usually related to chemotherapy
   2) Infectious granuloma
   3) Known infectious diseases, including herpes zoster
   4) Pregnancy (Category D) and lactation
 2. Platinum compounds
  a. General
   1) History of sensitivity to platinum-containing compounds
   2) Cautious use in pregnancy (Category D) and with other nephrotoxic drugs
   3) Impaired renal function and/or hearing
  b. Cisplatin (Platinol): history of gout and urate renal stones
  c. Carboplatin (Paraplatin): severe bone marrow depression (thrombocytopenia, leukopenia, and neutropenia)
 3. Nitrosourea: carmustine (BICNU)
  a. History of pulmonary function impairment
  b. Decreased platelets, leukocytes, or erythrocytes
  c. Safe use during pregnancy (Category D) not established

E. Significant drug interactions
 1. Nitrogen mustards
  a. Cyclophosphamide (Cytoxan)
   1) Multiple interactions, including a decreased serum level of digoxin if used concurrently
   2) Doxorubicin (Adriamycin): may increase cardiotoxicity
  b. Ifosfamide (Ifex)
   1) Barbiturates, phenytoin (Dilantin), and chloral hydrate (Aquachloral) may increase hepatic conversion of ifosfamide to active metabolite
   2) Corticosteroids may inhibit conversion to active metabolite
 2. Mechlorethamine (nitrogen mustard, Mustargen): may reduce effectiveness of antigout agents by raising serum uric acid levels
 3. Platinum compounds
  a. General
   1) Nephrotoxic drugs such as aminoglycosides, amphotericin-B, and vancomycin increase risk of nephrotoxicity
   2) Aminoglycosides and furosemide (Lasix) increase risk of ototoxicity
   3) Incompatible with 5% dextrose solutions, sodium bicarbonate, and metoclopramide (Reglan)
  b. Carboplatin (Paraplatin) may decrease phenytoin (Dilantin) levels
 4. Carmustine (BICNU): cimetidine may potentiate neutropenia and thrombocytopenia

F. Significant food interactions
 1. Are primarily for the miscellaneous alkylating agent procarbazine
 2. Avoid foods high in tyramine (e.g., beer, wine, cheese, brewer's yeast, chicken livers, and bananas) while taking procarbazine, since it may lead to hypertension and possible intracranial hemorrhage
 3. A disulfiram-like reaction can occur if client consumes alcohol and procarbazine

G. Significant assessment parameters

1. Nitrogen mustards

   a. Cyclophosphamide (Cytoxan)

   1) Determine total differential leukocyte count, platelet count, and hematocrit initially and at least every 2 weeks thereafter

   2) Obtain baseline and periodic determinations of liver and kidney function in addition to serum electrolytes

   3) Microscopic urine examinations are recommended after large doses

   b. Ifosfamide (Ifex)

   1) Monitor complete blood count (CBC) with differential before each dose; hold dose if WBC is below 2,000/mm^3 or platelet count is below 50,000/mm^3

   2) Monitor urine before and during each dose for microscopic hematuria

   3) Hydrate with at least 3,000 mL of fluid daily to reduce risk of **hemorrhagic cystitis** (excessive bleeding from bladder due to chemical irritation)

2. Platinum compounds

   a. Cisplatin (Platinol)

   1) Pretreatment ECG is indicated because of possible myocarditis or focal irritation

   2) Monitor urine output (UO) and specific gravity for 4 consecutive hours before therapy and for 24 hours after; report UO less than 100 mL/hr or a specific gravity of greater than 1.030; a UO of less than 75 mL/hr requires medical intervention

   3) Audiometric testing should be performed before initial dose

   4) Anaphylactic reactions may occur within minutes of drug administration

   5) Assess BUN, serum uric acid, serum creatinine, and urinary creatinine clearance before initiating therapy and every subsequent course

   6) Nephrotoxicity usually occurs within 2 weeks after drug administration and becomes more severe and prolonged with repeated courses

   7) Suspect ototoxicity if client manifests tinnitus or difficulty hearing in the high-frequency range

   8) Assess blood pressure (BP), mental status, pupils, and optic fundi every hour during therapy since hydration increases risk of elevated intracranial pressure

   9) Monitor and report abnormal bowel patterns since constipation may be an early sign of neurotoxicity

   b. Carboplatin (Paraplatin)

   1) Frequently monitor peripheral blood counts; nadir usually occurs at day 21

   2) Periodically monitor kidney function and creatinine clearance, although it has less renal toxicity than cisplatin

   3) Monitor for peripheral neuropathy, ototoxicity, and visual disturbances, although they occur less frequently than with cisplatin

   4) Monitor clients on diuretic therapy closely since carboplatin may also decrease serum sodium, potassium, calcium, and magnesium levels

3. Nitrosourea: carmustine (BICNU)

   a. Persistent nausea and vomiting may occur 2 hours after drug administration and persist up to 6 hours; prior administration of an antiemetic will help

   b. Monitor blood counts prior to beginning drug therapy and weekly for at least 6 weeks after last dose

   c. Assess results of pulmonary function studies prior to therapy and periodically thereafter

   d. Report symptoms of lung toxicity, such as cough, dyspnea, and fever

   e. Be alert to hepatic and renal insufficiency

H. Side effects/toxicity

1. Nitrogen mustards

   a. Cyclophosphamide (Cytoxan)

      1) Cardiotoxicity, acute cardiomegaly with high dose; prior radiation therapy and prior anthracycline therapy increases risk

      2) Hemorrhagic cystitis (occasionally chronic and severe)

      3) Metallic taste on administration

      4) Acute myelosuppression

      5) Acral erythema (palmar redness) and sloughing of skin on palms of hands and feet

      6) Decreased sperm production, which may be permanent

      7) Nausea and vomiting

   b. Ifosfamide (Ifex)

      1) Hemorrhagic cystitis, occasionally chronic and severe; mesna (Mesnex) is a chemoprotectant used with Ifex to minimize bladder damage

      2) Neutropenia and thrombocytopenia

      3) Nausea and vomiting

      4) Hepatic dysfunction and renal toxicity

      5) Somnolence, confusion, and hallucinations

2. Platinum compounds

   a. General

      1) Renal and hepatic toxicity

      2) Peripheral neuropathy; neurotoxicity

      3) Auditory toxicity: 8th cranial nerve damage

      4) Myelosuppression with pronounced thrombocytopenia

      5) Intense nausea and vomiting

3. Nitrosourea: carmustine (BICNU)

   a. Severe nausea and vomiting

   b. Ocular infarctions, retinal hemorrhage, suffusion of conjunctiva

   c. Delayed myelosuppression

   d. Pulmonary infiltration or fibrosis

I. Client and family education

1. Nitrogen mustards

   a. Cyclophosphamide (Cytoxan)

      1) Because of the drug's mutagenic potential, teach client to use adequate contraception during and for at least 4 months after termination of drug therapy

      2) Instruct client to void frequently and maintain hydration with oral fluids to at least 3,000 mL/24 hours for 4–5 days before and after therapy

   b. Ifosfamide (Ifex)

      1) Instruct client to void frequently and to maintain hydration

      2) Advise client that susceptibility to infection will increase

      3) Teach client to report any unusual bleeding or bruising

2. Platinum compounds

   a. Cisplatin (Platinol)

      1) Continue maintenance of adequate hydration with oral fluids to at least 3,000 mL/24 hr; report reduced UO, anorexia, nausea and vomiting uncontrolled by antiemetics, fluid retention, and weight gain

      2) Keep vestibular stimulation to a minimum to avoid dizziness or falling

      3) Tingling, numbness, tremors of extremities, loss of position sense and taste, and constipation are early warning signs of neurotoxicity

   b. Carboplatin (Paraplatin)

      1) Give special attention to strategies to prevent nausea

      2) Explain risk for infection and for hemorrhagic complications related to bone marrow suppression

Practice to Pass

List 3 measures to assist in the prevention of renal toxicity secondary to cisplatin (Platinol) administration.

   c. Instruct client to report paresthesias, visual disturbances, or symptoms of ototoxicity (hearing loss/tinnitus)
   3. Nitrosoureas
      a. Myelosuppression is severe and may be cumulative; teach neutropenic precautions and symptoms of sepsis
      b. Teach signs and symptoms of hypoglycemia when administering streptozocin
      c. Teach signs and symptoms of pulmonary toxicity when administering carmustine
      d. Stress need for central venous catheter (CVC) to prevent vascular damage, provide access for laboratory studies (blood draws), and promote ease of providing high-volume IV fluids with antineoplastic drugs

II. ANTIMETABOLITES

A. Action and use
   1. Inhibit protein synthesis, substitute erroneous metabolites or structural analogues during DNA synthesis, and inhibit DNA synthesis
   2. Cancer cells require nutrients to grow; use of antimetabolites disrupt these pathways causing cell death or slowed growth
   3. Most agents are **cell cycle specific**; that is, they exhibit a cytotoxic affect during a specific phase of the cell cycle, such as the S phase
   4. Used to treat leukemia, solid tumors, and lymphoma
   5. Most toxicity occurs in hematopoietic and GI systems; bone marrow toxicity is the primary adverse effect of drugs in this class

B. Common medications (Table 3-2)
C. Administration considerations
   1. Fluorouracil (5FU): usually for palliative treatment for inoperable neoplasms
   2. Cytarabine (Cytosar-U): blocks DNA synthesis, treating acute myelocytic leukemia

Table 3-2 **Common Antimetabolites**

Generic (Trade) Name	Route
Folic acid analogs	
Methotrexate (MTX, others)	IV, PO
Pemetrexed (Alimta)	IV
Pralatrexate (Folotyn)	IV
Purine analogs	
Cladribine (Leustatin)	IV
Clofarabine (Clolar)	IV
Fludarabine (Fludara)	IV
Mercaptopurine (Purinethol, 6-MP)	PO
Nelarabine (Arranon)	IV
Pentostatin (Nipent)	IV
Thioguanine (Tabloid, 6-TG)	PO
Pyrimidine analogs	
Capecitabine (Xeloda)	PO
Cytarabine (Cytosar-U, Depot-Cyt)	IV, IT
Floxuridine (FUDR)	Intra-arterial
Fluorouracil (Adrucil, 5-FU, others)	IV
Gemcitabine (Gemzar)	IV

Legend: PO, oral; IV, intravenous; IT, intrathecal

3. Methotrexate (Folex)
   a. Is a powerful immunosuppressant
   b. Avoid skin exposure and inhalation of drug during preparation
   c. Pregnancy Risk Category X
   d. Treatment of overdose: Leucovorin, which is a reduced form of folic acid

D. **Contraindications**
   1. Myelosuppression
   2. Pregnancy (Category D) and nursing women
   3. Concurrent administration of hepatotoxic drugs and hematopoietic depressants
   4. Cautious use in clients with hepatic, renal, or immune system impairment

E. **Significant drug interactions**
   1. Fluorouracil (5FU): cimetidine (Tagamet) increases pharmacological effects; thiazide diuretics increase risk of myelosuppression; leucovorin (Wellcovorin) increases cytotoxicity
   2. Cytarabine (Ara-C): decreases bioavailability of digoxin (Lanoxin)
   3. Methotrexate (Folex)
      a. Protein-bound drugs (i.e., aspirin, phenytoin, and tetracycline) increase toxicity
      b. Nonsteroidal inflammatory drugs (NSAIDS) increase and prolong methotrexate levels
   4. Mercaptopurine (Purinethol)
      a. Allopurinol (Zyloprim) increases 6-mercaptopurine levels
      b. Warfarin (Coumadin) affects prothrombin time (PT) levels
      c. Nondepolarizing muscle relaxants: decreased neuromuscular blockade
   5. Fludarabine (Fludara): fatal pulmonary toxicity can occur if administered concurrently with pentostatin (Nipent)
   6. Capecitabine (Xeloda): increased risk of excessive bleeding with anticoagulants; increased capecitabine levels and toxicity when combined with leucovorin

F. **Significant food interactions: none known**

G. **Significant assessment parameters**
   1. Assess baseline CBC, WBC differential, and platelet count prior to administration
   2. Notify health care provider if WBC is less than $3,500/mm^3$ or platelet count less than $100,000/mm^3$
   3. Assess for signs and symptoms of infection or bleeding

H. **Side effects/toxicity**
   1. General toxicities for this drug group
      a. Myelosuppression
      b. Nausea and vomiting
      c. Mucosal inflammation: stomatitis
      d. Photosensitivity with or without hyperpigmentation
      e. Diarrhea (most commonly associated with antimetabolites)
   2. Fluorouracil (5-FU): specific side effects/toxicity
      a. Cardiotoxicity mimicking an acute myocardial infarction (MI), angina, cardiogenic shock
      b. Photosensitivity and hyperpigmentation
      c. Cerebellar toxicity
   3. Methotrexate: specific side effects/toxicity
      a. Fatal bone marrow toxicity at high doses
      b. Low platelet counts can cause hemorrhage and bruising
      c. Use caution with OTC vitamins due to possibility of folic acid, which decreases response to methotrexate

Practice to Pass

What measures should the nurse take to prevent or decrease the severity of stomatitis secondary to the administration of fluorouracil (5-FU)?

4. Cytarabine (Ara-C): specific side effects/toxicity
    a. Maculopapular rash, with or without fever
    b. Cytarabine syndrome (rash with or without fever, myalgia, bone pain, malaise)
    c. Chemical conjunctivitis
    d. Acute neurotoxicity: cerebellar toxicity; clients over age 50 are at highest risk
    e. Hepatotoxicity
    f. Acral erythema

I. Client and family education
  1. Self-care measures are important to avoid infection and bleeding
    a. Avoid large crowds
    b. Avoid proximity to people with infections
    c. Avoid over-the-counter (OTC) aspirin-containing medications
    d. Report elevated temperature, fatigue, and other symptoms of infection
  2. Perform an oral assessment, maintain scheduled mouth care, and report development of stomatitis to prescriber
  3. Maintain a low residue diet after discharge and report excessive diarrhea (more than 3 loose stools in 24 hours) to prescriber
  4. Darkening of veins, mucous membranes, and fingernails may occur
  5. Follow photosensitivity precautions year-round
    a. Use sunscreen with a sun protection factor (SPF) of at least 15
    b. Avoid sun exposure between 10:00 a.m. and 2:00 p.m.
    c. Wear long sleeves and a large brimmed hat

III. ANTITUMOR ANTIBIOTICS

A. Action and use
  1. Interfere with nucleic acid synthesis and function, inhibit ribonucleic acid (RNA) synthesis, and inhibit DNA synthesis
  2. Most agents are cell cycle nonspecific and treat only a few specific types of cancer
  3. Major toxicities occur in hematopoietic, GI, reproductive, and cardiac systems (cumulative doses)
  4. Similar in action to alkylating agents, and side effects are also similar
  5. All antitumor antibiotics are administered intravenously or directly into a body cavity

B. Common medications (Table 3-3)

Table 3-3 Antitumor Antibiotics

Generic (Trade) Name	Route
Bleomycin (Blenoxane)	IV
Dactinomycin (Cosmegen, Actinomycin D)	IV
Daunorubicin (Cerubidine)	IV
Doxorubicin (Adriamycin)	IV
Epirubicin (Ellence)	IV
Idarubicin (Idamycin)	IV
Mitomycin (Mutamycin)	IV
Mitroxantrone (Novantrone)	IV
Valrubicin (Valstar)	IC

Legend: IV, intravenous; IC, intracavitary (bladder)

C. Administration considerations

1. Most antitumor antibiotics are severe vesicants except for bleomycin (see signs and symptoms of extravasation in Table 3-4 and antidotes for vesicant drugs in Table 3-5)

2. General principles of safe administration
   a. Administer slowly by IV push (IVP) via side-arm portal of a freely flowing IV
   b. Maintain clear view of injection site during administration
   c. IV catheter should have an excellent blood return, be recently placed, and not more than 48 hours old before administering vesicant therapy
   d. If possible, avoid use of antecubital veins, wrist or dorsum of hand, where extravasation could damage underlying tendons and nerves
   e. Avoid venous access in an extremity with compromised venous or lymphatic drainage
3. Doxorubicin (Adriamycin): extravasation, which can cause severe tissue damage and pain, should be treated with ice packs to the infiltrated area
4. Valrubicin (Valstar)
   a. Used to treat bladder cancer by instilling directly into the bladder
   b. Use aseptic technique to insert urinary catheter to maintain bladder drainage; use gravity to instill valrubicin (Valstar) slowly over several minutes intravesically
   c. Provide increased fluid intake (at least 2 L daily) to prevent urate calculi formation

Table 3-4   **Signs and Symptoms of Extravasation**

Assessment Parameter	Immediate Manifestations	Delayed Manifestations	Irritation of Vein	Flare Reaction
Pain	Severe pain or burning that lasts minutes to hours and eventually subsides; usually occurs while drug is being given around needle site	Up to 48 hours	Aching and tightness along vein	No pain
Redness	Blotchy redness around needle site; not always present at time of extravasation	Later occurrence	Full length of vein may be reddened or darkened	Immediate blotches or streaks along vein, which usually subside within 30 min with or without treatment
Ulceration	Develops insidiously; usually occurs 48 to 96 hours later	Later occurrence	Not usually	Not usually
Swelling	Severe swelling; usually occurs immediately	Up to 48 hours	Not likely	Wheals may appear along vein line
Blood Return	Inability to obtain a blood return	Good blood return during drug administration	Usually	Usually
Other	Change in quality of infusion	Local tingling and sensory deficits	NA	Urticaria

Table 3-5   **Antidotes for Vesicant Therapy**

Chemotherapeutic Drug	Antidote
Nitrogen mustard (Mustargen), cisplatin (Platinol)	Thiosulfate
Dactinomycin (Cosmegen)	Apply ice and elevate, heat may enhance tissue damage
Doxorubicin (Adriamycin)	Cold pack with circulating ice water first 24 to 48 hrs
Vinblastine (Velban), vincristine (Oncovin), vinorelbine (Navelbine)	Hyaluronidase; apply warm pack for first 24 to 48 hrs
Paclitaxel (Taxol)	Hyaluronidase; apply ice for first 24 hours

D. **Contraindications**
 1. General:
  a. Myelosuppression increasing the risk of bleeding and coagulation disorders
  b. Use cautiously in clients with compromised hepatic, renal or pulmonary function, or previous cytotoxic drug or radiation therapy
  c. Extreme caution with pregnant women (Risk Category D), lactating women, and women of childbearing age
  d. Hypersensitivity reactions
 2. Valrubicin (Valstar): perforated bladder and urinary tract infection
E. **Significant drug interactions**
 1. Serum digoxin (Lanoxin) levels and phenytoin (Dilantin) levels decreased with concurrent use
 2. Multiple incompatibilities, including other chemotherapeutic agents, antibiotics, and other commonly prescribed medications
F. **Significant food interactions: none known**
G. **Significant assessment parameters**
 1. General
  a. Assess hepatic, renal, hematopoietic, and cardiac function prior to administration and at regular intervals thereafter and report early signs of dysfunction
  b. Begin a flowchart to establish baseline data, including temperature, pulse, respiration, BP, body weight, laboratory values, intake and output (I & O) ratio and pattern, and cardiac ejection fraction
  c. Closely assess for symptoms of extravasation frequently during administration
 2. Doxorubicin (Adriamycin)
  a. Give prompt attention to reports of stinging or burning sensation at injection site
  b. Stomatitis is greatest at 2 weeks following therapy, begins with a burning sensation
  c. Nadir usually occurs 10 to 14 days after administration
  d. Radiation recall, erythema that develops in previously irradiated field, is common
 3. Valrubicin (Valstar)
  a. Assess I & O, reporting urine output less than 30 mL/hour
  b. Monitor temperature because fever could indicate beginning of infection
 4. Bleomycin (Blenoxane)
  a. Inject a test dose of 2 units or less deeply into muscle to assess anaphylactic response before IV administration
  b. Assess vital signs; a febrile reaction is relatively common
  c. Bone marrow toxicity is rare with bleomycin
  d. Pulmonary toxicity occurs in about 10% of clients, most usually in clients over age 70 years and when cumulative dose reaches 400 units (also called "Bleo lung")
  e. Radiation recall is common
H. **Side effects/toxicity**
 1. General
  a. Bone marrow suppression (neutropenia, anemia, thrombocytopenia)
  b. Severe GI issues, including severe nausea/vomiting, mucositis, stomatitis, and diarrhea
  c. Cardiotoxicity and pulmonary toxicity
   1) Cardiotoxicity leading to degenerative cardiomyopathy occurs over time
   2) Prior radiation therapy to chest wall may predispose client to enhanced cardiotoxicity
  d. Vesicant: flare reaction is common and may be difficult to distinguish from an extravasation
 2. Bleomycin (Blenoxane)
  a. Pulmonary toxicity that is dose and age related
  b. Anaphylactic reaction may occur

     c. Mild febrile reaction commonly occurs

     d. Diffuse **alopecia**, skin hyperpigmentation, vesiculation, acne, thickening of skin and nail beds

I. Client and family education

    1. General

      a. Alopecia, which may also involve eyelashes, eyebrows, beard and mustache, and pubic and axillary hair; regrowth of hair usually begins 2 to 3 months after completion of administration

      b. Report signs and symptoms of infection (such as fever and upper respiratory symptoms, as examples) and decreased platelet count (such as hemorrhage or bleeding)

      c. Use caution with OTC medications including herbal extracts

    2. Bleomycin: notify for changes in breathing, including shortness of breath

    3. Valrubicin (Valstar): report bladder irritation and passage of red-colored urine; increase fluid intake for 48 hours after administration

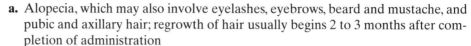

IV. PLANT-BASED ANTINEOPLASTIC AGENTS

A. Action and use

    1. Plant-based drugs that arrest or inhibit mitosis

    2. Most agents are cell cycle specific, M phase

    3. Major toxicities occur in hematopoietic, integumentary, neurologic, and reproductive systems; also, hypersensitivity reactions may occur

    4. Bone marrow suppression is the major dose-limiting factor

B. Common medications (Table 3-6)

C. Administration considerations

    1. Etoposide (VP-16)

      a. Inhibits an enzyme that helps repair DNA damage, thus damaging the tumor's DNA

      b. Administer by slow IV piggyback to avoid hypotension and bronchospasm

Practice to Pass

Before administration of a vesicant, list at least three steps the nurse should complete.

Table 3-6 Plant-Based Antineoplastic Agents	
Generic (Trade) Name	**Route**
Vinca alkaloids	
Vinblastine (Velban)	IV
Vincristine (Oncovin)	IV
Vinorelbine (Navelbine)	IV
Taxanes	
Cabazitaxel (Jevtana)	IV
Docetaxel (Taxotere)	IV
Paclitaxel (Taxol)	IV
Topoisomerase inhibitors	
Etoposide (VePesid)	IV
Ironotecan (Camptosar)	IV
Teniposide (Vumon)	IV
Topotecan (Hycamtin)	IV
Miscellaneous	
Eribulin (Halaven)	IV

Legend: IV, intravenous

2. Paclitaxel (Taxol)
   a. Is generally used for metastatic ovarian and breast cancer
   b. Do not use equipment or devices containing polyvinyl chloride (PVC)
   c. Tissue necrosis occurs with extravasation
   d. Administer via nitroglycerine tubing with an in-line filter of 0.22 micron or less
   e. Requires strict premedication (preferably with dexamethasone, diphenhydramine, and either cimetidine or ranitidine) per protocol order set before administration to prevent anaphylaxis
3. Vincristine (Oncovin)
   a. Major advantage: causes minimal immunosuppression
   b. Commonly used for pediatric leukemias, lymphomas, and other solid tumors
   c. Vesicant
      1) Administer into side arm portal of a freely flowing IV
      2) Hyaluronidase is the antidote should extravasation occur; also apply moderate heat to disperse drug and minimize sloughing

D. Contraindications
1. General
   a. Prior allergic reaction to any drugs in this class
   b. Pregnancy: Risk Category D–X
   c. Use cautiously in clients with hepatic, cardiac, or renal impairment
   d. Severe bone marrow depression including baseline neutropenia of less than 1,500 cells/mm^3
2. Vincristine (Oncovin)
   a. Obstructive jaundice
   b. Demyelinating neurological diseases, preexisting neuromuscular disease

E. Significant drug interactions
1. Etoposide (VP-16)
   a. Anticoagulants, antiplatelet agents, NSAIDS, and aspirin increase risk of bleeding
   b. Do not administer live vaccines
2. Paclitaxel (Taxol)
   a. Increased myelosuppression when administered with cisplatin
   b. Avoid using PVC bags and infusion sets due to leaching of DEPH (plasticizer)
3. Docetaxel (Taxotere): possible interaction with cyclosporine, erythromycin, ketoconazole, terfenadine, or troleandomycin
4. Vincristine (Oncovin): bronchospasm may occur in clients previously treated with mitomycin; hepatic metabolism of vincristine may be decreased when given with asparaginase (doses must separated by 12 to 24 hours)

F. Significant food interactions: none known

G. Significant assessment parameters
1. General
   a. Assess IV site before and after infusion; extravasation can cause thrombophlebitis and necrosis
   b. Assess frequently for symptoms of anaphylaxis
   c. Assess CBC, WBC and differential, and hepatic and renal function before administration and periodically during treatment
2. Etoposide (VP-16): monitor VS during and after infusion; if hypotension occurs, stop infusion
3. Paclitaxel (Taxol)
   a. Monitor for sensitivity reaction during first and second administration of drug; development of angioedema and generalized urticaria requires immediate discontinuation
   b. Monitor VS frequently; bradycardia occurs in 12% of clients who receive the drug
   c. Assess for peripheral neuropathy

4. Vincristine (Oncovin)
   a. Assess for leukopenia, which occurs in a significant number of clients
   b. Perform frequent neurological checks
      1) Symptoms of toxicity include numbness and tingling in limbs, loss of reflexes
      2) Assess hand grasps and deep tendon reflexes; depression of Achilles reflex is the earliest sign of neuropathy

H. **Side effects/toxicity**
   1. General
      a. Severe myelosuppression, including leukopenia, thrombocytopenia, neutropenia
      b. Severe mucositis and alopecia
   2. Etoposide (VP-16)
      a. Acral erythema and sloughing of skin on palms and soles
      b. Fever and chills during infusion
   3. Paclitaxel (Taxol)
      a. Transient bradycardia
      b. Peripheral neuropathy
      c. Neutropenia, thrombocytopenia
      d. Hypersensitivity reaction including hypotension, bronchospasm, urticaria, and angioedema
   4. Vincristine
      a. Neurotoxicity, loss of sensation on soles of feet and fingertips
      b. Severe constipation and paralytic ileus

I. **Client and family education**
   1. General
      a. Inspect mouth daily for ulcerations and bleeding and avoid obvious **irritants**
      b. Avoid use of products containing aspirin or ibuprofen, razors, or commercial mouthwash to decrease risk of bleeding
      c. Use nonhormonal contraceptive measures during therapy and more than 4 months after
      d. Inform of high probability of developing alopecia, which is reversible when therapy is completed
   2. Etoposide (VP-16): make position changes slowly, particularly from a recumbent position
   3. Paclitaxel (Taxol)
      a. Report dyspnea, chest pain, palpitations, or angioedema
      b. Be aware of and report signs of peripheral neuropathy
   4. Vincristine (Oncovin)
      a. Maintain a prophylactic regimen against constipation and paralytic ileus
      b. Report a change in bowel habits
      c. Report depression, double vision, paresthesias, pain, and motor problems

V. HORMONES AND HORMONE MODULATORS

A. **Action and use**
   1. Corticosteroids: lyse lymphoid malignancies and have an indirect effect on malignant cells
   2. Estrogens: suppress testosterone production in males and alter response of breast cancers to prolactin
   3. Progestins: promote palliation and tumor cell regression; exact mechanism of action is unknown
   4. Antiestrogens: compete with estrogens for binding with estrogen receptor sites on malignant cells

Practice to Pass

Constipation is a concern when administering vinca or plant alkaloid medications. What can the nurse do to prevent this treatment side effect?

5. Androgens: hormone therapy that has palliative use in metastatic/advanced carcinoma of breast; used if surgery and irradiation deemed inappropriate; otherwise, tamoxifen (Nolvadex) is drug of choice for this purpose
6. Androgen antagonists: inhibit binding of androgens at androgen receptor sites in target tissues; indicated for use in metastatic/advanced prostate cancer
B. Common medications (Table 3-7)
C. Administration considerations
    1. Corticosteroids
        a. Oral forms should be administered with meals and may be crushed
        b. IV form should be given slowly by IV piggyback to prevent vaginal and anal burning
    2. Estrogens
        a. Give orally immediately after solid food
        b. An exception is estramustine (Emcyt), which is a combination estrogen and nitrogen mustard compound; this must be taken with water an hour before meals, and requires that no milk, dairy products, or calcium-containing products be used concurrently

Table 3-7   **Hormones and Hormone Modulators**

Generic (Trade) Name	Route	Uses
Corticosteroids		
Prednisone (Deltasone)	PO	Inflammatory, allergic, and debilitating conditions related to autoimmune disorders, asthma, allergic reactions, and malignancies
Dexamethasone (Decadron)	PO, IV	
Hydrocortisone (SoluCortef)	PO	
Methylprednisolone (SoluMedrol)	IV	
Estrogens		
Diethylstilbestrol (DES)	PO	Hormone replacement therapy, oral contraceptive, atrophic vaginitis, female hypogonadism, primary ovarian failure, palliation of prostatic and mammary cancers
Ethinyl estradiol (Estinyl)	PO	
Polyestradiol (Estradurin)	IV	
Antiestrogens		
Tamoxifen (Nolvadex) Toremifene (Fareston) Anastrozole (Arimedex)	PO	Treatment of breast cancer in postmenopausal women, women without ovarian function, and treatment of prostatic cancer
Exemestane (Aromasin)	PO	
Fulvestrant (Faslodex)	IM	
Letrozole (Femara)		
Raloxifene (Evista)		
Progestins		
Medroxyprogesterone acetate (Depo-Provera)	PO, IM	Contraceptive, treatment of amenorrhea, palliative cancer therapy, fertility
Megestrol acetate (Megace)	PO	Appetite stimulant for anorexia
Antiandrogens (androgen receptor blockers)		
Bicalutamide (Casodex) Flutamide (Eulexin) Nilutamide (Nilandron)	PO PO PO	Advanced and metastatic prostate cancer, breast cancer, management of endometriosis
Androgens		
Testosterone (generic)	PO	Breast cancer in pre- and postmenopausal women
Fluoxymesterone (generic)	PO	

Legend: PO, oral; IM, intramuscular; IV, intravenous

    3. Progestins: give orally without regard to meals

    4. Estrogen antagonists: give orally; dosage may be decreased if side effects are severe

    5. Androgens and antiandrogens: give orally

D. Contraindications

    1. Corticosteroids

        a. Systemic infections

        b. Ulcerative colitis, diverticulitis, active or latent peptic ulcer disease

        c. Safe use in pregnancy (Category C) and nursing mothers has not been established

    2. Estrogens

        a. Known or suspected pregnancy

        b. Estrogen-dependent neoplasms

        c. History of thromboembolic disorders

    3. Progestins

        a. Severe dysrhythmias possible if client also takes a calcium-channel blocker

        b. Psychiatric depression

        c. Pregnancy (Category C), cautious use in lactation

    4. Antiestrogens: first trimester of pregnancy (Category C)

E. Significant drug interactions

    1. Corticosteroids

        a. Phenytoin (Dilantin) and rifampin (Rifadin) increase steroid metabolism

        b. Increased doses may be required when given with amphotericin-B

        c. Diuretics increase potassium loss

        d. May inhibit antibody response to vaccines and toxoids

    2. Estrogens: phenytoin (Dilantin) and rifampin (Rifadin) decrease estrogen effect by increasing its metabolism

    3. Progestins

        a. Can prolong cardiac conduction in clients taking beta blockers, calcium channel blockers, and possibly digoxin (Lanoxin)

        b. Quinine may decrease plasma levels

        c. Chloroquine may increase risk of seizures

    4. Antiestrogens: may enhance hypoprothombinemic effect of warfarin

F. Significant food interactions: none known

G. Significant assessment parameters

    1. Corticosteroids

        a. Establish baseline and continuing data on blood pressure, I & O, weight, and sleep patterns

        b. Measure 2-hour postprandial blood glucose, serum potassium, and serum calcium prior to therapy and at regular intervals thereafter

        c. Watch for changes in mood, emotional stability, and sleep patterns

    2. Estrogens

        a. Spotting or breakthrough bleeding may occur

        b. Severe hypercalcemia may occur

    3. Progestin

        a. Assess weight periodically

        b. Assess for allergic reactions, rash, urticaria, anaphylaxis, and tachypnea

    4. Antiestrogens: assess CBC, including platelet count, periodically

    5. Androgens: monitor serum calcium levels; hypercalcemia can result, requiring temporary termination of drug therapy and administration of large volumes of IV fluid

    6. Antiandrogens: monitor liver function studies periodically to detect rare complication of hepatitis

H. Side effects/toxicity

1. Corticosteroids
   a. Euphoria, headache, insomnia, psychosis
   b. Edema
   c. Muscle weakness, delayed wound healing, osteoporosis, spontaneous fractures
   d. Hyperglycemia
2. Estrogens
   a. Thromboembolic disorders
   b. Nausea
3. Progestins
   a. Vaginal bleeding and breast tenderness
   b. Abdominal pain, nausea, and vomiting
   c. Increased appetite and weight gain
4. Antiestrogens
   a. Thrombosis
   b. About 25% of clients experience nausea and vomiting
   c. Hot flashes, weight gain, changes in menstrual cycle, leaking from breasts
5. Androgens
   a. Virilization, including clitoral enlargement, increases in facial and body hair, deepened voice, increased libido, and male-pattern baldness
   b. Hypercalcemia
6. Antiandrogens
   a. Gynecomastia
   b. GI disturbances (nausea, vomiting, constipation, and diarrhea)
   c. Hepatitis

I. Client and family teaching: for all drug groups, teach clients about adverse effects and when to report them

VI. OTHER ANTINEOPLASTICS

A. Action and use

1. Asparaginase (Elspar) depletes extracellular supply of asparagine, an amino acid essential to DNA synthesis
2. Hydroxyurea (Hydrea) blocks incorporation of thymidine into DNA and may damage already formed DNA molecules

B. Common medications: asparaginase (also referred to as L-asparaginase) and hydroxyurea

C. Administration considerations

1. Asparaginase (Elspar)
   a. Administer intradermal (ID) skin test before initial dose because of the potential for anaphylaxis; a negative skin test does not preclude the possibility of an allergic reaction
   b. Fiber-like particles may develop in vial after reconstitution; use a 5-micron filter to remove particles (will not affect potency); do not use cloudy solutions
2. Hydroxyurea: capsule may be opened and mixed with water if client has difficulty swallowing

D. Contraindications

1. Asparaginase (Elspar)
   a. History of or existing pancreatitis
   b. Safe use during pregnancy (Category C) and nursing mothers is not established
2. Hydroxyurea: pregnancy (Category D)

E. **Significant drug interactions**
1. Asparaginase (Elspar)
    a. Causes decreased hypoglycemic effects of sulfonylureas and insulin
    b. Antitumor effect is blocked if administered concurrently with vincristine (Oncovin) or methotrexate (Folex)
2. Hydroxyurea (Hydrea): none established
F. **Significant food interactions**: none known
G. **Significant assessment parameters**
1. Asparaginase (Elspar)
    a. Prepare for anaphylaxis and have personnel, emergency medications, oxygen, and airway equipment readily available
    b. During administration, monitor vital signs and be alert for hypersensitivity or anaphylactic reaction, which usually occurs 30 to 60 minutes after medication administration
    c. Assess laboratory values prior to treatment and routinely thereafter, including CBC, amylase, serum calcium, coagulation factors, hepatic and renal function studies, and ammonia and uric acid levels
2. Hydroxyurea (Hydrea)
    a. Determine status of kidney, liver, and bone marrow function before and periodically during therapy
    b. Monitor I & O and increase fluid intake, especially in clients with high serum uric acid levels
H. **Side effects/toxicity**
1. Asparaginase (Elspar)
    a. Severe anaphylaxis is possible; crash cart should be readily available
    b. Severe nausea and vomiting
    c. Potential for bleeding because of reduced clotting factors, decreased circulating platelets, and decreased fibrinogen levels
2. Hydroxyurea (Hydrea)
    a. Bone marrow suppression
    b. Stomatitis
    c. Maculopapular rash
    d. Hyperuricemia

VII. SAFE HANDLING OF CHEMOTHERAPEUTIC AGENTS

A. **Drug preparation and administration**
1. All individuals preparing and administering cytotoxic drugs should be specially trained in safety procedures for handling of chemotherapeutic drugs and comply with agency standards, which in turn comply with government and professional practice standards
2. Chemotherapy doses are generally individualized according to body weight (kg) or body surface area (m^2)
3. Most chemotherapy protocol order sets consist of short, intermittent, high-dose courses of drugs (often in combination) to maximize cancer cell kill while allowing normal cells time to heal and recover
4. Chemotherapy drugs should be prepared for use in an air-vented space, such as a clean-air workstation or biohazard cabinet; access to this area should be limited
5. Wear a disposable, leak-proof gown, surgical latex gloves, a mask, and eye protection when preparing chemotherapeutic agents
6. Do not prepare or administer IV chemotherapy if pregnant because of possible risk to fetus; almost all chemotherapeutic agents are Pregnancy Risk Category D or X

B. Safe handling of antineoplastic agents and spill management

1. Use leak-proof, puncture-resistant containers to dispose of antineoplastic drugs and associated vials, needles, syringes, tubing, and other equipment; use double-bagging technique and identify container with a "biohazard" label
2. Do not separate needle from syringe or break needles to avoid leaking medication from them
3. If drug accidentally touches a nurse or client, wash area well with soap and water; immediately remove any contaminated clothing; copiously flush eyes if involved while keeping eyelids open
4. Double-glove to clean a drug spill, washing hands before and after
5. For powdered medications, wear a mask and eye protection as well
6. Place spilled substance in a plastic bag; wipe remaining area with a damp cloth and place it in same bag; place this bag into another plastic bag (double-bag) and label it as biohazardous
7. All materials used for drug preparation and administration must be disposed of by incineration

C. Disposal of client's body fluids

1. Handle all body substances cautiously, such as blood, urine, vomitus, stool, and others; carefully follow standard precautions and other procedures as designated by agency policy
2. Wear gloves when in contact with all body substances; carefully dispose of them in toilet; clean containers carefully and thoroughly

VIII. NURSING MANAGEMENT OF TREATMENT SIDE EFFECTS

A. Myelosuppression

1. Neutropenia
   a. Assessment
      1) Neutropenia is defined as an absolute neutrophil count of $1,500/mm^3$ or less
      2) Nadir (lowest point in WBC count reached after chemotherapy) most commonly occurs 7 to 14 days following chemotherapy administration
      3) Fever of more than 38°C or 100.4°F is the most reliable and often only sign of infection in clients with neutropenia
   b. Management
      1) Avoid exposure to these substances
         a) Fresh fruits, vegetables, flowers, and live plants
         b) People recently vaccinated with live organisms or viruses
         c) Pet excreta including fish tanks and aquariums
      2) Instruct clients to avoid contact with people who have a contagious illness
      3) Teach people who come in contact with client to wash hands prior to touching client
      4) Encourage client to practice good personal hygiene
      5) Prevent trauma to skin and mucous membranes
      6) Culture urine, peripheral blood, all lumens of CVCs and suspected sources of infection; obtain chest x-ray (CXR); administer antibiotics as ordered for empiric therapy
      7) Institute neutropenic precautions for hospitalized clients whose absolute neutrophil count drops as described above using previously described measures
      8) Administer filgrastim (Neupogen), a granulocyte colony-stimulating factor (G-CSF) that increases production of neutrophils, either IV or SubQ as ordered; client may report bone pain 1 to 3 days before blood count increases; this may be controlled with nonopioid analgesics

!

Practice to Pass

What measures should the nurse teach the client to decrease the potential for infection after chemotherapy administration?

!

!

    c. Client and family education
      1) Report temperature greater than 38°C or 100.4°F, shaking chills, dysuria, dyspnea, sputum production, or pain
      2) Reinforce need for meticulous hygiene
      3) Teach self-administration of G-CSF for neutropenia or granulocyte/macrophage colony-stimulating factor (GM-CSF) for treatment of blood-forming organ cancers as ordered

2. Thrombocytopenia
    a. Bone marrow suppression decreases platelet production
    b. Circulating platelets are diminished gradually because platelet life span is only 10 days
    c. Chemotherapy drugs accelerate platelet destruction
    d. Assessment
      1) Platelet count below 50,000/mm^3; risk significantly increases when platelet count falls below 20,000/mm^3
      2) Petechiae, bruising, and hemorrhage
      3) Neurological changes that may indicate intracranial bleeding
      4) Hypotension and tachycardia
    e. Management
      1) Institute bleeding precautions
      2) Decrease activity to prevent falls and maintain a safe environment
      3) Discourage heavy lifting and Valsalva maneuver, which may increase risk of intracranial bleeding
      4) Encourage client to eat a high-fiber diet and drink adequate liquids
      5) Daily care
        a) Avoid use of straight-edge razors; use an electric razor instead
        b) Avoid using nail clippers; use a nail file instead
        c) Avoid using vaginal douches, rectal suppositories, or enemas
        d) Use water-soluble lubricant for sexual intercourse
        e) Avoid intercourse when platelet count is below 50,000/mm^3
        f) Instruct menstruating women to monitor pad count and amount of saturation; tampon use should be avoided
        g) Encourage client to blow nose gently
        h) Instruct client to avoid dental floss and oral irrigation, and to use a soft toothbrush or sponge-tipped applicator for mouth care
        i) Avoid administration of aspirin or aspirin-containing products as well as NSAIDs
        j) Apply pressure for 5 to 10 minutes following venipuncture, bone marrow biopsy, or other invasive procedures; platelet transfusion prior to procedure may be indicated
    f. Client and family education
      1) Notify MD of symptoms of bleeding
      2) Test urine and stool for occult blood
      3) Teach other safety recommendations for daily management

B. Nausea and vomiting
  1. Anticipatory nausea: a conditioned response resulting from repeated association of chemotherapy-induced nausea and vomiting (N/V) and stimulus from environment
  2. Acute nausea: occurs 0 to 24 hours after chemotherapy administration
  3. Delayed nausea: persistent vomiting lasting 1 to 4 days after chemotherapy administration
  4. Assessment parameters
    a. Women have a higher incidence than men
    b. Younger clients experience more nausea than their older counterparts

c. A history of motion sickness can predispose some to experience chemotherapy-induced nausea

d. Dehydration may accelerate N/V

5. Administer antiemetics to cover the emetogenic period (see Table 3-8); these may include (but are not limited to) ondansetron (Zofran) and metoclopramide (Reglan), a prokinetic GI stimulant

6. Provide additional antiemetics to manage breakthrough nausea

7. Dexamethasone may be most effective agent in preventing anticipatory N/V

8. Client and family education

a. Eat small frequent meals and avoid fatty, sweet, salty, or spicy foods

b. Notify health care professional if vomiting persists more than 24 hours and client is unable to take oral hydration

c. Maintain antiemetic schedule for 48 to 72 hours to avoid delayed nausea

C. Diarrhea

1. Chemotherapy affects rapidly dividing cells of villae and micro-villae in GI mucosa

2. Combination chemotherapy and radiation therapy to pelvis can lead to additional cellular destruction

3. Monitor number of stools, amount, and consistency

4. Replace fluid and electrolytes, including potassium

5. Administer antidiarrheal medication to reduce peristalsis and frequency and volume of stools

Table 3-8 Emetogenic Potential, Onset, and Duration of Selected Chemotherapeutic Agents

Incidence	Agent	Onset (Hours)	Duration (Hours)
Very High	Cisplatin	1–6	24–72+
	Dacarbazine	1–3	1–12
	Mechlorethamine	0.5–2	8–24
	Melphalan	3–6	6–12
	Dactinomycin	1–2	4–20
High	Carmustine	2–4	4–24
	Cyclophosphamide	4–12	12–24
	Procarbazine	24–27	Variable
	Etoposide	4–6	24+
	Methotrexate	1–12	24–72
Moderate	Doxorubicin	4–6	6+
	Mitoxantrone	4–6	6+
	Fluorouracil	3–6	24+
	Mitomycin	1–4	48–72
	Carboplatin	4–6	12–24
	Ifosfamide	3–6	24–72
	Cytarabine	6–12	3–12
Low	Bleomycin	3–6	–
	Daunorubicin	1–2	–
	6-Mercaptopurine	4–8	–
	Methotrexate	4–12	–
	Vinblastine	4–8	–
	Lomustine	2–6	2–24
Very low	Vincristine	4–8	–
	Paclitaxel	4–8	–

6. Client and family education
  a. Consume low-residue, high-protein, high-calorie diet to promote bowel rest
  b. Eliminate irritating foods, such as alcohol, coffee, cold liquids, popcorn, and raw fruits and vegetables
  c. Drink 6 to 8 glasses of water per 24-hr period
  d. Implement a liquid diet if diarrhea is severe
  e. Avoid milk products and chocolate
  f. Decrease activity when diarrhea is severe to provide rest and decrease peristalsis
  g. Clean rectal area with mild soap after each bowel movement and apply moisture barrier
  h. Take warm sitz baths

D. Stomatitis
  1. Epithelial cells of oral mucosa are destroyed, causing an inflammatory response and denudation of oral mucosa
  2. Initial presentation: burning sensation with no physical changes in oral mucosa, sensitivity to heat and cold, and sensitivity to salty and spicy foods
  3. Promote a well-balanced intake, including a protein intake of greater than 1 gram/kg of body weight
  4. Promote consistent, thorough oral hygiene after each meal and at hour of sleep
  5. Administer antifungal or antiviral medication for prophylaxis as directed
  6. Client and family education
    a. Instruct in consistent oral hygiene
    b. Avoid using lemon/glycerin swabs, hydrogen peroxide, and products containing alcohol, which promote dryness and irritation

E. Constipation
  1. Neurotoxic effects of chemotherapy can decrease peristalsis or cause paralytic ileus
  2. Assess patterns of elimination including amount and frequency
  3. Assess usual fiber and fluid intake
  4. Determine laxative and cathartic use, including frequency and amounts taken
  5. Initiate a bowel maintenance program for clients receiving neurotoxic chemotherapeutic agents or those at high risk for constipation
  6. Recognize complications associated with constipation, such as fecal impaction
  7. Client and family education
    a. Drink warm liquids to stimulate bowel movement
    b. Increase fiber intake to increase peristalsis and stool bulk
    c. Drink at least 8 glasses of water per day
    d. Exercise regularly
    e. Develop a regular bowel program, avoiding use of laxatives if possible

F. Alopecia
  1. Cells responsible for hair growth have a high mitotic rate and are affected to some degree by most chemotherapeutic agents
  2. Hair loss begins approximately 2 weeks after drug administration and will continue until 3 to 5 months after last chemotherapy treatment is completed
  3. Devices to decrease circulation to scalp are contraindicated since they can also promote micrometastasis
  4. Provide emotional support to client who is experiencing body image change
  5. Client and family education
    a. Rationale and expected timeframe of hair loss and regrowth
    b. Provide gentle hair care, avoiding permanent waves, coloring, peroxide, electric rollers, and curling irons until regrowth has been reestablished long enough for 2 haircuts
    c. Hair prosthesis (wig)
    d. Emotional support strategies to cope with changing body image

G. Cardiotoxicity

1. May occur within 24 hr to up to 4 to 5 weeks after drug administration; is self-limiting; warrants immediate drug discontinuation
2. Higher doses over a shorter period of time increase its incidence
3. Baseline ejection fraction should be assessed before administration of cardiotoxic agents
4. Characteristics of cardiotoxicity are outlined in Table 3-9
5. Maintain ongoing documentation of client's cumulative dose
6. Cardioprotective iron chelating agents (e.g., dexrazoxane) may be administered to prevent cardiotoxicity in clients that have received three fourths of their lifetime dosage
7. Client and family education
   a. Cardiotoxicity is an expected side effect of some chemotherapy medications
   b. It is important to recognize signs of CHF and report them to health care provider as directed
   c. Chronic cardiotoxicity is dose-related and possibly irreversible

H. Pulmonary toxicity

1. Lung tissue is sensitive to toxic effects of chemotherapy, causing direct damage to alveoli and capillary endothelium
2. Dyspnea is the cardinal symptom
3. Deteriorating creatinine clearance (renal dysfunction) is an important predictor for pulmonary pneumonitis
4. High oxygen concentrations can enhance pulmonary toxicity of bleomycin
5. Risk of pulmonary toxicity increases significantly after age 70
6. Monitor pulmonary function studies as indicated
7. Client education
   a. Provide education regarding symptoms associated with pulmonary toxicity (e.g., dyspnea, chest pain, shallow breathing, chest wall discomfort)
   b. Teach pursed-lipped breathing and use a small fan to decrease symptoms of dyspnea
   c. Encourage use of opioid analgesia as prescribed to decrease fear of air hunger
   d. Review safety issues related to oxygen administration
   e. Explore with client and significant other their wishes for intubation and resuscitation; breastfeeding should be discontinued

Table 3-9 **Cardiotoxicity**

Drug	Characteristics	Comments
DNA Intercalators		
Doxorubicin (Adriamycin) Daunorubicin (DaunoXome) Dactinomycin (Cosmegen) Mitoxantrone (Novantrone)	EKG changes, nonspecific ST-T wave changes; premature ventricular and atrial contractions; low voltage QRS changes	Chronic effects seen with cumulative dosages greater than recommended
High-Dose Therapy		
Cylcophosphamide (Cytoxan)	Diminished QRS complexes on EKG, cardiomegaly, pulmonary congestion	May result in acute lethal pericarditis, hemorrhagic myocardial necrosis
Fluorouracil (5-FU)	Angina, palpitations, sweating and syncope	May treat prophylactically or therapeutically with long-acting nitrates or calcium channel blockers
Taxanes		
Paclitaxel (Taxol)	Asymptomatic bradycardia, hypotension, asymptomatic ventricular tachycardia, and atypical chest pain	A baseline EKG, client history, and cardiac assessment should be performed before treatment; routine cardiac monitoring not warranted

I. **Hemorrhagic cystitis**
1. Bladder mucosal irritation and inflammation results from contact with acrolein, the metabolic by-product of cyclophosphamide and ifosfamide
2. Prior radiation therapy to pelvis or bladder increases risk
3. It presents with dysuria, frequency, burning upon urination, and hematuria
4. A chemo-protectant agent (mesna), may be given to bind to acrolein in bladder, inactivating it and allowing excretion from bladder
5. Client education
   a. Instruct that hemorrhagic cystitis is a possible side effect of cyclophosphamide (Cytoxan) and ifosfamide (Ifex) therapy
   b. Report signs and symptoms of hemorrhagic cystitis
   c. Void every 4 to 6 hours and take medication early in the day
   d. Drink a minimum of 6 to 8 glasses of fluid daily

J. **Hepatotoxicity**
1. Is caused by direct toxic effect on liver when drugs are metabolized; see Table 3-10 for incidence
2. Prior liver infection, tumor involvement in liver, advanced age, total bilirubin greater than 2 mg/100 dL, or cirrhosis increase incidence
3. Clinical manifestations include jaundice, ascites, fatigue, anorexia, nausea, hyperpigmentation, upper right quadrant pain, hepatomegaly, and changes in urine and stool
4. Avoid hepatotoxic drugs if liver function tests are abnormal

Table 3-10 **Hepatotoxicity**

Classification	Incidence	Comments
Alkylating Agents		
Nitrogen Mustards		
Cyclophosphamide (Cytoxan)	Rare	Exception is greater than 3 grams used in bone marrow transplant (BMT)
Nitrosoureas		
Carmustine (BCNU) Lomustine (CeeNu) Streptozocin (Zanosar)	26% at low doses 26% 15–67%	Usually not clinically significant, however may be associated with veno-occlusive disease when used in BMT
Antimetabolites		
Methotrexate (Folex)	24% with oral administration	Cumulative dose is important Seen only when cumulative dosages exceed 2 mg/kg/day
Fluorouracil (Adrucil) Cytarabine (Cytosar)	Rare Unknown	
Antitumor Antibiotics		
Doxorubicin (Adriamycin)	Rare	May be lower than other anthracyclines
Mitoxantrone (Novantrone)	Rare	
Bleomycin (Blenoxane)	Rare	
Plicamycin (Mithracin)	16%	
Plant Based Agents		
Vincristine (Oncovin) Etoposide (VePesid) Paclitaxil (Taxol)	Rare Rare 7–22%	Rarely seen with standard dosages, higher dosages can cause irreversible liver enzyme changes
Miscellaneous		
Asparaginase (Elspar)	42–67%	Increases with higher doses

5. Client and family education
   a. Client should avoid alcohol-containing beverages
   b. Hepatotoxicity is a possible side effect of some chemotherapeutic medications
   c. Be aware of and report signs and symptoms of liver failure

K. **Nephrotoxicity**
   1. Is caused by direct damage to glomerulus, renal blood vessels, different parts of nephron, and/or precipitation of metabolites in acid environment of urine; leads to obstructive nephropathy
   2. Advancing age, preexisting renal disease, poor nutritional status, and administration of other nephrotoxic agents predispose client to nephrotoxicity
   3. It is manifested by increasing serum creatinine, declining creatinine clearance, hypomagnesemia, proteinuria, and hematuria
   4. Continuation of nephrotoxic agents should be reviewed if blood urea nitrogen (BUN) is greater than 22 mg/dL and/or creatinine is >2 mg/dL
   5. Institute hydration of 3,000 mL/day to prevent or minimize renal damage
   6. Induce diuresis with mannitol (Osmitrol) or furosemide (Lasix) when administering cisplatin
   7. Administer allopurinol (Zyloprim) to decrease uric acid production from high tumor-cell kill (e.g., leukemia, lymphoma, small cell lung cancer)
   8. Maintain alkalinization of urine with sodium bicarbonate to a pH level greater than 8 to prevent renal damage when giving high-dose methotrexate (Folex)
   9. Avoid administration of aspirin and NSAIDs
   10. Client and family education
       a. Instruct that nephrotoxicity is a possible side effect of selected chemotherapeutic agents
       b. Reinforce importance of compliance with measures to prevent nephrotoxicity
          1) Accurately obtain 12- or 24-hr urine for creatinine clearance
          2) Increase fluid intake
          3) Comply with instructions to alkalinize urine, complete leucovorin rescue, and/or allopurinol (Zyloprim) therapy

L. **Neurotoxicity**
   1. Caused by direct toxicity on nervous system, metabolic encephalopathy, or intracranial hemorrhage related to chemotherapy-induced coagulopathy
   2. Risk factors
      a. Administration of agents that cross blood–brain barrier
      b. Specified chemotherapeutic agents, especially cumulative doses of vinca alkaloids
      c. Concurrent radiation therapy to brain
      d. Incidence increases with age
      e. Impaired renal function
   3. Use assessment guidelines to determine fine motor losses, numbness, tingling, gait disturbance, constipation, and change in mentation, which are early warning signs
   4. Use measures outlined in Table 3-11 for collaborative management of neurotoxicity
   5. Client and family education
      a. Neurotoxicity is a possible side effect of some chemotherapy agents
      b. Be aware of early warning signs of neurotoxicity and importance of notifying provider if they occur

M. **Sexual and reproductive dysfunction**
   1. Infertility occurs in men primarily through depletion of germinal epithelium that lines seminiferous tubules
   2. Women experience reproductive dysfunction primarily as a result of hormonal alterations or direct effects that cause ovarian fibrosis and follicular destruction

Table 3-11	Neurotoxicity		
Area Affected	**Chemotherapy Agent**	**Assessment**	**Collaborative Management**
Cerebrum	Asparaginase Cisplatin Carboplatin Ifosfamide	Assess for confusion, memory loss, and level of consciousness	1. Use positive support and encouragement 2. Maintain a consistent schedule
Sensory	Cisplatin Carboplatin Cytarabine Etoposide Paclitaxil Vincristine	Assess for decreased deep tendon reflexes, numbness, decreased sensation, jaw pain, paresthesia of hands or feet	1. Avoid extreme temperatures 2. Use assistive devices as required 3. Use opioids, antidepressants, and antiepileptics for neuropathic pain
Autonomic	Vincristine	Assess for abdominal pain, constipation, ileus, bladder atony	1. Recommend a high-fiber diet 2. Increase fluid intake 3. Administer stool softeners and laxatives as required 4. Initiate a bowel management program ½ hour after meals 5. Monitor for bladder infection with urinary retention
Auditory	Cisplatin Prednisone	Assess for tinnitus, hearing loss	1. Report auditory changes 2. Reduce or discontinue chemotherapy

3. Chemotherapy compromises fertility by exerting cytotoxic effects on gametogenesis; degree is related to therapeutic agent and duration of treatment
4. Approximately 40 to 100% of clients experience some sexual dysfunction following treatment; it is frequently underreported because it is often not assessed by health care personnel
5. Males should be encouraged to bank sperm before starting treatment
6. Although expensive (and not always successful), females should be informed of opportunities to bank oocytes or cryopreserve embryos
7. Water-based lubricants or estrogen supplements may help to decrease vaginal dryness
8. Client education and counseling
    a. Provide an unbiased, sexually neutral environment that promotes open discussion
    b. Identify whether sexual issues pose a problem for client and/or partner
    c. Explain implications of treatments on sexuality
    d. Provide information related to contraception
    e. Discourage pregnancy during treatment
    f. Advise client of possible long-term side effects on reproductive function
    g. Encourage communication between client and significant other

Case Study

A 64-year-old male client is admitted for his first dose of chemotherapy. His wife died 6 months ago of a massive heart attack. He has 2 daughters who live out of state; 1 is a lawyer, while the other is a pediatrician. The client is the chief executive officer (CEO) of his own electronic business, is self-insured, and has no oncology supplement.

Chemotherapy orders include:

- Cytoxan 800 mg IVPB
- Methotrexate 160 mg IVPB
- Adriamycin 40 mg in 1,000 mL normal saline IV infusion over 24 hr times 2 doses
- Leucovorin 75 mg IVPB q6 hrs times 4 doses; begin Leucovorin 24 hr after methotrexate
- 5-FU 80 mg IVPB after second dose of leucovorin

Other medication orders include:

- Zofran 35 mg IVPB prior to starting chemotherapy and prior to the second liter of Adriamycin
- Zofran 15 mg IVPB 4 and 8 hr after each 35 mg loading dose
- Benadryl 12.5 mg, Reglan 5 mg, and Decadron 2 mg IVPB q6 hours around the clock

For suggested responses, see page 541.

Diagnostic studies include MUGA scan, ultrasound of the liver, CBC, and chemistry profile.

1. What are the most important nursing diagnoses, and what is your rationale for prioritizing them the way you did?
2. What important diagnostic and assessment values need to be obtained before initiating the chemotherapy?
3. Outline a pretreatment teaching plan for this client.
4. What orders need further clarification with the physician?
5. How will you prepare the client for discharge from the hospital?

POSTTEST

1 A client is receiving chemotherapy with carmustine (BiCNU), a nitrosourea, as treatment for cancer. The intravenous line infiltrates and extravasation occurs. The nurse should perform the following interventions in which order?

1. Discontinue carmustine infusion.
2. Consult plastic surgeon.
3. Treat site with local injections of sodium carbonate and normal saline.
4. Choose new site for continuation of administration.

2 The nurse makes it a priority to assess for hematuria and dysuria when a client is receiving which cancer chemotherapy agent?

1. Cyclophosphamide (Cytoxan)
2. Methotrexate (Mexate)
3. Streptozocin (Zanosar)
4. Cisplatin (Platinol)

3 Prior to administering 5-fluorouracil (5-FU), the nurse teaches the client that which of the following unique long-term disabling side effects may persist after administration ends?

1. Myelosuppression
2. Cerebellar syndrome
3. Nausea and vomiting
4. Alopecia

4 Prior to initiating chemotherapy, the nurse teaches clients the most common side effects associated with chemotherapy. In which order should the side effects be addressed?

1. Cardiotoxicity
2. Neurotoxicity
3. Myelosuppression
4. Hepatotoxicity

5 When preparing a client who has cancer and the client's family for the initiation of chemotherapy, in which order would the nurse complete the following interventions?

1. Clarify information and dispel misconceptions.
2. Obtain informed consent.
3. Evaluate client for chemotherapy-induced anemia and neutropenia.
4. Choose an appropriate venous access.
5. Demonstrate safe gloving, gowning, and administration of ordered chemotherapy.

6 A client receiving chemotherapy overheard the health care team use the term *cell-cycle specific* when discussing the chemotherapy. The client asks for an explanation of the term. Which of the following is the best response?

1. "It is medical jargon that is not related to your care."
2. "Chemotherapy drugs are lethal to certain types of cells."
3. "These drugs are aimed at cells that are dividing."
4. "This means the drugs work best after the cells have been through several cycles."

7 Several weeks after a health care provider changed the type of chemotherapy from an antimetabolite to an alkylating agent, the client is very anxious because of worsened fatigue, nausea and vomiting, and symptoms of peripheral neuropathy. Which of the following is the best response by the nurse to the client's concern?

1. "The new drug does not differentiate between normal and abnormal cells as well as the first drug."
2. "You are experiencing the side effects of both drugs."
3. "The lesion may not have responded to the first drug."
4. "I will obtain medication to relieve the signs and symptoms."

8 The nurse is providing care for several clients receiving chemotherapy. Which of the following clients is most likely to experience cardiotoxicity?

1. Female client receiving vincristine (Oncovin)
2. Older adult receiving doxorubicin (Adriamycin)
3. A reproductive-age male receiving mechlorethamine (Mustargen)
4. Native American receiving cisplatin (Platinol)

9 After the home health nurse notified the outpatient clinic that a client receiving chemotherapy has a serum neutrophil level of less than 2,300/mm^3, the nurse should expect to complete which collaborative and nursing interventions? Select all that apply.

1. Administer filgrastim (Neupogen) 5 mg/kg/day intravenously.
2. Prepare client for administration of whole blood transfusion.
3. Administer epoetin alfa (Epogen) 500 units/kg 3 times weekly subcutaneously.
4. Educate regarding proper hand hygiene techniques and food preparation.
5. Teach client to limit exposure to groups of people and those with any illness.

10 A client wants the dosage of chemotherapy doubled to assure maximum impact on a large inoperable lesion. Which is the most appropriate response by the nurse?

1. "I'll check with the health care provider."
2. "I don't know if this is realistic based on your history of previous treatments."
3. "The prescriber will gradually increase the dose as the lesion shrinks."
4. "The dosage is predetermined by the effect of the drug on the body."

➤ *See pages 116–118 for Answers and Rationales.*

ANSWERS & RATIONALES

Pretest

1 **Answer: 3** **Rationale:** The most profound adverse effects of plant (vinca) alkaloids such as vincristine lie in the peripheral nervous system. A decreased Achilles reflex is the earliest sign of neuropathy. There is no evidence of a significant change in level of consciousness or memory. Foot and hand drop (which would interfere with motor ability), along with paresthesia, occur later than impairment of the Achilles tendon. **Cognitive Level:** Analyzing **Client Need:** Pharmacological and Parenteral Therapies **Integrated Process:** Nursing Process: Assessment **Content Area:** Pharmacology **Strategy:** The core issue of the question is the ability to recognize an adverse effect of the plant alkaloids. Take time to review this information if this question was difficult. **Reference:** Adams, M., Holland, L., & Bostwick, P. (2011). *Pharmacology for nurses: A pathophysiologic approach* (3rd ed.). Upper Saddle River, NJ: Pearson Education, pp. 559–560.

2 **Answer: 3** **Rationale:** The combination of exercise and dexrazoxane (Zinecard) are the best interventions. Since the outcome of the toxicity results in decreased strength of the cardiac muscle, exercise is the best intervention because it strengthens cardiac muscle. Dexrazoxane protects the cardiac muscle against the toxic effects of doxorubicin. It interferes with iron-mediated free radicals thought to cause cardiomyopathy. Exercise and cessation of smoking would contribute to general health maintenance but would not protect the heart from cardiotoxicity. Smoking cessation and O_2 administration would be appropriate if the client developed CHF. A low-fat diet has no known contributory effects. **Cognitive Level:** Applying **Client Need:** Pharmacological and Parenteral Therapies **Integrated Process:** Nursing Process: Implementation **Content Area:** Pharmacology **Strategy:** A critical word in the question is *prevention*. Identify the category of dexrazoxane as a cytoprotective agent and associate it with outcomes of the drug. **Reference:** Wilson, B. A., Shannon, M. T., & Shields, K. M. (2011). *Pearson intravenous drug guide 2011-2012* (2nd ed.). Upper Saddle River, NJ: Pearson Education, pp. 224–225.

3 **Answer: 1, 2, 5** **Rationale:** Elevating the head of the bed will decrease the work of breathing. Pursed-lip breathing is the best respiratory technique, because it creates a back pressure that keeps the airways open longer, resulting in prolonged exhalation. This also facilitates removal of secretions from the bronchial tree. To manage normal life activities, the client needs to plan exercise and rest periods. Shallow, slow breathing would not maximize the client's pulmonary potential. Clients with hypoxia are likely to use accessory muscles in an attempt to "get more air in," rather than to exhale. The method is tiring and should not be taught; it is not as efficient as pursed-lip breathing. **Cognitive Level:** Analyzing **Client Need:** Pharmacological and Parenteral Therapies **Integrated Process:** Teaching and Learning **Content Area:** Pharmacology **Strategy:** Select the options most likely to promote perfusion and cellular ventilation as well as maximize utilization of available oxygen. **Reference:** LeMone, P., Burke, K., & Bauldoff, G. (2011). *Medical-surgical nursing: Critical thinking in patient care* (5th ed.). Upper Saddle River, NJ: Pearson Education, p. 1249.

4 **Answer: 2** **Rationale:** Pulmonary toxicity is a known adverse effect of bleomycin (Blenoxane). Primary side effects of 5-fluorouracil (5-FU) are GI (nausea and vomiting) and immune (leucopenia). Primary side effects of etoposide (Vepesid) are myelosuppression, anaphylaxis, and bronchospasms. Primary side effects of paclitaxel (Taxol) are neutropenia, thrombocytopenia, and peripheral neuropathy. **Cognitive Level:** Analyzing **Client Need:** Pharmacological and Parenteral Therapies **Integrated Process:** Nursing Process: Assessment **Content Area:** Pharmacology **Strategy:** It is helpful to think of "blue for bleomycin" to recall that it has significant respiratory adverse effects. **Reference:** Adams, M., Holland, L., & Bostwick, P. (2011). *Pharmacology for nurses: A pathophysiologic approach* (3rd ed.). Upper Saddle River, NJ: Pearson Education, p. 557. Wilson, B. A., Shannon, M. T., & Shields, K. M. (2011). *Pearson intravenous drug guide 2011–2012* (2nd ed.). Upper Saddle River, NJ: Pearson Education, pp. 94–96.

5 **Answer: 2** **Rationale:** Clients receiving chemotherapy have reduced immunity and are at greater risk for opportunistic infections. Intact skin and mucous membranes are the body's first defense against infection. The nurse should also work to prevent any alteration that could result in significant discomfort or change in body image, but they do not override the risk of an infection. Occurrence of mucositis has no relationship to cancer recurrence. **Cognitive Level:** Applying **Client Need:** Pharmacological and Parenteral Therapies **Integrated Process:** Nursing Process: Diagnosis **Content Area:** Pharmacology **Strategy:** Select the option that places the client at greatest risk. **Reference:** Adams, M., Holland, L., & Bostwick, P. (2011). *Pharmacology for nurses: A pathophysiologic approach* (3rd ed.). Upper Saddle River, NJ: Pearson Education, p. 552.

6 **Answer: 1** **Rationale:** Being female as well as having a positive history of non–disease-oriented nausea indicates the mother of 2 is more likely to experience chemotherapy-induced nausea. Because the pilot presents with only one of the predisposing factors (childhood motion sickness), this client is at risk to a lesser degree than a client with non–disease-oriented nausea. Since alcoholism predisposes to dehydration, the 38-year-old client presents with one predisposing factor. The female client without a history of non–disease-producing nausea is less likely to experience chemotherapy-induced nausea than a client with a history of morning sickness. **Cognitive Level:** Analyzing **Client Need:** Pharmacological and Parenteral Therapies **Integrated Process:** Nursing Process: Diagnosis **Content Area:** Pharmacology **Strategy:** Apply knowledge of characteristics of nausea experiences to clients receiving chemotherapy. **Reference:** Adams, M., Holland, L., & Bostwick, P. (2011). *Pharmacology for nurses: A pathophysiologic approach* (3rd ed.). Upper Saddle River, NJ: Pearson Education, pp. 552–555.

7 **Answer: 3** **Rationale:** Any activity that increases the potential for infection should be avoided. Since most clients become septic from organisms on their skin and in their environment, meticulous hygiene is the best way to prevent infection. An indwelling catheter is a source of infection and should only be used if the client is immobile and has a high risk for skin breakdown. Dressings should cover all open wounds to prevent contamination. Long-term catheters should be flushed after use or every 8 hours to prevent clotting; however, this will not decrease the client's risk for infection. **Cognitive Level:** Applying **Client Need:** Pharmacological and Parenteral Therapies **Integrated Process:** Nursing Process: Planning **Content Area:** Pharmacology **Strategy:** Associate the function of neutrophils (fighting infection) with the nursing care activity that also best fights infection. **Reference:** LeMone, P., Burke, K., & Bauldoff, G. (2011). *Medical-surgical nursing: Critical thinking in patient care* (5th ed.). Upper Saddle River, NJ: Pearson Education, pp. 1091–1092.

8 **Answer: 3** **Rationale:** Once stomatitis develops, meticulous oral hygiene must continue with a soft toothbrush and fluoride-containing toothpaste, and rinsing with a dilute baking soda solution. The nurse should provide cleansing along with rinsing during the night as well as during the day. Dilute hydrogen peroxide mouthwashes are not recommended since they can dry the mouth and inhibit granulation tissue formation. Commercial mouthwashes are never recommended since they usually contain alcohol, which is drying and can burn. **Cognitive Level:** Applying **Client Need:** Pharmacological and Parenteral Therapies **Integrated Process:** Nursing Process: Planning **Content Area:** Pharmacology **Strategy:** Evaluate each of the options in terms of how well they provide cleansing to reduce the bacteria count in the mouth, and by the gentleness of the products used to reduce the risk of further tissue breakdown. **Reference:** Adams, M., & Urban, C. (2013). *Pharmacology: Connections to nursing practice* (2nd ed.). Upper Saddle River, NJ: Pearson Education, p. 1048.

9 **Answer: 1, 2, 4** **Rationale:** Increasing fiber in the diet increases bulk and gastric motility, thereby decreasing constipation. Increasing activity along is likely to prevent constipation. Increased fluid intake could help reduce the occurrence by increasing the intestinal volume, which increases peristalsis. The use of stool softeners

should be encouraged, but laxative usage should be kept to a minimum to prevent becoming laxative dependent. Clients receiving chemotherapy are at risk for nutritional imbalance and should avoid ingesting anything that would increase loss of nutrients. The purpose of an antiflatulent is to reduce bloating, but this will not prevent constipation, although it would be helpful for clients following a meal high in gas-producing foods. **Cognitive Level:** Applying **Client Need:** Pharmacological and Parenteral Therapies **Integrated Process:** Nursing Process: Implementation **Content Area:** Pharmacology **Strategy:** Associate requirements for normal intestinal functioning with the threat of constipation. **Reference:** Wilson, B. A., Shannon, M. T., & Shields, K. M. (2011). *Pearson intravenous drug guide 2011–2012* (2nd ed.). Upper Saddle River, NJ: Pearson Education, pp. 682–684.

10 **Answer: 2** **Rationale:** Single-category chemotherapy leads to major tumor drug resistance. Most malignant tumors are comprised of cells at various stages of development. Because combination chemotherapy can attack cells at various stages of development, it has proven to be more successful in reducing tumor size and tumor resistance. Combined therapy can compound the nausea and vomiting response. The primary goal is reduce tumor size and treat any parallel side effects. Depending on the drugs, the effect on normal cells can be greater, but this is less relevant than tumor reduction. If drugs have an affinity for gonadal tissue, this will not be reduced by combination chemotherapy. **Cognitive Level:** Applying **Client Need:** Pharmacological and Parenteral Therapies **Integrated Process:** Nursing Process: Diagnosis **Content Area:** Pharmacology **Strategy:** Correlate the nature of cancerous growths with the nature and purpose of chemotherapy. **Reference:** Adams, M., Holland, L., & Bostwick, P. (2011). *Pharmacology for nurses: A pathophysiologic approach* (3rd ed.). Upper Saddle River, NJ: Pearson Education, p. 552.

Posttest

1 **Answer: 1, 4, 2, 3** **Rationale:** Discontinuation of medication is first priority in order to minimize the damage caused to the tissue. Vesicant therapy will cause tissue irritation with eventual sloughing without the appropriate antidote, which should be utilized immediately after discontinuing the infusion. Protocols should be in place to administer the antidote promptly to neutralize the vesicant and minimize tissue trauma. The priority is not choosing a new site for administration, but preventing tissue damage. However, the infusion should be completed at another intravenous site once the site is cared for. The site should be observed for 3 to 4 weeks, but a plastic surgeon need only be consulted if tissue damage actually occurs. **Cognitive Level:** Applying **Client Need:** Pharmacological and Parenteral Therapies **Integrated Process:** Nursing Process: Implementation **Content Area:** Adult Health **Strategy:** Recall that cancer chemotherapeutic drugs are more likely to be vesicants because of the nature in which they work. When an IV line infiltrates, consider this risk the priority and order the options that minimizes local tissue damage. **Reference:** Adams, M., Holland, L., & Bostwick, P. (2011). *Pharmacology for nurses: A pathophysiologic approach* (3rd ed.). Upper Saddle River, NJ: Pearson Education, p. 553.

2 Answer: 1 Rationale: Cystitis can occur in the urinary bladder after administration of cyclophosphamide or ifosfamide. This could lead to hematuria and dysuria. Damage to the renal tubules is more likely to occur after the administration of methotrexate (Mexate), streptozocin (Zanosar), and cisplatin (Platinol AQ), and signs would then reflect renal impairment rather than bladder symptoms. **Cognitive Level:** Analyzing **Client Need:** Pharmacological and Parenteral Therapies **Integrated Process:** Nursing Process: Assessment **Content Area:** Pharmacology **Strategy:** The core issue of the question is being able to identify which drug is most likely to cause damage to the urinary bladder. Associate the *cy* in the beginning of the word *cystitis* and the name *cyclophosphamide* as a strategy to remember the adverse effects of this drug. **Reference:** Wilson, B. A., Shannon, M. T., & Shields, K. M. (2011). *Pearson intravenous drug guide 2011–2012* (2nd ed.). Upper Saddle River, NJ: Pearson Education, pp. 187–190.

3 Answer: 2 Rationale: Cerebellar syndrome characterized by headache, disorientation, and nystagmus may persist after administration ceases. Myelosuppression is *not* unique to 5-fluorouracil (5-FU). Nausea and vomiting are common to most antineoplastic drugs and generally cease after administration ends. Alopecia is not unique to this drug and will resolve after treatment is completed. **Cognitive Level:** Applying **Client Need:** Pharmacological and Parenteral Therapies **Integrated Process:** Teaching and Learning **Content Area:** Pharmacology **Strategy:** Specific drug knowledge is needed to answer this question. Focus on the critical word *unique* in the question and select the most unusual adverse effect from those listed. **Reference:** Wilson, B. A., Shannon, M. T., & Shields, K. M. (2011). *Pearson intravenous drug guide 2011-2012* (2nd ed.). Upper Saddle River, NJ: Pearson Education, pp. 319–322.

4 Answer: 1, 4, 3, 2 Rationale: Cardiotoxicity is ranked first because this impaired the most relevant life-sustaining body function. Hepatotoxicity is ranked second because of the risk of bleeding and possible hemorrhage; also, the liver performs many life-sustaining activities. Myelosuppression ranks third because infection and generalized bleeding are important after heart function and the risk of hemorrhage are addressed. Neurotoxicity is not as common as myelosuppression and this toxic effect is not as life-threatening, making it fourth in priority. **Cognitive Level:** Analyzing **Client Need:** Pharmacological and Parenteral Therapies **Integrated Process:** Nursing Process: Planning **Content Area:** Pharmacology **Strategy:** Select the most significant side effect that that could

occur with antineoplastic agents (remember there is only one heart). Then rank the adverse effects according to the immediacy and magnitude of the effect(s) on the client. **Reference:** Adams, M., & Koch, R. (2010). *Pharmacology: Connections to nursing practice.* Upper Saddle River, NJ: Pearson Education., pp. 958–960.

5 Answer: 1, 2, 5, 3, 4 Rationale: Since fear and anxiety are commonly associated with management of a cancer diagnosis, clarifying information and dispelling the myths that surround cancer and cancer treatment should be the initial step in client and family education. Learning occurs more readily when the anxiety level is minimal. Informed consent helps the client anticipate the outcomes of the chemotherapy; the informed must be completed after initial education is performed. Safe gowning and gloving are nursing procedures that should be performed with administration of the chemotherapy to prevent injury to both the client and nurse. Bone marrow suppression, as evidenced by decreased platelet, WBC, and RBC counts, should be evaluated at the nadir postchemotherapy. The nadir occurs at different times depending on the chemotherapeutic agent administered. **Cognitive Level:** Analyzing **Client Need:** Safety and Infection Control **Integrated Process:** Nursing Process: Implementation **Content Area:** Adult Health **Strategy:** Visualize sequence of events in order to administer chemotherapy safely. **Reference:** LeMone, P., Burke, K., & Bauldoff, G. (2011). *Medical-surgical nursing: Critical thinking in patient care* (5th ed.). Upper Saddle River, NJ: Pearson Education, pp. 371–372. Adams, M., & Koch, R. (2010). *Pharmacology: Connections to nursing practice.* Upper Saddle River, NJ: Pearson Education, p. 958.

6 Answer: 3 Rationale: Drugs that are cell-cycle specific act preferentially on cells that are proliferating (dividing). Cells that are rapidly dividing tend to be more sensitive to these drugs. The statement about medical jargon that is not related to care violates a standard of practice that requires the nurse to provide clients with a reasonable response to their questions. The term addresses the phase of cell development rather than specific type. Cells move through one cycle rather than several. **Cognitive Level:** Applying **Client Need:** Pharmacological and Parenteral Therapies **Integrated Process:** Teaching and Learning **Content Area:** Pharmacology **Strategy:** Select the option that best describes the term *cell-cycle specific* as it relates to chemotherapy. **Reference:** Adams, M., Holland, L., & Bostwick, P. (2011). *Pharmacology for nurses: A pathophysiologic approach* (3rd ed.). Upper Saddle River, NJ: Pearson Education, pp. 550–552.

7 Answer: 1 Rationale: Because non–cell-cycle-specific drugs do not differentiate between normal and abnormal cells as well as cell-cycle-specific drugs, they tend to be more toxic. The side effects mentioned often cease after administration of the drugs end. There is no evidence that worsening of the signs and symptoms is related to the response of the lesion. This may unnecessarily increase the anxiety level. Because of the high level of anxiety, the nurse should help the client understand the reason for the change in the intensity of the signs and symptoms. **Cognitive Level:** Applying **Client Need:** Pharmacological and Parenteral Therapies **Integrated Process:** Communication and Documentation **Content Area:** Pharmacology **Strategy:** Compare and contrast the significant differences between the 2 drug groups. **Reference:** Adams, M., Holland, L., & Bostwick, P. (2011). *Pharmacology for nurses: A pathophysiologic approach* (3rd ed.). Upper Saddle River, NJ: Pearson Education, pp. 553–554.

8 **Answer: 2 Rationale:** Doxorubicin (Adriamycin) has a dose-limiting cardiotoxic effect that is more pronounced in the older adult clients and the pediatric clients. The major side effect of vincristine (Adriamycin) is peripheral neuropathy. There is no evidence that the side effect is gender related. The major side effects of nitrogen mustard are severe nausea and vomiting and thrombocytopenia. There are no known gender-related side effects. The major side effects of cisplatin (Platinol) are severe nausea, vomiting, and nephrotoxicity. There are no known culture-related side effects. **Cognitive Level:** Analyzing **Client Need:** Pharmacological and Parenteral Therapies **Integrated Process:** Nursing Process: Assessment **Content Area:** Pharmacology **Strategy:** Correlate client demographics, the antineoplastic category, and cardiotoxicity. **Reference:** Wilson, B. A., Shannon, M. T., & Shields, K. M. (2011). *Pearson intravenous drug guide 2011–2012* (2nd ed.). Upper Saddle River, NJ: Pearson Education, pp. 171–174, 259–264, 440–442, 682–684.

9 **Answer: 1, 4, 5 Rationale:** Filgrastim is a hematopoietic growth factor that increases the production of neutrophils. A client with a decreased neutrophil count does need to be educated about proper infection control practices. Also, exposure should be limited, since exposure to even a mild illness may cause sepsis and death in a client with decreased neutrophils. Whole blood transfusion contains RBCs and is not indicated at this time. Epogen is a hematopoietic growth factor that stimulates the production of RBCs and is not indicated based on the information given. **Cognitive Level:** Analyzing **Client Need:** Pharmacological and Parenteral Therapies **Integrated Process:** Nursing Process: Implementation **Content Area:** Adult Health **Strategy:** Correlate the drug with the remedy most likely to reverse or reduce the problem. **Reference:** Wilson, B. A., Shannon, M. T., & Shields, K. M. (2011). *Pearson intravenous drug guide 2011–2012* (2nd ed.). Upper Saddle River, NJ: Pearson Education, pp. 284–285, 311–313, 388–390.

10 **Answer: 4 Rationale:** Although a client's physical well-being and response to previous treatments are important to know, toxicities of the drug commonly determine the maximum amount of the drug that can be administered safely. The number of cancer cells in the body has little to do with the dose limitations of the medications. Checking with the health care provider will not resolve the problem. The primary health history feature most likely to determine dosage is influenced more by organs involved in metabolism and elimination. Because chemotherapy is systemic and can have a whole body effect, size of the lesion will not determine the maximum dosage. **Cognitive Level:** Applying **Client Need:** Pharmacological and Parenteral Therapies **Integrated Process:** Communication and Documentation **Content Area:** Pharmacology **Strategy:** Apply knowledge of the criteria used to determine chemotherapy dosages. **Reference:** Adams, M., Holland, L., & Bostwick, P. (2011). *Pharmacology for nurses: A pathophysiologic approach* (3rd ed.). Upper Saddle River, NJ: Pearson Education, p. 552.

References

Abrams, A. (2009). *Clinical drug therapy: Rationales for nursing practice* (9th ed.). Philadelphia, PA: Lippincott Williams & Wilkins.

Adams, M., Holland, L., & Bostwick, P. (2011). *Pharmacology for nurses: A pathophysiologic approach* (3rd ed.). Upper Saddle River, NJ: Pearson Education.

Adams, M., & Urban, C. (2013). *Pharmacology: Connections to nursing practice* (2nd ed.). Upper Saddle River, NJ: Pearson Education.

Aschenbrenner, D., & Venable, S. (2012). *Drug therapy in nursing* (4th ed.). Philadelphia, PA: Lippincott Williams & Wilkins.

Drug Facts & Comparisons® (Updated monthly). St. Louis, MO: A. Wolters Kluwer.

Karch, A. M. (2010). *Focus on nursing pharmacology* (5th ed.). Philadelphia, PA: Lippincott Williams & Wilkins.

Kee, J. (2009). *Laboratory and diagnostic tests and nursing implications* (8th ed.). Upper Saddle River, NJ: Pearson Education.

Lehne, R. (2010). *Pharmacology for nursing care* (7th ed.). St. Louis, MO: Mosby, Inc.

LeMone, P., Burke, K. M., & Bauldoff, G. (2011). *Medical-surgical nursing: Critical thinking in patient care* (5th ed.). Upper Saddle River, NJ: Pearson Education.

Wilson, B. A., Shannon, M. T., Shields, K. M. (2011). *Pearson intravenous drug guide 2011–2012* (2nd ed.). Upper Saddle River, NJ: Pearson Education.

Blood Modifying Agents

4

Chapter Outline

Anticoagulants
Antiplatelet Agents
Thrombolytics

Hemostatics
Medications to Treat Anemia

Medications to Lower Serum
Cholesterol

Objectives

➤ Describe goals of therapy related to the various blood-modifying medications.
➤ Identify significant nursing interventions for the client receiving an anticoagulant, antiplatelet, or thrombolytic medication.
➤ Identify antidotes for hemorrhage caused by various anticoagulants.
➤ Identify common side effects of medications used to lower serum cholesterol.
➤ Discuss nursing considerations related to administration of iron, vitamin B_{12}, or folic acid.
➤ Identify dietary sources of iron, vitamin B_{12}, and folic acid.
➤ Describe the action and use of epoetin alfa (Epogen, Procrit).
➤ List significant client education points related to various blood-modifying medications.

NCLEX-RN® Test Prep

Use the accompanying online resource, NursingReviewsandRationales, to test yourself with hundreds of NCLEX®-style practice questions.

Review at a Glance

activated partial thromboplastin time (APTT) a blood test used to determine intrinsic clotting response that is measured in seconds; used to monitor and evaluate a client's response to heparin

aggregation an accumulation of substances such as platelets in the blood that form a group or cluster

anticoagulants substances that prevent or delay the coagulation of blood

antithrombin III (ATIII) a specific substance in the clotting cascade that prevents the activation of three clotting factors (thrombin, activated IX, and activated X)

clotting cascade a coagulation pathway in which enzymes and specific blood factors interact to effectively maintain normal hemostasis in the body; includes both extrinsic and intrinsic

pathways and leads to conversion of prothrombin to thrombin

extrinsic pathway pathway in clotting cascade that acts within seconds to form fibrin; PT and INR measure extrinsic pathway function

fibrinolysis process whereby clot dissolution takes place utilizing specific plasminogen activators in the body to prevent excessive clotting that could lead to vascular obstruction

fibrinolytic system mechanism for releasing plasmin (through the use of plasminogen activators) to act on fibrin (blood) clot and cause it to dissolve

hemostatics substances, devices, or procedures that stop the flow of blood

heparin-induced platelet aggregation (HITT) a potentially fatal complication of heparin therapy, whereby the client develops new clot

formation with severe thrombocytopenia; it is also called white clot syndrome; HITT stands for heparin-induced thrombocytopenia and thrombosis

hypercoagulation a process whereby blood coagulates faster, leading to potential problems in the coagulation cascade

International Normalized Ratio (INR) a standard reference range used to establish consistency in reporting PT levels that accounts for normal variations seen in lab testing; INR leads to a better consensus of therapeutic management and ensures that evaluation of test results are based on common standards

intrinsic pathway pathway in clotting cascade that takes several minutes to form fibrin; intrinsic pathway function is measured by the APTT

PRETEST

low molecular weight heparin (LMWH) a term that refers to a group of heparin products that are comparable in molecular weight and have a higher bioavailability than traditional heparin

pernicious anemia a specific type of megaloblastic, macrocytic anemia that is related to the lack of intrinsic factor necessary for absorption of vitamin B_{12} in the GI tract

pica ingestion of nonfood substances, such as chalk, dirt, or paint, that can lead to nutritional deficiency states (and sometimes potential toxicity); it can be seen as a type of craving for these substances

protamine sulfate antidote used for heparin

prothrombin time (PT) a blood test used to measure in seconds extrinsic clotting response; a control level is run with the test to determine a standard

response; used to monitor and evaluate response to oral anticoagulation therapy

purple toe syndrome a complication of oral anticoagulation therapy, whereby vascular emboli are released leading to microemboli formation in the toes and disruption of circulation

thrombolytics a group of substances that break down existing clots in the vascular system to restore blood flow and circulation

PRETEST

1 A client diagnosed with iron deficiency anemia is taking iron supplements. The nurse should instruct the client to include which of the following foods to enhance the absorption of the medication?

1. Green leafy vegetables
2. Whole grain bread and cereals
3. Raisins at least 3 times per week
4. Orange juice or lemonade

2 After taking an antiplatelet medication for several weeks, a client presents with a noticeable bruise on the right arm. What assessment data is most significant to managing the client's health needs?

1. Whether the bruise is the result of a specific injury
2. Whether the client is taking the medication as prescribed
3. If the client self-monitors for skin manifestations
4. If the client's response to injury is different now

3 A client has been taking iron therapy for treatment of anemia. To evaluate drug effectiveness, the nurse reviews which laboratory test result as the best verification of iron stores in the body?

1. Ferritin level
2. Transferrin level
3. Hematocrit
4. Complete blood count (CBC)

4 When alteplase (Activase) is administered to a client diagnosed with a cerebrovascular accident (CVA or stroke) in the emergency department, the nurse determines that the priority nursing interventions in this client's care should include which of the following? Select all that apply.

1. After administration, assess vital signs every 15 minutes during the first hour.
2. Report dysrhythmias noted on the cardiac monitor.
3. Insert urinary catheter and maintain accurate hourly output measures.
4. Monitor client for hypothermia for first 8 hours after infusion.
5. Report increase in partial thromboplastin time (PTT).

5 A client is taking epoetin alfa (Epogen) for treatment of anemia related to chronic renal disease. The nurse uses which clinical finding as the best measure of the drug's therapeutic effectiveness?

1. The client is not experiencing any related bone pain when the medication is being administered.
2. The hemoglobin and hematocrit (H&H) levels are rising rapidly based on latest two daily blood draws.
3. The client's hemoglobin increases to 12 grams/dL.
4. The client maintains an afebrile state.

6 What information should the nurse present in an educational seminar for clients who are taking nicotinic acid (Niacin) for elevated cholesterol levels? Select all that apply.

1. Because niacin treatment is individualized, dose adjustments are correlated with lab values.
2. Facial flushing may occur immediately after ingesting dose.
3. Eat a diet high in niacin to ensure that the medication works effectively.
4. For maximum effect, niacin can be taken concurrently with lovastatin (Mevacor).
5. Taking an aspirin 30 minutes before taking niacin helps to reduce flushing.

7 A 69-year-old client, who is taking desmopressin (DDAVP) for von Willebrand's disease, asks the nurse to provide information about the drug. An appropriate response by the nurse includes which statements? Select all that apply.

1. "DDAVP helps restore and release deficient clotting factors (vW and VIII) that are reduced in von Willebrand's disease."
2. "You can ask your health care provider about using an intranasal preparation."
3. "You should monitor your fluid intake and output while taking this drug."
4. "Take your blood pressure every day while taking this drug."
5. "You will receive cryoprecipitate transfusions while you are taking this drug."

8 The home health nurse instructs the client to avoid taking ibuprofen (Motrin) after noting a decrease in which laboratory test result?

1. Ferritin level
2. Triglyceride level
3. Neutrophil count
4. Platelet count

9 The nurse is providing medication information about warfarin (Coumadin) to a client who is being discharged following a mechanical heart valve replacement. Which item of information would provide the best protection to the client? Select all that apply.

1. "Follow-up lab testing is required every 3 months."
2. "Use an electric razor and a soft toothbrush."
3. "Take this medication upon arising in the morning on an empty stomach."
4. "If a dose is missed, take the missed dose with the next scheduled dose."
5. "Eat a diet containing consistent but not large amounts of vitamin K."

10 The nurse received an order to start intravenous (IV) heparin (Liquaemin) on a client admitted with deep vein thrombosis (DVT). To implement this order appropriately, what action should the nurse take?

1. Place vitamin K at the bedside.
2. Tell client about need for being NPO while the medication is infusing.
3. Use an infusion pump to administer the drug.
4. Weigh the client twice weekly.

➤ *See pages 155–156 for Answers and Rationales.*

I. ANTICOAGULANTS

A. Oral medications

1. Action and use

    a. Oral **anticoagulants**, substances that prevent or delay blood coagulation, are used both to treat and prevent thromboembolic disorders in clients who are at risk; these disorders result from increased clotting activity, increased platelets, or both

    b. Vitamin K plays an active role in **extrinsic pathway** (a pathway that forms fibrin and acts within seconds) of **clotting cascade** (a coagulation pathway)

    c. Oral anticoagulants such as warfarin (Coumadin and its derivatives) prevent conversion of vitamin K, thereby decreasing its production in liver

    d. With vitamin K production reduced, several clotting factors (II, VII, IX, and X) are also reduced, thereby prolonging the clotting cascade

    e. Coumadin is bound to plasma proteins, most notably albumin, and is metabolized in liver

    f. Oral anticoagulants are used to manage clients with actual, potential, and recurrent health problems such as deep vein thrombosis (DVT), pulmonary embolism (PE), acute myocardial infarction (AMI), heart valve replacement (bioprosthetic and mechanical), atrial fibrillation, and antiphospholipid syndrome

    g. Selective factor Xa inhibitors inhibit thrombosis through specific action on just factor Xa in the clotting cascade

2. Common medications

    a. Coumarin derivative warfarin sodium (Coumadin) is probably the most frequently used oral anticoagulant in the United States

    b. Warfarin (Coumadin) is given orally at a usual dose of 1 to 15 mg daily, with dose titrated to keep INR 2 to 3

    c. Dabigatran (Pradaxa) is a direct thrombin inhibitor indicated for stroke prevention in clients with atrial fibrillation

    d. Rivaroxaban (Xarelto) is an anti-Xa inhibitor approved for stroke prevention in clients with atrial fibrillation

 3. Administration considerations

    a. Coumadin requires close monitoring (because of a narrow therapeutic range), frequent dose adjustments (because of individual dose response), and a high potential for the development of interactions (involving food and drug interactions) that can lead to ineffective therapy or toxicity

    b. Coumadin's onset of action is slow, and its full anticoagulant effect is not seen until after approximately 1 week; thus, the drug may be started while a client is still on heparin therapy and overlap as heparin is tapered once desirable anticoagulation has been reached

    c. **Prothrombin time (PT)**, a blood test used to measure extrinsic clotting response, and **International Normalized Ratio (INR)**, a standard reference range used to establish consistency in reporting PT levels, may be used to monitor client's response to therapy

    d. Coumadin is usually given in the evening after reviewing pertinent laboratory test results drawn earlier in day

    e. Depending on indication for therapy, desired range of PT or INR will vary; PT levels usually are felt to be effective when they are maintained at 1.5 to 2.5 times the control value; INR levels range from a usual 2.0 to 3.0 to a higher range of 3.0 to 4.5 if client has a mechanical cardiac valve replacement

    f. Duration of therapy can range from several months to lifelong depending on client's specific health problem

    g. Refer to agency protocol and provider's prescription for dose adjustments and monitoring of client's PT and INR levels

    h. Vitamin K is the antidote that reverses the action of Coumadin

4. Contraindications

    a. Oral anticoagulants are contraindicated in clients who are pregnant

    b. Lactating women can take warfarin as it will cross through in breast milk but there is little effect on an infant's PT; however, if infant were to require surgery, it would be advisable to obtain infant's PT as a baseline

    c. Oral anticoagulants should not be given to clients who are hemorrhaging or have bleeding tendencies, have malignant hypertension, or have a past history of allergic reaction to coumarin derivatives

    d. Clients with co-morbid conditions such as liver failure and congestive heart failure (CHF) may have problems with metabolism and utilization of the drug

    e. Dosage reduction for rivaroxaban and dabigatran are indicated in renal impairment

    f. A black box warning for rivaroxaban recommends use of another anticoagulant when rivaroxaban is stopped, since clients have an increased risk for stroke

5. Significant drug interactions

    a. Because Coumadin competes for binding sites in liver, there is a high potential for drug interactions relative to enzyme inhibitors and enzyme inducers; these chemical reactions will affect the serum concentration level of Coumadin

    b. Coumadin is considered to be a primary example of a medication that has complex interactions with a vast number of medications; it is 99% protein bound, contributing to these interactions

    c. Refer to Table 4-1 for a partial listing of medications that can potentiate and diminish the effect of Coumadin

    d. The use of herbal medications will be discussed in the next section because the Food and Drug Administration (FDA) considers these to be dietary supplements

6. Significant food interactions

    a. Increased effects are seen with chondroitin and garlic

    b. There is an increased bleeding risk seen with cayenne, feverfew, garlic, ginger, and Gingko biloba

    c. Decreased drug effectiveness is seen with use of green tea, ginseng, and goldenseal

    d. The action of oral anticoagulants can be dramatically diminished by an increase in dietary sources of vitamin K

    e. Foods high in vitamin K such as liver, cheese, egg yolk, leafy vegetables (broccoli, cabbage, spinach, and kale), and oils (peanut, corn, olive, or soybean) should be limited and sources should be taken regularly during therapy to help maintain steady blood levels

    f. Dietary supplements of vitamin K should be avoided

    g. Alcohol use should be restricted (if not avoided) to maintain effective drug therapy

Table 4-1	**Partial Listing of Coumadin Drug Interactions**
Drugs That Potentiate Action	**Drugs That Decrease Action**
Acetaminophen and acetylsalicylic acid (ASA)	Alcohol
Antibiotics	Barbiturates
H_2-histamine-receptor antagonists	Estrogens/oral contraceptives
Loop diuretics	Spironolactone
Nonsteroidal anti-inflammatory drugs (NSAIDs)	Thiazide diuretics
Sulfonamides	Thyroid drugs
Vitamin E	Vitamin K

  h. Increased effects due to prolonged excretion of warfarin may occur when taken with cranberry juice, fruit, or supplements

  i. Referral to a dietitian is always indicated for clients receiving Coumadin therapy because of the many potential dietary interactions and possibility of prolonged treatment with this type of medication

7. Significant laboratory studies

  a. Discoloration of urine (red-orange) can be seen with use of coumarin derivatives and may be of concern to client

  b. A hematologist should evaluate clients who are resistant to anticoagulation treatment with these types of medications for other specific underlying disorders of coagulation that might affect therapy

8. Side effects

  a. Ecchymosis of skin, or bleeding from any tissue or organ

  b. Gastrointestinal (GI) and dermatologic problems

  c. Hypotension

  d. Thrombocytopenia

9. Adverse effects/toxicity

  a. Bleeding is the major adverse effect and is usually seen at higher dosage levels

  b. GI: nausea, diarrhea, intestinal obstruction, anorexia, abdominal cramping

  c. Dermatologic manifestations: rash, urticaria, and **purple toe syndrome** (discoloration caused by decreased perfusion from release of microemboli)

  d. Increased serum transaminase levels, hepatitis, jaundice

  e. Burning sensation of feet

  f. Transient hair loss

10. Nursing considerations

  a. Monitor client's PT and INR with initiation and continuation of therapy

  b. Review client's medications and dietary history with regard to potential drug and food interactions; be sure to include nutritional and herbal supplements

  c. Notify prescriber of current PT and/or INR results, making note of client's current dose

  d. Communicate with dietitian regarding client's status and anticipate discharge planning needs as therapy continues

  e. Assess client's skin for bleeding tendencies and monitor for GI side effects

  f. Client teaching is critically important because of many potential interactions, length of therapy, and close follow-up monitoring required

  g. Vitamin K may be ordered to reverse effects of Coumadin depending on PT or INR; it can be ordered as a single-dose therapy if high PT and INR values persist; additional doses of vitamin K may be given, and the Coumadin dose may be withheld

  h. If the client experiences adverse effects or toxicity, withhold dose of Coumadin; depending on INR or client manifestations, administration of phytonadione (vitamin K) may be indicated

  i. If there is significant bleeding, prescriber may order transfusion of fresh frozen plasma (FFP) or prothrombin concentrate

11. Client education

  a. Establish individualized teaching goals that increase client's knowledge of disease process and improve compliance with long-term therapy

  b. Alert client to bleeding problems and how to respond

  c. Frequent follow-up blood tests will be required to make sure safe therapeutic therapy is maintained

  d. Point-of-care (POC) testing is available for self-monitoring of PT and INR; prescriber may establish a home protocol to help manage care and necessary dosage adjustments

        e. Dose must be taken on a daily basis; it cannot be stopped unless prescriber orders a dose to be withheld (pending PT or INR results) or client experiences a bleeding episode

        f. Communication between client and all health care team members is an essential part of therapeutic management

        g. Use a soft toothbrush and electric razor to minimize even mild trauma that could lead to bleeding

        h. Observe for bleeding gums, bruises, nosebleeds, tarry stools, hematuria, hematemesis, and petechiae; report these findings to prescriber

        i. Teach client to avoid excessive intake of foods high in vitamin K (see previous section)

        j. Teach clients importance of taking dabigatran and rivaroxaban on a daily basis and avoid skipping doses; these drugs have short half-lives and daily intake is important

B. Heparin and other related medications

    1. Action and use

        a. Heparin is a heterogeneous group of substances that exert anticoagulant effects; they have different molecular weights and other chemical properties that influence vascular system

        b. Heparin plays an active role in **intrinsic pathway** (where fibrin formation occurs and takes several minutes) in clotting cascade

        c. Heparin combines with a plasma heparin cofactor named **antithrombin III (ATIII)**, and this complex causes inactivation of specific clotting factors (II_a, X_a, XII_a, XI_a, and IX_a) in clotting cascade

        d. Heparin/ATIII complex has a very strong anticoagulant effect that inhibits conversion of fibrinogen to fibrin, prevents formation of a fibrin clot, and inhibits thrombin

        e. Molecular weight of the heparin molecule can range from 3,000 to 30,000 daltons (d), with average weight near 15,000 d; the standard measurement used is unfractionated heparin (UFH); **low molecular weight heparin (LMWH)** is also available with a molecular weight range of 4,000 to 6,500 d

        f. Because of its immediate effect, heparin is treatment of choice for clients who have DVT, PE, and embolism resulting from atrial fibrillation

        g. It is used as prophylaxis in clients at risk for developing thrombi as a result of surgical intervention

        h. It is used in a weak concentration as a flush solution to maintain patency and prevent thrombus formation in vascular access devices

        i. Direct thrombin inhibitors directly inhibit action of thrombin without the intermediate step of antithrombin III inhibition; they are administered IV using a 15–20 second bolus or by continuous infusion; they are indicated in treatment of heparin-induced thrombocytopenia (HIT), and to prevent associated thromboembolic events

    2. Common medications

        a. LMWH is a newer class of heparin molecule consisting of heparin fragments, with enoxaparin (Lovenox) being most commonly used

        b. Heparin (Liquaemin) sodium is the most commonly used anticoagulant for treatment and prevention of recurrent thromboembolic episodes

        c. Lepirudin (Refludan), argatroban (Argatroban), bivalirudin (Angiomax), and desirudin (Iprivask) are direct thrombin inhibitors used in the treatment of HIT

        d. Refer to Table 4-2 for a listing of heparin anticoagulants

    3. Administration considerations

        a. Heparin can be administered intravenously (IV) or by subcutaneous (subQ) injection

        b. Heparin bioavailability is influenced by its mode of administration and its chemical formulation; LMWH has a higher bioavailability when compared to standard UFH

Table 4-2	Heparin and Related Medications	
Generic (Trade) Names	**Route**	**Uses**
Heparins		
Heparin (Liquaemin)	IV, subQ	Diagnosis and treatment of deep intravascular clotting, prevention of clotting during dialysis, prevention of clot extension, deep vein thrombosis, pulmonary embolism, post-stroke, post–myocardial infarction, prophylactic in clients with a risk of thrombus formation, atrial fibrillation
Low Molecular Weight Heparins		
Ardeparin (Normiflo)	PO, IM, IV, subQ	Prevention of deep vein thrombosis after knee replacement, secondary prophylaxis for recurrent thromboembolic event
Dalteparin (Fragmin)	subQ	Unstable angina, non–Q-wave myocardial infarction, prevention of deep vein thrombosis that may lead to pulmonary embolism, status post–abdominal surgery or hip replacement, adjunct to antineoplastic chemotherapy
Danaparoid (Orgaran)	IV, subQ	Prevention of deep vein thrombosis, treatment of thromboembolism, anticoagulation during hemodialysis, hemofiltration, pregnant clients who are at risk for thromboembolism; used as a heparinoid in clients who develop heparin induced thrombocytopenia (HIT)
Enoxaparin (Lovenox)	subQ	Prevention of deep vein thrombosis, prevent development of thromboembolism following hip replacement, status post–abdominal surgery, treatment of deep vein thrombosis, prevention of ischemic complications of unstable angina, non–Q-wave myocardial infarction
Tinzaparin (Innohep)	subQ	Acute symptomatic deep vein thrombosis with or without pulmonary embolism when given with warfarin sodium
Direct Thrombin Inhibitors		
Lepirudin (Refludan)	IV	Treatment of active HIT and use in percutaneous coronary intervention procedures in clients at risk for HIT; unlabeled use: disseminated intravascular coagulopathy (DIC)
Argatroban (Argatroban)	IV	Used with ASA as an anticoagulant in clients undergoing percutaneous transluminal coronary angioplasty (PTCA), or clients at risk for HIT undergoing percutaneous coronary interventions
Bivalirudin (Angiomax)	IV	Prevention of deep vein thrombosis in clients undergoing joint replacement surgery, prevention of stroke in clients with nonvalvular atrial fibrillation
Dabigatran (Pradaxa)	IV	DVT prophylaxis in clients undergoing hip replacement surgery; off-label uses for prevention of thromboembolic events in clients with unstable angina or undergoing percutaneous coronary interventions
Desirudin (Iprivask)	IV	Prevention of deep vein thrombosis in clients undergoing joint replacement surgery, prevention of stroke in clients with nonvalvular atrial fibrillation
Selective Factor Xa Inhibitors		
Rivaroxaban (Xarelto)	PO	Prevention of deep vein thrombosis in clients undergoing joint replacement surgery and prevention of stroke in clients with nonvalvular atrial fibrillation

Legend: IM, intramuscular; IV, intravenous; PO, oral; subQ, subcutaneous

    c. Activated partial thromboplastin time (APTT) is a blood test that determines intrinsic clotting response and is measured in seconds; it is used to monitor a client who is receiving heparin therapy; results are trended over time to determine client response and therapeutic effect

    d. Low-dose UFH therapy is used as a prophylactic treatment for DVT; dosage ranges from 5,000 units subQ every 8–12 hours or 3 doses in immediate postoperative period per physician protocol; enoxaparin or Lovenox (a LMWH) is used clinically for this purpose and comes in prefilled syringes ready for individual use

Box 4-1	• Client weight should be obtained as a baseline for initiation of therapy.

**Heparin Weight-Based
Therapy Protocol
Management
Concerns**

- Client weight should be obtained as a baseline for initiation of therapy.
- Monitor daily weight and pertinent labs (aPTT).
- Hemoccult all stools to assess for possible adverse effect of bleeding.
- Titrate heparin dosage as needed based on results of aPTT.
- aPTT labs are usually ordered q6 hours until 2 consecutive therapeutic levels are obtained. At that time, aPTT can be ordered q24 hours.
- Once the client is stabilized, an oral anticoagulant such as Coumadin is usually added if client requires long-term therapy.
- Further monitoring of aPTT, PT, and INR is required as heparin is being discontinued and Coumadin being maintained as the method of anticoagulation.

! e. High-dose UFH therapy is done to achieve a therapeutic aPTT; aPTT levels should be stabilized at 1.5 to 2 times the control value

! f. An infusion pump is required for IV administration; it should be infused through a dedicated IV line because of its incompatibility profile

g. Heparin weight-based therapy protocol is a standard format used by prescribers in the clinical setting to effectively anticoagulate a client needing immediate intervention (refer to Box 4-1 for specific information relevant to protocol management)

h. Be sure to carefully identify strength on product label; several concentrations of IV heparin are available; some are used only as flushes for IV lines

! i. **Protamine sulfate** is the antidote to reverse heparin's action; dosage depends on dose of heparin given and time period elapsed following its administration; not more than 50 mg should be given in a 10-minute period; protamine sulfate is administered intravenous pyelogram (IVP)

j. Hypersensitivity or allergic reactions can be seen in clients receiving heparin, so epinephrine 1:1,000 should be readily available if a reaction develops

k. Thrombin inhibitors should not be administered to clients with active bleeding or those with an aPTT ratio of above 2.5

l. There is not a specific antidote for thrombin inhibitors, but since they have a very short half-life, discontinuation of an infusion leads to improved coagulation within a few hours

4. Contraindications

a. Uncontrolled bleeding, known hypersensitivity, and thrombocytopenia

b. Indirect (Heparin) and direct (Refludan) inhibitors should not be given with aspirin (ASA) and nonsteroidal anti-inflammatory drugs (NSAIDS), as this will increase risk of bleeding

c. LMWH are contraindicated in clients with active bleeding, thrombocytopenia, and/or heparin or pork allergy

! 5. Significant drug interactions: ASA, NSAIDS, and antiplatelet agents can potentiate anticoagulation effect and increase bleeding; herbal supplements such as ginger, garlic, feverfew, green tea, or gingko may increase risk of bleeding

! 6. Significant food interactions: Allergy to pork products may indicate a potential hypersensitivity to LMWH; green leafy vegetables (particularly those high in vitamin K, such as spinach) may be limited if adding warfarin therapy

7. Significant laboratory studies

a. Heparin prolongs aPPT level that is used to monitor oral anticoagulants

b. Elevations of serum transaminase levels have been seen

8. Side effects

a. Hemorrhage, hematuria, epistaxis, bleeding gums

b. Thrombocytopenia

9. Adverse effects/toxicity
   a. A serious form of thrombocytopenia called **heparin-induced platelet aggregation** (heparin-induced thrombocytopenia and thrombosis or HITT), also called white clot syndrome, can be fatal if not treated aggressively; thrombocytopenia is more pronounced (less than 100,000/mm^3) and begins 3–12 days after starting heparin therapy
   b. Clients on long-term heparin therapy (longer than 6 months' duration) are prone to develop osteoporosis

10. Nursing considerations
    a. Monitor client's baseline labs with regard to heparin protocol (specifically aPTT); trend results and titrate medication according to protocol; with continuous IV heparin infusion, aPTT is commonly measured every 6 hours; when level is critically high, infusion may be stopped for 1 or more hours and aPTT measured in 2–3 hours
    b. Obtain daily weight for client on weight-based heparin protocol
    c. Monitor client for signs of bleeding, perform a thorough skin assessment, hemoccult all stools to test for blood, and evaluate pertinent labs
    d. Verify with pharmacy or another RN the correct dosage of heparin before administering dose or adjusting heparin infusion
    e. Evaluate dosage for safety and therapeutic range based on normal adult dosage range of 20,000–40,000 units/24 hr; heparin is usually infused in units/hr
    f. Have antidote available (protamine sulfate) for heparin therapy
    g. SubQ administration of heparin requires site rotation; do not aspirate or rub injection site
    h. When administering heparin subQ, inject into abdomen using a small (5/8-inch, 25- to 27-gauge) needle at a 90° angle
    i. The preferred administration site for low molecular weight heparins, such as enoxaparin (Lovenox) is in antero- and posterolateral sides of the abdomen; do not administer enoxaparin (Lovenox) in deltoid area, as hematoma formation may result

11. Client education
    a. Establish specific goals to increase client's knowledge related to heparin administration
    b. Inform client that frequent blood work monitoring is required to ensure effective anticoagulation
    c. Teach client to be alert for bleeding problems and how to respond and to prevent injury
    d. Instruct client to observe for hematuria, nosebleeds, blood in stool, and petechiae
    e. Teach to decrease or maintain steady intake of green leafy vegetables if adding warfarin

II. ANTIPLATELET AGENTS

A. Action and use

1. Antiplatelet drugs are substances that inhibit the body's natural clotting mechanism; they prevent or disrupt **aggregation** (accumulation of substances in blood to form a group or cluster) of platelets needed to form a clot
2. Act at specific points in clotting cascade to prevent blood clot formation
3. Used to treat thrombi and are often used as adjunctive therapy to other anticoagulant medications such as warfarin (Coumadin)
4. Used as both preventive and treatment measures for clients with history of MI, stroke, and cardiac surgery
5. Inhibit or block certain enzyme pathways to prevent clot formation

Practice to Pass

What discharge instructions would you provide to a client who has been placed on anticoagulation therapy?

B. Common medications
1. Aspirin (or acetylsalicylic acid, ASA) is the most commonly used type of antiplatelet medication
2. Ticlopidine (Ticlid) can be used as an antiplatelet medication in clients who cannot take aspirin therapy
3. In addition to its utility as an antiplatelet agent, dipyridamole (Persantine) is also used in cardiac stress testing
4. ASA has many other therapeutic properties such as analgesic, anti-inflammatory, and antipyretic action
5. Clopidogrel bisulfate (Plavix) is used as a form of secondary prevention for clients who have had MI, stroke, and peripheral arterial disease
6. Abciximab (ReoPro) is a fab fragment of a specific monoclonal antibody
7. Refer to Table 4-3 for a listing of common antiplatelet medications and their uses

Table 4-3   **Antiplatelet Agents**

Generic (Trade) Name	Route	Uses
ASA		
Aspirin	PO	Reduce incidence of transient ischemic attacks, reduce the risk of nonfatal myocardial infarction in clients with a history of myocardial infarctions
Adenosine ADP Inhibitors		
Dipyridamole (Persantine)	PO	Prevention of thromboembolism in client with heart valves, combination therapy with warfarin sodium, coronary artery disease, angina pectoris
Glycoproteins		
Abciximab (ReoPro)	IV	Used in combination with heparin and aspirin in prevention of cardiac attacks during transluminal coronary angioplasty
Clopidogrel bisulfate (Plavix)	PO	Treat clients who are at risk for ischemic events, history of myocardial infarction, ischemic stroke, or peripheral arterial disease
Eptifibatide (Integrelin)	IV	Acute coronary syndrome, prevention of ischemic attacks during percutaneous coronary interventions
Tirofiban (Aggrastat)	IV	In conjunction with heparin to treat acute coronary syndrome, prevent cardiac ischemic events during percutaneous coronary care
Miscellaneous		
Ticagrelor (Brilinta)	PO	Prevention of thrombotic events in clients with acute coronary syndrome or myocardial infarction with ST elevation
Anagrelide (Agrylin)	PO	Essential thrombocytopenia to decrease platelet count and reduce risk of thrombosis
Cilostazol (Pletal)	PO	Reduce symptoms related to intermittent claudication
Prasugrel (Effient)	PO	Treatment of unstable angina, non-ST elevation myocardial infarction, reduction of thrombosis in clients with acute coronary syndrome (ACS) or undergoing percutaneous coronary interventions
Sulfinpyrazone (Anturane)	PO	Prevent reinfarction following myocardial infarction by inhibiting degranulation of platelets, reduce incidence of systemic emboli with rheumatic mitral stenosis; primary use is in treatment of gouty arthritis and tophaceous gout
Ticlopidine (Ticlid)	PO	Reduce thrombotic stroke in transient ischemic attack clients who cannot tolerate aspirin therapy, sickle cell disease, primary glomerulonephritis, arterial peripheral vascular occlusive disease

Legend: IV, intravenous; PO, oral

C. Administration considerations
1. ASA is administered in dosages ranging from 81 to 325 mg/day (baby ASA to adult strength); it can also be given as an enteric-coated preparation to minimize GI upset
2. Dipyridamole (Persantine) has a better profile when used with clients who have prosthetic mechanical heart valves
3. Ticlopidine (Ticlid) has been used effectively as a preventive measure in clients who are at risk for MI
4. Abciximab (ReoPro) is administered parenterally and client can receive a bolus dose as well as a constant infusion

D. Contraindications
1. ASA is contraindicated with known hypersensitivity to salicylates, bleeding disorders, asthma, or when gastrointestinal (GI) bleeding is present; ASA should not be given to children because it can be associated with development of Reye syndrome
2. Dipyridamole (Persantine) is contraindicated during pregnancy or lactation
3. Abciximab (ReoPro) is contraindicated in clients with evidence of current or recent bleeding, cerebrovascular accident (CVA) or stroke within past 2 years with deficit, and thrombocytopenia
4. Ticlopidine (Ticlid) is contraindicated during pregnancy, with a known hypersensitivity, liver disease, or evidence of blood dyscrasias
5. Clopidogrel bisulfate (Plavix) is contraindicated with known hypersensitivity or active bleeding as a result of intracranial hemorrhage or peptic ulcer disease

E. Significant drug interactions
1. With ASA, increased effects are seen with use of ETOH, anticoagulants, methotrexate, and sulfonylureas; decreased effects are seen with use of angiotensin converting enzyme (ACE) inhibitors, beta-blockers, and diuretics
2. Dipyridamole/ASA can lead to additive effects and lead to an increased risk for bleeding
3. Ticlopidine (Ticlid) can increase levels of theophylline and phenytoin; cimetidine can lead to increased levels of Ticlid
4. Clopidogrel bisulfate (Plavix)/NSAIDs may increase risk of bleeding episodes

F. Significant food interactions
1. Ticlopidine is best taken on a full stomach to help maximize absorption and not in the presence of antacids
2. ASA is usually taken on a full stomach to minimize GI upset
3. Avoid these herbal treatments, which can increase risk of bleeding: angelica, cat's claw, chamomile, chondroitin, feverfew, garlic, gingko, golden seal, grape seed extract, green leaf tea, horse chestnut seed, psyllium, or turmeric

G. Significant laboratory studies
1. ASA can cause false-negative or false-positive results for urine glucose and increase uric acid levels
2. Ticlopidine has a potential to cause blood dyscrasias and a rise in serum cholesterol levels

H. Side effects
1. ASA: blood dyscrasias, hemorrhage, GI symptoms, as well as central nervous system (CNS) alterations, increased bleeding tendencies, hemorrhage, nausea and vomiting, dizziness, and confusion
2. Persantine: GI complaints, nausea and vomiting (N/V), CNS alterations, headache, and dizziness
3. Ticlopidine: serious blood dyscrasias such as agranulocytosis and neutropenia; GI symptoms, such as nausea, vomiting, and jaundice
4. Clopidogrel: flulike symptoms, chest pain, edema, and hypertension
5. In general: bruising, hematuria, tarry stools

I. **Adverse effects/toxicity**
1. ASA toxicity: tinnitus and ototoxicity
2. Abciximab: allergic reaction
3. Ticlid: potentially life-threatening decrease in platelets, leading to thrombotic thrombocytopenic purpura (TTP)

J. **Nursing considerations**
1. A baseline level of pertinent hematologic labs should be included at time of client admission
2. Monitor vital signs
3. Monitor bleeding time
4. Monitor client for side effects related to bleeding
5. Use of antiplatelet medications should be stopped for at least 7 days prior to a planned surgery
6. Older adult clients may require closer monitoring with antiplatelet therapy to avoid toxicity because it may be harder to assess for tinnitus and ototoxicity if a client's baseline hearing is already diminished
7. Life span concerns: Children, pregnant women, and lactating women should not take antiplatelet medications; used in pregnancy only when benefit to mother outweighs risk to fetus; lactating women should be informed of risks to infant if this therapy is considered

K. **Client education**
1. Instruct client to carry a MedicAlert bracelet
2. Establish specific individualized goals to increase client's knowledge of therapy and need for continued compliance
3. Instruct client to monitor for side effects related to bleeding and report them
4. Inform client that communication between client and health care team members is critical
5. Inform client that adults should not use aspirin for self-medication of pain longer than 5 days without consulting a health care provider
6. Instruct to maintain adequate fluid intake to prevent salicylate crystalluria
7. Inform female clients that prolonged use of ASA can lead to iron deficiency anemia
8. Instruct client and family of measures to prevent bleeding and actions to take if bleeding occurs
9. Instruct clients taking Ticlid to report fever, chills, sore throat, or other signs of infection immediately

Practice to Pass

A client has been told by his physician to "take an aspirin a day to thin the blood" but is unsure as to the type and dosage. What information would you provide to the client with regard to this dilemma?

III. THROMBOLYTICS

A. **Action and use**
1. **Thrombolytics**: substances that dissolve or break down a thrombus or blood clot
2. After a thrombus is broken down, blood flow is reestablished to area (increased perfusion) to maintain vascular integrity and prevent ischemia
3. Thrombolytics help activate the **fibrinolytic system** that breaks down a thrombus or blood clot
4. Conversion of plasminogen to plasmin aids clot breakdown by digesting fibrin and degrading fibrinogen and other procoagulant proteins into soluble fragments; plasminogen must be present for thrombolytics to work
5. Process of **fibrinolysis** is activated naturally in the body to prevent excessive clotting or vascular compromise
6. Thrombolytic therapy is indicated for clients at risk for developing thrombus with resultant ischemia such as acute MI, arterial thrombosis, DVT, pulmonary embolism, and occlusion of catheters or shunts
7. Thrombolytic medications are mostly given in emergency and critical care areas

Table 4-4	Thrombolytics	
Generic (Trade) Name	**Route**	**Uses**
Alteplase (Activase)	IV	Myocardial infarction (MI) acute pulmonary embolism, acute ischemic stroke
Anistreplase (Eminase)	IV	Immediately after onset of acute MI
Reteplase (Retavase)	IV	Coronary artery thrombosis associated with MI
Tenecteplase (TNKase)	IV	Reduce mortality associated with acute MI

B. Common medications
1. Streptokinase (Streptase) is isolated from group-A beta-hemolytic streptococci (bacteria) and is considered to be antigenic; its action is systemic in nature
2. Alteplase (Activase) is a natural substance secreted by vascular endothelial cells in body and therefore does not cause an antigenic response; its action is specific in nature
3. Refer to Table 4-4 for a listing of common thrombolytics

C. Administration considerations
1. Thrombolytics are usually given to clients who are acutely ill in emergency and critical care settings where stabilization is the primary goal of intervention
2. Alteplase has a very short half-life (5 minutes), which may require repeat administration and/or administration with heparin to prevent reocclusion of blood vessels
3. Baseline vital signs and pertinent coagulation studies are necessary
4. IV administration is carried out using specific protocols and guidelines to maintain safe and therapeutic effects; monitor IV sites for signs and symptoms of infiltration and/or phlebitis
5. If IV site is not patent or if symptoms suggesting infiltration or phlebitis develop, site should be changed to opposite extremity

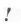

6. Continuous monitoring of blood pressure (BP), mental status, and neurological signs, and response to therapy should be documented; report any signs of chest pain, dizziness, headache, or evidence of bleeding to the health care provider

7. Place client on a cardiac monitor during administration of thrombolytics

8. The antidote to streptokinase is aminocaproic acid (Amicar)

D. Contraindications
1. Pregnancy
2. Not for use in clients who are actively bleeding, have a recent history of CVA/stroke, severe uncontrolled hypertension, recent trauma, or neoplasm

3. IM route for medication administration is contraindicated when using thrombolytics

E. Significant drug interactions: increased risk of bleeding with anticoagulant and antiplatelet drugs

F. Significant food interactions: none reported

G. Significant laboratory studies
1. Reductions in plasminogen and fibrinogen levels are seen with use of thrombolytic agents
2. Monitoring coagulation profile such as bleeding time, aPTT, and PT is required to ensure safe and therapeutic treatment

H. Side effects

1. Hemorrhage
2. Hypersensitivity reactions; allergic reactions with vascular collapse occur more frequently with streptokinase
3. Nausea, vomiting, and hypotension; streptokinase may cause first-dose hypotension
4. Cardiac dysrhythmias

I. Adverse effects/toxicity
1. Side effects of thrombolytic agents are dose-related
2. Dysrhythmias as a consequence of therapy may pose further problems for the client who is already in an acute situation, such as when administered via an intracoronary catheter

 J. Nursing considerations
1. Monitor pertinent baseline labs and continue to assess client during therapy
2. Monitor client for vital sign changes, as there may be variations in pulse, BP, and temperature caused by thrombolytic administration; watch for signs of impending shock; neurological checks should be done frequently
3. Maintain adequate IV site for medication administration; observe closely for signs and symptoms of infiltration
4. Limit invasive procedures when a client is on thrombolytic therapy to reduce risk of bleeding
5. Assess frequently for signs of bleeding, both obvious and occult
6. If client is found to be bleeding, the medication should be stopped; fresh frozen plasma (FFP) and packed red blood cells (PRBCs) may be prescribed
7. Monitor client closely for development of dysrhythmias
8. Maintain aseptic technique to prevent infection
 9. Antidote: aminocaproic acid (Amicar) should be readily available on clinical unit
10. Provide adequate nutrition and rest in order to support client during treatment
11. Support client and family members during acute care management period
12. Maintain effective, open, and therapeutic communication among client, family, and all health care team members

K. Client education
1. Treatment methods and medication administration
 2. Use methods to reduce risk of bleeding
   a. Use electric razor to reduce risk of bleeding
   b. Brush teeth gently using a soft toothbrush to reduce risk of bleeding
   c. Avoid trauma to skin and other areas of body to reduce risk of bleeding
3. Lifestyle changes may be instituted in order to prevent further occurrences of abnormal clotting
4. Measurable signs of clinical response may not occur for 6–8 hours after therapy is started
 5. Avoid taking aspirin or NSAIDs during therapy because risk of bleeding is enhanced
6. Discontinue medication if bleeding occurs and notify health care provider

IV. HEMOSTATICS

A. Systemic hemostatics
1. Action and use
   a. Systemic **hemostatics** are substances that inhibit bleeding after an injury to maintain hematologic balance
   b. Used to stop/or prevent bleeding in clients who are at risk due to injury
   c. Vitamin K is also used as mandatory treatment to prevent hemorrhagic disease of newborn
   d. Vitamin K works in liver to formulate specific clotting factors (II, VII, IX, and X) that are necessary in coagulation cascade
2. Common medications
   a. Aminocaproic acid (Amicar) and tranexamic acid (Cyklokapron) both impede fibrinolysis

Table 4-5	Systemic Hemostatics	
Generic (Trade) Name	**Route**	**Uses**
Aminocaproic acid (Amicar)	PO, IV	Excessive bleeding from cardiac surgery, trauma, abruption placentae, thrombolytic agent antidote
Aprotinin (Trasylol)	IV	Excessive bleeding from cardiac surgery
DDAVP (Desmopressin)	IV, intranasal	Spontaneous bleeding and trauma-induced hemorrhage
Phytonadine Vitamin K_1 (AquaMEPHYTON)	PO, subQ, IM	Promotes liver synthesis of clotting factors; antidote for coumarin overdosage; reverses hypoprothrombinemia secondary to oral antibiotic, quinidine, quinine, salicylate, sulfonamide, and vitamin A; prophylaxis therapy for neonatal hemorrhagic disease
Menadiol sodium diphosphate, Vitamin K_4 (Synkavite)	PO, subQ, IM, IV	Vitamin K deficiency, promote blood clotting
Tranexamic acid (Cyklokapron)	PO, IV	Prevent tooth hemorrhage during and after tooth extraction in hemophiliac clients

    b. Aminocaproic acid is used to treat postoperative hyperfibrinolysis-induced hemorrhage and for hematologic disorders such as aplastic anemia, hepatic cirrhosis, and some neoplastic disease states; it is also an antidote to thrombolytic drugs

    c. Tranexamic acid is used 1 day before and 2–8 days after dental or other surgery in clients with hemophilia

    d. Phytonadione, vitamin K_1 (Aquamephyton) is the antidote to warfarin and is fat soluble; it reverses excess effects of oral anticoagulants

    e. Menadiol sodium diphosphate, vitamin K_4 (Synkayvite) is a water-soluble compound

    f. Refer to Table 4-5 for a listing of common systemic hemostatics

3. Administration considerations

    a. Aminocaproic acid and tranexamic acid are administered via oral or IV route; close continuous monitoring of the client is required

    b. Phytonadione is usually given IM to newborns in the delivery room for treatment and prophylaxis of hemorrhagic disease of the newborn

    c. Vitamin K preparations can be given PO, IM, subQ, or IV

    d. Monitoring of PT levels will provide information relative to dosing and therapeutic management of client

    e. DDAVP (Desmopressin) may be used to treat spontaneous bleeding and trauma induced hemorrhage

4. Contraindications

    a. Aminocaproic acid is contraindicated in clients who have disseminated intravascular coagulopathy (DIC), postpartum bleeding, upper urinary tract bleeding, or new burns

    b. Contraindicated in any client with a known hypersensitivity

    c. Vitamin K is contraindicated during last few weeks of pregnancy and in clients with liver disease

    d. Tranexamic acid is contraindicated in subarachnoid bleed

    e. Megadoses of iron are contraindicated in first trimester of pregnancy because of risk of fetal teratogenic effects

5. Significant drug interactions

    a. Concurrent use of aminocaproic acid and tranexamic acid with estrogen and oral contraceptives (OCT) can lead to increased coagulation

    b. Use of aminocaproic acid and certain antibiotics can lead to ototoxicity and nephrotoxicity; check individual antibiotic product literature

      c. Use of antibiotic therapy may lead to a decrease in vitamin K synthesis due to destruction of intestinal bacteria, and supplementation may be required

      d. Mineral oil can decrease absorption of vitamin K

  6. Significant food interactions

      a. Dietary sources of vitamin K are found in green leafy vegetables, milk and meats

      b. Vitamin K is a fat-soluble vitamin and can be synthesized by intestinal flora; deficiency states are usually not identified solely with diet, but are more likely caused by malabsorption problems linked to liver disease or alcohol abuse

      c. The addition of yogurt in diet helps to provide a medium for bacterial growth that can lead to maintenance of intestinal flora

  7. Significant laboratory studies

      a. PT level is an indicator of response to vitamin K administration

      b. Amicar can cause a decrease in potassium levels when used in clients with decreased renal function

  8. Side effects

      a. GI: N/V, diarrhea, and abdominal cramps

      b. Headache, dizziness, and flushing

      c. Localized reaction at injection site with vitamin K administration

      d. Allergic response with vitamin K products

  9. Adverse effects/toxicity

      a. Most drug effects are mild and are usually dose related

      b. Overdose with vitamin K can lead to a serious problem if client is a newborn because of its effect on coagulation cascade

  10. Nursing considerations

      a. Monitor client for baseline labs related to renal and liver function

      b. Monitor PT levels and response to therapy for vitamin K administration

      c. Monitor client's coagulation profile as antifibrinolytics can cause a **hypercoagulation** or rapid coagulation of blood

      d. Rotate injection sites for administration of vitamin K; assess client for signs of local irritation

      e. Monitor client closely for signs of hypersensitivity and allergic reactions

      f. Monitor client closely during administration via parenteral infusion as there is risk for volume overload and adverse reactions

      g. Use of an infusion pump for IV administration is required

  11. Client education

      a. Dietary sources of vitamin K previously discussed

      b. Periodic PT levels will be drawn to monitor response to therapy

      c. Monitor for signs and symptoms of bleeding

      d. Use of dietary yogurt and buttermilk products can help restore normal intestinal flora that will aid in vitamin K synthesis; clients who are on antibiotic therapy or who have intestinal problems may benefit from this supportive therapy

      e. Report difficulty urinating or reddish-brown urine (caused by myoglobinuria) while taking aminocaproic acid

      f. Report chest pain, arm or leg pain, or difficulty breathing

B. Local absorbable hemostatic agents

  1. Action and use

      a. Localized hemostatics are utilized to stop or inhibit bleeding at a specific site

      b. The use of topical local hemostatics leads to absorption of blood in a controlled manner

      c. Thrombin can be used following dental extraction procedures to stop bleeding

Box 4-2	• Absorbable gelatin sponge (Gelfoam): a sterile gelatin that absorbs blood when placed in surgical wound and is absorbed within 4–6 weeks

Local Hemostatics

- Absorbable gelatin sponge (Gelfoam): a sterile gelatin that absorbs blood when placed in surgical wound and is absorbed within 4–6 weeks
- Absorbable gelatin film (Gelfilm): a sterile absorbable gelatin film often used in neurosurgery, thoracic surgery, or ocular surgery to absorb blood in tissues, act as dural substitute (neurosurgery), or repair pleural defect (thoracic surgery)
- Epinephrine: a medication that reduces bleeding by causing vasoconstriction
- Oxidized cellulose (Oxycel): a specially treated form of surgical gauze or cotton that is hemostatic and is absorbable in 2–7 days usually; controls bleeding during surgery involving liver, pancreas, spleen, kidney, thyroid, and prostate
- Oxidized regenerated cellulose (Surgicel): see oxidized cellulose noted previously
- Microfibrillar collagen hemostat (Avitene): an absorbable topical hemostatic substance that attracts platelets and causes platelet aggregation on a bleeding surface
- Thrombin (Fibrindex): a sterile powder treated with thromboplastin in the presence of calcium; catalyzes conversion of fibrinogen to fibrin and may cause platelet aggregation; used topically for capillary bleeding or in combination with absorbable gelatins (previously listed) during surgery

2. Common medications
   a. Gelatin products, oxidized cellulose, thrombin, and epinephrine are all examples of topical hemostatic agents
   b. Refer to Box 4-2 for a listing of common local hemostatics
3. Administration considerations
   a. Topical hemostatics are available in pads, powder, sponge, film, and liquid forms
   b. Application involves adherence of the form to a local bleeding site and the material is allowed to remain in place to establish hemostasis
   c. Depending on type of local hemostatic used, removal may be done as early as 24–48 hours
   d. Irrigation with normal saline may be necessary to prevent further tissue destruction as the topical is removed
   e. If product is a sponge or film, it may be completely reabsorbed into body
4. Contraindications
   a. Contraindicated if client has a previous allergy to animal protein products or gelatin, since they are composed of animal protein
   b. Contraindicated in the presence of infection
5. Significant drug interactions: none reported
6. Significant food interactions: none reported
7. Significant laboratory studies: none reported
8. Side effects: hypersensitivity reactions at site of application, erythema, pruritus, and localized irritations
9. Adverse effects/toxicity: same as previously noted
10. Nursing considerations
    a. Application of topical hemostatics must be done according to prescriber protocol and within guidelines of product information
    b. Assess local site for signs of hypersensitivity and document findings
    c. Remove topical hemostatics as indicated by product guidelines; irrigation of site with normal saline may be required to prevent further tissue destruction; document site appearance in medical record
    d. If client develops an allergic reaction to product or if a reaction is anticipated, an antihistamine such as diphenhydramine (Benadryl) may be given
    e. Switching from one material to another may facilitate a better response

!

Practice to Pass

A topical hemostatic agent used on the client now has to be removed. What nursing interventions would you employ to perform this action?

11. Client education
    a. Removal of topical hemostatics: It is important not to pull off dry materials as this could cause further skin damage and pain
    b. Treatment with local hemostatics may occur over a number of days and weeks
    c. Compliance with treatment regimen is necessary to achieve a good outcome
    d. Monitor site for signs of potential infection

C. **Clotting factor replacement therapy**
    1. Action and use
       a. Refers to specific restoration of blood components necessary for body to regain hemostasis and maintain hematologic integrity
       b. Congenital deficiencies of specific clotting factors can lead to serious (if not fatal) consequences unless there is adequate replacement therapy
       c. Functional platelet and plasma abnormalities can lead to coagulation problems that include specific syndromes, such as hemophilia and von Willebrand disease
       d. Used to stop and prevent hemorrhage in clients who have specific identified factor deficiencies
       e. Used to support clients with specific factor deficiencies who are undergoing a surgical procedure
    2. Common medications or blood products
       a. Cryoprecipitate provides a concentrated form of fibrinogen and is a blood product obtained from fresh frozen plasma (FFP)
       b. Antithrombin III (Atnativ, Thromvate III) works with heparin to provide an anticoagulant effect
       c. Desmopressin acetate (DDAVP) is classified as an antidiuretic hormone, but it has adjunctive effects on increasing factor VIII in body
       d. Refer to Box 4-3 for a listing of replacement therapy medications
    3. Administration considerations
       a. Antihemophilic factor (AHF) medications, such as Hemofil, are administered via IV route; dosage is individualized based on client's weight, bleeding status, factor deficiency, presence of factor inhibitor and results of pertinent coagulation lab studies
       b. DDAVP can be administered intranasally; alternate nares when administering drug and document appropriately on medication record
       c. AHF medications are usually refrigerated
       d. Administration of AHF should be done according to protocol; premedicate with antihistamines if ordered; document vital signs during the first 15 minutes of therapy to determine that they stay within client's baseline
    4. Contraindications
       a. Clients with a hypersensitivity to bovine, hamster, or mouse protein
       b. Antithrombin III may cause possible infection and hepatitis in pediatric clients and therefore should be used cautiously

Box 4-3	Antihemophilic factor (Hemofil M, Koate-HP)
	Cryoprecipitated antihemophilic factor-human
Clotting Factor	Antihemophilic factor-porcine (Hyate C)
Replacement Therapy	Antihemophilic factor-recombinant (Helixate, Kogenate)
	Antithrombin III (ATnativ, Thrombate III)
	Desmopressin (DDAVP)
	Factor IX complex, human (Bebulin VH, Konyne-80)
	Coagulation Factor IX, recombinant (BeneFIX)

    c. DDAVP is contraindicated in pregnant or lactating clients or clients with known hypersensitivity to drug; it should be used with caution in pediatric or older adult clients due to its antidiuretic effect and potential to develop hyponatremia

5. Significant drug interactions

    a. Concurrent use of antithrombin III and heparin leads to an increased anticoagulant effect

    b. The effects of DDAVP can be potentiated with use of chlorpropamide, clofibrate, and carbamazepine

6. Significant food interactions: none reported

7. Significant laboratory studies: sodium levels may need to be monitored with DDAVP therapy because of its effect on this electrolyte

8. Side effects

    a. AHF: hypersensitivity, lethargy, fatigue, nausea, and hypotension

    b. Antithrombin III: none reported

    c. DDAVP: headaches, nausea, nasal congestion, facial flushing, and chills

9. Adverse effects/toxicity

    a. AHF: developing AIDS and hepatitis, as certain AHF products are derived from human plasma

    b. DDAVP overdose: increased symptoms noted previously and dyspnea

10. Nursing considerations

    a. Proper reconstitution and administration of dose is required according to protocol

    b. Monitoring of pertinent baseline hematologic labs is required

    c. Document baseline vital signs during first 15 minutes of therapy and then according to protocol to monitor client's continued response

    d. Observe client closely for signs of hypersensitivity

    e. Infusion may have to be slowed down or discontinued if client develops increased allergic symptoms

    f. Review client's medication profile for use of concurrent medications that could interfere with clotting

    g. Clients with defined factor deficiencies and their families will need anticipatory support and guidance during a lifetime of therapy

    h. A collaborative health care team approach should be instituted to provide continued care to client and family

    i. Clients who have hereditary factor antithrombin III deficiency and become pregnant or require surgery are at risk of developing thrombosis; monitor closely during obstetric and postsurgical time periods

11. Client education

    a. Medication storage and administration if therapy is to be given at home

    b. Disease process and genetic transmission issues; referral to a genetic counselor may be indicated in clients of childbearing age

    c. Refer client to support groups for assistance and strengthening of coping mechanisms

    d. Since client is at risk for bleeding because of factor deficiencies, review concepts of safety as related to lifestyle and job/employment

V. MEDICATIONS TO TREAT ANEMIA

A. Iron salts

1. Action and use

    a. Iron is an essential trace element that participates in oxygen transport, tissue respiration, and enzyme reactions

    b. Iron is stored as ferritin in body; ferritin levels reflect visceral stores of iron that are available to body; transferrin levels reflect how iron is transported in body

    c. Iron deficiency anemia (IDA) is one of the most common nutritional deficiencies in United States

    d. IDA is classified as a microcytic anemia; iron preparations are indicated for treatment of this type of anemia

    e. The use of ferrous salts is indicated for treatment of iron deficiency

    f. Iron medications are available through prescription and over the counter (OTC)

2. Common medications

    a. Ferrous iron salts provide the largest amount of elemental iron and are available as oral medications

    b. Ferrous fumarate, ferrous gluconate, and ferrous sulfate are 3 oral iron preparations available; they all are equally effective but require different doses to provide an equivalent amount of iron

    c. Iron dextran is available as an injection when a client cannot tolerate oral administration or if oral therapy is ineffective

    d. Refer to Table 4-6 for a listing of common iron preparations

3. Administration considerations

    a. Oral iron is given with meals in order to decrease gastric upset

    b. Z-track administration of iron dextran is required to minimize client discomfort, prevent tissue discoloration, and ensure absorption

    c. There is a risk of anaphylactic reaction following iron dextran administration; therefore, a test dose may be ordered over 5 minutes to monitor client response; have epinephrine ready to use if hypersensitivity occurs

    d. Iron can be found in vitamins and nutritional supplements; monitor client for alternate sources of iron so as to avoid potential overdosing and toxicity

    e. Be aware of potential drug interactions that may limit or increase oral iron medications

    f. Liquid (elixir) iron is administered by straw to avoid discoloration of tooth enamel

4. Contraindications

    a. Contraindicated in clients with ulcerative colitis, peptic ulcer disease, cirrhosis, and hemolytic anemia

    b. Contraindicated in clients with iron overload syndromes (hemosiderosis and hemochromatosis)

    c. Prior history of reaction could lead to a contraindication for use of iron dextran injection (hypersensitivity including anaphylaxis can occur)

    d. Megadoses of iron are contraindicated during first trimester of pregnancy because of risk for teratogenic effects

Table 4-6   **Iron Salts**

Generic (Trade) Name	Route	Uses
Ferrous fumarate (Femiron)	PO	Correct simple iron deficiency (microcytic, hypochromic anemia) Periods of increased iron needs such as infancy, childhood, and pregnancy
Ferrous gluconate (Fergon)	PO	Correct simple iron deficiency (microcytic, hypochromic anemia) Periods of increased iron needs such as infancy, childhood, and pregnancy
Ferrous sulfate (Feosol)	PO	Correct simple iron deficiency (microcytic, hypochromic anemia) Periods of increased iron needs such as infancy, childhood, and pregnancy
Iron dextran injection (DexFerrum)	IV, IM	Iron deficiency anemia when oral administration of iron is unsatisfactory or impossible

5. Significant drug interactions
   a. Antacids, antibiotics (quinolones and tetracycline), and thyroid drugs decrease absorption of iron; therefore, oral iron medication should not be administered at same time
   b. Decreased effect of tetracycline and penicillamine
   c. Vitamin C can increase absorption of oral iron medications
6. Significant food interactions
   a. Iron is composed of both heme (animal) and non-heme (plant) sources in the diet; heme sources have a higher bioavailability and are more beneficial in maintaining iron levels
   b. Clients on a strict vegetarian diet may require supplementation to ensure adequate iron levels
   c. Taking iron with vitamin C can lead to increased absorption
   d. Foods that are high in phytates (grains and cereals) can cause a decreased absorption of dietary iron
   e. Iron should not be taken with milk, as decreased absorption will occur
7. Significant laboratory studies
   a. Monitor client's reticulocyte count, which will increase if bone marrow is responding and RBC production is increasing
   b. If hemoglobin and hematocrit levels do not rise following iron therapy, additional testing may be required to determine exact type of anemia
8. Side effects
   a. GI: upset stomach, N/V, diarrhea, and constipation
   b. Dark and tarry stools
   c. Dermatologic: discoloration of skin and pain upon injection
9. Adverse effects/toxicity
   a. **Pica** (ingestion of nonfood items in diet) can interfere with iron levels in body, causing individuals to become anemic; pregnant women are the client group most likely to be involved with pica
   b. Iron can accumulate in body, leading to potentially toxic levels
   c. Symptoms of iron overdose can lead a client to progress to shock, seizures, or coma; serum iron levels evaluated greater than 300 mcg/dL is serious and should be treated aggressively
   d. Removal of iron from body during iron overdose is necessary; poison control should be notified if iron overdose is suspected
   e. Chelation therapy should be instituted to remove iron from body in addition to supportive measures such as airway maintenance, correction of acidosis and administration of IV fluids
10. Nursing considerations
    a. Monitor client for expected side effects related to iron administration, such as tarry stools
    b. Give oral medication on a full stomach to minimize GI upset
    c. Since anemia is often a symptom of a disease, assess for underlying cause; monitor client lab findings to confirm a diagnosis of IDA
    d. If client does not show a clinical response to iron therapy, notify prescriber
    e. Referral to a dietitian may be indicated to support client's food choices in maintaining adequate iron levels
    f. Evaluate client for pica if there is a high index of suspicion
11. Client education
    a. Proper administration of oral iron medications
    b. Importance of adequate food sources to maintain iron levels; these include foods such as lean meats, liver, egg yolks, dried beans, green vegetables (e.g., spinach)
    c. Expected changes in the characteristics of stool (black, tarry)

B. Vitamin B$_{12}$ (Cyanocobalamin)

1. Action and use
   a. Vitamin B$_{12}$ is a water-soluble vitamin that is utilized as part of many coenzyme reactions during metabolism of carbohydrate, protein, and fat; is also essential for DNA synthesis
   b. Vitamin B$_{12}$ is found primarily in foods of animal origin (liver, meat, shellfish, and dairy food items)
   c. Deficiency of vitamin B$_{12}$ affects neurological, hematological, and GI systems
   d. Vitamin B$_{12}$ is considered to be the extrinsic factor whereas the intrinsic factor is released by parietal cells in stomach
   e. Clients with GI surgeries that result in partial or complete removal and/or anastomosis of stomach and end the release of intrinsic factor will require injections of vitamin B$_{12}$ on a lifelong basis
   f. **Pernicious anemia** is the anemia that results from vitamin B$_{12}$ deficiency
   g. Vitamin B$_{12}$ deficiency is classified as a megaloblastic macrocytic anemia
   h. Atrophic gastritis is associated with vitamin B$_{12}$ deficiency
   i. Because B-complex vitamins work together, there is likelihood that there is more than one deficiency existing at the same time

2. Common medications
   a. Cyanocobalamin is available as both prescription and OTC
   b. Cyanocobalamin is contained in many multivitamin preparations in addition to being sold as a separate vitamin unit
   c. Vitamin B$_{12}$ is available in oral and injectable forms
   d. Refer to Table 4-7 for a listing of common Vitamin B$_{12}$ preparations

3. Administration considerations
   a. Vitamin B$_{12}$ must be administered parenterally in clients who cannot manufacture intrinsic factor
   b. Therapeutic level for vitamin B$_{12}$ is Schilling test result greater than 30%
   c. Rotation sites with injection of this medication; use Z-track method to minimize burning and local irritation
   d. Cyanocobalamin injection should be protected from light, as light will inactivate drug; it should not be mixed with other medications but given as a separate injection

4. Contraindications: known prior hypersensitivity

5. Significant drug interactions
   a. Medications such as antiepileptics, aminoglycosides, cholestyramine, colchicine, neomycin, and potassium timed-release products will cause decreased absorption of vitamin B$_{12}$
   b. Monitor potassium levels as use of cyanocobalamin can cause hypokalemia
   c. Chloramphenicol antagonizes the hematologic action of this vitamin
   d. Decreased effectiveness with methotrexate and excessive alcohol use

6. Significant food interactions
   a. Clients with malabsorption problems may be prone to develop vitamin B$_{12}$ deficiency

Table 4-7   **Vitamin B$_{12}$ Preparations**

Generic (Trade) Name	Route	Uses
Vitamin B$_{12A}$ (Hydroxocobalamin)	IM	Vitamin B$_{12}$ malabsorption, thyrotoxicosis, hemolytic anemia, gluten enteropathy, small bowel bacterial overgrowth, folic acid deficiency
Vitamin B$_{12}$ (Cyanocobalamin, Rubramin PC)	IM, deep subQ	Pernicious anemia, inadequate secretion of intrinsic factor, dietary deficiency, Vitamin B$_{12}$ malabsorption

       b. Clients with alcoholism are more likely to have malabsorption problems and therefore are likely to have many vitamin deficiencies

       c. A strict vegetarian diet without adequate supplementation may increase a client's risk for developing this vitamin deficiency

  7. Significant laboratory studies

       a. Monitor pertinent hematologic labs to confirm diagnosis of pernicious anemia

       b. Monitor client for potential hypokalemia

  8. Side effects

       a. Flushing

       b. GI: diarrhea with resultant hypokalemia

       c. Dermatologic: itching and pain at the injection site

  9. Adverse effects/toxicity

       a. Vitamin B_{12} is a water-soluble vitamin and as such should not reach toxic levels in body

       b. Some clients can have more serious cardiac effects such as development of CHF and pulmonary edema

  10. Nursing considerations

       a. Review client's medications, both prescription and OTC, for potential drug interactions

       b. Rotate injection site and document appropriately on medication record

       c. Establish baseline pertinent labs and monitor as needed to document response to treatment

       d. Assess client's pulses and vascular status to determine baseline

       e. Clients with pernicious anemia cannot take oral vitamin therapy alone to correct the problem; medication must be administered via parenteral route

       f. If client's lab values do not indicate a positive response to treatment, notify prescriber and further investigate to determine underlying cause

       g. Refer to dietitian for supportive diet management; foods high in vitamin B_{12} (for those who can absorb it) include liver, kidney, fish, and milk

  11. Client education

       a. Lifelong nature of therapy if diagnosed with pernicious anemia

       b. Food sources of vitamin B_{12} for inclusion in diet (see previous section)

       c. Effects of alcohol on the absorption of vitamin B_{12}

       d. Monitor for signs and symptoms of B_{12} deficiency (numbness and tingling in lower extremities, weakness, fatigue, anorexia, loss of taste, diarrhea, memory loss, and mood changes)

       e. If diarrhea is significant, a change in drug dosage may be required

C. Folic acid

  1. Action and use

       a. Folic acid (vitamin B_9) is a water-soluble vitamin needed for DNA synthesis and cellular division

       b. Folic acid may be used either to treat deficiency states, or as prophylaxis against a deficiency state, such as in pregnancy

       c. Deficiency states have been associated with neural tube defects in developing fetus and with hematologic manifestations such as megaloblastic macrocytic anemia

       d. Folic acid helps to break down homocysteine (an amino acid) in body; if there is a folic acid deficiency state, then levels of homocysteine can elevate; high homocysteine levels are associated with heart disease

       e. Dietary sources of folic acid are found in fresh green vegetables, yellow fruits and vegetables, liver, yeast and meats

       f. Folic acid supplements in addition to dietary sources are used to treat deficiency states; supplementation is recommended during pregnancy and lactation

2. Common medications
   a. Folic acid (Folvite) can be obtained as an OTC medication; therapeutic oral dose is less than 1 mg per day and maintenance dose is less than 0.4 mg per day
   b. Nutritional supplements and/or multivitamin preparations can contain folic acid
   c. Leucovorin calcium (Wellcovorin) may be given IM or IV at a usual adult dose of not more than 1 mg per day; this form of folic acid is reserved for use as an adjunct to cancer chemotherapy, not folic acid deficiency
3. Administration considerations
   a. Route of administration can be oral, subQ, IM, or IV depending on formulation; folic acid can be given IVP or added to an infusion; IV rate should not exceed 5 mcg/minute
   b. Folic acid (0.4 mg) is recommended daily for all pregnant women in the United States to prevent folate deficiency; it is suggested that therapy start 1 month prior to conception and continue throughout first trimester
   c. Regardless of client's age, daily dose should not be less than 0.1 mg/day
   d. Folic acid should not be mixed with any other medication and should be given as a separate injection
   e. Clients may experience a rash or hypersensitivity at site of injection; rotate injection sites
   f. If client has neurological deficits, use of folic acid will not correct the problem; attention must be directed to other B vitamins, and appropriate therapy must be instituted to correct neurological compromise
4. Contraindications
   a. Contraindicated for treatment of other anemias not caused by folic acid deficiency
   b. Folic acid injections may contain benzyl alcohol and therefore should not be given to neonates; the use of this preservative is contraindicated in neonates
   c. Use cautiously during lactation
5. Significant drug interactions
   a. ASA, phenytoin, and sulfonamides cause decreased folic acid levels
   b. There is increased likelihood of seizure activity when used concurrently with phenytoin
   c. Oral contraceptives can increase the risk of folic acid deficiency
   d. Steroid use increases the need for folic acid in body
   e. Methotrexate, pyrimethamine, triamterene, and trimethoprim act as folic acid antagonists
   f. Alcohol use can lead to folic acid deficiency because it increases folic acid requirements
   g. Continued use of folic acid may interfere with findings associated with vitamin B_{12} deficiency states
6. Significant food interactions
   a. Dietary sources of folic acid should be identified for client
   b. Prolonged cooking of vegetables may destroy the folic acid present
   c. Heating can destroy the vitamin, leading to decreased bioavailability
7. Significant laboratory studies: none specific
8. Side effects: yellow discoloration of urine, nausea, altered sleep, depression, rash, and bronchospasm
9. Adverse effects/toxicity
   a. No toxic effects are reported with oral folic acid
   b. Toxicity can occur if client is on antiepileptic therapy concurrently with vitamin B_{12} because of competition for binding sites
   c. Hemolytic anemia can occur as a result of increased utilization

10. Nursing considerations

    a. Clients who are pregnant should take 0.4 mg of folic acid on a daily basis as neural tube defect prophylaxis

    b. Review client medications for potential drug interactions

    c. Assess and monitor pertinent hematologic labs related to folic acid

    d. Referral to dietitian for dietary support and maintenance of folic acid levels

    e. Counsel client as to the effect that alcohol can have on folic acid levels

    f. Monitor client for potential allergic reactions to medication

    g. Therapeutic effects include improvement in lab studies and reversal of symptoms of folic acid deficiency (diarrhea, constipation, restless legs, fatigue, diffuse muscular pain, forgetfulness, and mental depression)

11. Client education

    a. Importance of neural tube prophylaxis during pregnancy

    b. Potential for increased drug interactions exist with this vitamin

    c. Repeated lab tests are necessary to monitor response to therapy

    d. Remain under close medical supervision while taking folic acid

    e. Food sources high in folic acid include such foods as green leafy vegetables, yellow fruits and vegetables, yeast, and meats

D. Epoetin alfa (Epogen, Procrit)

1. Action and use

    a. Epoetin is a recombinant form of erythropoietin that stimulates RBC production; it is chemically identical to erythropoietin produced in kidneys and serves the same function, to promote RBC growth

    b. Used to treat clients with anemia from various causes such as renal failure, HIV infection, and nonmyeloid malignancies with associated chemotherapy-induced anemia

    c. Used as a treatment measure to reduce need for blood transfusions because of its growth potential effect in clients who are undergoing surgery

    d. Ferritin and transferrin saturation levels must be adequate in order to support RBC formation

    e. Darbopoetin alfa (Aranesp) is closely related to Epogen and is indicated in treatment of anemia associated with cancer chemotherapy or chronic renal failure

2. Common medications

    a. Epogen dosage varies with client's situation and is calculated in units/kg; dose may range from 3 to 500 units/kg/dose three times/wk and is given subQ or IV

    b. Aranesp has an extended duration of action, allowing it to be administered once weekly

3. Administration considerations

    a. Medication is refrigerated; let warm to room temperature before administration

    b. Do not use medication that is discolored or contains particulate matter

    c. Do not administer with any other solutions; medication can be administered subQ or IV; vial contains no preservative, so unused portion must be discarded

    d. Do not shake medication as this will lead to inactivation

    e. Administration of Epogen must adhere to physician protocol to avoid overdose

    f. Dosages are individualized depending on clinical condition and whether or not dialysis has been instituted

    g. Hemoglobin (Hgb) indicates client response; prescriber identifies target levels (10–12 grams/dL) and therapy is titrated to achieve target; if Hgb level rises too quickly or passes target goal, client may be at risk for developing hypertension and seizures; if Hgb does not rise in response to therapy, dose will be increased depending on adequacy of iron stores; initial effects are usually seen in 1–2 weeks, while achievement of target goal usually takes 2–3 months

    h. Hemoglobin levels should be maintained below 12 grams/dL in clients with renal failure and less than 10 g/dL in clients with cancer to reduce risk of serious cardiovascular adverse events

    i. Therapy should be discontinued when Hgb levels are greater than 12 grams/dL in renal failure clients and when at 10 grams/dL in clients with cancer

4. Contraindications

    a. Uncontrolled hypertension or known hypersensitivity to human albumin

    b. Complicated anemia from multiple etiologies

    c. Epogen should not be used in pregnant clients unless benefits outweigh potential risks

5. Significant drug interactions

    a. The use of myelosuppressive agents can interfere with ability of Epogen to work because they have an antagonistic effect; Epogen is usually given following chemotherapy to avoid this effect

    b. The use of Epogen is limited in that it cannot correct underlying problem associated with specific type of anemia; continued use of Epogen leads to potential long-term ineffectiveness as body tries to compensate

6. Significant food interactions: Use of iron supplementation is recommended with this medication and can include dietary sources and oral medications

7. Significant laboratory studies

    a. Expected to have an effect on the RBC lineage and raise the serum level, as well as the hematocrit and hemoglobin concentrations

    b. Adjustment of dosage is related to pertinent lab values such as hematocrit, and adequate iron stores; dose is usually adjusted when hematocrit is between 30 and 36%

8. Side effects

    a. Hypertension and edema

    b. Diarrhea, constipation, N/V

    c. Fever, joint pain, and pain at injection site

    d. Thrombocytosis, iron deficiency, sweating, and arthralgias

9. Adverse effects/toxicity

    a. Overcorrection can result in toxic levels leading to development of polycythemia

    b. Clients can develop hypertension and seizures with toxic levels or a too rapid therapeutic response

10. Nursing considerations

    a. Closely monitor client's baseline hematologic labs to provide information relative to treatment response

    b. Monitor BP before initiating therapy and monitor closely during therapy

    c. Rotate injection sites to minimize discomfort

    d. Monitor client for the risk of thrombotic events, such as MI, CVA/stroke, and transient ischemic accident (TIA), especially for clients with chronic renal failure (CRF)

    e. Follow administration protocols and monitor ongoing pertinent labs

    f. Clients who are on dialysis may require adjusted dosages caused by stress of the hemodynamic process

    g. Monitor client's iron stores (ferritin) and transferrin levels; use of additional supplementation and/or medication may be required to support effects on RBC maturation

    h. Refer to dietitian for nutritional support

    i. Monitor client's baseline vital signs and continue to monitor BP following drug administration

11. Client education
    a. Need for continued lab follow-up and possible dosage adjustment
    b. Possible side effects
    c. Premedicate if necessary with analgesics if bone pain is present or client becomes febrile
    d. Medication can be given in home setting; client can be taught to self-administer dose
    e. Importance of keeping follow-up appointments
    f. Do not drive or be involved in other hazardous activity during the first 90 days of therapy because of possible seizure activity
    g. Importance of compliance with dietary and drug therapy

VI. MEDICATIONS TO LOWER SERUM CHOLESTEROL

A. HMG-Coenzyme A (HMG-CoA) reductase inhibitors

1. Action and use
   a. Belong to the class of "statins" that work in liver to inhibit cholesterol synthesis
   b. Competitively inhibit this rate-limiting enzyme in the liver, which leads to a decrease in cholesterol concentration
   c. Used to lower LDL cholesterol levels in clients with significant cholesterol elevations and for whom diet therapy has not been effective
   d. Also have an effect on HDL cholesterol that is somewhat dose dependent; lipoprotein levels are not affected by use of statins

2. Common medications
   a. Lovastatin (Mevacor), simvastatin (Zocor), pravastatin (Pravachol), and rosuvastatin (Crestor) are similar in nature and are isolated from fungal cultures
   b. Fluvastatin (Lescol) and atorvastatin (Lipitor) are produced synthetically
   c. Refer to Table 4-8 for a listing and dosage recommendations for common medications

3. Administration considerations
   a. Administration is usually done at night
   b. This dosing schedule increases drug's effectiveness, as cholesterol synthesis normally occurs during evening hours

Table 4-8 HMG-CoA Reductase Inhibitors

Generic (Trade) Name	Route	Uses
Atorvastatin (Lipitor)	PO	Adjunctive therapy to reduce cholesterol, low-density lipoprotein, and triglycerides
Fluvastatin (Lescol)	PO	Adjunctive therapy to reduce cholesterol, low-density lipoprotein, and triglycerides, slow the progression of coronary artery disease
Lovastatin (Mevacor)	PO	Adjunctive therapy to reduce cholesterol, low-density lipoprotein, and triglycerides
Pitavastatin (Livalo)	PO	Adjunctive therapy to reduce cholesterol, low-density lipoprotein, and triglycerides
Pravastatin (Pravachol)	PO	Prevention of myocardial infarction in clients who have no increase in cholesterol, slow progression of coronary artery disease; adjunctive therapy to reduce cholesterol, low-density lipoprotein, and triglycerides
Rosuvastatin (Crestor)	PO	Adjunctive therapy to reduce cholesterol, low-density lipoprotein, and triglycerides
Simvastatin (Zocor)	PO	Prevention of myocardial infarction in clients who have no increase in cholesterol, slow progression of coronary artery disease; adjunctive therapy to reduce cholesterol, low-density lipoprotein, and triglycerides

      c. An FDA advisory was released in 2011 recommending simvastatin 80 mg should only be used in clients who have been taking this dose for 12 or more months without evidence of myopathy; clients being started on this drug should be started on lower doses

4. Contraindications

      a. Clients with active liver disease and abnormal serum transaminase levels

      b. Pregnant and nursing mothers

5. Significant drug interactions

      a. Increased risk of myositis when used concurrently with immunosuppressives, antifungal agents, fibric acid derivatives, nicotinic acid, and erythromycin

      b. Additive effects are seen when used with cholestyramine (Questran)

      c. Spironolactone and cimetidine can cause decreased levels of HMG-CoA reductase inhibitors

      d. Rosuvastatin (Crestor) increases serum levels and toxic risk when administered with cyclosporine or gemfibrozil; increased risk of bleeding with sodium warfarin (Coumadin)

      e. Simvastatin at any dose is contraindicated with these drugs: itraconazole, ketoconazole, posaconazole, erythromycin, clarithromycin, telithromycin, HIV protease inhibitors, nefazodone, gemfibrozil, cyclosporine, and danazol

      f. Do not exceed 10 mg of simvastatin daily with concurrent use of amiodarone, verapamil, or diltiazem; do not exceed 20 mg with concurrent use of amlodipine or ranolazine

6. Significant food interactions: none reported

7. Significant laboratory studies

      a. Baseline liver function tests (LFTs) should be obtained before starting therapy

      b. LFTs should continue to be monitored at predetermined intervals (12 weeks and with dose adjustment) to confirm response to treatment and prevent possible adverse/toxic reactions

      c. Creatinine phosphokinase (CPK) levels may be monitored to evaluate possible development of myositis

      d. Digoxin level should be monitored if taking concurrently

8. Side effects

      a. GI upset, dyspepsia, flatulence

      b. Pain and myalgias

      c. Headache, rash, dizziness

      d. Sinusitis

9. Adverse effects/toxicity

      a. Altered liver function tests (elevated serum transaminase levels)

      b. Clients with uncontrolled hypothyroidism are at increased risk for muscle-related statin side effects

10. Nursing considerations

      a. Drug selection depends on prescriber preference and client tolerance

      b. They are not recommended for use in clients younger than age 20 years

      c. Administer dose with evening meal to coincide with body's timing of cholesterol production

      d. Monitor results of baseline and periodically drawn LFTs

      e. Monitor lipid levels within 2–4 weeks after initiation of therapy

      f. Arrange for consult, if needed, with a dietitian or nutritionist about need for a low-fat diet

11. Client education

      a. Proper self-administration (at evening meal) in order to promote biochemical activity

  b. Lab monitoring is required to maintain compliance and assess client response

  c. Report immediately to prescriber any unexplained muscle pain, tenderness, yellowing of skin or eyes, or loss of appetite

  d. Alcohol intake should be minimized or avoided

  e. Women of childbearing age should use contraceptives while taking a "statin"

B. Bile acid sequestrants

  1. Action and use

  a. Bile acid sequestrants are a group of nonabsorbable amine compounds that work in GI tract to bind with bile acids

  b. This binding leads liver cells to respond by sending cholesterol to maintain bile acid synthesis, thereby causing plasma levels of LDL cholesterol to decrease

  c. Indications for use include elevated cholesterol levels with or without high triglyceride levels

  d. Also used as an adjunctive therapy to dietary management of cholesterol elevations

  2. Common medications

  a. Cholestyramine (Questran) and colestipol (Colestid) are similar in their ability to lower LDL levels

  b. Colestipol is available as a tablet or powder, 5–30 grams/day in 2 to 4 doses before meals and at bedtime

  c. Cholestyramine is available as a powder, 4 grams bid to qid before meal times and at bedtime; a client may need up to 24 grams/day

  d. Colesevelan hydrochloride (Welchol) binds with bile acids to allow excretion in feces, which lowers cholesterol; dose is up to six 625 mg tablets daily

  3. Administration considerations

  a. Colestipol tablets should not be crushed, chewed, or cut; they should be taken with adequate fluids

  b. Powdered drug forms should be mixed at bedside to prevent overthickening and esophageal obstruction; they may be unflavored or orange flavored; because cholestyramine powder contains phenylalanine, it should not be used in clients who have phenylketonuria (PKU)

  c. Bile acid sequestrants should be administered alone due to potential for increased binding effects with other medications; give other drugs 1–2 hours before or 4–6 hours after bile acid administration

  d. Contents of one packet should be mixed with at least 120–180 mL of water or other preferred liquid; undissolved medication is irritating to mucous membranes

  4. Contraindications

  a. Colestipol is not recommended for use in pediatric clients

  b. Contraindicated in clients with complete biliary obstruction

  5. Significant drug interactions

  a. Bile acid sequestrants can bind to many other medications such as thyroxine, digoxin, diuretics, antibiotics and warfarin; because of this, they should not be given concurrently with other medications

  b. Additive effects are seen with use of bile acids and HMG-CoA reductase inhibitors and nicotinic acid

  c. Colesevelam (Welchol) is contraindicated with fat-soluble vitamins

  6. Significant food interactions: Powdered forms must be mixed in appropriate food or fluid to maximize absorption and prevent obstruction

  7. Significant laboratory studies

  a. Monitor baseline labs relative to cholesterol and triglyceride levels before starting therapy; continue to trend results to determine client response

  b. Decreased levels of LDL cholesterol should be seen within 1 month of therapy

8. Side effects
   a. Abdominal pain, bloating, reflux, constipation, steatorrhea, and hemorrhoids
   b. Associated vitamin deficiencies (A, D, K)
   c. Rash irritations of skin, tongue, and perianal areas
9. Adverse effects/toxicity
   a. Hypoprothrombinemia
   b. Decreased erythrocyte folate levels

! 10. Nursing considerations
   a. Properly mix and administer medication according to schedule to maximize biochemical activity (see also previous comments on mixing)
   b. Assess and monitor client for side effects of medication
   c. Bile acid sequestrants are not usually used as a first line therapy to treat elevated cholesterol levels because of poor client tolerance
   d. Vitamin deficiencies may require supplementation, if not discontinuation of bile acid sequestrants, to restore normal levels
   e. Problems related to hemorrhoids and/or constipation may require intervention to provide client comfort
   f. If the client develops GI complaints, a lower dosage may be necessary in order to maintain client compliance with this drug regimen
   g. Serum cholesterol levels are reduced within 24–48 hours after initiation of therapy
   h. Long-term use of cholestyramine can increase bleeding tendency

! 11. Client education
   a. Properly administer and schedule medication to maximize effect
   b. Be alert for signs and symptoms indicating side effects of these agents
   c. Follow-up blood work will be done to monitor cholesterol levels
   d. Increase high-bulk diet with adequate fluid intake
   e. Do not omit doses
   f. Report constipation immediately
   g. Eat small, frequent meals when experiencing heartburn, nausea, or loss of appetite with colesevelam (Welchol)

C. Fibric acid derivatives

1. Action and use
   a. They are a group of compounds that affect lipoproteins
   b. They act on very low density lipoproteins (VLDL) and chylomicrons leading to a reduction of triglyceride levels
   c. HDL cholesterol levels are increased but this is not the primary effect; there is also a variable effect on LDL levels
   d. Fibric acid derivatives are indicated for treatment of elevated triglyceride levels and elevated cholesterol level that is resistant to dietary management
2. Common medications
   a. Fibric acid derivatives decrease triglyceride and LDL levels and increase HDL levels
   b. Gemfibrozil (Lopid) is also indicated when there is an increased risk for a client to develop pancreatitis
   c. Refer to Table 4-9 for a listing of fibric acid derivatives
3. Administration considerations: Dose is usually given in divided doses, 30 minutes prior to morning and evening meals
4. Contraindications
   a. Gallbladder disease, renal problems, liver or biliary cirrhosis
   b. Pregnant or nursing women

Table 4-9 **Fibric Acid Derivatives**

Generic (Trade) Name	Route	Uses
Clofibrate (Atromid-S)	PO	Reduce cholesterol, VLDL, and triglycerides
Fenofibrate (Tricor)	PO	Type IV and V hyperlipidemia and hypertriglyceridemia
Gemfibrozil (Lopid)	PO	Reduce VLDL and triglycerides

5. Significant drug interactions
   a. Drug interactions can be seen with use of anticoagulants; monitor PT or INR levels
   b. Do not use fibric acid derivatives with statins (HMG-CoA reductase inhibitors) as rhabdomyolysis can occur
   c. Clofibrate increases hypoglycemic effect of sulfonylureas and should not be used in type 2 diabetes mellitus
6. Significant food interactions: fibric acid derivatives can cause altered taste perception
7. Significant laboratory studies
   a. Obtain baseline lipid levels prior to starting therapy; monitor ongoing labs periodically to document response to treatment
   b. If LFTs are persistently abnormal after 3 months, then therapy should be discontinued
   c. Hypokalemia may be seen in response to therapy
   d. Decreased hemoglobin, hematocrit, and white blood cell (WBC) count may be seen with the use of gemfibrozil
8. Side effects
   a. Abdominal or epigastric pain
   b. Jaundice, blurred vision, headache, and depression
   c. Rash, dermatitis, pruritus with gemfibrozil
   d. Back pain, muscle cramps, myalgia, and swollen joints
9. Adverse effects/toxicity
   a. Client may develop gallbladder disease and acute appendicitis
   b. Eosinophilia
   c. Hypokalemia
10. Nursing considerations
    a. Monitor baseline labs and perform ongoing assessments according to protocol
    b. If there is no response to therapy after 3 months, notify prescriber because the medication should be discontinued
    c. Monitor client for potential side effects and adverse effects
    d. Monitor closely for right upper quadrant (RUQ) abdominal pain or vomiting
11. Client education
    a. Lab work will be ongoing in nature to determine client response and evaluate for potential side effects
    b. Report immediately unexplained bleeding
    c. Restrict carbohydrate and alcohol intake
    d. Notify prescriber immediately if any serious side effects, such as acute appendicitis or gallbladder disease, should occur

D. **Nicotinic acid (niacin, vitamin B₃)**
   1. Action and use
      a. Is the active form of vitamin B_3 (niacin) in body and is water soluble
      b. Works to lower most lipoprotein levels (total cholesterol, LDL, triglyceride and lipoproteins) and increase HDL levels

    c. Indicated for clients with high cholesterol levels and as adjunctive therapy for clients where diet management is ineffective; dosage is usually started at 1 gram tid in adults

    d. It causes peripheral vasodilation and can be used to treat clients with peripheral vascular disease

    e. Pellagra (dermatitis, diarrhea, and dementia) is the clinical deficiency state associated with niacin deficiency; the required dosage of niacin to treat pellagra is 300 to 500 mg/day orally in divided doses

2. Common medications

    a. Vitamin B_3 is available both as a prescription and OTC medication

    b. The dosage for lowering cholesterol is higher (more than 3 grams/day) than the normal vitamin dose (500 mg/day in adults)

    c. Nicotinic acid is available in an immediate release form as well as a sustained-release preparation

3. Administration considerations

    a. Tablets should be taken whole; do not crush or divide the pill

    b. Medication can be taken with meals to prevent GI upset

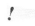   **c.** Flushing is a common side effect of niacin caused by its vasodilator properties

    d. Oral nicotinic acid should be taken with cold water

4. Contraindications

    a. Liver disease and/or unexplained levels of elevated serum transaminases and with active peptic ulcer disease

    b. Severe hypotension

5. Significant drug interactions

    a. Nicotinic acid should not be taken concurrently with statins, as there can be an increase in the occurrence of rhabdomyolysis

    b. Nicotinic acid may potentiate action of other drugs, such as antihypertensive and vasoactive drugs

    c. Nicotinic acid should be used cautiously with clients who are on anticoagulant therapy

    d. Clients with diabetes may need adjustment of their antidiabetic agents when taking nicotinic acid

    e. Niacin can decrease uricosuric effect of probenecid and sulfinpyrazone, leading to increased uric acid levels

    f. Niacin is often used in conjunction with bile resins to enhance effects

6. Significant food interactions

    a. Since niacin is available in OTC preparations, there is an increased likelihood of higher dosing

    b. 60 mg of dietary tryptophan (amino acid) is necessary to convert to 1 mg of niacin in body

    c. Corn in the diet interferes with conversion of tryptophan to niacin in body

7. Significant laboratory studies: nicotinic acid leads to increases in blood glucose, uric acid, and serum transaminase levels

8. Side effects

    a. Flushing

    b. Postural hypotension, vasovagal attacks

    c. Pruritus, increased sebaceous gland activity

    d. Dyspepsia, epigastric pain, and nausea

9. Adverse effects/toxicity

    a. Clients who report GI symptoms should be monitored closely for possibility of adverse reactions

b. Shortness of breath or edema

c. Megadose therapy has been associated with liver damage, hyperglycemia, hyperuricemia, and cardiac dysrhythmias

10. Nursing considerations

a. Administer dose as ordered to maximize absorption and minimize potential side effects

b. Dose is variable depending on whether it is prescribed to reduce cholesterol levels or as a vitamin supplement; be aware of specific dosing levels

c. Expect side effect of flushing when administering medication

d. Evaluate client for food sources that are high in niacin (dairy, meats, tuna, and egg) and assess dietary intake

e. Review list of medications with client and determine if there are any possible drug interactions

11. Client education

a. Change position slowly to avoid sudden BP drop

b. Avoid direct exposure to sunlight

c. Flushing in face, neck, and ears may occur within 2 hours after oral ingestion and immediately after IV dose and may last several hours

d. Follow up lab work will be ongoing to determine response to therapy

e. Alcohol and niacin cause increased flushing

f. Do not self-medicate with additional sources of niacin as this can lead to overdose

E. Cholesterol Absorption Inhibitors

1. Action and uses

a. Ezetimibe (Zetia) blocks absorption of cholesterol in intestinal lumen, thereby decreasing serum cholesterol

b. Since the liver may compensate by increasing production of cholesterol, a statin is often administered concurrently

c. Results in decrease of total cholesterol, LDL cholesterol, and triglycerides; these effects are enhanced when taken with a statin

d. Indicated in treatment of hypercholesterolemia

2. Common medications

a. The only drug in this class is ezetimibe (Zetia), given once daily orally

b. The drug Vytorin is a fixed combination of ezetimibe and simvastatin

3. Administration considerations: Avoid administering at same time as a bile acid sequestrant; administer ezetimibe 2 hours before or 4 hours following

4. Contraindications

a. It is extensively metabolized in liver and so contraindicated in clients with severe liver impairment or elevated serum transaminases

b. Hypersensitivity to ezetimibe

c. Children younger than 10 years

5. Significant drug interactions

a. Bile acid sequestrants will interfere with absorption of ezetimibe

b. Fibric acid derivatives and cyclosporine can increase ezitimibe drug levels

6. Significant food interactions; none reported

7. Significant laboratory studies

a. Monitor baseline and periodic lipid profile, Hgb and Hct, and platelet count

b. Monitor baseline and periodic liver function tests when used in conjunction with a statin

8. Side effects

a. Abdominal pain, back pain, diarrhea, and arthralgia

b. Fatigue, angioedema, myopathy, dizziness, and headache

9. Adverse effects/toxicity: increased risk for myopathy when given with statins

Practice to Pass

Why should cholesterol-lowering medications be taken at bedtime?

10. Nursing considerations
    a. Administer no sooner than 2 hours before or 4 hours after a bile acid sequestrant
    b. Assess for and report unexplained muscle pain
11. Client education
    a. Teach clients to store the drug at 15–30°C
    b. Report unexplained muscle pain, weakness, or tenderness
    c. Females need to prevent pregnancy while taking the medication

F. **Combination agents: Some drugs contain fixed combinations of lipid-lowering agents**
    1. Vytorin contains simvastatin and ezetimibe
    2. Advicor contains lovastatin and niacin
    3. Simcore contains various combinations of simvastatin and niacin

---

Case Study

C. W., a 48-year-old male client, is being admitted for deep vein thrombosis (DVT) of the left lower extremity and is to be placed on a weight-based heparin protocol. You are the nurse that has been assigned to take care of this client.

1. Why is the weight-based heparin protocol being utilized for this client?

2. What pertinent lab values and diagnostic tests would help to establish therapeutic care of this client?

3. C. W. does not understand why blood tests are done so frequently, and he is becoming quite anxious. What measures can you employ to decrease C. W.'s anxiety?

4. Coumadin is now being added to the treatment regimen and within a few days, C.W. is being discharged. C. W. is concerned about "all the possible risks" associated with Coumadin. What collaborative measures could you include in developing a plan of care with regard to Coumadin therapy?

For suggested responses, see pages 541–542.

POSTTEST

1 The nurse checks the laboratory values of a client receiving chemotherapy who is scheduled to receive epoetin alfa (Epogen) subcutaneously. Upon finding the hemoglobin is 12.2 grams/dL, the nurse takes which action? Select all that apply.

1. Administer the medication as ordered.
2. Withhold the medication dose.
3. Check the client's platelet count before administering the epoetin alfa (Epogen).
4. Notify the primary care provider of the client's laboratory value.
5. Assess the client for signs of internal bleeding.

2 When the client with pernicious anemia asked why vitamin B_{12} injections are necessary, the nurse should provide which of the following responses?

1. "They contribute to the increased production of red blood cells (RBCs) after a significant blood loss."
2. "Vitamin B_{12} is needed to prevent the red blood cells from sickling."
3. "Your stomach does not produce a substance needed for intestinal absorption of vitamin B_{12}."
4. "Vitamin B_{12} is needed to prevent excessive production of red blood cells (RBCs)."

POSTTEST

3 When managing the care of a client receiving intravenous (IV) anistreplase (Eminase), the nurse should take which of the following actions? Select all that apply.

1. Instruct client to avoid activities that could lead to bruising or bleeding.
2. Handle client gently when turning and positioning in bed.
3. Post sign at bedside that states, "No intramuscular injections."
4. Anticipate medicating the client with ibuprofen (Motrin) for joint pain prn.
5. Monitor laboratory results for 50% decrease in bleeding time.

---

4 A client is ordered to receive enoxaparin (Lovenox) 0.5 mg/kg subcutaneously. The client weighs 110 pounds and the enoxaparin comes in a pre-filled syringe containing 40 mg/mL. The nurse prepares the correct dose of how many mL?

_____ mL

---

5 The home health nurse is scheduling appointments for several clients who are taking folic acid (Folvite) for treatment of folic acid anemia. Which of the following clients should have the *first* appointment?

1. Client taking vitamin B_{12} (hydroxycobalamin) 100 mcg daily by subcutaneous injection for pernicious anemia
2. Client taking tetracycline (Sumycin) 500 mg PO qid for gonorrhea
3. Client taking allopurinol (Zyloprim) 100 mg PO daily for hyperuricemia
4. Client taking an oral contraceptive daily

---

6 Because a client treated with heparin therapy exhibited signs and symptoms of a heparin overdose or toxicity, the nurse should place priority on initiating which action?

1. Administer standard dose of 50 mg of protamine sulfate over a 10-minute period.
2. Draw client's activated partial thromboplastin time (aPTT) level during injection of protamine sulfate.
3. Determine amount of heparin infused along with time frame associated with the infusion.
4. Administer protamine sulfate concurrently with vitamin K to increase its therapeutic effect.

---

7 A surgical client has suddenly begun to bleed excessively while in the operating room. The nurse should prepare which of the following medications for possible injection?

1. Alteplase (Activase)
2. Aminocaproic acid (Amicar)
3. Dipyridamole (Persantine)
4. Heparin (Liquaemin)

---

8 The nurse anticipates an order to administer which of the following drugs to a client with aplastic anemia?

1. Dipyridamole (Persantine)
2. Allopurinol (Zyloprim)
3. Acetylsalicylic acid (Aspirin)
4. Cyclosporine (Sandimmune)

---

9 The nurse should teach which item of information to a client being discharged on long-term warfarin (Coumadin) therapy following cardiac valve replacement surgery?

1. Eat lettuce and tomatoes for lunch only a few times per week.
2. Limit dietary intake of yellow wax beans to twice weekly.
3. Use aspirin for minor aches and pains.
4. Wear shoes that completely enclose the feet.

10 The nurse is monitoring the activated partial thromboplastin time (aPTT) for a client receiving heparin therapy. When the latest aPTT is 2.0 times the normal aPTT, the nurse should perform which of the following actions specific to this result?

1. Assess for bleeding gums after tooth brushing is complete.
2. Perform a test for occult blood on stool.
3. Assess client for abnormal bruising.
4. Report the value during intershift report.

➤ *See pages 157–158 for Answers and Rationales.*

ANSWERS & RATIONALES

Pretest

1 **Answer: 4** **Rationale:** Oranges and lemons are high in vitamin C, which will enhance absorption of the iron supplement. Leafy green vegetables, whole grain breads, and raisins are high in iron, but would not enhance the absorption of the medication. **Cognitive Level:** Applying **Client Need:** Pharmacological and Parenteral Therapies **Integrated Process:** Nursing Process: Planning **Content Area:** Pharmacology **Strategy:** Note the critical words in the question are *enhance absorption*. Differentiate the foods that may be sources of iron from the one that is most likely to promote absorption of the iron supplements. **Reference:** Adams, M., & Holland, L. (2011). *Pharmacology for nurses: A pathophysiologic approach* (3rd ed.). Upper Saddle River, NJ: Pearson Education, p. 404.

2 **Answer: 4** **Rationale:** A change in clotting is a side effect of antiplatelet drugs. Clients may bruise from minor injuries more readily while receiving antiplatelet therapy. It is important to know how the client previously responded to injury and how he or she does now in order to determine whether the risk for bleeding is increased. Adherence is important but not as relevant as the client's response to therapy. Self-monitoring is an important general safety measure, but data indicating whether bruising has changed helps the nurse determine if the client is at risk. **Cognitive Level:** Applying **Client Need:** Pharmacological and Parenteral Therapies **Integrated Process:** Nursing Process: Assessment **Content Area:** Pharmacology **Strategy:** To choose correctly, you need to determine if the bruise is related to the drug. **Reference:** Adams, M., & Holland, L. (2011). *Pharmacology for nurses: A pathophysiologic approach* (3rd ed.). Upper Saddle River, NJ: Pearson Education, pp. 376–378.

3 **Answer: 1** **Rationale:** Ferritin levels reflect the visceral stores of iron in the body and transferrin levels reflect how iron is transported in the body. Hemoglobin and hematocrit refer to concentration and proportion of red blood cells (RBCs). The CBC will provide information about blood concentration of all three cell lines (red blood cells, white blood cells, and platelets). **Cognitive Level:** Applying **Client Need:** Pharmacological and Parenteral Therapies **Integrated Process:** Nursing Process: Assessment **Content Area:** Pharmacology **Strategy:** Recall concepts related to physiology and associated drug therapy to choose correctly. **Reference:** Adams, M., & Holland, L. (2011). *Pharmacology for nurses: A pathophysiologic approach* (3rd ed.). Upper Saddle River, NJ: Pearson Education, pp. 399–400.

4 **Answer: 1, 2, 5** **Rationale:** Alteplase (Activase) is a thrombolytic drug that can cause internal bleeding, and vital signs should be monitored closely in the first hour following administration. After dissolution of clots, the heart may respond to reperfusion by developing dysrhythmias, so the client should be placed on a cardiac monitor. Alteplase interferes with clot formation and would produce an increase in the partial thromboplastin time (PTT), which should be reported to monitor effects on coagulation. Hourly urinary outputs are not necessary when administering alteplase. Hourly urinary outputs are not necessary when administering alteplase. **Cognitive Level:** Applying **Client Need:** Pharmacological and Parenteral Therapies **Integrated Process:** Nursing Process: Planning **Content Area:** Pharmacology **Strategy:** Recall first that this drug dissolves clots and evaluate each option to determine the likelihood of each as a consequence of the drug's action. Choose options that relate to bleeding as a primary adverse effect, pertinent effects on cardiac rhythm, and laboratory test results. **Reference:** Wilson, B. A., Shannon, M., & Shields, K. (2012). *Pearson nurse's drug guide 2012.* Upper Saddle River, NJ: Pearson Education, pp. 51–54.

5 **Answer: 3** **Rationale:** The target goal with epoetin alfa (Epogen) therapy is a hemoglobin level of 10–12 grams/dL and reflects effectiveness of therapy. Bone pain is an adverse effect to epoetin alfa therapy, but the absence of bone pain does not guarantee drug efficacy. A rapid rise in hemoglobin and hematocrit (H&H) is undesirable as it can lead to hypertension and seizures, and it would not reflect an effective therapeutic response. Fever is an adverse response to epoetin alfa, but being afebrile does not guarantee the drug is effective at raising the client's H&H. **Cognitive Level:** Analyzing **Client Need:** Pharmacological and Parenteral Therapies **Integrated Process:** Nursing Process: Evaluation **Content Area:** Pharmacology **Strategy:** Since erythropoietin is produced by the kidneys, *poetin* is an important suffix that should help guide your thinking toward altered hematology. **Reference:** Lehne, R. (2010). *Pharmacology for nursing care* (7th ed.). St. Louis, MO: Mosby, Inc., pp. 647–649.

6 **Answer: 2, 5** **Rationale:** Facial flushing is a common side effect of niacin and it occurs shortly after ingesting the drug. Administering aspirin 30 minutes prior to taking niacin can help to reduce this effect. Over time, the flushing will be reduced, but taking the aspirin can help to reduce this very bothersome side effect. Dosages may be adjusted if the client develops side effects; they are not based on lab values. It is not necessary to eat a diet high in niacin in order for the medication to be effective. The medication is given to improve lipid levels, but taking niacin with lovastatin (Mevacor) can increase the risk for myopathy and should be avoided. **Cognitive Level:** Applying **Client Need:** Pharmacological and Parenteral Therapies **Integrated Process:** Teaching and Learning **Content Area:** Pharmacology **Strategy:** The wording of the question indicates that the correct response provides true information related to niacin use. Recall the drug's action and side effects to choose correctly. **Reference:** Wilson, B. A., Shannon, M., & Shields, K. (2012). *Pearson nurse's drug guide 2012*. Upper Saddle River, NJ: Pearson Education, pp. 49–52.

7 **Answer: 1, 2, 3, 4** **Rationale:** In the treatment of von Willebrand's disease, desmopressin (DDAVP) stimulates an increase in clotting factors vW and VIII. DDAVP is the hormone vasopressin, or antidiuretic hormone (ADH), which promotes water reabsorption in the renal tubules. If an excessive amount of drug is used, the client may retain water, and urine output will decrease while the blood pressure could increase. Cryoprecipitate is not used to treat von Willebrand's disease since it cannot be filtered safely for HIV. **Cognitive Level:** Analyzing **Client Need:** Pharmacological and Parenteral Therapies **Integrated Process:** Communication and Documentation **Content Area:** Pharmacology **Strategy:** The wording of the question indicates the correct options are true statements. Specific drug knowledge is needed to answer this question, so review it now if needed. **Reference:** Wilson, B. A., Shannon, M., & Shields, K. (2012). *Pearson nurse's drug guide 2012*. Upper Saddle River, NJ: Pearson Education, pp. 432–435.

8 **Answer: 4** **Rationale:** Ibuprofen (Motrin) has an antiplatelet effect and can lead to bleeding as an adverse effect; this would further decrease the platelet count and increase risk of bleeding. Ibuprofen does not affect ferritin levels, although low ferritin levels reflect iron stores, which could indirectly affect bleeding risk. Ibuprofen may be taken when triglyceride levels

are low. Low neutrophil counts will affect immune response, but does not necessitate a need to avoid using ibuprofen. **Cognitive Level:** Analyzing **Client Need:** Pharmacological and Parenteral Therapies **Integrated Process:** Teaching and Learning **Content Area:** Pharmacology **Strategy:** Correlate the adverse effect (bleeding) of ibuprofen (Motrin) with the function of platelets to make the correct selection. **Reference:** Wilson, B. A., Shannon, M., & Shields, K. (2012). *Pearson nurse's drug guide 2012*. Upper Saddle River, NJ: Pearson Education, pp. 753–756.

9 **Answer: 2, 5** **Rationale:** After cardiac valve replacement surgery, safe management requires life-long anticoagulation therapy. Clients must be instructed regarding bleeding risks as well as how to modify their environment and activities of daily living accordingly. Follow-up lab testing is required but initially would be weekly or every other week, rather than every 3 months. Coumadin should be taken at the same time of day. Clients are instructed not to double-up doses and to take the medication as specifically ordered to ensure safe and therapeutic effects. Clients should eat a consistent amount of foods containing vitamin K daily. Large amounts of foods high in vitamin K can interfere with the action of warfarin and reduce effectiveness. **Cognitive Level:** Applying **Client Need:** Pharmacological and Parenteral Therapies **Integrated Process:** Teaching and Learning **Content Area:** Pharmacology **Strategy:** Recall that the major adverse effect of anticoagulants is bleeding. With this in mind, select the option that minimizes the risk of bleeding, which is also directly related to the critical term *protection* in the question. **Reference:** Wilson, B. A., Shannon, M., & Shields, K. (2012). *Pearson nurse's drug guide 2012*. Upper Saddle River, NJ: Pearson Education, pp. 1590–1593.

10 **Answer: 3** **Rationale:** The rate of administration must be closely monitored since heparin (Liquaemin) affects blood clotting. The client could receive a subtherapeutic dose or be at increased risk for bleeding if the infusion was infused too slowly or too quickly, respectively. Vitamin K is the antidote for warfarin (Coumadin) therapy, not heparin, and it is not standard policy in most institutions to leave medications at the bedside. Heparin does not require the client to be NPO during IV infusion. Heparin infusion therapies are weight based, and daily weights provide a more accurate dosing. **Cognitive Level:** Applying **Client Need:** Pharmacological and Parenteral Therapies **Integrated Process:** Nursing Process: Planning **Content Area:** Pharmacology **Strategy:** Identify the drug action and the risk to the client, and then determine the nursing action that would best protect the client. The core underlying issue is safety during administration of this medication. **Reference:** Wilson, B. A., Shannon, M., & Shields, K. (2012). *Pearson nurse's drug guide 2012*. Upper Saddle River, NJ: Pearson Education, pp. 726–729.

Posttest

1 **Answer: 2, 4** **Rationale:** The dose should not be administered as the hemoglobin has surpassed the target level. When hemoglobin levels are above 12 grams/dL in clients with renal failure and above 10 grams/dL in clients receiving chemotherapy, and epoetin alfa is continued, the client is at greater risk to experience serious adverse events, such as heart attack, stroke, and death. The primary care provider should be notified that the hemoglobin level is above target level. Epoetin alfa (Epogen) does not affect platelet levels. **Cognitive Level:** Analyzing **Client Need:** Pharmacological and Parenteral Therapies **Integrated Process:** Nursing Process: Assessment **Content Area:** Pharmacology **Strategy:** First recall the target hemoglobin levels for a client on chemotherapy who is receiving epoetin alfa (Epogen). Then determine if it is safe to administer the medication to this client. **Reference:** Lilley, L. L, Collins, S. R., Harrington, S., & Snyder, J. S. (2011). *Pharmacology and the nursing process* (6th ed.). St. Louis, MO: Mosby Elsevier, pp. 666–667.

2 **Answer: 3** **Rationale:** Intrinsic factor, produced in the stomach, is needed for absorption of vitamin B_{12}. Because vitamin B_{12} activates an enzyme that moves folic acid into the cells to contribute to the production of RBCs, deficiencies of the intrinsic factor results in anemia. Pernicious anemia is due to this absence of intrinsic factor. Significant blood losses are usually replaced with blood transfusions and iron supplements. Sickle cell anemia is treated with hydroxyurea (Droxia) rather than vitamin B_{12}. Vitamin B_{12} does not prevent excessive production of RBCs. **Cognitive Level:** Applying **Client Need:** Pharmacological and Parenteral Therapies **Integrated Process:** Teaching and Learning **Content Area:** Pharmacology **Strategy:** Select the option that remedies the interruption caused by the disease. **Reference:** Ignatavicius, D., & Workman, L. (2010). *Medical-surgical nursing: Critical thinking for collaborative care* (6th ed.). Philadelphia: W. B. Saunders, pp. 887–896.

3 **Answer: 1, 2, 3** **Rationale:** Because of the risk of bleeding with infusion of thrombolytic drugs such as anistreplase, vigorous activities or activities that could cause bleeding are discouraged. Internal injury is unseen and places the client at extreme risk. Because of the risk of bleeding, IM injections should be avoided. The client needs to avoid drugs that would prolong bleeding time, such as ibuprofen and aspirin. The client's bleeding time would be increased rather than decreased following administration of a thrombolytic medication. **Cognitive Level:** Applying **Client Need:** Pharmacological and Parenteral Therapies **Integrated Process:** Teaching and Learning **Content Area:** Pharmacology **Strategy:** Associate the drug's action with the greatest risks to the client. **Reference:** Adams, M., & Holland, L. (2011). *Pharmacology for nurses: A pathophysiologic approach* (3rd ed.). Upper Saddle River, NJ: Pearson Education, Inc., pp. 383–386.

4 **Answer: 0.63** **Rationale:** The dose is ordered in mg/kg, so the weight of 110 lbs is divided by 2.2 kg/lb, to yield a weight of 50 kg. The ordered dose is 0.5 mg/kg, so 50 multiplied by 0.5 mg = 25 mg. Using the equation

$$\frac{\text{Desired}}{\text{Have}} \times 1 \text{ mL}$$

$$\frac{25 \text{ mg}}{40 \text{ mg}} \times 1 = \frac{25}{40}$$

$$= 25x = 40$$

$$x = .625$$

Round appropriately to 2 decimal places to obtain 0.63 mL **Cognitive Level:** Applying **Client Need:** Pharmacological and Parenteral Therapies **Integrated Process:** Nursing Process: Implementation **Content Area:** Pharmacology **Strategy:** First recognize the need to convert the client's weight in pounds to kilograms. Then use the "desired over have times quantity" equation to calculate the correct dose. **Reference:** Adams, M. P., & Koch R. W. (2010). *Pharmacology: Connections to nursing practice.* Upper Saddle River, NJ: Pearson Education, pp. 645, 647.

5 **Answer: 4** **Rationale:** Oral contraceptives taken concurrently with folic acid will diminish the effectiveness of the folic acid. Therefore, this client needs the first appointment to determine that drug therapy is effective. Vitamin B_{12} enhances the effects of folic acid, so this client is likely to have a more optimal outcome initially. There are no known negative drug interactions between tetracycline and folic acid or allopurinol and folic acid. **Cognitive Level:** Applying **Client Need:** Pharmacological and Parenteral Therapies **Integrated Process:** Nursing Process: Planning **Content Area:** Pharmacology **Strategy:** The client who should be seen first is the one who is less likely to have a good outcome of therapy or is more at risk for drug interactions. Select the client who correlates best with negative outcomes associated with the drug. **Reference:** Wilson, B. A., Shannon, M., & Shields, K. (2012). *Pearson nurse's drug guide 2012.* Upper Saddle River, NJ: Pearson Education, pp. 666–668.

6 **Answer: 3** **Rationale:** Because protamine has a longer half-life than heparin (protamine 2 hrs and heparin 90 minutes) and also has some anticoagulant qualities, the dose of protamine needs to be titrated according to the amount and length of time the heparin was administered. This intervention *precedes* relevant assessment parameters. Monitoring aPTT levels *after* injection of protamine sulfate is the appropriate method for determining effectiveness. Protamine sulfate is the antidote for heparin and vitamin K is the antidote for warfarin; both medications would not be given together. **Cognitive Level:** Analyzing **Client Need:** Pharmacological and Parenteral Therapies **Integrated Process:** Nursing Process: Implementation **Content Area:** Pharmacology **Strategy:** The critical issue of the question is the need to know the antidote specifically associated with heparin, which is protamine sulfate and data needed for proper dosing. **Reference:** Wilson, B. A., Shannon, M., &

Shields, K. (2012). *Pearson nurse's drug guide 2012.* Upper Saddle River, NJ: Pearson Education, pp. 1289–1290.

7 **Answer: 2** **Rationale:** Hemostatics such as aminocaproic acid are used to control excessive bleeding. They may be applied topically to stop a local hemorrhage, or they can be administered parenterally to stop a systemic hemorrhage. Alteplase (Activase) is a thrombolytic agent and would cause further bleeding. Dipyridamole (Persantine) is an antiplatelet agent used to prevent platelet aggregation and could increase the risk of bleeding. Heparin (Liquaemin) is an anticoagulant given to prolong the time it takes for blood to clot; it would be contraindicated in a client who is actively bleeding. **Cognitive Level:** Applying **Client Need:** Pharmacological and Parenteral Therapies **Integrated Process:** Nursing Process: Planning **Content Area:** Pharmacology **Strategy:** Differentiate between drugs that cause bleeding and drugs that would reduce bleeding. The correct answer is the drug that reduces bleeding. **Reference:** Wilson, B. A., Shannon, M., & Shields, K. (2012). *Pearson nurse's drug guide 2012.* Upper Saddle River, NJ: Pearson Education, pp. 51–54, 66–67, 480–481, 726–729.

8 **Answer: 4** **Rationale:** Cyclosporine (Sandimmune) is used in the treatment of aplastic anemia. It works by preventing destruction of the stem cells by lymphocytes. Dipyridamole (Persantine) is prescribed for clients with *polycythemia vera* to prevent the increased viscosity resulting from the excessively high numbers of RBCs. Allopurinol (Zyloprim) is administered to treat the signs and symptoms of gout associated with *polycythemia vera.* Acetylsalicylic acid (Aspirin) would be contraindicated in the treatment of anemia since it interferes with platelets and can cause gastric bleeding. **Cognitive Level:** Applying **Client Need:** Pharmacological and Parenteral Therapies **Integrated Process:** Nursing Process: Planning **Content Area:** Pharmacology **Strategy:** Correlate the drug with the nature of the disease. **Reference:** Wilson, B. A., Shannon, M., & Shields, K. (2012). *Pearson nurse's drug*

guide 2012. Upper Saddle River, NJ: Pearson Education, pp. 41–43, 119–122, 385–387, 480–481.

9 **Answer: 4** **Rationale:** Clients on oral anticoagulant therapy are at increased risk of bleeding and should wear shoes to protect them from possible injury. Lettuce, tomatoes, and yellow wax beans do not contain enough vitamin K to interact negatively with warfarin (Coumadin), so they do not need to be limited. Aspirin increases the risk of bleeding and therefore should not be used while taking an anticoagulant such as warfarin. **Cognitive Level:** Analyzing **Client Need:** Pharmacological and Parenteral Therapies **Integrated Process:** Teaching and Learning **Content Area:** Pharmacology **Strategy:** Recall that warfarin is an anticoagulant that carries an increased risk of bleeding. Select the option that provides the client with the greatest amount of protection against this risk. **Reference:** Wilson, B. A., Shannon, M., & Shields, K. (2012). *Pearson nurse's drug guide 2012.* Upper Saddle River, NJ: Pearson Education, pp. 1590–1593.

10 **Answer: 4** **Rationale:** Since the therapeutic range for APTT level should be 1.5 to 2.5 times the control value, no action is necessary and the nurse would provide routine care, including reporting the expected value to the oncoming shift. Monitoring for bleeding gums and excessive or abnormal bruising should be done without regard to the aPTT. Testing for occult blood is a preventive mechanism that would not be related to the therapeutic aPTT range. **Cognitive Level:** Applying **Client Need:** Pharmacological and Parenteral Therapies **Integrated Process:** Nursing Process: Implementation **Content Area:** Pharmacology **Strategy:** The core issue of the question is the appropriate range for activated partial thromboplastin time (aPTT) during anticoagulant therapy. Recall the normal range and use the process of elimination to select the option that reflects ordinary care. **Reference:** Wilson, B. A., Shannon, M., & Shields, K. (2012). *Pearson nurse's drug guide 2012.* Upper Saddle River, NJ: Pearson Education, pp. 726–729.

References

Abrams, A. (2009). *Clinical drug therapy: Rationales for nursing practice* (9th ed.). Philadelphia, PA: Lippincott Williams & Wilkins.

Adams, M., Holland, L., & Bostwick, P. (2011). *Pharmacology for nurses: A pathophysiologic approach* (3rd ed.). Upper Saddle River, NJ: Pearson Education.

Adams, M., Koch R. (2010). *Pharmacology: Connections to nursing practice.* Upper Saddle River, NJ: Pearson Education.

Aschenbrenner, D., & Venable, S. (2012). *Drug therapy in nursing* (4th ed.). Philadelphia, PA: Lippincott Williams & Wilkins.

Drug Facts & Comparisons® (Updated monthly). St. Louis, MO: A. Wolters Kluwer.

Ignatavicius, D., & Workman, M. (2010). *Medical-surgical nursing: Critical thinking for collaborative care* (6th ed.). Philadelphia, PA: W. B. Saunders.

Karch, A. M. (2010). *Focus on nursing pharmacology* (5th ed.). Philadelphia, PA: Lippincott Williams & Wilkins.

Kee, J. (2009). *Laboratory and diagnostic tests and nursing implications* (8th ed.). Upper Saddle River, NJ: Pearson Education.

Lehne, R. (2010). *Pharmacology for nursing care* (7th ed.). St. Louis, MO: Mosby, Inc.

LeMone, P., Burke, K., & Bauldoff, G. (2011). *Medical-surgical nursing: Critical thinking in patient care* (5th ed.). Upper Saddle River, NJ: Pearson Education.

Lilley, L., Collins, Harrington, S., & Snyder, J. (2011). *Pharmacology and the nursing process* (6th ed.). St. Louis, MO: Mosby, Inc.

Wilson, B. A., Shannon, M. T, & Shields, K. M. (2012). *Pearson nurse's drug guide 2012.* Upper Saddle River, NJ: Pearson Education.

Cardiac Medications

5

Chapter Outline

Nitrates and Nitrites
Beta-Adrenergic Blockers
Calcium Channel Blockers
Peripheral Vasodilators
Cardiac Glycosides

Phosphodiesterase III
   Inhibitors
Atrial Natriuretic Peptide
   Hormone
Antidysrhythmics

Antihypertensives,
   Antihypotensives,
   Diuretics, and Potassium
   Supplements

Objectives

➤ Describe general goals of therapy when administering cardiovascular medications.
➤ Identify specific nursing interventions related to administering digoxin (Lanoxin).
➤ Identify signs and symptoms of digitalis toxicity.
➤ List side effects of the most commonly used antidysrhythmics.
➤ Identify the nursing considerations when administering antidysrhythmics.
➤ Discuss side effects and adverse reactions of beta-adrenergic blockers, calcium channel blockers, and nitrates.
➤ Identify specific client teaching points related to the administration of nitroglycerin.
➤ List significant client education points related to the various cardiovascular medications.

NCLEX-RN® Test Prep

Use the accompanying online resource, NursingReviewsandRationales, to test yourself with hundreds of NCLEX®-style practice questions.

Review at a Glance

afterload resistance to blood being ejected from left ventricle; resistance in great vessels that the heart pumps against

automaticity ability of heart to initiate impulses on its own without external stimulation

cardiac output amount of blood ejected in liters/minute by heart; consists of input from preload, afterload, contractility, and heart rate

chronotropic affecting heart rate (HR); positive chronotropic medications increase HR; negative chronotropic medications decrease HR

conductivity ability of impulses to spread throughout cardiac muscle fibers despite absence of specialized conduction tissue

contractility amount of force and pressure to pump blood from ventricles;

amount of or ability of ventricles to "squeeze"

dromotropic affecting speed with which impulses pass through conduction system; positive dromotropic medications increase speed of impulses, while negative dromotropic medications decrease speed of impulses

dysrhythmia a general term that refers to abnormalities in electrocardiogram (EKG, ECG) pattern; these refer to electrical activity and not mechanical pumping action (contraction) of heart

inotropic affecting force of contraction; positive inotropic medications increase force of contraction and therefore increase cardiac output (CO); negative inotropic medications decrease force of contraction and therefore decrease CO

irritability a state in which heart muscle responds to a variety of external stimuli, including hypoxia, ischemia, abnormal electrolyte levels, particular hormones, medications, and physical trauma

preload degree to which ventricles are filled with blood and myocardial fibers are stretched prior to contraction

refractory period either relative (able to respond only to a strong stimulus) or absolute refractory period (unable to respond even to a strong stimulus); refers to recovery period in cardiac cycle when heart varies in its depolarization (electrical activity leading to contraction)

titrate act of adjusting medication (usually intravenous) according to a predetermined parameter

PRETEST

1 The nurse is preparing to teach the client newly diagnosed with angina pectoris how to self-administer nitroglycerine (NTG) tablets. What client teaching should the nurse emphasize? Select all that apply.

1. "Stop all activities immediately and sit down if chest pain occurs."
2. "If the pain is unrelieved after taking one NTG tablet, continue to rest, take another tablet in 5 minutes, and call the prescriber."
3. "After discharge to home, keep NTG tablets on your bedside table day and night."
4. "Immediately after chest pain begins, notify your personal physician."
5. "The NTG tablet should tingle when placed under the tongue."

2 The client states, "I always put my nitroglycerin (NTG) patch in the same place so I do not forget to take it off." Which of the following is the best response by the nurse?

1. "Change the patch every 24 hours."
2. "Take 2 acetaminophen tablets 30 minutes prior to applying the patch."
3. "Rotate the NTG patch to a different hairless area each day."
4. "After removing the patch, scrub the area vigorously with soap and water."

3 A client hospitalized for heart failure is receiving digoxin (Lanoxin) IV push. The nurse obtains the following data on the client. Place the data in order from that of highest concern to least concern to the nurse.

1. Potassium (K+) level is 3.2 mEq/L
2. Apical pulse is 53 beats per minute
3. Client has been taking furosemide (Lasix) 20 mg daily for 2 days
4. Client enjoys orange juice with breakfast

4 A health care provider orders nitroglycerin (NTG) to be administered by IV drip. The nurse places priority on monitoring the client for which of the following?

1. Shortness of breath
2. Urine output
3. Blood pressure and heart rate
4. Headache and facial flushing

5 Before a client receives metoprolol (Lopressor) for hypertension, the nurse should ask the client about a history of which of the following?

1. Bronchospasm
2. Seizures
3. Peripheral vascular disease
4. Myasthenia gravis

6 A nurse assesses a 75-year-old client for side effects of verapamil (Calan-SR). Which of the following side effects would be of most concern regarding this client?

1. Hypertension
2. Angina
3. Skin rash
4. Constipation

7 The client is receiving intravenous lidocaine through an infusion pump at a rate of 2 mg per minute. The nurse should discontinue the infusion and notify the health care provider immediately if which of the following occurs? Place the elements in order of priority.

1. Demonstrates slurred speech
2. Regular heart rate of 64/min
3. Respiratory rate of 12/min
4. Electrocardiogram (ECG) reveals prolonged PR interval

8 A client is admitted to the emergency department in acute heart failure. Blood pressure is 116/86 and heart rate is 98. The nurse ensures that which medication is available for immediate use once it is ordered?

1. Atropine sulfate
2. Digoxin (Lanoxin)
3. Propranolol (Inderal)
4. Verapamil (Calan)

9 A client asks the nurse to explain why she is receiving lidocaine (Xylocaine) in her IV when her dentist injects it into her gums to numb the teeth before a filling. The nurse includes which information about lidocaine in a response? Select all that apply.

1. It regulates electrical activity in the heart.
2. It acts as local anesthetic on nerve endings of the cardiac muscles.
3. It reduces irritability of the cardiac cells.
4. It increases the heart rate.
5. It primarily treats dysrhythmias originating in the ventricles.

10 The nurse provides discharge instructions to a client about the use of amiodarone (Cordarone). Which statement indicates that the client has the knowledge necessary to safely self-administer the drug?

1. "As soon as the physician says I can stop taking this medication, I will be able to enjoy the sun again."
2. "The side effects of this medication may not begin to show up for several weeks or even months after I start taking it."
3. "If my pulse drops below 100 beats per minute, I should call the primary care provider right away."
4. "If I miss a dose of medication I will take two pills the next day."

➤ *See pages 186–187 for Answers and Rationales.*

I. NITRATES AND NITRITES

A. Action and use
1. Increase oxygenated blood flow to myocardium by dilating coronary and systemic blood vessels to relieve chest pain
2. Prophylactic treatment of angina in clients with coronary artery disease (CAD)
3. Dilation of systemic vascular bed leads to pooling of blood in peripheral vascular system; this reduces left ventricle workload by reducing both **preload** (volume in left ventricle just prior to contraction) and **afterload** (resistance to blood being ejected by left ventricle) and ultimately reducing myocardial oxygen (O_2) demand
4. Short acting nitrates are used to treat angina episodes; long acting nitrates are used to prevent angina and treat symptoms of heart failure

B. Common medications (Table 5-1)

C. Administration considerations
1. Client's mucous membranes should be moist when taking sublingual (SL) tablets
2. Intravenous (IV) nitroglycerin (NTG) must be delivered as a continuous or intermittent infusion (not IV push) and given via an infusion pump

Table 5-1	Common Nitrates and Nitrites	

Generic (Trade) Name	Route	Uses
Isosorbide Dinitrate (Dilatrate-SR, Isordil)	PO	Prevention of angina pectoris; symptomatic treatment of heart failure
Isosorbide mononitrate (Imdur, ISMO, Monoket)	PO	Prevention of angina pectoris; symptomatic treatment of heart failure
Nitroglycerin SL (Nitrostat)	SL	Prophylaxis or treatment of angina pectoris
Nitroglycerin SR (Nitrong, Nitro-Bid)	SL	Prophylaxis or treatment of angina pectoris
Nitroglycerin Topical (Nitrol)	Topical	Prophylaxis or treatment of angina pectoris
Nitroglycerin Transdermal (Transderm-Nitro)	Topical	

3. NTG for IV use must be diluted in 5% dextrose or 0.9% sodium chloride (NaCl) solution

4. Intravenous NTG should be mixed in glass bottles and only manufacturer-supplied IV tubing should be used; regular IV tubing can absorb 40–80% of NTG because of polyvinyl chloride plastic

5. Administer regular form of isosorbide on empty stomach; if chewable form used, tell client to chew thoroughly before swallowing; do not crush sustained-release tablets

6. Nitroglycerine drips are often ordered to control or treat client's chest pain; nurse should **titrate** (adjust medication according to a predetermined parameter) medication accordingly

7. Monitor blood pressure (BP) and heart rate (HR) every 15 minutes when using IV NTG and titrating the medication; be prepared to treat hypotension by decreasing or stopping the NTG infusion

8. Wear gloves or use applicator when applying NTG ointment to avoid absorption of medication into nurse's skin

9. Rotate location of NTG paste or patch to reduce skin irritation and enhance absorption; place on hairless areas for predictable absorption and avoid areas with scar tissue; appropriate areas include chest, upper abdomen, anterior thigh, or upper arm

10. For a hospitalized client, keep tablets at bedside only if policy allows; instruct client to report all attacks; count tablets daily if kept at bedside

11. The dosing regimen should allow for a 6- to 8-hour nitrate-free period to prevent the body's development of tolerance; NTG patch should be applied in the morning and removed at 10 p.m.

D. **Contraindications**
1. Hypersensitivity to nitrates
2. Hypotension and/or hypovolemia
3. Severe bradycardia or severe tachycardia
4. Right ventricular myocardial infarction
5. Use of sildenafil (Viagra) or other phosphodiesterase-5 inhibitors for erectile dysfunction within 24 hours

E. **Significant drug interactions**
1. Do not mix with any other medications in the bottle or IV tubing
2. Use of phosphodiesterase-5 inhibitors within 24 hours leads to profound hypotension
3. All other antihypertensive and vasodilator medications may interact to cause profound hypotension
4. Intravenous NTG may antagonize heparin anticoagulation
5. Alcohol consumption should be avoided

F. **Significant food interactions: none reported but alcohol may enhance hypotensive effect**

G. Significant laboratory studies
1. Nitroglycerine may increase urinary catecholamines
2. It may cause a false report of decrease in serum cholesterol
3. Prolonged high-dose use of NTG may lead to methemoglobinemia

H. Side effects
1. Headache
2. Postural hypotension
3. Flushing
4. Local burning or tingling sensation
5. GI upset with oral form
6. Contact dermatitis with topical use

I. Adverse reactions/toxicity
1. Blurred vision and dry mouth
2. Central nervous system (CNS): weakness, dizziness, vertigo, and faintness
3. Cardiovascular (CV): severe postural hypotension with resulting tachycardia; when BP falls, heart rate increases to sustain **cardiac output** (amount of blood ejected in liters/minute by heart)
4. Gastrointestinal (GI): nausea, vomiting, fecal and urinary incontinence, abdominal pain, and dry mouth

J. Nursing considerations
1. Drug forms appropriate for angina prophylaxis include NTG paste, NTG patch, spray, SL tablet, and oral sustained-release forms
2. Drug forms appropriate for acute angina include NTG spray, SL tablet, or IV infusion
3. Ensure that client is sitting or lying down when taking NTG to prevent dizziness or fainting
4. Allow tablet to dissolve naturally under tongue; if mouth is dry, instruct client to take a sip of water before placing tablet under the tongue
5. If pain is not relieved after the first dose, notify health care provider or emergency services; doses can be repeated up to 3 times every 5 minutes
6. Store ointment in a cool, dry place with the cap attached tightly
7. Check NTG IV infusion concentration carefully, as many different dilutions are possible
8. See also previous section on administration considerations
9. Monitor vital signs closely, especially for hypotension; measure BP prior to each NTG tablet

K. Client education
1. All forms of NTG might cause dizziness and headache; rest for at least 15 minutes after taking SL NTG to avoid dizziness; headaches decrease in intensity and frequency with continued therapy and respond to acetaminophen
2. Report to health care provider if symptoms become worse or increase in frequency when taking NTG
3. If pain is not relieved after first dose, call 911, as this could indicate an impending myocardial infarction (MI); may repeat dose up to 3 times while awaiting treatment
4. Write down emergency phone numbers and place them next to phone; tell client to sit near phone when taking NTG in case of need to call for help
5. Take a sublingual or spray NTG before an event that might cause angina, such as exercise or sexual intercourse; keep NTG on hand for prn use
6. Keep a written record for prescriber of times, dates, amount of medication required for relief of each attack and possible precipitating factors
7. NTG tablets degrade in heat, light, or moisture, so store in original dark container in a cool, dry place; replace every 3–6 months after opening; tablets should cause tingling or slight stinging sensation under tongue if fresh (potent)

Practice to Pass

An overweight female client has just told you she is planning to take OTC diet pills to lose 50 pounds. The client is also taking Transderm-Nitro. How would you address this issue? What client teaching is needed related to this medication?

8. Change position slowly, especially older adults, to avoid postural hypotension and falls
9. Shake aerosol spray well prior to use as this affects the metered dose; spray 1–2 sprays onto or under tongue at onset of angina; repeat as needed for a maximum of 3 sprays in 15 minutes
10. If wearing an NTG patch or paste and experiencing an angina attack, take an SL NTG tablet using the safety measures previously outlined
11. Client may swim or bathe with an NTG patch in place
12. Frequent and prolonged use of NTG may reduce efficacy, requiring a medication adjustment
13. Avoid over-the-counter (OTC) medications or herbal products without consulting prescriber
14. Avoid alcohol use after taking nitroglycerin, as it can cause a sharp drop in blood pressure
15. Report blurred vision, dry mouth, chest pain, or fainting to provider, as these may warrant discontinuation of drug

II. BETA-ADRENERGIC BLOCKERS

A. Action and use

1. Decrease effects of sympathetic nervous system by blocking action of circulating catecholamines (epinephrine and norepinephrine)
2. In therapeutic doses, they block beta-adrenergic receptors (remember b_1—you have one heart) that are found chiefly in cardiac muscle; also referred to as *cardioselective*
3. In higher doses, they may block beta-adrenergic receptors in airways (remember b_2—you have two lungs) leading to increased airway resistance, especially in clients with asthma or chronic obstructive pulmonary disease (COPD); also referred to as *noncardioselective*
4. Blocking beta-adrenergic receptors leads to reduction in renin activity, with resulting suppression of renin–angiotensin–aldosterone system; this results in:
   a. Competition for binding of catecholamines at beta-adrenergic receptor sites
   b. Reduction in systolic and diastolic BP
   c. A negative **inotropic** (force of contraction) and **chronotropic** (heart rate) effect
5. Are used therapeutically to manage hypertension, angina pectoris, acute myocardial infarction (AMI), and supraventricular tachycardia
6. Should be administered to all clients with suspected myocardial infarction (MI) and unstable angina in the absence of complications such as heart failure (HF); they also help prevent ventricular fibrillation
7. They block cardiac effects of beta-adrenergic stimulation resulting in:
   a. Reductions in HR, myocardial **irritability** (cardiac muscle response to a variety of external stimuli such as hypoxia), and force of contraction
   b. Depression of **automaticity** (heart's ability to initiate impulses on its own without any external stimulation) of the sinoatrial (SA) node
   c. Reduction in atrioventricular (AV) node and intraventricular **dromotropic** (conduction velocity) effect
8. Are also useful in controlling panic attacks and stage fright in some clients

B. Common medications (Table 5-2)

C. Administration considerations

1. Assess client before, during, and after initial dose
   a. Monitor BP, HR, and cardiac rhythm frequently during initial administration; if given orally, assess client 30 minutes before and 60 minutes after initial dose
   b. Subsequent to the next dose, reassess BP, heart rate, and rhythm

Table 5-2	Common Beta-Adrenergic Blocker Medications	
Generic (Trade) Name	**Route**	**Uses**
Acebutolol (Sectral)	PO	PVCs, reduction of exercise-induced tachycardia
Atenolol (Tenormin)	PO	Angina pectoris related to coronary atherosclerosis, hypertension, MI, migraine headache, alcohol withdrawal syndrome, ventricular and supraventricular dysrhythmias
Esmolol (Brevibloc)	IV	Immediate termination of atrial tachydysrhythmias, noncompensatory sinus tachycardia, atrial flutter or fibrillation
Sotalol (Betapace)	PO	Ventricular dysrhythmias, maintenance of normal sinus rhythm, delay recurrence of atrial fibrillation or flutter
Metoprolol (Lopressor, Toprol XL)	PO	HF, hypertension, prevention of recurrent MI
Nadolol (Corgard)	PO	Hypertension, angina pectoris, ventricular dysrhythmias, migraine headaches, lithium-induced tremors, essential tremors
Propranolol (Inderal)	PO	Hypertension, migraine headaches, pheochromocytoma, essential tremor, tardive dyskinesia, cardiac dysrhythmias, angina pectoris, 5–21 days post MI to prevent reinfarction
Timolol (Blocadren)	PO	Hypertension, prevent reinfarction post MI, migraine headaches, reduce intraocular pressure in glaucoma

2. Give medication at consistent times with or without meals; it is recommended to take medication before meals and at bedtime

3. Beta-adrenergic blockers are not the same as calcium channel blockers; simultaneous use of beta-adrenergic blockers and calcium channel blockers may increase adverse effects, including bradycardia and hypotension

4. Tablets may be crushed as needed (prn) before administration and taken with fluid of choice

5. Intravenous administration: for IV push (IVP) give 1 mg/minute either undiluted or diluted in up to 50 mL of 5% dextrose or 0.9% NaCl and give as an infusion over 15–30 minutes

6. Be alert for unintended drug effects precipitated by comorbid conditions, such as masking of hypoglycemia in diabetes mellitus and bronchoconstriction in asthma or COPD

7. Do not discontinue therapy abruptly; dosage is reduced gradually over 1–2 weeks, and observe client for paradoxical reactions such as hypertension and tachycardia

D. **Contraindications**

1. Greater than first-degree heart block (a consistent PR interval longer than 0.20 second)

2. Right ventricular failure secondary to pulmonary hypertension

3. Sinus bradycardia

4. Cardiogenic shock

5. Significant aortic or mitral valve disease

6. Hyperreactive airway syndrome (asthma or bronchospasm)

7. Severe seasonal allergies (allergic rhinitis during pollen season)

8. Concurrent use of psychotropic drugs that use an adrenergic augmentation or within 2 weeks of a monoamine oxidase (MAO) inhibitor

9. Use cautiously in client with systemic allergies to insect stings and major surgery, renal or hepatic impairment, diabetes mellitus, myasthenia gravis, or Wolff–Parkinson–White (WPW) syndrome

E. **Significant drug interactions**
1. Phenothiazines have an additive effect, worsening hypotension
2. Beta-adrenergic agonists (e.g., albuterol) antagonize effects (cancel each other)
3. Atropine and tricyclic antidepressants block bradycardia
4. Diuretics and other antihypertensive medications increase hypotension
5. High doses of tubocurarine (a neuromuscular agent used as an adjunct to anesthesia to relax skeletal muscles) may potentiate neuromuscular blockade
6. Cimetidine (Tagamet) decreases clearance and increases effect
7. Antacids may decrease absorption

F. **Significant food interactions: none reported**

G. **Significant laboratory studies**
1. May cause false negative test results in exercise tolerance electrocardiogram (ECG)
2. May cause false positive test results with glucose tolerance test
3. Elevations in serum potassium, platelet count, uric acid, serum transaminase, alkaline phosphatase, lactate dehydrogenase (LDH), serum creatinine, and blood urea nitrogen (BUN)
4. Increase or decrease in blood glucose levels of diabetic clients

H. **Side effects**
1. Bradycardia, atrioventricular block, and hypotension
2. Bronchospasm, wheezing, dyspnea
3. Impotence
4. Weight gain or worsening HF
5. Dizziness, fatigue, and lethargy
6. GI upset
7. Masked cardiovascular signs of hypoglycemia in clients with diabetes mellitus

I. **Adverse reactions/toxicity**
1. CNS: sleep disturbances, depression, confusion, agitation, or psychosis
2. CV: hypotension, profound bradycardia, heart block, acute HF, and peripheral paresthesias resembling Raynaud phenomenon
3. Laryngospasm or bronchospasm
4. Dry eyes with a gritty sensation, blurred vision, tinnitus, or hearing loss
5. GI: dry mouth, nausea and vomiting (N/V), heartburn, diarrhea, constipation, abdominal cramps, and flatulence
6. Agranulocytosis, hypoglycemia, hyperglycemia and hypocalcemia in clients with hyperthyroidism

J. **Nursing considerations**
1. Take apical pulse and BP before administering drug; evaluate client for fluid volume overload as it may indicate HF
2. Monitor intake and output (I & O) and daily weight
3. Withhold dose if HR is less than 60 beats per minute (bpm) or if systolic BP is less than 90 mmHg
4. Perform a head to toe physical exam and assess client thoroughly for a history of asthma, allergies, or COPD; beta blockers may lead to bronchospasm in clients with no history of pulmonary disease
5. Assess HR, BP, and respiratory status carefully during periods of dosage adjustment; maintain effective communication with prescriber
6. The most common adverse reaction is bradycardia; clients with digitalis toxicity and WPW syndrome are most at risk

Practice to Pass

Your client is taking a beta-adrenergic blocker medication. Upon auscultation of the lungs, you hear diffuse wheezing throughout the lung fields. What are the appropriate actions to take? What are your rationales for these interventions?

7. With IV beta-blocker use, monitor client's ECG rhythm and rate, BP, and occasionally pulmonary capillary wedge pressure (left ventricular end-diastolic pressure or LVEDP) in the intensive care unit (ICU); reduction in sympathetic stimulation may lead to cardiac standstill

8. When beginning therapy with sotalol, client should be on continuous cardiac monitoring for at least first 3 days

9. Adverse reactions are most likely to occur after IV form of beta blockers are administered, but may occur in older adults and clients with impaired renal function taking oral doses soon after therapy is initiated

10. Dietary sodium is usually restricted to prevent fluid volume overload; check with prescriber regarding sodium restriction or concurrent use of a diuretic

11. Fasting longer than 12 hours may induce hypoglycemia, which is worsened by beta-blocker therapy because signs are masked

12. Periodic evaluations of renal, hepatic, cardiac, and hematologic functions should be made in clients receiving prolonged medication therapy

K. **Client education**

1. How to check pulse and BP; be aware of desired range for these values and keep a record of daily measurements; call prescriber if outside prescribed parameters, such as pulse rate less than 60

2. Abrupt medication withdrawal can lead to severe paradoxical or rebound reactions, including sweating, tremulousness, severe headache, malaise, palpitations, hypertension, MI, and life-threatening heart rhythm disturbances

3. Establish a routine for taking medication and strive to comply with prescriptive plan for best results (write out a daily schedule for medication)

4. Take metoprolol (Toprol XL) with food to enhance absorption

5. Change position slowly to avoid postural hypotension

6. Notify prescriber if dizziness or lightheadedness occurs; avoid driving or operating machinery until these symptoms are relieved

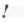
7. Stop smoking as this might offset desired outcomes of controlled heart rate, BP, and prevention of angina; smoking also increases hepatic metabolism of beta blockers, leading to unpredictable or diminished drug effects

8. Avoid OTC medications or herbal supplements without consulting prescriber

9. Notify all health care providers regarding use of beta-adrenergic blockers

10. Notify ophthalmologist or optometrist while taking this medication as it may lower intraocular pressures

III. CALCIUM CHANNEL BLOCKERS

A. **Action and use**

1. Are Class IV antidysrhythmic drugs that inhibit calcium ion influx through slow channels into cells of myocardial and arterial smooth muscle (both cardiac and peripheral blood vessels); normal role of calcium is to activate myocardial contraction, which increases cardiac workload

2. Intracellular calcium remains below levels needed to stimulate cell

3. Dilate coronary arteries and arterioles and prevent coronary artery spasm

4. Myocardial O_2 delivery is increased, preventing angina

5. Slow conduction through SA and AV nodes, resulting in a lower heart rate and decreased strength of cardiac muscle contraction (negative inotropic effect)

6. Decrease automaticity and **conductivity** (amount of force and pressure to pump blood out of ventricles) by blocking flow of calcium into cell

     7. Decrease systemic vascular resistance (SVR) and thus afterload by dilating peripheral arterioles
     8. Reduce arterial BP (antihypertensive effect) and heart rate
     9. Are used for vasospastic angina (Prinzmetal, variant), angina at rest, chronic stable (classic and activity-induced) angina, and essential hypertension; the IV form is useful in treating atrial fibrillation, atrial flutter, and supraventricular tachycardia

B. Common medications (Table 5-3)

C. Administration considerations
     1. Administer oral diltiazem before meals and at bedtime and oral verapamil with food to reduce gastric irritation
     2. Evaluate BP and ECG before initiation of therapy
     3. Monitor for headache; an analgesic may be required
     4. Intravenous forms of diltiazem: give undiluted IVP over 2 minutes and repeat in 15 minutes or dilute in D_5W, NS or $D_5\frac{1}{2}$ NaCl; continuous infusion may be given via infusion pump at a rate of 5–15 mg/hr; infusions over 24 hours and greater than 15 mg/h are not recommended
     5. Verapamil may be given IVP when diluted in 5 mL of sterile water for injection at a rate of 10 mg/min
     6. Withhold medication if BP less than 90/60
     7. Use caution when administering diltiazem to clients with HF

D. Contraindications
     1. Avoid use when there is known hypersensitivity to drug
     2. Sick sinus syndrome (unless pacemaker is in place)
     3. Second- or third-degree heart blocks
        a. Second-degree Type I or Wenckebach: progressive PR prolongation until a QRS complex is dropped on electrocardiogram
        b. Second-degree Type II: P waves are constant until a QRS is dropped on electrocardiogram
        c. Third-degree heart block: no association between P waves and QRS, usually ventricular HR is usually 20 to 40 bpm
     4. Severe hypotension, BP less than 90/60

E. Significant drug interactions
     1. Beta blockers and digoxin may have an additive effect in prolonging AV node conduction
     2. They may increase digoxin or quinidine levels leading to toxicity
     3. Cimetidine may increase serum levels of calcium channel blockers

Table 5-3   **Common Calcium Channel Blocker Medications**

Generic (Trade) Name	Route	Uses
Amlodipine (Norvasc)	PO	Mild to moderate hypertension or angina pectoris
Diltiazem (Cardizem, others)	PO, IV	Angina pectoris, vasospastic angina, prevention of reinfarction in non–Q wave MI, essential hypertension
Felodipine (Plendil)	PO	Chronic angina pectoris and hypertension
Isradipine (DynaCirc)	PO	Hypertension
Nicardipine (Cardene, Cardene SR)	PO	Angina pectoris and hypertension
Nifedipine (Procardia, others)	PO	Angina pectoris and hypertension
Nisoldipine (Nisocor)	PO	Angina pectoris and hypertension
Verapamil HCl (Calan, Isoptin)	PO	Angina pectoris, cardiac dysrhythmias, and hypertension

4. Calcium channel blockers may increase serum levels of cyclosporine (an immunosuppressant)
5. Furosemide is incompatible in IV solution

! F. **Significant food interactions:** do not administer calcium channel blockers with grapefruit or grapefruit juice

G. **Significant laboratory studies**
1. Total serum calcium levels are not altered
2. Monitor baseline and periodic lab tests of hepatic and renal function
3. Monitor diabetics closely; may induce hyperglycemia
4. Cyclosporine levels may become elevated
5. Digoxin and quinidine levels may become elevated

! H. **Side effects**
1. Headache
2. Fatigue
3. Constipation (especially with oral and sustained-release forms)
4. Postural hypotension
5. Peripheral edema

I. **Adverse effects/toxicity**
1. CNS: dizziness, nervousness, insomnia, confusion, tremor, and gait disturbance
2. CV: heart block and profound bradycardia, HF, profound hypotension with syncope, palpitations, and fluid volume overload
3. GI: N/V and impaired taste
4. Skin rash
5. Altered liver and kidney function
6. In high doses, nifedipine has been associated with increased incidence of sudden cardiac death

J. **Nursing considerations**
1. Evaluate BP and ECG before beginning treatment and monitor them closely during medication adjustment; withhold dose and notify prescriber for BP less than 90/60; monitor heart rhythm for sick sinus syndrome and second- or third-degree AV block
2. Monitor hepatic and renal lab test results
3. Monitor for headache
4. May induce hyperglycemia; monitor diabetic clients closely
! 5. Advise client to report gradual weight gain and evidence of edema; may indicate onset of HF
6. Avoid smoking and alcohol intake

K. **Client education**
! 1. It is important to take radial pulse before each dose (especially verapamil); an irregular pulse or one slower than baseline level should be reported
2. Withhold dose and notify prescriber if BP is less than 90 mmHg systolic or less than 60 mmHg diastolic
! 3. Change position slowly to prevent postural hypotension
4. Avoid driving if dizziness or faintness occur; report these symptoms immediately
5. Take medication exactly as prescribed and avoid skipping or doubling doses; do not stop therapy without approval of prescriber
6. Do not crush or chew sustained-release tablets
7. Follow-up care is important to monitor drug effectiveness
8. Avoid OTC medications and herbal supplements without consulting prescriber
! 9. Client should stop smoking and avoid alcohol consumption
10. Client should report easy bruising, petechiae, or unexplained bleeding

Practice to Pass

Your client is receiving a diltiazem (Cardizem) infusion. The ECG technician notifies you that the PR intervals are becoming progressively longer and occasionally an entire QRS is dropped. What is the most appropriate action for you to take? What is the possible cause of the cardiac rhythm disturbance?

IV. PERIPHERAL VASODILATORS

A. Action and use
1. Potent, non-nitrate hypotensive agents that reduce BP by direct effects on vascular smooth muscle of arteries (some vasodilators such as sodium nitroprusside work equally in all vessel beds)
2. Act directly on vascular smooth muscle to produce peripheral vasodilation, resulting in lowered arterial BP, increased heart rate, and increased cardiac output (CO)
3. Most commonly used to treat hypertension and as an adjunct in treating HF
4. Certain vasodilators may be ordered to treat peripheral vascular disease (PVD) to increase blood flow to extremities, such as in Raynaud disease

B. Common medications (Table 5-4)

C. Administration considerations
1. Take oral forms of medications with food to increase bioavailability
2. IV hydralazine may be given undiluted via direct IV push at a rate of 10 mg/min
3. IV sodium nitroprusside is diluted by dissolving 50 mg in 2–3 mL of D_5W and then diluted in 250 mL D_5W (200 mcg/mL); it should be infused cautiously through an IV pump; when mixed, it appears orange and must be covered in a foil pouch to avoid exposure to light during infusion
4. Do not mix with other IV solutions
5. All vasodilators should be discontinued slowly to avoid paradoxical hypertensive effects
6. Store medication in light-resistant container
7. Monitor HR and BP closely during administration to prevent sudden hypotension
8. Reflex tachycardia may occur as a compensatory response to sudden decrease in BP
9. Salt and water retention may occur as a compensatory increase in aldosterone secretion triggered by drop in BP

D. Contraindications
1. When client has a compensatory hypertension, as in an arteriovenous shunt or coarctation of the aorta
2. Inadequate cerebral perfusion leading to a decreased cerebral perfusion pressure (CPP)
3. Hypovolemia
4. Clients with systemic lupus erythematosus (SLE) (hydralazine only)
5. Use cautiously with coronary heart disease (CHD); hydralazine can precipitate angina attacks

Table 5-4 Common Peripheral Vasodilator Medications

Generic (Trade) Name	Route	Uses
Diazoxide (Hyperstat IV)	IV	Reduce peripheral vascular resistance and blood pressure by vasodilation
Hydralazine (Apresoline)	PO, IV, IM	Vasodilation, which reduces peripheral resistance to improve cardiac output
Minoxidil (Loniten, Rogaine)	PO Topical	Vasodilator with a greater hypotensive effect by blocking calcium uptake through the cell membrane Male pattern baldness
Nitroprusside sodium (Nipride)	IV	Acts on vascular smooth muscle to produce vasodilation
Prazosin hydrochloride (Minipress)	PO	Lowers blood pressure
Combination Therapies		
Hydralazine and hydrochlorothiazide (Apresazide)	PO	Moderate to severe hypertension
Hydralazine and isosorbide dinitrate (BiDil)	PO	Treatment of HF in African Americans

E. Significant drug interactions
1. All antihypertensive medications, vasodilators (e.g., nitroglycerine), and diuretics may interact to induce profound hypotension
2. Beta blockers and calcium channel blockers will compound hypotensive effects but may be used concurrently to prevent reflex tachycardia
3. No additional medication should be infused through same IV line if given as an infusion
4. NSAIDS may decrease hypotensive effects
5. Hawthorne may increase hypotensive effects

F. Significant food interactions: none reported

G. Significant laboratory studies
1. Various vasodilators have differing laboratory data that is significant; review product literature of individual drugs prior to administration
2. When administering hydralazine hydrochloride:
    a. Positive direct Coomb's tests can reveal hydralazine-induced systemic lupus erythematosus (SLE); this condition mimics SLE and is potentially reversible if identified early
    b. Hydralazine interferes with urinary 17-OHCS (modified Glenn-Nelson techniques)
    c. Do baseline and periodic LE cell prep and antinuclear antibody (ANA) titer, BUN, creatinine, uric acid, serum potassium, and blood glucose levels
3. During administration of sodium nitroprusside
    a. Measure baseline and periodic BUN, creatinine, uric acid, serum potassium, and blood glucose levels
    b. Monitor serum thiocyanate levels with prolonged IV infusion and in clients with impaired renal function
    c. Monitor plasma cyanogen levels with prolonged infusion longer than 2 days or with impaired hepatic function
    d. There are increased or decreased serum cobalamin levels

H. Side effects
1. CNS: headache
2. CV: palpitations and tachycardia
3. SLE-like syndrome (with hydralazine)
4. Salt and water retention

I. Adverse effects/toxicity
1. CNS: dizziness, tremors, apprehension, and muscle twitching
2. CV: angina, tachycardia or bradycardia, flushing, paradoxical pressor response (sudden unexpected elevation in BP and HR), ECG changes, profound hypotension, shock, and dysrhythmias
3. GI: anorexia, N/V, constipation or diarrhea, abdominal pain, and paralytic ileus
4. GU: difficulty urinating and glomerulonephritis
5. Hematologic: decreased hematocrit and hemoglobin, anemia, agranulocytosis (rare)
6. Skin: rash, irritation at IV site, urticaria, pruritus, fever, chills, arthralgia, eosinophilia, and cholangiitis
7. SLE-like syndrome, edema
8. When administering sodium nitroprusside, monitor for signs and symptoms of thiocyanate toxicity: profound hypotension, tinnitus, fatigue, pink skin color, metabolic acidosis, and loss of consciousness

J. Nursing considerations
1. Assess carefully baseline vital signs including HR, cardiac rhythm, ECG, and neurological status
2. When administering IV vasodilators:
    a. Establish a large, stable IV site for infusions because they are irritating to tissue; administer using an IV infusion pump

Practice to Pass

Your client is receiving a sodium nitroprusside infusion. Upon assessment, you notice a BP of 80/50 and HR of 134 bpm. The client is less responsive. What do you do first? What possible clinical manifestation would you conclude is an adverse effect of this medication?

      b. Monitor BP every 5–15 minutes with an automatic external BP machine or with an arterial line during initial infusion and during medication adjustment

      c. Monitor I & O

       d. If adverse response is noted (e.g., hypotension), decrease infusion and monitor client closely; if sudden severe hypotension occurs, discontinue medication; maintain airway, breathing, and circulation (ABCs); establish IV site; contact prescriber, and initiate emergency protocols as necessary

   3. Obtain baseline vital signs and check BP, heart rate, and cardiac rhythm before each dose when administering orally

K. Client education

   1. Monitor pulse and BP

   2. Headaches and palpitations are possible within 2–4 hours after first oral dose

   3. Follow-up care is important

   4. Write down questions to ask prescriber on each follow-up visit

   5. Avoid all OTC medications and herbal supplements unless approved by prescriber

    6. Stop smoking and avoid alcohol intake, which may negate positive drug effects

   7. Monitor weight daily and report edema

    8. Change position slowly and avoid hot tubs and hot baths that might induce profound vasodilation and hypotension

V. CARDIAC GLYCOSIDE

A. Action and use

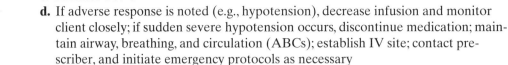   **1.** Used primarily in treatment of HF, although survival rates are not extended

   2. Used for treatment of atrial **dysrhythmias** (abnormalities in electrical activity of heart), such as atrial fibrillation

   3. Increase **contractility** (ability to contract) and efficiency of myocardial contraction

   4. Produce a positive inotropic action, which increases force of myocardial contraction

   5. Decrease conduction velocity through AV node

B. Common medications: digoxin (Lanoxin)

C. Administration considerations

   1. May be given with or without food

   2. Tablet may be crushed and mixed with fluid or food as desired; pediatric elixir is also available

   3. IV administration: IVP digoxin may be administered undiluted or diluted in 4 mL of sterile water, 5% dextrose, or NS; administer each direct IV dose over 5 minutes; client may receive a loading dose (digitalization) to achieve adequate serum drug levels

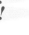   **4.** Never administer digoxin intramuscularly (IM) because it would cause tissue irritation and great variation in bioavailability

   5. Infiltration into subcutaneous tissue can cause local irritation and tissue sloughing

D. Contraindications

   1. Avoid use in clients with known hypersensitivity to drug

   2. Full digitalizing dose should not be given if client has received digoxin in the previous week

   3. Presence of digoxin toxicity

   4. Use cautiously in the following conditions:

      a. Renal insufficiency

      b. Hypokalemia

      c. Advanced heart disease, acute MI, heart block, and cor pulmonale

      d. Hypothyroidism

      e. Lung disease

Practice to Pass

A client is receiving digoxin 0.125 mg PO every morning. Upon arrival to the office, you notice that the HR is 44 bpm. The client reports feeling weak and nauseated. Based on the clinical data, what might cause the low heart rate? What are the priority nursing assessments? ❗

    f. Pregnant or nursing mothers

    g. Children or premature infants

    h. Older adults

E. Significant drug interactions

    1. Antacids, cholestyramine, and colestipol decrease digoxin absorption

    2. Diuretics, corticosteroids, amphotericin B, laxatives, and sodium polystyrene sulfonate may cause hypokalemia, which increases risk of toxicity

    3. IV calcium when given with digoxin may increase risk of cardiac dysrhythmias

    4. Quinidine, verapamil, alprazolam, and amiodarone significantly increase digoxin levels, and digoxin dose should be decreased by 50%

    5. Erythromycin and nefazodone may increase digoxin levels

    6. Succinylcholine may potentiate dysrhythmias

    7. Dobutamine or doxapram should not be injected in same IV line or mixed in solution with digoxin

    8. Ginseng may increase risk of toxicity

F. Significant food interactions: none reported

G. Significant laboratory studies

    1. Before initiating cardiac glycoside therapy, baseline labs should be drawn, including potassium, magnesium, and calcium

    2. Draw serum digoxin level periodically during therapy and if client develops symptoms of toxicity; draw sample at least 6 hours after daily dose and preferably just before next scheduled daily dose

    3. Therapeutic range of serum digoxin is 0.8–2 ng/mL, and toxic levels are greater than 2 ng/mL

    4. Closely monitor potassium levels; hypokalemia potentiates digoxin toxicity

H. Side effects

    1. Nausea

    2. Loss of "usual appetite"

    3. Headache or blurred yellow vision

I. Adverse reactions/toxicity

    1. CNS: fatigue, muscle weakness, headache, facial neuralgia, depression, paresthesias, hallucinations, confusion, drowsiness, agitation, dizziness, and malaise

    2. CV: dysrhythmias, hypotension, AV heart block, and diaphoresis

    3. GI: anorexia, N/V, diarrhea, and dysphagia

    4. Visual disturbances (blurred, green or yellow vision, or halo effect)

    5. Digoxin toxicity may be unrecognized, since it may have same manifestations as a "flu"; these include anorexia, N/V, diarrhea, or visual disturbances

J. Nursing considerations

    1. Obtain baseline data and perform ongoing physical assessments, including neurological status, HR, BP, and cardiac rhythm

    2. Check baseline serum digoxin level prior to initiating digoxin therapy:

        a. Blood level is 0 if no digoxin has been taken before

        b. Therapeutic levels are 0.8 to 2 ng/mL

        c. Toxic levels are greater than 2 ng/mL

    3. Assess baseline and ongoing laboratory values, including serum electrolytes, creatinine clearance, magnesium, and calcium

    4. Monitor closely for digoxin toxicity in older adults taking digoxin and a diuretic for HF or atrial fibrillation

    5. Take the apical pulse for 1 full minute prior to administering digoxin, noting rate, rhythm, and quality; if any changes are noted, withhold dose, and notify the prescriber; an ECG will likely be ordered

6. Withhold the medication if client has symptoms of digoxin toxicity (anorexia, N/V, diarrhea, or visual disturbances)

7. In children, early signs of toxicity include cardiac dysrhythmias; children rarely demonstrate anorexia, N/V, diarrhea, or visual disturbances

8. Advise client to eat foods high in potassium such as oranges, bananas, fruit juices, vegetables, and potatoes if taking loop diuretics

9. Monitor I & O and daily weight especially in clients with impaired renal failure; auscultate breath sounds for crackles; assess extremities for edema because it indicates fluid volume overload

10. Antidote: digoxin immune Fab (Digibind) is used in extreme toxicity

11. Concurrent antibiotic and digoxin therapy can precipitate toxicity because of alterations in intestinal flora

12. Monitor client closely when being switched from one administration route to another; often a dose adjustment is required (if tablet form is replaced by elixir, potential for toxicity increases)

K. Client education

1. Check pulse for 1 full minute prior to taking digoxin; advise to contact prescriber before taking dose if pulse is below 60 bpm or above 110 or if skipped beats are present

2. Suspect toxicity if any of the following occur: N/V, anorexia, diarrhea, or visual disturbances (halos, green or yellow lights)

3. Withhold next dose if digoxin toxicity is suspected and contact the prescriber immediately

4. Weigh self daily with same clothes and at same time; report weight gain greater than 2 lb/day

5. Take digoxin as ordered; do not skip or add additional dose if experiencing chest discomfort (a common report from clients admitted with digoxin toxicity is that they take digoxin as a "heart pill" when experiencing chest pain)

6. Do not take OTC medications or herbal supplements without consulting prescriber because they might have direct adverse effects on absorption of digoxin

7. Insist on original brand of digoxin ordered by prescriber to avoid errors in dosing; bioavailability may differ between brands

VI. PHOSPHODIESTERASE III INHIBITORS

A. Action and use

1. Block the enzyme phosphodiesterase III in cardiac and smooth muscle, leading to increased amounts of calcium available for cardiac contraction; a positive inotropic action and vasodilation occur and cardiac output is increased

2. Used to treat acute HF resistant to treatment with ACE inhibitors, digoxin and other therapies, and short-term therapy of serious and decompensated HF

B. Common medications (Table 5-5)

C. Administration considerations

1. Continuous monitoring for ventricular dysrhythmias is necessary

2. Therapy is limited to 2–3 days

3. Peak effects can occur within 2–3 minutes of IV administration

Table 5-5 Phosphodiesterase III Inhibitors

Generic (Trade) Name	Route	Uses
Inamrinone (Inocor)	IV	Short-term treatment of acute decompensated heart failure (HF)
Milrinone (Primacor)	IV	Short-term treatment of acute decompensated heart failure (HF)

4. Overdose of milrinone may cause hypotension, which can be treated with normal saline or a vasopressor
5. Hypovolemia or electrolyte imbalances should be corrected before initiating infusion
6. Dosage should be reduced in client with renal impairment
7. Use cautiously with liver impairment (inamrinone)

D. Contraindications
1. Severe valvular heart disease (milrinone)
2. Use with caution with preexisting dysrhythmias
3. Known drug allergy

E. Significant drug interactions
1. Additive effects may be seen when given with digoxin, dobutamine, or other inotropic drugs
2. Concurrent use of diuretics can cause significant hypotension
3. Concurrent administration with furosemide will form a precipitate
4. Mixing inamirinone with glucose-containing solutions results in loss of inamrinone activity over 24 hours

F. Significant food interactions: ginger may contribute to cardiac actions of milrinone

G. Significant laboratory studies
1. Complete blood count (CBC), electrolytes, renal function tests
2. Thromboytopenia may occur with inamrinone

H. Side effects
1. Ventricular dysrhythmia, hypotension, angina
2. Headache, N/V
3. Hypokalemia, tremor

I. Adverse reactions/toxicity
1. Severe hypotension
2. Ventricular dysrhythmias
3. Thrombocytopenia (inamrinone)

J. Nursing considerations
1. Assess client before, during, and after initial dose
   a. Monitor BP and HR frequently during initial administration
   b. Cardiac monitoring is necessary throughout treatment
2. Slow or stop infusion if severe hypotension develops
3. Check for hypokalemia and notify provider if present

K. Client education: instruct client to immediately report chest pain should it occur during infusion

VII. ATRIAL NATRIURETIC PEPTIDE HORMONE

A. Action and use
1. A small peptide hormone produced through recombinant DNA technology
2. Is structurally identical to endogenous beta-type natriuretic peptide (hBNP), which is secreted by right atrium in response to increased pressure of blood in atria
3. Promotes diuresis by inhibiting ADH, vasodilation, and reduces preload
4. Should be reserved for treatment of acutely decompensated HF in clients who have dyspnea at rest

B. Common medication: nesiritide (Natrecor) is the only drug in this new class

C. Administration considerations: administer by IV bolus followed by IV infusion for up to 48 hours

D. Contraindications
1. Allergy to nesiritide
2. Hypotension with systolic BP lower than 90 mmHg
3. Clients with low cardiac filling pressures

E. **Significant drug interactions: possible additive hypotension if used concurrently with antihypertensives such as angiotensin converting enzyme (ACE) inhibitors**
F. **Significant food interactions: none reported**
G. **Significant laboratory studies: baseline and periodic serum creatinine**
H. **Side effects**
1. Lightheadedness or dizziness
2. Confusion or weakness
3. Headache, back pain, injection site pain
4. Insomnia and anxiety
5. Abdominal pain, N/V, fever
I. **Adverse reactions/toxicity**
1. Hypotension
2. Chest pain
3. Dysrhythmias
J. **Nursing considerations**
1. Monitor IV infusion frequently
2. Monitor BP and other hemodynamic parameters closely and be aware that if hypotension occurs, it may persist for several hours after drug is discontinued
3. Monitor cardiac rhythm during administration
4. Observe for intended drug effects of improvement in heart failure and increased diuresis
K. **Client education: drug is for short-term IV use (up to 48 hours) and client will be monitored closely throughout therapy**

VIII. ANTIDYSRHYTHMICS

A. **Class I-A (fast sodium channel blockers)**
1. Action and use
   a. Used to treat both atrial and ventricular dysrhythmias; prevent recurrence of premature ventricular contractions (PVCs) and ventricular tachycardia that are not severe enough to require cardioversion
   b. Depress myocardial contractility and excitability and prolong **refractory period** (ability to respond only to a strong stimulus)
   c. Reduce rate of spontaneous diastolic depolarization in pacemaker cells, thereby suppressing ectopic focal activity
   d. Disopyramide shortens sinus node recovery time and increases atrial and ventricular effective refractory period
   e. Quinidine is classified as a chemical cardioversion agent useful to convert atrial fibrillation to normal sinus rhythm
2. Common medications (Table 5-6)

Table 5-6 **Common Antidysrhythmic Medications: Class I–A: Fast Sodium Channel Blockers**

Generic (Trade) Name	Route	Uses
Disopyramide (Norpace)	PO	Life-threatening ventricular dysrhythmias, paroxysmal supraventricular tachycardia (PSVT), decreases rate of diastolic repolarization, increases action potential and prolongs refractory period
Procainamide hydrochloride (Pronestyl, Pronestyl SR)	PO, IV	Life-threatening ventricular dysrhythmias, conversion of atrial fibrillation or flutter to normal sinus rhythm
Quinidine gluconate (Quinaglute, others); Quinidine sulfate (Quinidex, others)	PO, IV	Atrial dysrhythmias, chronic atrial tachycardia, life-threatening *Plasmodium falciparum* infections when IV therapy with quinidine gluconate is indicated

3. Administration considerations
   a. Give first dose of disopyramide 6–12 hours after last quinidine dose and 3–6 hours after last procainamide dose
   b. Do not administer controlled-release capsules when giving a loading dose, when rapid control is required, or when creatinine clearance is less than 40 mL/min
   c. Do not crush or open controlled-release capsules as it may deliver a potentially toxic dose of medication
   d. Start controlled-release form of capsule 6 hours after last dose of conventional capsule when switching from a conventional capsule to a controlled-release form
4. Contraindications
   a. Cardiogenic shock
   b. Second- or third-degree heart block
   c. Severe heart failure
   d. Hypotension
   e. Caution should be used when administering disopyramide in the presence of:
      1) Sick sinus syndrome
      2) WPW syndrome
      3) Bundle branch block
      4) Myocarditis or other cardiomyopathy
      5) Hepatic or renal impairment
      6) Urinary tract disease (especially prostatic hyperplasia)
      7) Myasthenia gravis
      8) Angle closure (narrow angle) glaucoma
5. Significant drug interactions
   a. Do not inject quinidine with anticholinergic drugs such as tricyclic antidepressants and antihistamines
   b. Antidysrhythmics compound toxicities
   c. Phenytoin and rifampin may increase metabolism of disopyramide and decrease blood level
   d. Disopyramide may increase warfarin-induced hypoprothrombinemia
6. Significant food interactions: drug metabolism is decreased and risk of toxic sodium channel blocker effect is increased with grapefruit juice
7. Significant laboratory studies
   a. Determine baseline hepatic and renal function and monitor periodically during therapy
   b. Assess blood glucose levels and serum potassium levels because hyperkalemia worsens toxic effects; hypokalemia and other electrolyte imbalances should be corrected before therapy is initiated
   c. Monitor ECG closely; notify prescriber immediately if these changes occur:
      1) Prolonged QT interval
      2) Worsening of dysrhythmias
      3) Widening of the QRS, greater than 25%
      4) HR less than 60 bpm or greater than 120 bpm
      5) Unusual change in rate, rhythm, or quality of pulse
   d. Serum quinidine levels are inaccurate in clients taking triamterene
8. Side effects
   a. Mild hypotension
   b. Blurred vision
   c. Dry mouth
   d. Urinary hesitancy or retention
   e. Constipation
   f. Abdominal cramping, N/V

9. Adverse effects/toxicity
   a. CNS: dizziness, headache, fatigue, muscle weakness, seizures, paresthesias, nervousness, acute psychosis, and peripheral neuropathy

   b. CV: severe hypotension, chest pain, edema, dyspnea, syncope, bradycardia, tachycardia, increased dysrhythmias, HF, cardiogenic shock, and heart block
   c. GI: epigastric and abdominal pain, jaundice
   d. GU: profound urinary retention, frequency, urgency, and renal insufficiency
   e. Skin: pruritis, urticaria, rash, photosensitivity, and laryngospasm
   f. Drying of nose, throat and bronchial secretions
   g. Uterine contraction during pregnancy, precipitation of myasthenia gravis, agranulocytosis (decreased granulocytes), and thrombocytopenia

10. Nursing considerations

    a. Check apical pulse before administering dose
    b. Monitor ECG and report any changes to prescriber immediately
    c. Monitor BP especially during dosage adjustment and if receiving high doses of medication

    d. Monitor I & O especially in older adults and clients with impaired renal function, prostatic hyperplasia, and urinary retention/hesitancy
    e. Monitor labs results as appropriate
    f. Assess for peripheral neuritis

11. Client education

    a. Measure daily weight and report weight gain greater than 2–4 lb/week
    b. Inspect ankles and tibia daily for edema
    c. Change position slowly to avoid dizziness and syncope; avoid prolonged periods of standing and lie down if feeling lightheaded; avoid driving or other hazardous activities if dizzy or lightheaded
    d. Take medication as prescribed and do not skip doses
    e. Do not stop taking medication abruptly
    f. Do not take OTC medications or drink alcohol without contacting prescriber
    g. Avoid exposure to sunlight or ultraviolet radiation

    h. Notify all other health care providers of medication and have regular eye exams for glaucoma
    i. Clients taking procainamide (Pronestyl) should watch for lupus-like symptoms

B. Class I-B
   1. Action and use
      a. Decreases the refractory period
      b. Suppresses automaticity in Bundle of His–Purkinje system
      c. Elevates electrical stimulation threshold of ventricle during diastole
      d. Treats or prevents ventricular dysrhythmias
   2. Common medications (Table 5-7)
   3. Administration considerations

      a. Bolus dose of lidocaine may be given undiluted via IVP at a rate of 25–50 mg/min
      b. Add 1 gram lidocaine to 250 to 500 mL of D_5W for infusion; flow rate should not be more than 4 mg/mL
      c. Use microdropper and infusion pump for an infusion
      d. Discontinue IV infusion as soon as client's basic cardiac rhythm stabilizes
      e. Hypokalemia should be corrected prior to initiating tocainide
      f. Administer phenytoin undiluted clear without precipitate
   4. Contraindications
      a. History of hypersensitivity to amide-type anesthetics
      b. Stokes-Adams syndrome
      c. Untreated sinus bradycardia

Table 5-7   **Common Antidysrhythmic Medications: Class I–B**

Generic (Trade) Name	Route	Uses
Lidocaine (Xylocaine)	IV	Suppresses Bundle of His–Purkinje system, elevating ventricular electrical stimulation threshold during diastole, rapid control of ventricular dysrhythmias during acute MI or cardiac catheterization
Mexiletine (Mexitil)	PO	Modest suppression of SA and AV node, acute and chronic ventricular dysrhythmias, severe tachydysrhythmias
Phenytoin (Dilantin)	IV	Dysrhythmias (including digitalis-induced)
Tocainide (Tonocard)	PO	Refractory ventricular dysrhythmias, prevention of ventricular tachyarrhythmia, shortens the effective refractory period of atria, AV node, and ventricles without affecting AV conduction

   d. Severe degrees of SA, AV, and intraventricular heart block
   e. Use cautiously with:
      1) Hepatic or renal disease
      2) HF
      3) Hypovolemia or shock
      4) Myasthenia gravis
      5) Debilitated clients or older adults
      6) Family history of malignant hyperthermia
5. Significant drug interactions
   a. Barbiturates decrease lidocaine activity
   b. Beta blockers, quinidine, phenytoin, and procainamide increase effect of lidocaine
   c. Phenytoin and cefazolin are incompatible with lidocaine infusion
   d. Decreased absorption of phenytoin and increased metabolism with concurrent oral anticoagulant use
   e. Phenytoin is incompatible with nisoldipine, amiodarone, chloramphenicol, omeprazole, and ticlopidine
6. Significant food interactions: none reported
7. Significant laboratory studies
   a. Lidocaine levels should be assessed
      1) Therapeutic level is 1.5–6 mcg/mL
      2) Potentially toxic level is greater than 7 mcg/mL
   b. Assess electrolytes and correct hypokalemia before treating with antidysrhythmics
   c. Check baseline hepatic and renal blood studies
8. Side effects
   a. Drowsiness
   b. Lightheadedness
   c. Mild hypotension
9. Adverse effects/toxicity
   a. CNS: restlessness, confusion, disorientation, irritability, apprehension, euphoria, wild excitement, numbness of lips or tongue and other paresthesias, chest heaviness, and difficulty speaking
   b. Dyspnea and difficulty swallowing, muscular twitching, tremors, psychosis, seizures, and respiratory depression with high doses
   c. CV: hypotension, bradycardia, heart block, cardiovascular collapse, and cardiac arrest
   d. Ear: tinnitus and decreased hearing
   e. Eye: severe blurred vision, double vision, and impaired color perception
   f. GI: anorexia, N/V, and excessive perspiration
   g. Skin: urticaria, rash, edema, and anaphylactoid reactions

10. Nursing considerations
    a. Assess ECG for changes including prolonged PR interval, widened QRS, aggravation of dysrhythmias, and heart block
    b. Monitor BP frequently
    c. Assess CNS status at baseline and frequently during infusion
    d. Administer via infusion pump and observe rate carefully
    e. Administer oral drug with food to decrease GI upset
    f. Auscultate breath sounds for crackles and monitor respiratory rate
    g. Assess serum blood levels
11. Client education
    a. Notify prescriber if lightheadedness; dizziness; confusion; numbness or tingling of lips, tongue, or fingers occur; and notify for visual changes or ringing in ears
    b. Notify prescriber if unusual CNS changes occur, or nausea, vomiting, or yellowish changes in whites of eyes or skin (jaundice) when taking oral forms of medication
    c. Do not take any OTC medications or herbal supplements without consulting prescriber
    d. Take medications as prescribed without skipping doses

C. **Class I-C**
1. Action and use
    a. Decrease automaticity and conductivity through AV node and ventricles
    b. Are used to treat life-threatening ventricular dysrhythmias
2. Common medications (Table 5-8)
3. Administration considerations
    a. Medications are available in oral forms
    b. Increasing dosages are not recommended more frequently than every 4 days especially with older adults or clients with previous extensive myocardial damage
    c. Dosage reduction should be considered in severe liver dysfunction and with significant widening of QRS complex
4. Contraindications
    a. Hypersensitivity to flecainide
    b. Severe degrees of heart block
    c. Intraventricular blocks
    d. Cardiogenic shock
    e. Hepatic failure
5. Significant drug interactions
    a. Cimetidine may increase flecainide levels
    b. Flecainide may increase digoxin levels by 25%
    c. Beta blockers enhance negative inotropic effects
6. Significant food interactions: none reported
7. Significant laboratory studies
    a. Assess baseline electrolytes
    b. Monitor serum levels
        1) Effective trough level is 0.7 to 1 mcg/mL
        2) Toxic trough level is greater than 1 mcg/mL
    c. Monitor blood levels frequently if client is taking digoxin or has severe HF or renal failure

Table 5-8 Common Antidysrhythmic Medications: Class I–C

Generic (Trade) Name	Route	Uses
Flecainide (Tambocor)	PO	Life-threatening ventricular dysrhythmias
Propafenone (Rythmol)	PO	Ventricular tachycardia

8. Side effects
   a. Slight dizziness
   b. Blurred vision
   c. Nausea
9. Adverse effects/toxicity
   a. CNS: headache, prolonged lightheadedness, unsteadiness, paresthesias, fatigue, and fever
   b. CV: worsening dysrhythmias, chest pain, HF, edema, and dyspnea
   c. Eye: prolonged blurred vision and spots before eyes
   d. GI: prolonged nausea, constipation, and changes in taste perception
10. Nursing considerations
    a. Assess laboratory data and treat hypokalemia/hyperkalemia before initiating therapy
    b. Monitor ECG rhythm for changes, including worsening of dysrhythmias; client may need Holter monitoring for ambulatory assessment
    c. Determine threshold levels of pacemaker before initiating medication and at regular intervals thereafter
11. Client education
    a. Take medications as prescribed without skipping doses
    b. Report any visual changes
    c. Do not take any OTC medications or herbal supplements without consulting health care provider
    d. Follow-up care is important
D. **Class II (beta blockers): see previous section II**
E. **Class III (potassium channel blockers)**
   1. Action and use
      a. Prolong repolarization and refractory period
      b. Decreases intraventricular conduction
      c. Used to treat ventricular tachycardia and ventricular fibrillation
      d. May also be used to treat supraventricular tachycardias
   2. Common medications: (Table 5-9)
   3. Administration considerations
      a. Gastroenteritis symptoms may occur with high oral dose therapy and loading dose
      b. Use infusion pump when administering IV dose; central line should be used if rate exceeds 2 mg/mL
      c. Dofetilide does not have as negative an inotropic effect as amiodarone, but has significant dose-related prodysrhythmic effects including heart block, ventricular tachycardia, and torsades de pointes
      d. Continuously monitor ECG when infusing ibutilide and dofetilide and for at least 4 hours following infusion
      e. Correct hypokalemia and hypomagnesemia prior to initiating therapy with ibutilide and dofetilide to reduce risk for dysrhythmias

Table 5-9 **Common Antidysrhythmic Medications: Class III—Potassium Channel Blockers**

Generic (Trade) Name	Route	Uses
Amiodarone (Cordarone)	PO, IV	Atrial dysrhythmias in HF, ventricular tachycardia, atrial fibrillation, ventricular fibrillation
Dofetilide (Tikosyn)	PO	Rapid conversion of atrial flutter or fibrillation to normal sinus rhythm
Ibutilide (Corvert)	IV	Rapid conversion of atrial flutter or fibrillation to normal sinus rhythm

4. Contraindications
  a. Hypersensitivity to amiodarone
  b. Cardiogenic shock
  c. Severe sinus bradycardia or severe degrees of heart block
  d. Hepatic disease
  e. Use cautiously in: Hashimoto's thyroiditis, goiter, hyperthyroidism or hypothyroidism, HF, electrolyte imbalance, preexisting pulmonary disease, cardiac surgery, and sensitivity to iodine

5. Significant drug interactions
  a. Increases digoxin levels
  b. Enhances effects and toxicities of disopyramide, procainamide, quinidine, flecainide, lidocaine, cyclosporine
  c. Enhances anticoagulant effects
  d. Bradycardia effects are greater when used with verapamil, diltiazem, and beta-adrenergic blockers
  e. Increases phenytoin blood levels two- to three-fold
  f. Cimetidine and ritonavir may increase amiodarone levels and toxicity
  g. Cholestyramine may decrease amiodarone levels
  h. Other Class Ia and Class III antidysrhythmic drugs can increase risk for prolonged QT interval and life-threatening dysrhythmias

6. Significant food interactions: none reported

7. Significant laboratory studies
  a. Thyroid function test abnormalities (in the absence of thyroid function impairments)
  b. Baseline and periodic serum assessments of:
    1) Liver enzymes: aspartate aminotransferase (AST) and alanine aminotransferase (ALT)
    2) Lung: pulmonary function tests, ABGs
    3) Thyroid hormone levels
    4) Creatinine and electrolyte levels with dofetilide

8. Side effects
  a. Skin and corneal pigmentation (lipofuscinosis) in client receiving drug longer than 2 months; reversible in 7 months after discontinuing drug (amiodarone)
  b. Muscle weakness
  c. Hypotension, dizziness
  d. Mild anorexia, nausea, and constipation

9. Adverse reactions/toxicity
  a. CNS: peripheral neuropathy, muscle wasting, weakness, fatigue, abnormal gait, dyskinesia, dizziness, paresthesias, and headache
  b. CV: bradycardia, severe hypotension, sinus arrest, cardiogenic shock, CHF, worsening dysrhythmias, and heart block
  c. Eye: corneal microdeposits, blurred vision, optic neuritis, optic neuropathy, permanent blindness, corneal degeneration, macular degeneration, and photosensitivity
  d. Respiratory: alveolitis, pneumonitis, and interstitial pulmonary fibrosis
  e. Skin: slate-blue pigmentation to skin and rash
  f. GI: severe anorexia, nausea, vomiting, and constipation
  g. Angioedema, hyperthyroidism or hypothyroidism, and hepatotoxicity
  h. Torsades de pointes, supraventricular dysrhythmias (ibutilide and dofetilide)

10. Nursing considerations
  a. Monitor BP during IV infusion and titrate to prevent hypotension and bradycardia
  b. Monitor client continually due to unusually long half-life of drug (10–55 days)

    c. Check laboratory and other reports for liver, lung, thyroid, GI, and neurological dysfunction

    d. Baseline and regular ophthalmic examinations with a slit-lamp are recommended throughout therapy

    e. Report adverse reactions promptly

    f. Be alert to signs of pulmonary toxicity: dyspnea, fatigue, cough, pleuritic pain, or fever; auscultate breath sounds for adventitious sounds

    g. Monitor client for CNS changes, which generally develop within a week after amiodarone therapy begins; muscle weakness and tremors are a potential safety risk

    h. Observe client already receiving other antiarrhythmic therapy for adverse effects, especially heart block and worsening dysrhythmias

  11. Client education

    a. Assess pulse daily and report a HR less than 60 bpm

    b. Notify all health care providers of medication

    c. Have regular ophthalmic examinations

    d. Photophobia may be eased by wearing darkened glasses but some clients should avoid daylight entirely

    e. Erythema and pruritus may develop when exposed to ultraviolet radiation; avoid sunlight, tanning beds, and sunlamps

    f. Wear protective clothing and a barrier-type sunblock to avoid sun exposure (zinc-oxide or titanium-oxide preparations)

    g. Blue-gray skin pigmentation may slowly disappear after medication is stopped; may take months to resolve (amiodarone)

    h. Take medication as prescribed without skipping doses

    i. Avoid taking OTC medications or herbal supplements without consulting prescriber

    j. Follow-up care is important

    k. Instruct client to report any chest pain, cough, or shortness of breath to provider

F. Class IV (calcium channel blockers): see previous section III

G. Other antidysrhythmics (miscellaneous)

  1. Action and use

    a. Slow conduction through SA and AV nodes

    b. Interrupt reentry pathways through AV node

    c. Depress left ventricular function (very temporary)

    d. Treat supraventricular dysrhythmias

  2. Common medication: adenosine (Adenocard, Adenoscan)

  3. Administration considerations

    a. Give by rapid IV bolus (over 1–2 seconds) followed by rapid normal saline flush; administer directly into vein as proximal to insertion site as possible; half-life is only 10 seconds

    b. Solution contains no preservatives so it must be clear; discard any unused portion

    c. Expect sudden slowing of the HR or even asystole for a brief period of time; do not repeat dose if a high grade of AV heart block develops after the first dose

    d. Must be stored at room temperature to avoid crystallization; if crystals appear, dissolve by warming to room temperature

  4. Contraindications

    a. Severe degrees of heart block

    b. Sick sinus syndrome (without a pacemaker)

    c. Atrial fibrillation or atrial flutter

    d. Ventricular tachycardia

    e. Use cautiously with asthma, pregnancy, hepatic failure, and renal failure

5. Significant drug interactions
    a. Dipyridamole can potentiate effects of adenosine
    b. Theophylline will block electrophysiological effects of adenosine
    c. Carbamazepine may increase risk of heart block
6. Significant food interactions: none reported
7. Significant laboratory studies: none reported
8. Side effects
    a. During conversion to sinus rhythm (SR) many dysrhythmias can occur
        1) Sinus bradycardia or arrest
        2) Sinus tachycardia
        3) PVCs
        4) Premature atrial contractions (PACs)
        5) Various degrees of heart block
    b. Facial flushing
9. Adverse effects/toxicity: transient dyspnea, dysrhythmias, hypotension
10. Nursing considerations
    a. Monitor ECG continuously
    b. Evaluate baseline BP, HR, and respiration
    c. Must be administered very quickly over 1–2 seconds and followed by a rapid NS flush; if given too slowly, it will have no effect
    d. Monitor HR and BP every 15 minutes after administration until stable
    e. Monitor carefully for bronchospasm especially in clients with asthma
11. Client education
    a. Various forms of monitoring are needed during medication administration
    b. Transient facial flushing may occur

IX. ANTIHYPERTENSIVES, ANTIHYPOTENSIVES, DIURETICS, AND POTASSIUM SUPPLEMENTS: Refer to Chapter 12

Case Study

A 56-year-old male client is admitted to the intensive care unit with a diagnosis of acute myocardial infarction. He has a T wave inversion and elevation of the ST segment. The EKG indicates myocardial ischemia and necrosis. He is started on lidocaine hydrochloride by IV infusion. He is also given aspirin 325 mg PO, heparin subcutaneous 5,000 units bid, and atenolol (Tenormin) 50 mg PO daily. It should be noted the client received morphine 10 mg IV to relieve chest pain in the emergency room.

1. What assessments should be made prior to administration of these medications?

2. What is the action of each of the medications listed and what is the rationale for their administration?

For suggested responses, see page 542.

3. What nursing implications should be implemented with each of the medications?

4. What information about the medications should be explained to the client?

5. What adverse effects of the medications should the nurse be alert and assess for?

POSTTEST

1 The nurse would monitor a client beginning drug therapy with sotalol (Betapace) for which life-threatening manifestations of an adverse drug reaction?

1. Slight drop in systolic blood pressure and fatigue
2. Early signs of a cerebrovascular accident (CVA)
3. Hives and wheezing
4. Bradycardia and dyspnea

2 A client with a history of mild congestive heart failure (CHF) is receiving diltiazem (Cardizem) for hypertension. The nurse should give priority to which of the following assessments?

1. Tachycardia and rebound hypertension
2. Weight loss and euphoria
3. Bradycardia and peripheral edema
4. Increased ability to perform activities of daily living (ADLs)

3 The nurse has just administered a dose of hydralazine (Apresoline) intravenously to a client. After the initial dose, which of the following assessments is the priority?

1. Cardiac rhythm
2. Oxygen saturation
3. Blood pressure
4. Respiratory rate

4 After initiating a continuous infusion of nitroglycerin (Nitrostat) intravenously, the nurse would use which data to conclude that the client is experiencing an unintended effect? Select all that apply.

1. Pulmonary capillary wedge pressure (PCWP) falling from 13 to 11 mmHg
2. Tachycardia
3. Heart rate (HR) falling from 96 to 78
4. Blood pressure (BP) falling from 130/80 to 90/64
5. Headache

5 A nurse is assigned to the care of a client who will be starting drug therapy with amlodipine (Norvasc) for chronic stable angina. The nurse should include which appropriate information in the teaching plan?

1. This drug has also been utilized for relief of migraine headaches.
2. Dizziness may occur if rising from a sitting position too rapidly.
3. Report urinary retention if it occurs.
4. Call the prescriber if the respiratory rate slows excessively.

6 A client taking atenolol (Tenormin) for hypertension tells the nurse, "Since I have been taking that medicine I feel so tired." The nurse formulates which most appropriate nursing diagnosis?

1. Risk for Activity Intolerance
2. Decreased Cardiac Output
3. Ineffective Health Maintenance
4. Self-Care Deficit

7 The nurse is scheduled to administer a dose of digoxin (Lanoxin) to an adult client with atrial fibrillation. The client has a potassium level of 4.3 mEq/L. The nurse should perform which of the following activities next?

1. Withhold dose only for that day.
2. Obtain order for dose of potassium before giving digoxin.
3. Withhold dose and notify prescriber.
4. Administer dose as ordered.

8 The nurse has prepared nitroprusside 50 mg in 250 mL of 5% Dextrose in water. The client is to receive 1.5 mg/min. What rate should the nurse set the infusion to administer per minute? Record your answer rounding to one decimal place.

_____ mL

POSTTEST

9 After a health care provider prescribed propranolol (Inderal) for a client with frequent premature ventricular contractions (PVCs), the nurse should include which of the following in the care plan?

1. Inform the client that breathing will be improved with exercise.
2. Measure heart rate daily before taking dose.
3. Client will have increased resistance to infection.
4. Skin rashes are rare side effects.

10 The nurse should prepare which of the following medications for chemical cardioversion for a client in atrial fibrillation?

1. Amiodarone (Cordarone)
2. Verapamil (Calan)
3. Nifedipine (Procardia)
4. Lidocaine (Xylocard)

➤ *See pages 187–189 for Answers and Rationales.*

ANSWERS & RATIONALES

Pretest

1 **Answer: 1, 2, 5** **Rationale:** Since chest pain of cardiac origin is related to inadequate coronary oxygen supply, the client needs to decrease the oxygen demand by stopping all activities. An absence of relief from chest pain indicates the NTG is ineffective. The client should seek emergency cardiac care if there is no relief after taking 1 tablet. When tablets are potent, they should sting or tingle when placed under the tongue. NTG should be kept with the client, not on the bedside table. The physician does not need to be contacted for each episode of chest pain; instead the client should take the NTG first as ordered. **Cognitive Level:** Applying **Client Need:** Pharmacological and Parenteral Therapies **Integrated Process:** Teaching and Learning **Content Area:** Pharmacology **Strategy:** The core issue of the question is information that should be included when teaching a client about nitroglycerin as treatment for angina pectoris. Evaluate each option in terms of its truth, and select the options that are true statements. **Reference:** Wilson, B. A., Shannon, M., Shields, K., & Stang, C. (2012). *Pearson nurse's drug guide 2012.* Upper Saddle River, NJ: Pearson Education, pp. 1079–1082.

2 **Answer: 3** **Rationale:** Nitroglycerin patches and ointments must be rotated daily to a hairless area to reduce skin irritation and should be removed after 12 hours to decrease the risk of tolerance. The area should be cleansed gently after removal but does not require vigorous scrubbing. Acetaminophen may be used if headaches develop as a side effect, but it does not need to be used prophylactically. **Cognitive Level:** Applying **Client Need:** Pharmacological and Parenteral Therapies **Integrated Process:** Teaching and Learning **Content Area:** Pharmacology **Strategy:** The critical words in the question are *best response*. With this in mind, select the option that is a true statement. **Reference:** Wilson, B.A., Shannon, M., Shields, K., & Stang, C. (2012). *Pearson nurse's drug guide 2012.* Upper Saddle River, NJ: Pearson Education, pp. 1079–1082.

3 **Answer: 2, 1, 3, 4** **Rationale:** The normal pulse for an adult is 60 to 100 beats per minute, and an adverse effect of digoxin is a low pulse rate. For this reason, the apical rate is assessed before each dose and the dose is withheld (and the prescriber is notified) as the first priority if the pulse rate falls below 60. A low potassium level (normal 3.5 to 5.1 mEq/L) increases the risk of digoxin toxicity so this is of concern second because it increases the potential for digoxin toxicity. Although furosemide can cause hypokalemia, this would be the third concern since the other data indicate actual risk, not potential risk, to the client. Orange juice is of no concern with this medication and is therefore lowest in priority. **Cognitive Level:** Analyzing **Client Need:** Pharmacological and Parenteral Therapies **Integrated Process:** Nursing Process: Diagnosis **Content Area:** Pharmacology **Strategy:** Analyze the data and determine which element could cause the greatest harm most rapidly. Then discriminate between potential risks and normal data of no concern. **Reference:** Wilson, B. A., Shannon, M., & Shields, K., & Stang, C. (2012). *Pearson nurse's drug guide 2012*. Upper Saddle River, NJ: Pearson Education, pp. 463–465.

4 **Answer: 3** **Rationale:** Because nitroglycerin (NTG) is a vasodilator, the blood pressure and heart rate must be monitored closely during titration to prevent hypotension and tachycardia. Shortness of breath is generally important but is not directly related to NTG infusion. Measurement of urinary output is relevant to the client's care but is not related directly to NTG administration. Because of the cerebrovascular dilation, headache frequently occurs and is treated commonly with acetaminophen or another mild analgesic. **Cognitive Level:** Applying **Client Need:** Pharmacological and Parenteral Therapies **Integrated Process:** Nursing Process: Assessment **Content Area:** Pharmacology **Strategy:** Recall the action of NTG as a vasodilator and select the option that focuses directly on cardiovascular status. **Reference:** Wilson, B. A.,

Shannon, M. T., & Shields, K. M. (2012). *Pearson nurse's drug guide 2012.* Upper Saddle River, NJ; Pearson Education, pp. 1079–1082.

5 **Answer: 1** **Rationale:** Metoprolol is a beta-blocking agent that blocks the effects of both beta$_1$ and beta$_2$ receptors, leading to a reduction in systemic vascular resistance. This effect also may lead to bronchospasm (from bronchoconstriction secondary to beta$_2$ blockade). Metoprolol would not be contraindicated with a history of seizures, peripheral vascular disease or myasthenia gravis. **Cognitive Level:** Applying **Client Need:** Pharmacological and Parenteral Therapies **Integrated Process:** Nursing Process: Assessment **Content Area:** Pharmacology **Strategy:** Consider the sites of action of this drug and use this information to choose the option that matches a risk with its blockade. **Reference:** Wilson, B. A., Shannon, M., & Shields, K. (2012) *Pearson nurse's drug guide 2012.* Upper Saddle River, NJ: Pearson Education, pp. 985–988.

6 **Answer: 4** **Rationale:** Verapamil is a calcium channel blocker used to treat angina. Significant constipation is a frequent complaint of clients taking the sustained-release form of verapamil. Many older adults have difficulty with this, and the nurse must anticipate the need for teaching about increasing fiber and fluid intake. Hypotension is an adverse reaction to verapamil. Since the drug dilates coronary arteries, it is not likely that angina will occur. **Cognitive Level:** Applying **Client Need:** Pharmacological and Parenteral Therapies **Integrated Process:** Nursing Process: Assessment **Content Area:** Pharmacology **Strategy:** It may help to remember that verapamil causes constipation by recalling it is a calcium channel blocker (both begin with the letter *c*). Note the age of the client to further prioritize constipation as a key concern since this can be an age-related concern of older adults anyway. **Reference:** Wilson, B.A., Shannon, M., & Shields, K. (2012) *Pearson nurse's drug guide 2012.* Upper Saddle River, NJ: Pearson Education, pp. 1576–1579.

7 **Answer: 1, 4, 3, 2** **Rationale:** Early indications of lidocaine toxicity include various central nervous system (CNS) complications. These may include slurred speech, dizziness, confusion, and paresthesias. If they are ignored, the client can develop seizures that are often difficult to stop and death may ensue. The nurse would be concerned second with a prolonged PR interval, which could indicate excessive drug dose. The respiratory rate of 12 is at the low end of normal for an adult, which is 12–20 breaths per minute. Since this is technically within normal limits, it would be third in priority. A heart rate of 64/min is within the adult normal range of 60–100, making it the lowest priority. **Cognitive Level:** Analyzing **Client Need:** Pharmacological and Parenteral Therapies **Integrated Process:** Nursing Process: Diagnosis **Content Area:** Pharmacology **Strategy:** Rank the options according to immediacy, irreversibility, magnitude, and predictability of the threat. **Reference:** Wilson, B. A., Shannon, M., & Shields, K. (2012). *Pearson nurse's drug guide 2012.* Upper Saddle River, NJ: Pearson Education, pp. 875–878.

8 **Answer: 2** **Rationale:** Because it increases contractility (inotropy) of the heart, digoxin is classified as a positive inotropic drug. Because the primary problem associated with heart failure is decreased contractility, digoxin is the drug of choice. Atropine is utilized for sinus bradycardia. Propranolol, a beta-blocker, is used for hypertension and angina. Verapamil, a calcium channel blocker, is a negative inotropic medication and is used for hypertension, tachycardia, and angina. By virtue of their action, calcium channel blockers can also cause heart failure if taken in excessive doses. **Cognitive Level:** Applying **Client Need:** Pharmacological and Parenteral Therapies **Integrated Process:** Nursing Process: Planning **Content Area:** Pharmacology **Strategy:** Correlate the altered cardiac function with the primary actions of the drug. **Reference:** Wilson, B. A., Shannon, M., & Shields, K. (2012). *Pearson nurse's drug guide 2012.* Upper Saddle River, NJ: Pearson Education, pp. 134–136, 469–471, 1064–1066, 1284–1287.

9 **Answer: 1, 3, 5** **Rationale:** Intravenous lidocaine reduces dysrhythmias by raising the electrical threshold of cardiac cells, reduces the automaticity of cardiac tissue, and is used to treat ventricular dysrhythmias. Local anesthetic activity occurs when the drug is injected directly into tissue such as the skin. The drug is more likely to decrease heart rate than to increase it. **Cognitive Level:** Analyzing **Client Need:** Pharmacological and Parenteral Therapies **Integrated Process:** Teaching and Learning **Content Area:** Pharmacology **Strategy:** The wording of the question tells you the correct options are those that contain correct statements. Use the process of elimination to discard options that contain false information. **Reference:** Wilson, B. A., Shannon, M., & Shields, K. (2012). *Pearson nurse's drug guide 2012.* Upper Saddle River, NJ: Pearson Education, pp. 875–878.

10 **Answer: 2** **Rationale:** The side effects of amiodarone take several weeks or longer to manifest themselves. Sometimes they persist for up to 4 months, and because photosensitivity is a continuing concern, the client should avoid tanning and excessive sunlight. The pulse should be monitored and if it remains above 100 (not below) the primary care provider should be notified. **Cognitive Level:** Analyzing **Client Need:** Pharmacological and Parenteral Therapies **Integrated Process:** Nursing Process: Evaluation **Content Area:** Pharmacology **Strategy:** Specific drug knowledge is needed to answer this question. The wording of the question tells you the correct option will be a true statement of fact. **Reference:** Wilson, B. A., Shannon, M., & Shields, K. (2012). *Pearson nurse's drug guide 2012.* Upper Saddle River, NJ: Pearson Education, pp. 72–75.

Posttest

1 **Answer: 4** **Rationale:** Sotalol is a beta-adrenergic blocking agent which has negative inotropic and chronotropic effects on the heart and may block beta$_2$ receptors in the lung resulting in side effects such as bradycardia, dyspnea, and chest pain, which can be life-threatening complications. CNS side effects are fatigue and dizziness. Hives and wheezing are signs of anaphylaxis, but this is not commonly associated with sotalol. **Cognitive Level:** Applying **Client Need:** Pharmacological and Parenteral Therapies **Integrated Process:** Nursing Process: Assessment **Content Area:** Pharmacology **Strategy:** Note that the drug ends in *-olol*, indicating that it is a beta-adrenergic blocker. Since these drugs reduce cardiac rate, associate this with bradycardia in the correct option. As an added assurance, note that dyspnea is another sign, which can also result from blockade of the beta receptors in the lungs. **Reference:** Wilson, B. A., Shannon, M., & Shields, K. (2012). *Pearson nurse's drug guide 2012.* Upper Saddle River, NJ: Pearson Education, pp. 1405–1407.

2 **Answer: 3 Rationale:** Because calcium channel blocker agents decrease the contraction of cardiac muscle, drugs such as diltiazem (Cardizem) should be used cautiously in clients with congestive heart failure (CHF). An excessive dosage could actually worsen the state of heart failure. Bradycardia and peripheral edema signal adverse effects of this drug group. Although reflex tachycardia could occur because of sudden hypotension, rebound hypertension is not likely. Weight gain and drowsiness may occur rather than weight loss and euphoria. Instead of increased ability to perform activities of daily living (ADLs), the client is more likely to experience fatigue, drowsiness, and weakness as side effects of this drug. **Cognitive Level:** Applying **Client Need:** Pharmacological and Parenteral Therapies **Integrated Process:** Nursing Process: Assessment **Content Area:** Pharmacology **Strategy:** Correlate the adverse effects of the drug with the primary alteration associated with congestive heart failure (CHF). Recall that the drug reduces the force of contraction and so could worsen the CHF state, making signs of CHF the answer to the question. **Reference:** Wilson, B. A., Shannon, M., & Shields, K. (2012). *Pearson nurse's drug guide 2012.* Upper Saddle River, NJ: Pearson Education, pp. 1405–1407.

3 **Answer: 3 Rationale:** Hydralazine (Apresoline) is a powerful vasodilator that exerts its action on the smooth muscle walls of arterioles. After a parenteral dose, blood pressure is checked every 15 minutes until stable and then every hour. Normal dosage may result in tachycardia but not dysrhythmia. Decreased blood pressure could result in decreased oxygenation, but is not the primary focus of the therapy. **Cognitive Level:** Applying **Client Need:** Pharmacological and Parenteral Therapies **Integrated Process:** Nursing Process: Assessment **Content Area:** Pharmacology **Strategy:** To answer this question correctly, it is necessary to understand that this drug is a powerful vasodilator that exerts an antihypertensive action. With this in mind, select the option that focuses on tracking the client's blood pressure.

Reference: Wilson, B. A., Shannon, M., & Shields, K. (2012). *Pearson nurse's drug guide 2012.* Upper Saddle River, NJ: Pearson Education, pp. 733–735.

4 **Answer: 2, 4, 5 Rationale:** Tachycardia may result because of the decreased cardiac output. Nitroglycerin (NTG) is a vasodilator resulting in redistribution of central circulating volume. A decrease in BP from 130/80 to 90/64 is excessive, and warrants further assessment by the nurse to determine whether perfusion to major organs is adequate. Because of the vasodilation of blood vessels in the cranium, headache and flushing may occur. Pulmonary capillary wedge pressure (PCWP) is an indirect measurement of left ventricular end diastolic pressure. Because nitroglycerin causes a reduction in peripheral resistance, left ventricular preload and left ventricular afterload are reduced. Therefore, a decrease in PCWP and central venous pressure (CVP) is expected. **Cognitive Level:** Applying **Client Need:** Pharmacological and Parenteral Therapies **Integrated Process:** Nursing Process: Planning **Content Area:** Pharmacology **Strategy:** Recall first that this drug is a powerful vasodilator, especially when given by the IV route. Note the critical words *unintended effect* in the question. Think through the physiological effects of this drug's action, and select the options that are excessive or unexpected. **Reference:** Wilson, B. A., Shannon, M., & Shields, K. (2012). *Pearson nurse's drug guide 2012.* Upper Saddle River, NJ: Pearson Education, pp. 1079–1082.

5 **Answer: 2 Rationale:** Amlodipine (Norvasc) is a calcium channel blocker. Adverse or toxic reactions from overdosage may produce excessive peripheral vasodilation and marked hypotension with reflex tachycardia and headaches. For this reason, the client may experience dizziness when rising from a recumbent or sitting position. This drug is more likely to cause urinary frequency than retention. The client is more likely to have dyspnea from pulmonary congestion secondary to reduced cardiac pumping action rather than a decrease in respiratory rate. **Cognitive Level:** Applying **Client Need:** Pharmacological and Parenteral Therapies **Integrated Process:** Teaching and Learning **Content Area:** Pharmacology **Strategy:** Select the option that includes the adverse effect that is most likely to place the client at greatest risk as well as the most likely to occur. **Reference:** Wilson, B. A., Shannon, M., & Shields, K. (2012). *Pearson nurse's drug guide 2012.* Upper Saddle River, NJ: Pearson Education, pp. 78–79.

6 **Answer: 2 Rationale:** Decreased cardiac output is an outcome of the drug therapy. Because atenolol, a beta adrenergic blocker, causes decreased heart rate, blood pressure, and cardiac output, fatigue is a most common side effect. Activity intolerance is the state in which an individual has insufficient energy to complete activities of daily living. The client reported feeling tired, but did not address being unable to perform activities. There is no evidence that the client is unable to perform health maintenance activities or is unable to perform self-care.

Cognitive Level: Analyzing **Client Need**: Pharmacological and Parenteral Therapies **Integrated Process**: Nursing Process: Diagnosis **Content Area**: Pharmacology **Strategy**: The critical word in the question is *tired*. Consider the nature of the drug and the effect it has on the heart, and from there consider that fatigue could result from the decreased pumping action of the heart to choose correctly. **Reference**: Wilson, B. A., Shannon, M., & Shields, K. (2012) *Pearson nurse's drug guide 2012*. Upper Saddle River, NJ: Pearson Education, pp. 125–126.

7 **Answer: 4** **Rationale**: Hypokalemia is a common electrolyte imbalance commonly associated with digoxin therapy. The normal adult reference range for potassium is 3.5 to 5.1 mEq/L. Reduced potassium levels will result in an increased risk of digitalis toxicity. The client's level is within normal limits and the dose should be administered. There is no reason to withhold the dose, administer additional potassium, or to notify the prescriber. **Cognitive Level**: Applying **Client Need**: Pharmacological and Parenteral Therapies **Integrated Process**: Nursing Process: Planning **Content Area**: Pharmacology **Strategy**: To answer this question correctly, it is necessary to understand the nature of the drug and the normal potassium level. Use this knowledge and the process of elimination to make a selection. **Reference**: Wilson, B. A., Shannon, M., & Shields, K. (2012). *Pearson nurse's drug guide 2012*. Upper Saddle River, NJ: Pearson Education, pp. 463–465.

8 **Answer: 7.5** **Rationale**: Use the equation

$$\frac{Desired}{Have} \times Quantity\ available$$

$$\frac{1.5\ mg}{50\ mg} \times 250\ mL$$

$$1.5 \times 250 = 50x$$
$$375 = 50x$$
$$x = 7.5\ mL$$

Cognitive Level: Applying **Client Need**: Pharmacological and Parenteral therapies **Integrated Process**: Implementation **Content Area**: Pharmacology **Strategy**: Using the equation Desired/Have × Quantity available, calculate the correct

dose. **Reference**: Wilson, B. A., Shannon, M., & Shields, K. (2012). *Pearson nurse's drug guide 2012*. Upper Saddle River, NJ: Pearson Education, pp. 1082–1083.

9 **Answer: 2** **Rationale**: Because the drug is a beta-adrenergic blocker, bradycardia is a common side effect. For this reason, the client should be taught to self-monitor the heart rate daily. Agranulocytosis is a side effect that could result in decreased resistance to infection. Many serious skin eruptions are associated with the drug. **Cognitive Level**: Analyzing **Client Need**: Pharmacological and Parenteral Therapies **Integrated Process**: Nursing Process: Planning **Content Area**: Pharmacology **Strategy**: First recall that the drug is a beta-adrenergic blocking agent. Then select the option that most represents the drug characteristics. **Reference**: Wilson, B. A., Shannon, M., & Shields, K. (2012). *Pearson nurse's drug guide 2012*. Upper Saddle River, NJ: Pearson Education, pp. 1284–1287.

10 **Answer: 1** **Rationale**: Amiodarone is a Class III antidysrhythmic agent which prolong the duration of action potential and refractory period of the heart. It slows conduction through the AV node and is effective in suppressing supraventricular arrhythmias, particularly atrial fibrillation. Verapamil is a calcium channel blocker that primarily influences the dilation of coronary arteries and has secondary effects on cardiac conduction. Although nifedipine is a calcium channel blocker, it has no effect on SA-AV node conduction. It causes greater dilation of coronary and peripheral vessels than verapamil. Lidocaine is used predominantly for treatment of ventricular dysrhythmias. **Cognitive Level**: Analyzing **Client Need**: Pharmacological and Parenteral Therapies **Integrated Process**: Nursing Process: Planning **Content Area**: Pharmacology **Strategy**: Specific drug knowledge is needed to answer the question. First consider which drug group would exert a therapeutic effect for this dysrhythmia, and then associate the electrical activity in the heart with the action of the drug. **Reference**: Wilson, B. A., Shannon, M., & Shields, K. (2012). *Pearson nurse's drug guide 2012*. Upper Saddle River, NJ: Pearson Education, pp. 72–75.

References

Abrams, A. (2009). *Clinical drug therapy: Rationales for nursing practice* (9th ed.). Philadelphia, PA: Lippincott Williams & Wilkins.

Adams, M., Holland, L., & Bostwick, P. (2011). *Pharmacology for nurses: A pathophysiologic approach* (3rd ed.). Upper Saddle River, NJ: Pearson Education.

Adams. M. P., & Koch R.W. (2010). *Pharmacology: Connections to nursing practice*. Upper Saddle River, NJ: Pearson Education.

Aschenbrenner, D., & Venable, S. (2012). *Drug therapy in nursing* (4th ed.).

Philadelphia, PA: Lippincott Williams & Wilkins.

Drug Facts & Comparisons® (Updated monthly). St. Louis, MO: Wolters Kluwer.

Ignatavicius, D., & Workman, M L. (2010). *Medical-surgical nursing: Critical thinking for collaborative care* (6th ed.). Philadelphia, PA: W. B. Saunders.

Karch, A. M. (2010). *Focus on nursing pharmacology* (5th ed.). Philadelphia, PA: Lippincott Williams & Wilkins.

Kee, J. (2009). *Laboratory and diagnostic tests and nursing implications* (8th ed.). Upper Saddle River, NJ: Pearson Education.

Lehne, R. (2010). *Pharmacology for nursing care* (7th ed.). St. Louis, MO: Mosby, Inc.

LeMone, P., Burke, K. M., & Bauldoff, G. (2011). *Medical-surgical nursing: Critical thinking in patient care* (5th ed.). Upper Saddle River, NJ: Pearson Education.

Lilley, L. L., Collins, S. R., et al. (2011). *Pharmacology and the nursing process* (6th ed.). St. Louis, MO: Mosby, Inc.

Wilson, B. A., Shannon, M. T, & Shields, K. M. (2012). *Pearson nurse's drug guide 2012*. Upper Saddle River, NJ: Pearson Education.

ANSWERS & RATIONALES

6

Endocrine System Medications

Chapter Outline

Medications Affecting the
  Pituitary Gland
Medications Affecting the
  Adrenal Glands

Medications Affecting the
  Thyroid Glands
Medications Affecting the
  Parathyroid Glands

Medications Used to Treat
  Diabetes Mellitus

NCLEX-RN® Test Prep

Use the accompanying online resource, NursingReviewsandRationales, to test yourself with hundreds of NCLEX®-style practice questions.

Objectives

➤ Describe the general goals of therapy when administering endocrine system medications.
➤ Describe the action, use, and nursing considerations related to the administration of medications used to treat diabetes insipidus.
➤ Identify the nursing considerations related to the administration of thyroid replacement medications.
➤ Discuss the medications used to treat hyperthyroidism.
➤ List the client teaching points related to the administration of calcium and vitamin D supplements.
➤ Identify the characteristics of various types of insulin.
➤ Identify the side effects and complications associated with the use of glucocorticoids.
➤ Discuss the nursing considerations related to the administration of insulin.
➤ Describe the significant client teaching points related to the administration of medications used to treat diabetes mellitus.
➤ List the significant client education points related to various endocrine system medications.

Review at a Glance

Addison disease life-threatening disease caused by partial or complete failure of adrenocortical function
adrenal crisis an acute, life-threatening state of profound adrenocortical insufficiency requiring immediate therapy
adrenal insufficiency a condition in which adrenal glands are unable to produce adequate amounts of adreno-cortical hormones
catecholamine any one of a group of sympathomimetic compounds

composed of a catechol molecule and the aliphatic portion of an amine; some are produced naturally by the body and function as key neurologic chemicals
cushingoid state having the habitus and facies characteristic of Cushing disease, including fat pads on the upper back and face, ruddy complexion, striae on trunk, thin legs, and excess facial hair
glucocorticoid an adrenocortical steroid hormone that increases glycogenesis, exerts an anti-inflammatory effect, and influences many body functions

glycosylated hemoglobin concentration representative of the average blood glucose level over the previous several weeks
Graves' disease a disorder characterized by pronounced hyperthyroidism usually associated with an enlarged thyroid gland and exophthalmos; also called thyrotoxicosis
hypercalciuria presence of abnormally large amounts of calcium in the urine resulting from conditions characterized by augmented bone resorption

hyperglycemia a greater than normal amount of glucose in the blood most frequently associated with diabetes mellitus, post-administration of glucocorticoids, and with excessive infusion of glucose-containing intravenous solutions

hyperthyroidism a condition characterized by hyperactivity of the thyroid gland; the gland is usually enlarged, secreting greater than normal amounts of thyroid hormones, and the metabolic processes of the body are accelerated

hypoglycemia a less than normal amount of glucose in the blood, usually caused by administration of too much insulin, excessive secretion of insulin by the islet cells of the pancreas, or dietary deficiency

hypoparathyroidism a condition of insufficient secretion of parathyroid glands caused by primary parathyroid dysfunction or by elevated serum calcium level

hypothyroidism a condition characterized by decreased activity of the thyroid gland caused by surgical removal of all or part of the thyroid gland, over-dosage with antithyroid medication, decreased effect of thyroid releasing hormone secreted by the hypothalamus, decreased secretion of thyroid stimulating hormone by the pituitary gland, or atrophy of the thyroid gland itself

lipodystrophy any abnormality in the metabolism or deposition of fats

mineralocorticoid a steroid hormone that acts on the kidney to promote retention of sodium and water and excretion of potassium and hydrogen

myxedema most severe form of hypothyroidism characterized by swelling of the hands, face, feet, and periorbital tissues and may lead to coma and death

osteomalacia an abnormal condition of the lamellar bone, characterized by a loss of calcification of the matrix resulting in softening of the bone and accompanied by weakness, fracture, pain, anorexia, and weight loss

osteoporosis a disorder characterized by abnormal loss of bone density most frequently seen in postmenopausal women, sedentary or immobilized individuals, and clients receiving long-term steroid therapy

Paget disease a common nonmetabolic disease of bone of unknown cause, usually affecting middle-aged people and older adults, characterized by excessive bone destruction and unorganized bone repair

PRETEST

1 Parents are concerned that their 5-year-old son is not growing fast enough and ask the nurse if he should be receiving growth hormone (GH). Which of the following is the best response by the nurse?

1. "Growth hormone will only affect your child's short bones."
2. "Can your son swallow pills easily?"
3. "Scientific evidence is required before growth hormone can be administered to children."
4. "How tall do you think your son should be?"

2 After ingesting high dosages of glucocorticoids for several weeks, the client asks the nurse about termination of the drug. Which of the following is the nurse's best response?

1. "Even at high doses, adverse reactions are unlikely if the medication is abruptly withdrawn."
2. "It is dangerous for steroids to be withdrawn suddenly."
3. "You may experience severe psychological symptoms when the medication is withdrawn."
4. "Tapering of the medication requires daily blood work to measure serum chemistries."

3 A nurse is providing education to the client who is prescribed intranasal desmopressin (DDAVP). The nurse should include which of the following pieces of information during the teaching session? Select all that apply.

1. Shake the drug rigorously prior to use.
2. Keep a record of each night's sleep and record incidents of bed-wetting.
3. Angle the tip of the nasal spray low into the cavity when administering this drug.
4. A rapid weight gain should be reported to the prescriber immediately.
5. Report drowsiness to the prescriber.

4 Because a client is taking a high dose of fludrocortisone (Florinef) for treatment of Addison disease, the nurse should include which of the following in the client education program?

1. Keep a log of weekly early-morning weights.
2. Report weight loss greater than 5 pounds per week.
3. There will be reduced ability to resist infection.
4. It is important to measure postural blood pressures.

5 The nurse is reviewing a client's medication record and notes that levothyroxine (Synthroid) is ordered. The nurse is aware this drug may be used for a variety of conditions, including which of the following? Select all that apply.

1. Cretinism
2. Thyroid cancer
3. Myxedema coma
4. Adrenal insufficiency
5. Type 2 diabetes mellitus

6 After liotrix (Thyrolar) is prescribed for a client with hypothyroidism, the nurse should make which important statement as part of client teaching in preparing for discharge?

1. "Measure the body temperature every morning."
2. "Report chest pain or palpitations to your health care provider immediately."
3. "You may experience sleepiness while taking this drug."
4. "You may experience nervousness while taking this drug."

7 After taking propylthiouracil (PTU) for 6 weeks, a client with Graves' disease reports a sore throat and fever. What should the nurse at the outpatient clinic do next as a priority?

1. Ask client about exposure to the common cold.
2. Measure client's body temperature and ask about history of fever over last few weeks.
3. Review laboratory report for client's white blood cell (WBC) count with differential.
4. Ask about current mental stressors that could be weakening the immune system.

8 Several weeks ago calcitonin (Calcimar) was prescribed for a client with Paget disease. To determine therapeutic effectiveness, the nurse should review the medical record for which of the following?

1. Decreased alkaline phosphatase levels
2. Increased serum calcium levels
3. Bone x-rays for return of bones to normal
4. Magnetic resonance imagery (MRI) results of skull deformities

9 When caring for a male client who has been receiving insulin for 2 weeks, the home health nurse should include which of the following statements in client teaching? Select all that apply.

1. "I will need to be sure that a family member also learns how to administer insulin injections."
2. "Visual changes can occur over time if your blood glucose is not sufficiently controlled with insulin."
3. "You may experience impotence as an effect of the disease process."
4. "Loss of sight and the loss of lower legs are common in clients with diabetes who take insulin."
5. "A high glucose level is not always an indication for an increase in insulin dosage."

10 The nurse is evaluating a client's knowledge of the treatment of an insulin reaction. The nurse would place highest priority on determining that the client understands which of the following points?

1. Symptoms indicating the need to notify the health care provider
2. When to schedule fasting (serum) blood glucose level
3. When to ingest orange juice and peanut butter on crackers
4. Importance of maintaining sufficient oral fluid intake

➤ *See pages 217–218 for Answers and Rationales.*

I. MEDICATIONS AFFECTING THE PITUITARY GLAND

A. Growth hormone (GH) or GH suppressants

1. Action and use of GH
   a. Stimulates growth and metabolism of all body cells
   b. Action: determines adult physical size by regulating growth of organs and tissues, specifically length of long bones
   c. Use: approved only for use in children to treat GH deficiency or inadequate GH secretion related to documented lack of GH
2. Action and use of GH suppressants: reduce GH levels; bromocriptine may manage amenorrhea associated with prolactinemia, symptoms of Parkinson's disease, or acromegaly
3. Common medications (Table 6-1)
4. Administration considerations
   a. Is only given parenterally (IM or subQ); oral route is inactivated by digestive enzymes
   b. Is packaged in powder form and is reconstituted for administration with 1 to 5 mL of approved diluent; mixture must be clear and not cloudy or contain any undissolved particles; label date of reconstitution and discard refrigerated drug according to manufacturer's directions
   c. Rotate IM sites and use appropriate needle length to inject into muscle layer
5. Contraindications
   a. To stimulate growth in children who are short unrelated to GH deficiency; during or after closure of epiphyseal plates in long bones; or with secondary intracranial tumors
   b. Use cautiously if there is diabetes or family history of same, hypothyroidism, or concurrent or previous use of thyroid hormones in males before puberty
   c. Known sensitivity to benzyl alcohol (a preservative in bacteriostatic water that may also be harmful to newborns); preferred diluent is sterile water, especially for newborns
6. Significant drug interactions
   a. Adrenocorticotropic hormone (ACTH) or corticosteroids may slow the action of growth hormone

Table 6-1 **Drugs that Influence Growth Hormone**

Generic (Trade) Name	Route	Uses
Growth Hormone Suppressants		
Bromocriptine (Parlodel)	PO	Suppresses growth hormone levels.
Octreotide (Sandostatin)	subQ, IM, IV	Suppresses intestinal peptide hormones, insulin, glucagons, and growth hormone. Promotes fluid and electrolyte reabsorption.
Lanreotide (Somatuline Depot)	subQ	Suppresses GH level in clients with acromegaly who have not responded to radiation therapy or are unable to tolerate surgery.
Pegvisomant (Somavert)	subQ	GH receptor antagonist
Growth Hormone		
Mecasermin (Increlex)	subQ	Recombinant DNA insulin-like growth factor (IGF) with same actions as GH; used for growth failure in children only (before bone epiphyses close)
Somatropin (Humatrope, others)	IM, subQ	Used as replacement therapy.

       b. Octreotide acetate may decrease cyclosporine levels

       c. Thyroid hormone, anabolic steroids, androgens, or estrogens may hasten closure of epiphyseal plates of long bones

  7. Significant food interactions: none

  8. Significant laboratory studies

       a. Plasma GH levels to confirm deficiency (less than 5 to 7 ng/mL)

       b. Regular measurement of thyroid levels to detect undiagnosed hypothyroidism

       c. Blood or urine glucose levels to detect glucose intolerance in diabetic clients or those with significant family history of diabetes

  9. Side effects

       a. Metabolic: glucose intolerance, ACTH deficiency, or hypothyroidism

       b. Renal: **hypercalciuria** (excess calcium excretion in the urine) during first 2 to 3 months of treatment; risk of renal calculi with complaints of flank pain, colic, GI upset, urinary frequency, chills, fever, and hematuria

       c. Other: recurrent intracranial tumor growth or presence of GH antibodies

 10. Adverse effects/toxicity

       a. Local allergic reaction: pain and edema at injection site

       b. Systemic allergic reaction: peripheral edema, headache, myalgia, and weakness

       c. Excess dosage: diabetes mellitus, atherosclerosis, enlarged organs, hypertension, and features related to acromegaly

 11. Nursing considerations

       a. Make sure there is documentation of growth rate for at least 6 to 12 months prior to initiating treatment

       b. Assess client for any adverse effects or toxicities related to drug administration

       c. Make sure annual bone age assessments are performed, especially for clients undergoing thyroid, androgen, or estrogen replacement therapy

 12. Client education

       a. Advise parents or caregivers to have regular bone age assessments done at specific times

       b. Tell parents or caregivers that a 3- to 5-inch growth rate is expected in the 1st year and less in the 2nd year, with normal growth rate subsequent years; subcutaneous fat is diminished during treatment, but will return later

       c. Teach parents or caregivers how to accurately document monthly height and weight measurements and to report any less-than-expected growth to the prescriber

       d. Teach parents or caregivers signs and symptoms of slipped femoral epiphysis (hip or knee pain and limp) and to notify prescriber of same

       e. Advise parents or caregivers that treatment is discontinued when adequate adult height reached, when epiphyseal plates are fused, or when client fails to respond to growth hormone

       f. Instruct client and caregivers how to administer subQ or IM injections

B. Antidiuretic hormone (ADH)

  1. Action and use

       a. Action: on renal tubules to promote reabsorption of water; vasopressor effect due to constriction of smooth muscle; increases aggregation of platelets

       b. Use: is a posterior pituitary hormone for replacement therapy for clients with diabetes insipidus; also for use in hemophilia A, von Willebrand disease Type 1

  2. Common medications (Table 6-2)

  3. Administration considerations

       a. Give intranasally, intravenously (IV), subcutaneously (subQ), intramuscularly (IM), or intra-arterially according to order and preparation

       b. Infusion pump is needed for intravenous or intra-arterial routes

Table 6-2 **Drugs to Treat Diabetes Insipidus (DI)**

Generic (Trade) Name	Route	Uses
Desmopressin (DDAVP)	Intranasal, IV, subQ, PO	Used as replacement therapy, in DI; relieve polyuria and polydipsia associated with trauma or pituitary surgery.
Vasopressin (Pitressin)	IM, IV, subQ, intra-arterial	Used as replacement therapy in DI or dispel gas in abdominal x-ray.

4. Contraindications: clients with coronary artery or vascular disease; blood pressure (BP) elevation is caused by vasoconstriction
5. Significant drug interactions
   a. Demeclocycline and lithium carbonate may inhibit action and promote continuation of diuresis
   b. Carbamazepine, chlorpropamide, and clofibrate may also extend action of antidiuretics
   c. Epinephrine, heparin, and phenytoin may decrease ADH effects of vasopressin
   d. Guanethidine and neostigmine increase vasopressor actions
6. Significant food interactions: none known
7. Significant laboratory studies
   a. Serum osmolality and plasma osmolality with diabetes insipidus
   b. Factor VIII coagulation level for hemostasis
8. Side effects
   a. CNS: drowsiness, headache, lethargy
   b. EENT: nasal congestion and irritation; rhinitis
   c. GI: abdominal cramps, nausea, and heartburn
   d. GU: pain in vulva
   e. CV: elevated BP
9. Adverse effects/toxicity
   a. IV route may cause anaphylaxis
   b. Overdose may produce symptoms of water intoxication
10. Nursing considerations
    a. Check client's alertness to rule out water intoxication disorientation, lethargy, and behavioral changes
    b. Initial dose is given in the evening and amount is increased until uninterrupted sleep is noted
    c. Check vital signs (BP and pulse) before giving by the IV and subQ routes
    d. Measure daily I & O to monitor water retention and sodium depletion; assess edema in extremities
    e. Weigh daily to monitor water retention
    f. For nasal spray, make sure nasal mucosa is intact by inspecting nares prior to dose; use alternate nares for alternate doses
    g. IV dose may be given undiluted over 1 minute
    h. Store nasal spray at room temperature; all other solutions need refrigeration
11. Client education
    a. Proper technique for nasal instillation (tube inserted into nostril to instill)
    b. Avoid over-the-counter (OTC) meds containing epinephrine that can decrease drug's action
    c. Avoid alcohol use when taking drug
    d. Wear MedicAlert identification
    e. Do not double dose if dose missed; may take skipped dose up to one hour before next dose
    f. Report any nasal congestion or upper respiratory tract infection

Practice to Pass

A female client who is taking antidiuretic hormone (ADH) intranasally calls to tell you that she has a cold and flulike symptoms. What will you advise her to do?

II. MEDICATIONS AFFECTING THE ADRENAL GLANDS

A. Minera locorticoids

1. Action and use

   a. A **mineralocorticoid** is a steroid hormone that acts on kidneys to retain sodium and water and release potassium

   b. Synthesis is regulated by the renin-angiotensin system

   c. Replacement hormone therapy is required with missing mineralocorticoid action, which occurs in adrenal gland failure or hypofunction

2. Common medications (Table 6-3)

3. Administration considerations

   a. Fludrocortisone acetate is drug of choice

   b. Is given orally from 0.1 mg 3 times/week to 0.2 mg/day

4. Contraindications: hypersensitivity to glucocorticoids; idiopathic thrombocytopenic purpura (ITP); acute glomerulonephritis; viral or bacterial skin infections or infections not being treated with antibiotics; amebiasis; Cushing syndrome; vaccinations and immunologic procedures, osteoporosis

5. Drug interactions

   a. Hypokalemic effect may potentiate action of other drugs

   b. Hypernatremia may result if given with high-sodium drugs

   c. Higher dosage may be needed if given with hepatic metabolic enzymes (such as rifampin and phenytoin)

   d. Increased therapeutic and toxic effects of cortisone if taken with troleandomycin

   e. Decreased steroid blood levels with phenytoin, phenobarbital, and rifampin

6. Food interactions: high-sodium foods

7. Significant laboratory studies: monitor serum electrolyte levels

8. Side effects: sodium and fluid retention, nausea, acne, and impaired wound healing

9. Adverse effects/toxicity

   a. Adverse reactions occur rarely, but use cautiously in clients with heart disease, congestive heart failure (CHF), or hypertension

   b. Thromboembolism

   c. Aggravation or masking of infection

   d. Anaphylactoid reactions are rare but may occur in clients hypersensitive to glucocorticoids

10. Nursing considerations

    a. Is used with glucocorticoids for replacement therapy

    b. Monitor serum electrolyte levels

    c. Monitor weight and I & O and report weight gain of 5 lb/week

Practice to Pass

A client taking mineralocorticoid therapy tells you that she has gained 5½ pounds in the last 2 days. What action will you take?

Table 6-3 Drugs for Adrenal Replacement Therapy (Mineralocorticoids)

Generic (Trade) Names	Route	Uses
Cortisone (Cortone)	PO	Ulcerative colitis, multiple sclerosis (MS), leukemia, lymphoma, thrombocytopenia, inflammatory diseases such as rheumatoid arthritis and asthma, hypercalcemia related to cancer, replacement therapy in adrenal cortical insufficiency
Fludrocortisone (Florinef)	PO	Replacement therapy in primary and secondary adrenocortical insufficiency, treatment of salt-losing adrenogenital syndrome, management of orthostatic hypotension
Hydrocortisone (Cortof)	PO	Replacement therapy in adrenal cortical insufficiency, allergic reactions, hypercalcemia related to cancer, inflammatory diseases such as rheumatoid arthritis and asthma, thrombocytopenia, trichinosis, ulcerative colitis, MS, anorectal cream to relieve hemorrhoids

      d. Monitor and record BP daily and more frequently during periods of dosage adjustment

      e. Check for signs of overdosage related to hypercorticism (psychosis, excess weight gain, edema, CHF, increased appetite, severe insomnia, and elevated BP)

      f. Give daily doses before 9 a.m. to mimic peak corticosteroid blood levels

      g. Check for signs of under dosage: weight loss, poor appetite, nausea, vomiting, diarrhea, muscular weakness, increased fatigue, and low BP

  11. Client education

      a. Report signs of low potassium associated with high sodium (muscle weakness, paresthesias, circumoral numbness, fatigue, anorexia, nausea, depression, delirium, diminished reflexes, polyuria, irregular heart rate, CHF, ileus)

      b. Utilize range-of-motion exercises to decrease musculoskeletal effects

      c. Eat foods high in potassium

      d. Salt intake regulates drug's effect, so report signs of edema

      e. Weigh self daily and report consistent weight gain

      f. Report any infections, trauma, or unexpected stress

      g. Wear or carry medical identification alert including drug use and MD's name

      h. Call prescriber to increase dosage if client is under stress

B. Glucocorticoids

  1. Action and use

      a. A **glucocorticoid** is a steroid hormone that affects carbohydrate, protein, and fat metabolism, and has anti-inflammatory and immunosuppressive activity; its synthesis is regulated by the pituitary gland via negative feedback loop; may regulate metabolism of skeletal and connective tissues

      b. Is used in acute **adrenal insufficiency** (inability of adrenal glands to produce sufficient adrenocortical hormones) caused by trauma or thrombosis; chronic primary adrenal insufficiency (also known as **Addison disease**); and secondary adrenal insufficiency (diseased or destroyed adenohypophysis with inadequate production of ACTH)

      c. In allergic conditions (asthma, angioedema, transfusion reactions, and serum sickness)

      d. In dermatological conditions, such as dermatitis and pemphigus

      e. In inflammatory GI disorders, such as Crohn disease and ulcerative colitis

      f. In hematologic disorders, such as autoimmune hemolytic anemia and thrombocytopenia

      g. In joint inflammation, bursitis

      h. With antineoplastic agents in leukemias and lymphomas

      i. In ophthalmic diseases, such as allergic conjunctivitis, chorioretinitis, iritis, iridocyclitis, and keratitis

      j. Rheumatic disease (acute inflammatory states of arthritis and systemic lupus erythematosus)

  2. Common medications (Table 6-4)

  3. Administration considerations

      a. Routes of administration for systemic use to treat inflammatory conditions include IV, IM, and PO

      b. Routes of administration for nonsystemic use include inhalation, nasal, ophthalmic, otic, and topical

  4. Contraindications: systemic fungal infections and known hypersensitivity

  5. Significant drug interactions

      a. Antibiotics, cyclosporine, estrogen and ketoconazole slow metabolism or clearance of glucocorticoids

Table 6-4 **Drugs for Adrenal Replacement Therapy (Glucocorticoids)**

Generic (Trade) Name	Route	Notes	Uses
Betamethasone (Celestone)	PO	Has little or no mineralocorticoid action	Hypercalcemia associated with cancer, inflammatory and allergic disorders, thrombocytopenia, ulcerative colitis, MS, leukemia, lymphoma, trichinosis, prevention of respiratory distress syndrome in premature neonates, relief of psoriatic plaques
Cortisone (Cortone)	PO	Has both mineralocorticoid and glucocorticoid action	Ulcerative colitis, MS, leukemia, lymphoma, thrombocytopenia, inflammatory diseases such as rheumatoid arthritis and asthma, hypercalcemia related to cancer, replacement therapy in adrenal cortical insufficiency
Hydrocortisone (Cortef)	PO	Has both mineralocorticoid and glucocorticoid action	Adrenal cortical insufficiency, allergic disorders, hypercalcemia related to cancer, inflammatory and allergic disorders, thrombocytopenia, trichinosis, ulcerative colitis, MS, leukemia, lymphoma, psoriatic plaques, anorectal cream, and suppositories to relieve inflammation related to hemorrhoids

    b. Aminoglutethimide, carbamazepine, cholestyramine, phenobarbital, phenytoin, and rifampin increase metabolism

    c. Antianxiety agents, antipsychotics, anticholinesterases, anticoagulants, antihypertensives, hypoglycemics, vaccines, pancuronium, salicylates, and sympathomimetics also affect metabolism or clearance

6. Significant food interactions: none identified

7. Significant laboratory studies

    a. CBC and differential, serum electrolytes, and blood glucose

    b. With long-term therapy monitor hypothalamic–pituitary–adrenal axis function to check adrenal function

8. Side effects: few if high doses given for only a few days

9. Adverse effects/toxicity

    a. Higher doses and prolonged therapy may alter metabolism of tissues and organs leading to muscle wasting, and increased fat deposits in the central portion of the body and face; emotional lability or changes in behavior and personality may also occur

    b. Prolonged therapy may cause growth suppression in children and osteoporosis in adults; impaired glucose tolerance and frank diabetes mellitus may also result

    c. Prolonged therapy can suppress the hypothalamic–pituitary–adrenal axis; **adrenal crisis** (an acute, life-threatening state of profound adrenocortical insufficiency) may result if drug is abruptly withdrawn, so always taper doses

    d. Toxicity may include anaphylactoid reactions, hypertriglyceridemia, peptic ulcers, acute pancreatitis, aseptic necrosis of bone, cataracts, glaucoma, hypertension, and opportunistic infections

10. Nursing considerations

    a. Check vital signs including BP, lung sounds, weight (including history of gain or loss), nausea and vomiting, and signs of dependent edema

    b. Conduct mental status exam and assess for signs of depression, withdrawal, insomnia, and anorexia

    c. Check skin for striae, thinning, bruising, change in color, change in hair growth, and acne

    d. In children on prolonged therapy, monitor height and growth pattern

    e. Advise regular ophthalmic examinations with long-term therapy

    f. Check stool for occult blood periodically

g. With prolonged therapy, move and reposition immobilized clients carefully and limit use of adhesive tape on skin because skin may become fragile and damaged more easily

11. Client education

    a. Benefits and possible side effects with long-term use; report any new side effects

    b. Take oral doses with meals and avoid use of alcohol

    c. If ordered every other day, take any missed dose as soon as remembered if on same day; if remembered the next day, then take dose and readjust schedule to be every other day; do not double up missed doses

    d. Implement weight reduction diet, limit sodium intake, and increase potassium intake if excessive weight gain occurs

    e. For clients with diabetes mellitus, carefully monitor blood glucose levels for elevation

    f. Report any blood in stool or black, tarry stools, mood changes or insomnia, vision changes or headache, weight gain of more than 5 pounds per week, irregular menses or pregnancy, irregular heart rate, excessive fatigue, severe abdominal pain, serious injury, or infection

    g. Avoid strenuous activities if skin is fragile and bruises easily

    h. With long-term therapy, take prescribed doses every day and do not discontinue medication without notifying prescriber; do not increase or decrease dose on own; tapering of dose is necessary

    i. Avoid immunizations during therapy and for 3 months after; avoid contact with anyone with measles or chicken pox or anyone receiving oral polio vaccine

    j. Avoid skin testing during therapy

    k. Wear specific medical identification during therapy

    l. With long-term therapy, report any fever, cough, sore throat, malaise, and unhealed injuries; avoid contact with anyone who has an active infection

    m. Review drug and teach specific administration and that client should not share drug with others

C. Adrenocorticotropic hormone (ACTH)

1. Action and use

    a. Directly stimulates adrenal cortex to synthesize adrenal steroids

    b. Used to diagnose adrenal disorders such as Addison disease and secondary adrenal insufficiency caused by pituitary dysfunction

    c. Used in treatment of adrenocorticoid-responsive diseases, such as MS

    d. Limited use in treatment of adrenal insufficiency

2. Common medications (Table 6-5)

3. Administration considerations

    a. Agents may be given IV, IM, subQ, or PO

    b. Administer drug according to manufacturer's instructions

    c. Incompatible if mixed with aminophylline or sodium bicarbonate

4. Contraindications

    a. Ocular herpes simplex; recent surgery

    b. Disorders such as CHF, scleroderma, osteoporosis, systemic fungoid infections, hypertension

    c. Sensitivity to porcine proteins

    d. Conditions related to adrenocortical insufficiency or hyperfunction

5. Significant drug interactions: aspirin, nonsteroidal anti-inflammatory drugs (NSAIDs), barbiturates, phenytoin, rifampin, estrogens, amphotericin B, and diuretics

Practice to Pass

A client taking glucocorticoid therapy asks the nurse about wearing some sort of MedicAlert identification. How should the nurse respond?

Table 6-5	Drugs Used in Diagnosing Adrenal Gland Disorders	
Generic (Trade) Name	**Route**	**Uses**
Corticotropin (Acthar)	IV, subQ	Evaluates adrenal function, nonsuppurative thyroiditis, hypercalcemia related to cancer, MS, trichinosis, tuberculosis meningitis, leukemia, lymphoma, infantile spasms, or rheumatic, collagen, or allergic reaction
Cosyntropin (Cortrosyn)	IV, IM, subQ	Assists in diagnosing adrenocortical insufficiency, bronchial asthma, bronchospasm, allergic rhinitis, allergic disorders of the eye, mastocytosis (orphan drug use), prevention of GI and systemic food allergies
Metyrapone (Metopirone)	PO	Evaluates hypothalamic and pituitary function; blocks cortisol synthesis in adrenals (may cause acute adrenal insufficiency)

6. Significant food interactions: none
7. Significant laboratory studies: baseline electrolyte levels, and baseline plasma cortisol level
8. Side effects: nausea and vomiting, dizziness, drowsiness, or light-headedness
9. Adverse effects/toxicity
   a. Hypersensitivity including urticaria, pruritus, dizziness, vomiting, and anaphylactic shock
   b. Cataracts or glaucoma; peptic ulcer with perforation; hirsutism and amenorrhea
   c. Sodium and water retention, potassium and calcium loss, and hyperglycemia
   d. Acne, impaired wound healing, fragile skin, petechiae, ecchymosis
   e. **Osteoporosis** (abnormal loss of bone density), decreased muscle mass, **cushingoid state** (having the appearance and facies characteristic of Cushing disease), activation of latent tuberculosis or diabetes mellitus, vertebral compression fractures
10. Nursing considerations
    a. Individualized dosage and gradual dosage changes should be made only after apparent full effect from drug is seen
    b. Shake liquid drug well before injecting into deep gluteal muscle; after administration observe closely for 15 minutes for any hypersensitivity reactions; prolonged treatment may increase risk of hypersensitivity reactions
    c. Monitor vital signs and BP and assess for dizziness, fever, flushing, rash, and urticaria
    d. Monitor plasma or urinary cortisol levels and serum electrolytes
    e. Be aware that agents may suppress signs and symptoms of chronic disease; new infections may appear during treatment
    f. At high dosage levels, drug must be gradually tapered
    g. Carefully monitor growth and development in children
    h. Clients with diabetes mellitus may require increased doses of oral antidiabetic agents or insulin during corticosteroid therapy
11. Client education
    a. Do not discontinue drug before notifying prescriber
    b. Low-salt or potassium-rich diet if ordered
    c. Take oral doses with food, milk, or meals
    d. If dizziness, drowsiness or light-headedness occurs, avoid driving or operating hazardous equipment
    e. Avoid exposure to communicable diseases or people with infections

III. MEDICATIONS AFFECTING THE THYROID GLANDS

A. Thyroid hormones

1. Action and use

   a. As replacement hormone therapy for **hypothyroidism** (decreased activity of thyroid gland with a variety of specific causes); have same action as thyroid hormones produced in body to increase metabolic rate

   b. Used to diagnose and treat thyroid deficiency and **myxedema** (most severe form of hypothyroidism characterized by swelling of face, feet, and periorbital tissues; may lead to coma and death), and to control goiter or thyroid carcinoma

2. Common medications (Table 6-6)

3. Administration considerations

   a. May be given IV, IM, subQ, or PO

   b. Administer drug according to manufacturer's instructions

4. Contraindications

   a. Thyrotoxicosis, acute MI and cardiovascular disease, morphologic hypogonadism, nephrosis, and uncorrected hypoadrenalism

   b. Cautious use with angina pectoris; hypertension; older adults with cardiac disease; renal insufficiency; pregnancy; concurrent use of **catecholamines** (drugs that mimic effects of sympathetic nervous system); diabetes mellitus; **hyperthyroidism** (hyperactivity of thyroid gland), and malabsorption states

5. Significant drug interactions: thyroid hormones given with oral anticoagulants, insulin and sulfonylureas, epinephrine, and cholestyramine

6. Significant food interactions: none noted

7. Significant laboratory studies: serum T_4, free thyroxine, T_3 uptake, serum T_3, serum thyroid stimulating hormone (TSH), protirelin test, thyroid uptake of radioiodine, TSH test, and thyroid suppression test

8. Side effects: weight loss, vomiting, and tachycardia

9. Adverse effects/toxicity

   a. Angina pectoris, coronary occlusion, or stroke in elderly or predisposed clients

   b. Relative adrenal insufficiency in clients with inadequate pituitary function related to secondary hypothyroidism and secondary adrenal insufficiency; adrenal crisis

   c. Overdosage causing signs of hyperthyroidism related to thyroid storm with shock and coma; thyrotoxicosis with CHF, angina, cardiac dysrhythmias, and shock

   d. Reactions to thioamides include fever, itching, and skin rash; blood dyscrasias and peripheral neuropathy; pain and swelling of joints or lupus-like syndrome; dizziness; or alterations in taste

   e. Overdosage of thioamides causes hypothyroidism

Practice to Pass

A client taking thyroid hormone is also receiving sodium warfarin (Coumadin). What laboratory test should the nurse monitor?

Table 6-6	Drugs for Diagnosing Thyroid Disorders or Replacement Therapy	
Generic (Trade) Name	**Route**	**Uses**
Levothyroxine (Synthroid, others)	PO, IV	Chemically pure form of T_4 and preferred therapy for hypothyroidism. Given IV for myxedema coma.
Liothyronine (Cytomel)	PO, IV	Chemically pure form of T_3; for adult hypothyroidism; not used for cretinism since T_3 does not cross blood–brain barrier as well as T_4 does.
Liotrix (Thyrolar, Euthroid)	PO	Chemically pure T_4 and T_3 in 4:1 ratio; used for hypothyroidism.
Thyrotropin (Thyrogen)	IM, subQ	Natural TSH extracted from animals. Used to differentiate primary hypothyroidism from secondary.

10. Nursing considerations
    a. Assess vital signs, BP, weight and history of weight change, normal diet, energy level, mood, subjective feeling, and response to temperature
    b. In children, check height
    c. Monitor thyroid function test results and blood glucose levels
    d. TSH may be frequently checked, high TSH indicates hormone replacement level is low; low TSH may indicate hormone replacement is too high
    e. Start older adults on lower doses of thyroid hormones and increase dose by small increments; assess for symptoms of stress that could lead to angina or stroke
11. Client education
    a. How to monitor pulse, weight, and height
    b. Adhere to hormone replacement dosage schedule and intervals; realize that therapy is life-long; do not change brand of thyroid medication without discussing with prescriber because of differences in bioavailability
    c. Immediately report any chest pain or other signs of aggravated cardiovascular disease
    d. With juvenile hypothyroidism therapy, dramatic weight loss and catch-up growth may occur
    e. Do not discontinue drug and do carry medical alert identification
    f. With radioactive iodine, most clients become hypothyroid and require replacement therapy with thyroid hormones; urge periodic thyroid evaluation
    g. Explain side effects and related treatment if changes in insulin or anticoagulants are needed

B. Antithyroid medications
1. Action and use: treatment of hyperthyroidism and **Graves' disease** (pronounced hyperthyroidism often associated with enlarged thyroid gland and exophthalmos; also called thyrotoxicosis)
2. Common medications (Table 6-7)
3. Administration considerations
    a. Is given orally
    b. Administer drug according to manufacturer's instructions
4. Contraindications
    a. Previous allergic or other severe reactions to thioamides
    b. Impaired hepatic function may require reduced doses

Table 6-7 Drugs Used to Treat Hyperthyroidism and Graves' Disease

Generic (Trade) Name	Route	Notes
Thioamides		
Methimazole (Tapazole)	PO	Inhibits thyroid hormone synthesis but not release.
Propylthiouracil (PTU)	PO	Inhibits thyroid hormone synthesis but not release; in peripheral tissues inhibits conversion of T_4 to T_3
Iodine		
Potassium Iodide and Iodine (Lugol's solution, Thyro-Block)	PO	Has direct action on thyroid and used for short-term inhibition of thyroid hormone synthesis.
131I as NaI (Iodotope)	PO	Radionuclide concentrated in thyroid. Releases radiation and destroys tissue.
Beta-Adrenergic Blockers		
Propranolol (Inderal)	PO	Does not lower T_4 and T_3 release from thyroid. Decreases pulse and BP related to hyperthyroidism.

5. Significant drug interactions
    a. Thioamides given with any iodine preparations including amiodarone, iodine solution, potassium iodide, and some contrast imaging dyes or radioactive iodine uptake
    b. Coumarin and other anticoagulants; digitalis
6. Significant food interactions: none noted
7. Significant laboratory studies: serum T_4, serum T_3, free T_4, free T_3, T_3 resin uptake, serum thyroid uptake of radioiodine, and thyroid suppression test; TSH diagnoses primary versus secondary hypothyroidism
8. Side effects: fever, itching, and skin rash
9. Adverse effects/toxicity
    a. Blood dyscrasias and peripheral neuropathy
    b. Pain and swelling of joints or lupus-like syndrome
    c. Dizziness and alteration in taste
    d. Overdosage results in hypothyroidism
    e. Rare instances of agranulocytosis
10. Nursing considerations
    a. Assess for tingling of fingers and toes
    b. Monitor weight and check for hair loss and skin changes
    c. Check CBC, differential count and thyroid and liver function tests
     d. Dilute oral iodine solutions well in milk, juice, or other beverage
    e. Assess for metallic taste in mouth, sneezing, edematous thyroid, vomiting, and bloody diarrhea
11. Client education
    a. Explain need to wear medical identification tag or bracelet
    b. Explain goals and side effects of medications (side effects may not appear for days or weeks after treatment begun)
     c. Advise to report any fever, chills, sore throat, and unusual bleeding or bruising
     d. Instruct to take med at same time of day and with meals or snack; space additional daily doses throughout the day

IV. MEDICATIONS AFFECTING THE PARATHYROID GLANDS

A. Medications to treat hypocalcemia

1. Action and use
    a. Consist of calcium supplements
    b. Replaces calcium to supply body's metabolic needs
    c. Helps prevent calcium loss from bones and maintain bone strength
    d. Used to treat mild hypocalcemia and supplementation of dietary calcium
    e. Has additional use as an antacid
2. Common medications (Table 6-8)

Table 6-8 Drugs Used to Treat Mild Calcium Deficiency

Generic (Trade) Name	Route	Calcium Content
Calcium acetate (Phos-Ex, PhosLo)	PO	25%
Calcium carbonate (various names)	PO	40%
Calcium citrate (Citracal)	PO	21%
Calcium glubionate (Neo-Calglucon)	PO	6.6%
Calcium phosphate tribasic (Posture)	PO	39%

3. Administration considerations
   a. Oral route
   b. Dosage differs among the different oral calcium salts
   c. Must be taken with large glass of water with or after meals
   d. When used as antacid, should be taken 1 hour after meals and at bedtime
4. Contraindications: hypercalcemia, renal calculi, and hypophosphatemia
5. Significant drug interactions
   a. Glucocorticoids reduce calcium absorption
   b. Absorption of tetracyclines and quinolones is reduced if given with calcium
   c. Thiazide diuretics decrease renal excretion of calcium
   d. May enhance inotropic and toxic effects of digoxin
6. Significant food interactions: spinach, Swiss chard, beets, and bran and whole-grain cereals can reduce calcium absorption
7. Significant laboratory studies: serum calcium level
8. Side effects: constipation and flatulence
9. Adverse effects/toxicity
   a. Hypercalcemia may occur if frequent or high doses
   b. May also occur in clients being treated with calcium as part of renal dysfunction therapy
10. Nursing considerations
   a. Take 1 to 1½ hours after meals
   b. Space additional daily doses throughout the day
   c. Note number and consistency of stools; if constipation a problem, then a laxative or stool softener may be ordered
   d. With prolonged therapy, monitor weekly serum and urine calcium levels
   e. Observe for signs of hypercalcemia if receiving frequent or high doses
   f. Monitor for acid rebound if used as an antacid on repeated basis for more than 1 to 2 weeks
11. Client education
   a. Signs of hypercalcemia; report any nausea, vomiting, constipation, frequent urination, lethargy, or depression
   b. Do not take with cereals or other foods high in oxalates that form insoluble, nonabsorbable compounds with calcium
   c. Potential dangers of repeated use as an antacid for more than 2 weeks

B. Vitamin D
1. Action and use
   a. Vitamin D is needed for proper absorption of calcium, is a fat-soluble vitamin that can accumulate in the body
   b. Used to control hypocalcemia or vitamin D deficiency
   c. Used to treat rickets, **osteomalacia** (abnormal loss of calcification of the matrix in lamellar bone, leading to bone softening and fracture), and **hypoparathyroidism** (insufficient secretion of parathyroid glands caused by primary parathyroid dysfunction or elevated serum calcium level)
2. Common medications (Table 6-9)
3. Administration considerations
   a. Given orally (all) or IV (calcitriol)
   b. Adequate calcium is needed for optimal response to treatment
4. Contraindications: clients with hypercalcemia or vitamin D toxicity and malabsorption syndrome
5. Significant drug interactions
   a. Antacids or other preparations containing magnesium may cause high serum magnesium levels
   b. Digitalis glycosides

Practice to Pass

A client taking long-term calcium supplements also takes digoxin. What type of drug interaction should the client be prepared to monitor for?

Table 6-9	Drugs Used to Treat Vitamin D Deficiency	
Generic (Trade) Name	**Route**	**Uses**
Calcitriol (Rocaltrol)	PO, IV	Hypoparathyroidism or chronic renal failure
Doxercalciferol (Hectoral)	PO	Hypoparathyroidism or chronic renal failure
Ergocalciferol (Calciferol, Drisdol)	PO	Hypoparathyroidism and to treat and prevent vitamin D deficiency

6. Significant food interactions: none noted
7. Significant laboratory studies
   a. Serum calcium and phosphorus levels
   b. BUN, serum creatinine levels, serum alkaline phosphatase
   c. Urinary calcium and urinalysis
8. Side effects: hypercalcemia related to overdosage; signs include ataxia, fatigue, irritability, seizures, somnolence, tinnitus, hypertension, GI tract distress or constipation, and hypotonia in infants
9. Adverse effects/toxicity
   a. Vitamin D hypercalcemia may lead to dysrhythmias in clients taking digoxin
   b. Hypervitaminosis D caused by large therapeutic doses may lead to hypercalcemia, hypercalciuria, bone decalcification, and calcium deposits in soft tissues
10. Nursing considerations
    a. Assess for any CNS problems
    b. Monitor BP, pulse, and I & O
    c. Monitor BUN, serum creatinine levels, serum calcium and phosphorus levels, serum alkaline phosphatase and urinalysis
    d. If vitamin D toxicity occurs, make sure client stops drug immediately, forces fluid, and eats a low-calcium diet
11. Client education
    a. Make sure oral dose is swallowed intact without crushing or chewing tablet
    b. Do not increase or decrease dosage before notifying prescriber
    c. Check with prescriber before taking any OTC meds containing calcium, phosphorus, or vitamin D, and any excessive amounts of any substances containing vitamin D
    d. Do not drive or use heavy equipment if client develops fatigue, somnolence, vertigo, or weakness
    e. Avoid magnesium-containing antacids

C. **Medications to treat hypercalcemia**
   1. Action and use
      a. Promote urinary excretion of calcium
      b. Decrease mobilization of calcium from bone
      c. Decrease intestinal absorption of calcium
      d. Form complexes with free calcium in blood
      e. Achieve rapid lowering of blood calcium levels
      f. Used in emergency treatment of hypercalcemia, and to control hypercalcemia resulting from malignancies of the bone
   2. Common medications (Table 6-10)
   3. Administration considerations
      a. May be given subQ, IM, IV or PO
      b. Give IM doses at bedtime to minimize effects of flushing following injection
      c. In emergency situations, dilute IV dose before administration to prevent extravasation; infuse over prescribed period of time
   4. Contraindications: known hypersensitivity or with impaired renal function

Table 6-10	Drugs Used to Treat Hypercalcemia	
Generic (Trade) Name	**Route**	**Uses**
Edetate disodium (Disotate, Endrate)	IV	Strong chelating agent; used on short-term basis to remove excess calcium.
Gallium nitrate (Ganite)	IV	Used for hypercalcemia caused by cancer.
Pamidronate (Aredia)	IV	Acts directly on bone by slowing bone reabsorption and lowering release of calcium; also used for Paget disease.

5. Significant drug interactions
   a. Antacids, mineral supplements, calcium salts, and vitamin D
   b. Decreased effects of digitalis when serum calcium is reduced
   c. Nephrotoxic medications
6. Significant food interactions: calcium-rich dairy products
7. Significant laboratory studies
   a. CBC with differential count
   b. Serum electrolytes, alkaline phosphatase, and creatinine
   c. Liver function tests
   d. Urinalysis
8. Side effects
   a. Nausea, vomiting, diarrhea, and dyspepsia with oral route
   b. Facial flushing and occasional inflammatory reaction at injection site
   c. Transient influenza-like symptoms with IV route
   d. Nasal dryness and irritation with intranasal spray
9. Adverse effects/toxicity
   a. Allergic reactions with calcitonin salmon
   b. IV administration may cause venous irritation, thrombophlebitis, and nephrotoxicity
   c. Varying effects of hypocalcemia
   d. Toxicity with higher doses causes more severe GI distress, such as esophagitis, severe nephrotoxicity, and severe hypocalcemia

Practice to Pass

A client with osteoporosis is complaining of severe bone pain. What assessment criteria should the nurse employ?

10. Nursing considerations
    a. Assess for hypercalcemia and hypocalcemia
    b. Monitor weight and I & O if vomiting and diarrhea occur
    c. Monitor serum electrolytes, serum alkaline phosphatase, serum creatinine, BUN, and liver function tests
    d. Monitor vital signs and assess for dysrhythmias with IV infusion
    e. Provide emotional support as needed
11. Client education
    a. How to self-administer subQ injection (use return demonstration)
    b. Do not discontinue therapy without notifying prescriber
    c. Taking doses in evening may lessen flushing
    d. Take oral doses on empty stomach
    e. Wear medical alert identification if on long-term therapy
    f. Low-calcium and low-vitamin D diet (decrease in dairy products, for example)
    g. Drink sufficient fluids (at least 6–8 glasses of water per day and possibly more if not contraindicated by other health problems)

D. **Medications to treat osteoporosis and Paget disease**
   1. Action and use
      a. Reduce calcium release from bone
      b. Slow bone resorption and remodeling

    c. Prevent high serum calcium concentrations

    d. Used long-term for **Paget disease** (a non-metabolic disease of bone) and post-menopausal osteoporosis (abnormal loss of bone density)

    e. Also used to treat heterotropic ossification after spinal cord injury and hip replacement

2. Common medications (Table 6-11)

3. Administration considerations

    a. Is given subQ, IM, PO, IV, and intranasal

    b. Nasal spray is given once daily in alternate nostrils

4. Contraindications: do not give to clients with known hypersensitivity to salmon calcitonin or fish products, esophageal disorders, or during lactation; use cautiously with renal insufficiency, osteoporosis, and pernicious anemia

5. Significant drug interactions: antacids, mineral supplements, calcium salts, and vitamin D

6. Significant food interactions: calcium-rich dairy products

7. Significant laboratory studies

    a. Serum electrolytes, serum alkaline phosphatase, calcium and phosphorus and 24-hour urinary hydroxyproline prior to therapy, during first 3 months, and then every 3 to 6 months

    b. Baseline values of bone mineral density (BMD) in hip, vertebrae, and forearm

8. Side effects

    a. Nausea, vomiting, diarrhea, and dyspepsia with oral route

    b. Facial flushing and occasional inflammatory reaction at injection site

    c. Transient influenza-like symptoms with IV route

    d. Muscle spasms, leukopenia with chills, fever, or sore throat

    e. Nasal dryness and irritation with intranasal spray

9. Adverse effects/toxicity

    a. Allergic reactions with calcitonin salmon

    b. IV administration may cause venous irritation, thrombophlebitis and nephrotoxicity

    c. Varying effects of hypocalcemia

    d. Toxicity with higher doses causes more severe hypocalcemia, GI distress such as severe esophagitis with ulceration, and severe nephrotoxicity

Table 6-11   **Drugs Used to Treat Osteoporosis and Other Bone Disorders**

Generic (Trade) Name	Route
Bisphosphonates	
Alendroate (Fosamax)	PO
Etidronate (Didronel)	PO
Ibandronate (Boniva)	PO, IV
Pamidronate (Aredia)	IV
Risedronate (Actonel)	PO
Tiludronate (Skelid)	PO
Zolendronate (Reclast, Zometa)	IV
Miscellaneous Agents	
Calcitonin salmon (Calcimar, Miacalcin)	IM, SubQ
Cinacalcet (Sensipar)	PO
Raloxifene (Evista)	PO
Teriparatide (Forteo)	subQ

    10. Nursing considerations

        a. Assess for hypercalcemia and hypocalcemia

        b. Monitor weight and I & O if vomiting and diarrhea occur

        c. Monitor serum electrolytes, serum alkaline phosphatase, calcium and phosphorus and 24-hour urinary hydroxyproline

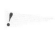
        d. Monitor BMD values; in some clients therapy may be discontinued when symptoms are relieved

        e. Monitor bone pain in clients with Paget disease

        f. Ensure parenteral calcium is available to treat hypocalcemic tetany if it occurs

    11. Client education

        a. How to self-administer subcutaneous injection (obtain return demonstration) and rotate sites

        b. Do not discontinue therapy without notifying prescriber

        c. Taking doses in evening may lessen flushing

        d. Take PO doses on empty stomach and remain upright for 30 minutes after taking

        e. Recognize signs of esophagitis and discontinue drug and notify prescriber if difficulty swallowing or worsening heartburn occur

        f. Wear MedicAlert identification if on long-term therapy

        g. How to follow low-calcium and low-vitamin D diet

        h. Sufficient fluid intake is important

        i. How to activate and administer metered dose pump for nasal spray use

V. MEDICATIONS USED TO TREAT DIABETES MELLITUS

A. Insulin

    1. Action and use

        a. Restores ability of cells to use glucose as an energy source

        b. Corrects **hyperglycemia** (greater than normal amount of glucose circulating in blood)

        c. Corrects many associated metabolic derangements

        d. Is used to treat both type 1 and type 2 diabetes mellitus and diabetic ketoacidosis

        e. Also lowers plasma potassium levels and is used as emergency treatment of hyperkalemia

    2. Types of insulin (Table 6-12)

    3. Administration considerations

        a. Is given only by injection; is inactivated by digestive system enzymes if given orally

        b. May be given subQ, IM, or IV; only *regular insulin* may be given IV

        c. All insulins (except lispro and regular) are mixed in suspension so particles must be dispersed before insulin is drawn up into syringe

        d. Injection sites include: upper arms, thighs, and abdomen, and back in scapular area

        e. One general location is used at one time to maintain consistent absorption rates although sites within each general location are used only once each month; American Diabetes Association (ADA) currently recommends rotating on abdominal sites

        f. Only mix insulins that are compatible with one another and use according to manufacturer's guidelines

        g. Store unopened vials in refrigerator; opened vials can remain at room temperature for up to 1 month; label vial with date and time opened and/or due to expire according to agency policy

Table 6-12 Types of Insulin Preparations

Insulin Type	Trade Name	Action	Notes
Lispro	Humalog	**Onset:** 5–15 min **Peak:** 1–1.5 hr **Duration:** 3–4 hr	Rapid-acting
Aspart	Novalog	**Onset:** 10–20 min **Peak:** 1–3 hr **Duration:** 3–5 hr	Rapid-acting
Glulisine	Apidra	**Onset:** 15–30 min **Peak:** 1 hr **Duration:** 3–4 hr	Rapid-acting
Regular	Humulin R Novolin R	**Onset:** 0.5–1 hr **Peak:** 1–5 hr **Duration:** 6–10 hr	Short-acting
NPH (Isophane) Insulin	NPH, Humulin N	**Onset:** 1–2 hr **Peak:** 6–14 hr **Duration:** 16–24 hr	Intermediate-acting
Insulin detemir	(Levemir)	**Onset:** 3–8 hr **Peak:** none **Duration:** 24 hr	Long acting
Insulin glargine	Lantus	**Onset:** 2–4 hr **Peak:** none **Duration:** 24 hr	Long-acting.
NPH/Regular Mixture (70–30%)	Humulin 70/30 Novolin 70/30	**Onset:** 0.5–1 hr **Peak:** 5–10 hr **Duration:** 6–8 hr	Combination Isophane Insulin Suspension and Regular Insulin

    h. Alternate methods of delivery include: jet injectors, pen injectors, portable insulin pumps, implantable pumps, and insulin by inhalation; an intranasal form is undergoing study

    i. Dosage must be monitored and linked with insulin needs

    j. Dosing schedules include the following:

        1) Conventional therapy: short-acting and intermediate-acting insulin is given twice a day on a fixed regimen

        2) Intensified therapy: long-acting insulin taken in the evening and a fast-acting insulin given before meals according to blood glucose levels

        3) Continuous subQ insulin infusion: a portable infusion pump is connected to a catheter and infuses regular insulin at a steady rate

        4) A variety of schedules are evolving including use of rapid-acting insulin and multiple dosing schedules to maintain euglycemia

  4. Contraindications: previous allergic response to local or systemic use of drug

  5. Significant drug interactions

    a. Hypoglycemic agents that lower blood glucose levels, such as sulfonylureas; acute use of alcohol; and beta-adrenergic blocking agents

    b. Hyperglycemic agents that increase blood glucose levels, such as thiazide diuretic agents, glucocorticoids, and sympathomimetics

    c. Beta-adrenergic blocking agents that delay response of insulin-related hypoglycemia and mask signs of sympathetic nervous system stimulation (tachycardia and palpitations)

6. Significant food interactions: moderate to high alcohol consumption without food enhances hypoglycemic action
7. Significant laboratory studies: random blood glucose (BG), fasting BG, glucose tolerance test, **glycosylated hemoglobin** A1c, (a blood test representative of the average BG level over the past several weeks), urinary glucose and ketones, and serum electrolytes
8. Side effects
   a. Hypoglycemic reactions when blood glucose levels drop below 50 mg/dL
   b. Signs of hypoglycemic reaction include anxiety, confusion, nervousness, hunger, diaphoresis, and cool, clammy skin
9. Adverse effects/toxicity
   a. Somogyi phenomenon: a rapid decrease in blood glucose level at night
   b. Coma related to inadequate dosage caused by uncontrolled diabetic derangements with high blood glucose levels and ketoacidosis
   c. Hyperosmolar coma (nonketotic hyperglycemia)
   d. Coma related to insulin overdosage caused by inadequate food intake, excessive exercise, or excessive insulin administration; may be life-threatening if prolonged

10. Complications
    a. Presence of insulin antibodies that can lead to insulin resistance
    b. **Lipodystrophy** (abnormal deposition of subcutaneous fat at injection sites)
    c. Local allergic reaction related to a contaminant in the insulin preparation
    d. Systemic allergic reaction related to insulin itself and not to any contaminant
11. Nursing considerations
    a. Assess vital signs, weight, condition of skin and nails, serum and urine glucose levels, glycosylated hemoglobin (and electrolyte and arterial blood gas levels) when appropriate
    b. Assess for long-term complications related to acceleration of atherosclerosis (hypertension, heart disease, stroke); retinopathy leading to possible blindness, nephropathy leading to possible renal failure; neuropathy leading to lower limb ulcerations and amputation, impotence, and gastroparesis
    c. Consult with prescriber regarding insulin management when there is insufficient food intake or when client is NPO for surgery
    d. Adhere to agency policy regarding insulin administration
12. Client education
    a. Individualized teaching plan regarding insulin management
    b. All aspects of insulin administration including syringe use, mixing of insulins, stability of mixture, injection technique and sites
    c. Do not switch type or source of insulin or brand of syringe and avoid taking any new drug before notifying prescriber
    d. Signs and symptoms of hyperglycemia and hypoglycemia (client and family)
    e. How to test blood glucose levels
    f. Dietary restrictions and weight control; refer to dietitian for individualized instruction and meal planning
    g. Regular exercise helps achieve euglycemia
    h. Foot care and related aspects of personal hygiene
    i. Sick-day management of diabetes and insulin administration (continue to eat and take liquids as able, check blood glucose, maintain insulin schedule, and call prescriber if blood glucose is >250 mg/dL)
    j. Obtain and wear a MedicAlert tag or bracelet
    k. Avoid smoking or drinking alcoholic beverages
    l. Female clients should consult with health care provider before conceiving
    m. Refer to local home care agency and to ADA for additional follow-up and access to community-based resources

B. Oral antidiabetic (hypoglycemic) agents—sulfonylureas

1. Action and use
   a. Stimulate release of insulin from pancreatic islets and increase sensitivity of insulin receptors on cells
   b. Are used as an adjunct to nondrug therapy to reduce BG levels in type 2 diabetes mellitus
2. Common medications (Table 6-13); note tolbutamide (Orinase) has shortest duration of action and is quickly converted to inactive metabolites
3. Administration considerations
   a. Dose is given orally 1 to 3 times a day
   b. Different agents possess different durations of action
   c. May be used alone or in combination with insulin
4. Contraindications
   a. During pregnancy related to teratogenicity in animals
   b. In women who are nursing or lactating
   c. In clients with allergy to sulfa or urea
5. Significant drug interactions
   a. Nonsteroidal anti-inflammatory drugs (NSAIDS), sulfonamide antibiotics, acute use of ethanol, salicylates, phenothiazines, thiazides, ranitidine, and cimetidine
   b. Beta-adrenergic blocking agents can suppress insulin release and delay response to hypoglycemia
6. Significant food interactions: none noted
7. Significant laboratory studies
   a. CBC with differential, platelet count
   b. Liver function tests
   c. Blood glucose
8. Side effects: GI distress and neurologic symptoms such as dizziness, drowsiness, or headache
9. Adverse effects/toxicity
   a. Alcohol may cause a disulfiram-like reaction causing flushing, palpitations, and nausea
   b. Allergy related to skin reaction
   c. Hypoglycemia related to drug overdosage, drug interactions, altered drug metabolism, or inadequate food intake
   d. Hypoglycemic reactions are most likely to occur in presence of renal or hepatic dysfunction

Practice to Pass

A client with type 2 diabetes mellitus has been sick at home for several days with a fever and flulike symptoms. What instructions should the nurse give to the client regarding sick-day diabetes management?

Table 6-13 Oral Antidiabetics/Hypoglycemics (Sulfonylureas)

Generic (Trade) Name	Duration of Action
First generation	
Tolbutamide (Orinase)	6–12 hr
Tolazamide (Tolinase)	12–24 hr
Chlorpropamide (Diabinese)	24–72 hr
Second generation	
Glipizide Standard (Glucotrol)	12–24 hr
Glipizide Sustained release (Glucotrol XL)	24 hr
Glyburide Nonmicronized (Diabeta, Micronase)	12–24 hr
Glyburide Micronized (Glynase, Pres Tab)	24 hr
Glimepiride (Amaryl)	24 hr

10. Nursing considerations
    a. Assess vital signs, weight, condition of skin and nails, serum and urine glucose levels, glycosylated hemoglobin and electrolyte and arterial blood gas levels when appropriate
    b. Assess for long-term complications of diabetes as noted in previous section regarding nursing considerations with insulin
    c. Consult with prescriber regarding management when client has insufficient food intake or is NPO for surgery
    d. Discuss psychosocial factors and lifestyle as they relate to adherence with therapy
11. Client education
    a. Individualized teaching plan based on client's previous knowledge, educational level, motivation to learn, and cultural considerations
    b. All aspects of drug therapy; take with food if GI upset occurs
    c. Take medication even if not feeling well
    d. Take dose with first daily meal and take any missed dose as soon as remembered unless time for next dose; do not double doses
    e. Signs and symptoms of hypoglycemia (client and family) and notify prescriber if they occur
    f. How to test blood glucose levels
    g. Dietary restrictions and weight control; refer to dietitian (very helpful for developing effective meal and weight management plans)
    h. Regular aerobic exercise in amount suited to client's health and abilities will help control BG levels
    i. Foot care and related aspects of personal hygiene
    j. Sick-day management of diabetes and prn insulin administration
    k. Obtain and wear MedicAlert tag or bracelet
    l. Avoid smoking or drinking alcoholic beverages
    m. Female clients should consult with prescriber before conceiving and discontinue drug during pregnancy and lactation
    n. Refer to local home care agency and to ADA for additional follow-up and access to community-based resources

C. Oral antidiabetics (hypoglycemic) agents—nonsulfonylureas

1. Action and use
    a. Biguanides lower blood glucose by decreasing production of glucose by the liver
    b. Alpha-glucosidase inhibitors delay absorption of dietary carbohydrates and reduce blood glucose
    c. Both are used to decrease blood glucose levels after meals in clients with type 2 DM not controlled by diet modification and exercise
2. Common medications (Table 6-14)
3. Administration considerations
    a. Orally 1 to 3 times a day
    b. Biguanides are used alone or in combination with a sulfonylurea
    c. Alpha-glucose inhibitors are used alone or in combination with insulin or a sulfonylurea
    d. Metformin increases peripheral utilization of glucose and decreases hepatic glucose
    e. Repaglinide and nateglinide close potassium channels and open calcium channels in beta cells to increase insulin release
    f. Acarbose delays digestion of ingested carbohydrates leading to decreased BG postprandial (after meals); is an additive to sulfonylureas in BG control
    g. Pioglitazone stimulates insulin receptor sites to lower BG and increase insulin action; also decreases gluconeogenesis
    h. Rosiglitazone resensitizes tissues to insulin and decreases hepatic gluconeogenesis

Table 6-14 Oral Antidiabetics/Hypoglycemics (Nonsulfonylureas)

Generic (Trade) Name	Route	Classification
Nateglinide (Starlix)	PO	Meglitinide
Repaglinide (Prandin)	PO	Meglitinide
Acarbose (Precose)	PO	Alpha-glucosidase inhibitor
Migitol (Glyset)	PO	Alpha-glucosidase inhibitor
Pioglitazone (Actos)	PO	Thiazolidinedione
Rosiglitazone (Avandia)	PO	Thiazolidinedione
Metformin (Glucophage)	PO	Biguanide
Exenatide (Byetta)	SC	Incretin Enhancer (GLP-1 Agonist)
Liraglutide (Victoza)	SC	Incretin Enhancer (GLP-1 Agonist)
Linagliptin (Tradjenta)	PO	Incretin Enhancer (DPP-4 Agonist)
Saxagliptin (Onglyza)	PO	Incretin Enhancer (DPP-4 Agonist)
Sitagliptin (Januvia)	PO	Incretin Enhancer (DPP-4 Agonist)

4. Contraindications: renal insufficiency and kidney disease
5. Significant drug interactions
   a. Both forms should not be taken together because of the incidence of significant GI distress
   b. Amiloride, cimetidine, digoxin, morphine, procainamide, quinidine, quinine, ranitidine, triamterene, trimethoprim, and vancomycin may decrease renal secretion of antidiabetic agent
6. Significant food interactions: alcohol may increase risk of hypoglycemia or lactic acidosis
7. Significant laboratory studies
   a. CBC with differential, platelet count
   b. Liver function tests
   c. Blood glucose
8. Side effects
   a. Biguanides may cause decreased appetite, nausea, and diarrhea that usually subside over time; also increased absorption of vitamin B_{12} and folic acid may occur
   b. Alpha-glucosidase inhibitors cause flatulence, cramps, abdominal distention, borborygmus ("stomach growling"), and diarrhea; also may decrease absorption of iron, leading to anemia
   c. Thiazolidinediones may lead to anemia and edema
9. Adverse effects/toxicity
   a. Biguanides with hypoglycemia and lactic acidosis result in a mortality rate of 50%
   b. Alpha-glucosidase inhibitors may lead to hypoglycemia if given with insulin or a sulfonylurea
   c. Thiazolidinediones (rosiglitazone) may cause CHF or angioedema
10. Nursing considerations
    a. Assess vital signs, weight, condition of skin and nails, serum and urine glucose levels, glycosylated hemoglobin, and electrolyte and arterial blood gas levels when appropriate
    b. Assess renal function and evidence of renal insufficiency
    c. Assess for early sign of lactic acidosis
    d. Assess for long-term complications of diabetes mellitus
    e. Consult with prescriber regarding management when client has insufficient food intake or is NPO for surgery

11. Client education
    a. All aspects of diabetic management as outlined in previous client education section for sulfonylureas
    b. Early signs of hypoglycemia and lactic acidosis (hyperventilation, myalgia, malaise, unusual somnolence) and notify prescriber immediately if occur

D. Glucose-elevating medications—glucagon

1. Action and use
    a. Promotes breakdown of glycogen, reduces glycogen synthesis, and stimulates synthesis of glucose
    b. Emergency treatment of severe **hypoglycemia** (lower than normal circulating glucose level) in unconscious clients or those unable to swallow and in clients receiving insulin shock therapy
2. Common medication: glucagon (GlucaGen)
3. Administration considerations
    a. Reconstitute according to manufacturer's directions
    b. Given subQ, IM, or direct IVP; flush IV line with 5% dextrose instead of NaCl solution
    c. Incompatible in syringe with any other medication
4. Contraindications
    a. Hypersensitivity to glucagon or protein compounds
    b. Cautious use in insulinoma and pheochromocytoma
5. Significant drug interactions: incompatible with sodium chloride solutions or additives
6. Significant food interactions: none noted
7. Significant laboratory studies: blood glucose levels
8. Side effects: nausea and vomiting
9. Adverse effects/toxicity: hypersensitivity reactions, hyperglycemia and hypokalemia
10. Nursing considerations
    a. Client usually responds or awakens within 5 to 20 minutes after administration
    b. Give 50% glucose IV if no response to glucagon
    c. After client awakens and is able to swallow, give oral carbohydrate
    d. After recovery assess for persistent headache, nausea, and weakness
11. Client education
    a. How to test blood glucose levels
    b. Teach responsible family member how to administer subQ or IM in the presence of frequent hypoglycemic reactions
    c. Notify prescriber immediately after reaction to determine cause

Practice to Pass

A client who has been experiencing frequent hypoglycemic (insulin) reactions at home calls and says that he cannot afford to buy any more blood glucose testing equipment. What should the nurse do?

Case Study

A 20-year-old female is diagnosed with type 1 diabetes mellitus (DM). She is hospitalized to establish a proper insulin dosage in the morning and afternoon, and to be educated on her diabetic care. The health care provider has prescribed NPH insulin 35 units and Regular insulin 10 units in the morning and NPH insulin 25 units and Regular insulin 8 units in the evening before her meal. She is on a 2,000-calorie diabetic diet with 3 meals and 2 snacks. Identify what is appropriate to teach this woman about her diabetic care.

1. What do you need to teach this client about the onset and pathophysiology of type 1 DM?

2. How would you explain the clinical manifestations of DM?

3. What would you teach the client about hyperglycemia and hypoglycemia and the treatment for each condition?

4. What would you teach the client about managing insulin therapy to prevent hyperglycemia and hypoglycemia?

For suggested responses, see pages 542–543.

POSTTEST

❶ Before a child begins drug therapy with growth hormone, the nurse should stress which of the following teaching points with the parents?

1. "Your child's expected growth rate is 3 to 5 inches during the first year of treatment."
2. "You need to measure your child's height and weight daily."
3. "Growth hormone therapy, once started, must be taken until the child reaches the age of 21."
4. "The amount of subcutaneous fat your child has will increase during the treatment period."

❷ When the nurse teaches a client about insulin administration, which of the following pieces of client information alerts the nurse that special instruction is needed?

1. Client closely restricts foods high in carbohydrates
2. Client wants spouse to learn to administer insulin
3. Client performs 30 minutes of aerobic exercise every other day
4. Client takes nap each day in the afternoon

❸ A client recently diagnosed with type 2 diabetes mellitus is taking tolbutamide (Orinase). The nurse should conduct a drug history with special emphasis on which of the following drugs? Select all that apply.

1. Ginseng, which increases hypoglycemic effects
2. Alcoholic beverages, which cause a disulfiram-like (Antabuse) reaction
3. Thiazide diuretics, which increase risk for aplastic anemia
4. Beta blockers, which mask signs and symptoms of hypoglycemic reaction
5. Garlic, which increases risk of bleeding

4 A female client with a tumor on the posterior pituitary gland is taking cabergoline (Dostinex) 0.25 mg PO twice weekly. The nurse should monitor for which of the following therapeutic outcomes?

1. Normal serum calcium levels
2. Reduced number of hot flashes per day
3. Lowering of blood pressure
4. Relief from inappropriate lactation

5 A client who has received metyrapone (Metopirone) experiences an adrenal crisis. The nurse considers that which of the following most likely predisposed the client to this occurrence?

1. Client has hyperaldosteronism
2. Client has adrenal insufficiency
3. Client has pheochromocytoma
4. Client has type 1 diabetes mellitus

6 A client with adrenal insufficiency is prescribed to take hydrocortisone (Cortef) 3 times daily on a long-term basis. What should the nurse include in client teaching? Select all that apply.

1. "Immediately stop taking this medication if weight gain or diarrhea occurs."
2. "Alcohol and caffeine should be avoided while taking this medication."
3. "You will likely notice an improvement in your daily blood glucose levels and hemoglobin A1C levels."
4. "Report symptoms of persistent heartburn or indigestion."
5. "Report any wound that will not heal or is healing very slowly."

7 A client who recently started taking desmopressin (DDAVP) reports onset of a headache, lethargy, and drowsiness. The nurse makes which assessment of the client next?

1. History of recent streptococcal infection
2. Whether client also takes carbamazepine (Tegretol)
3. If client has developed hypertension
4. Signs and symptoms of dehydration

8 Before surgery, propranolol (Inderal) is prescribed for a client with hyperthyroidism. The nurse should assess for which of the following intended outcomes?

1. Change in heart rate, reduced anxiety, reduced sweating
2. Regrowth of scalp hair, increased tolerance of extreme temperature changes
3. Weight gain, improved respiratory status
4. Decreased insomnia, decreased restlessness

9 A client taking digoxin (Lanoxin) is scheduled to receive an injection of intravenous calcium. The nurse should prepare to intervene if which of the following drug interactions occurs?

1. Hypertension and tingling around the mouth
2. Sustained, significant bradycardia
3. Nausea, vomiting, and diarrhea
4. Sloughing of tissue at the injection site

10 Because a client with hypocalcemia needs to increase the level of calcium absorption, the nurse performs which of the following activities as part of the therapeutic plan of care?

1. Administer magnesium sulfate PO.
2. Encourage increase in exercise.
3. Administer verapamil (Calan) 80 mg PO q8h.
4. Administer ergocalciferol (vitamin D).

➤ *See pages 218–220 for Answers and Rationales.*

ANSWERS & RATIONALES

Pretest

1 **Answer: 3** **Rationale:** Growth hormone (GH) is only approved for use in children to treat a documented lack of growth hormone. It is available as a parenteral medication only, to be given IM or subcutaneously. Only long bones are affected. The nurse should answer the parent's question before exploring other areas. **Cognitive Level:** Analyzing **Client Need:** Pharmacological and Parenteral Therapies **Integrated Process:** Communication and Documentation **Content Area:** Pharmacology **Strategy:** Recall first the guidelines for prescribing growth hormone. Then compare this information to the statement in each option and use the process of elimination to make a selection. **Reference:** Wilson, B. A., Shannon, M., & Shields, K. (2010). *Pearson nurse's drug guide 2010.* Upper Saddle River, NJ: Pearson Education, pp. 1424–1426.

2 **Answer: 2** **Rationale:** Abrupt cessation of long-term steroid therapy can cause acute adrenal insufficiency, which could lead to death. Signs and symptoms include nausea and vomiting, lethargy, confusion, and coma. Because long-term glucocorticoid therapy results in shrinkage of the adrenal gland, it cannot produce an adequate level of the hormone. Abrupt withdrawal can cause problems. Central nervous system symptoms such as confusion and psychosis are adverse effects of steroids such as prednisone. Gradual reduction of dosages decreases the severity of the withdrawal signs and symptoms without blood work. **Cognitive Level:** Applying **Client Need:** Pharmacological and Parenteral Therapies **Integrated Process:** Communication and Documentation **Content Area:** Pharmacology **Strategy:** Determine the time frame associated with safe withdrawal of corticosteroids. Then select the option that best matches this information. **Reference:** Wilson, B. A., Shannon, M., & Shields, K. (2010). *Pearson nurse's drug guide 2010.* Upper Saddle River, NJ: Pearson Education, p. 1281.

3 **Answer: 2, 4** **Rationale:** A record of nocturnal enuresis should be maintained and discussed with the prescriber. Rapid increases in weight, heart rate, blood pressure, and shortness of breath should be reported to the prescriber because they may indicate water retention. Drowsiness, lethargy, or confusion may be signs of water intoxication and should be reported to the prescriber. The drug should not be shaken, as this may lead to drug breakdown. Desmopressin (DDAVP) nasal spray should be administered high up into the nasal cavity and not down the throat. **Cognitive Level:** Applying **Client Need:** Pharmacological and Parenteral Therapies **Integrated Process:** Nursing Process: Implementation **Content Area:** Pharmacology **Strategy:** Specific drug information is needed to answer the question. Consider all aspects of drug administration and note the wording of the question indicates that more than one option will be correct. **Reference:** Adams, M. P., & Koch, R. W. (2010). *Pharmacology: Connections to nursing practice.* Upper Saddle River, NJ: Pearson Education, p. 1115.

4 **Answer: 1** **Rationale:** High doses of fludrocortisone (Florinef) may result in excess retention of sodium and water resulting in excessive weight gain. Because outcomes include sodium and fluid retention, the client is more likely to gain weight than lose it. A reduced ability to resist infection is associated with Cushing's disease rather than Addison's disease. Because of the risk of excess fluid retention, the client is not likely to experience hypovolemia. **Cognitive Level:** Applying **Client Need:** Pharmacological and Parenteral Therapies **Integrated Process:** Nursing Process: Planning **Content Area:** Pharmacology **Strategy:** Recall first that the drug is a mineralocorticoid. Therefore, the drug's action will involve sodium retention. Next recall that sodium retention leads to water retention and associate this with the need to measure weight as an indicator of fluid volume status. **Reference:** Wilson, B. A., Shannon, M., & Shields, K. (2010). *Pearson nurse's drug guide 2010.* Upper Saddle River, NJ: Pearson Education, pp. 659–661.

5 **Answer: 1, 2, 3** **Rationale:** Levothyroxine (Synthroid) is indicated for use in clients with cretinism, congenital hypothyroidism, and for some types of thyroid cancer that contribute to hypothyroidism. Myxedema coma occurs in clients who have very low thyroid hormone levels. The use of levothyroxine (Synthroid) and other forms of thyroid hormone replacement would be indicated. Glucocorticoid and mineralocorticoid replacement is expected for adrenal insufficiency. Oral and injectable hypoglycemic agents are used to treat type 2 diabetes mellitus. **Cognitive Level:** Analyzing **Client Need:** Pharmacological and Parenteral Therapies **Integrated Process:** Nursing Process: Planning **Content Area:** Pharmacology **Strategy:** Consider options that have some relationship to the thyroid gland to make your selections. Note the wording of the question indicates that more than one option is correct. **Reference:** Adams, M. P., & Koch, R. W. (2010). *Pharmacology: Connections to nursing practice.* Upper Saddle River, NJ: Pearson Education, p. 1152.

6 **Answer: 2** **Rationale:** Symptoms of adverse effects of liotrix (Thyrolar) include tachycardia and angina. Without treatment, these symptoms can result in cardiac damage. Assessing the heart rate is the most important assessment. Toxicity can result in slight hyperthermia, but this will have minimal impact on the client's health. Thus, temperature does not have to be monitored. Sleepiness is a sign or symptom of the disease, which should decrease or resolve once drug therapy is started. Nervousness is a side effect of this drug, but this is less threatening than cardiac alterations. **Cognitive Level:** Applying **Client Need:** Pharmacological and Parenteral Therapies **Integrated Process:** Communication and Documentation **Content Area:** Pharmacology **Strategy:** Select the option that could place the client at risk the most rapidly and the most significantly. Oxygenation and circulation should be considered first when the items ask for priority setting. As a separate strategy to eliminate sleepiness being a side effect, differentiate the disease profile from the characteristics of the drug. **Reference:** Wilson, B. A., Shannon, M., & Shields, K. (2010). *Pearson nurse's drug guide 2010*. Upper Saddle River, NJ: Pearson Education, pp. 908–909.

7 **Answer: 3** **Rationale:** Agranulocytosis is the most serious toxic effect of this drug, and it can predispose the client to a variety of infections. Attempts to determine the risk for infection are important, but are not as important as reviewing the white blood cell count as an indicator of current ability to fight infection. Although stress can predispose the client to infection, the immediate concern is the client's actual condition and ability to combat infection, as evidenced by the WBC count. **Cognitive Level:** Applying **Client Need:** Pharmacological and Parenteral Therapies **Integrated Process:** Nursing Process: Implementation **Content Area:** Pharmacology **Strategy:** To answer the question correctly, it is necessary to be aware of the risk for agranulocytosis with this drug. From there, associate the drug side effects with the option that directly assesses this parameter. **Reference:** Wilson, B. A., Shannon, M., & Shields, K. (2010). *Pearson nurse's drug guide 2010*. Upper Saddle River, NJ: Pearson Education, pp. 1312–1314.

8 **Answer: 1** **Rationale:** Paget disease is characterized by overactive osteoblasts (cells that break down the bone), which stimulates an increase in alkaline phosphatase levels. Calcitonin (Calcimar) decreases the cell turnover. This is evident in the reduced alkaline phosphate level. Calcitonin would decrease the calcium level rather than increase it. Bone deformity is permanent, not temporary, so bones will not return to normal. Skull deformities are common with Paget but are unrelated to therapeutic effectiveness. **Cognitive Level:** Applying **Client Need:** Pharmacological and Parenteral Therapies **Integrated Process:** Nursing Process: Implementation **Content Area:** Pharmacology **Strategy:** The critical words in the question are *therapeutic effectiveness*. This tells you that the correct option is one that illustrates the expected effect of the drug. Use this knowledge and the process of elimination to make a selection. **Reference:** Wilson, B. A., Shannon, M., & Shields, K. (2010). *Pearson nurse's drug guide 2010*. Upper Saddle River, NJ: Pearson Education, pp. 217–219.

9 **Answer: 2, 3, 5** **Rationale:** Visual changes can occur because of diabetic retinopathy, particularly in clients whose blood glucose is not well controlled. Changes in penile vasculature may cause impotence prior to diagnosis of diabetes mellitus; initial insulin therapy may increase this problem. Some clients experience a rebound hyperglycemia (Somogyi effect). It is helpful for a family member to be able to inject insulin, but the initial focus should be on teaching the client. With control of serum glucose levels, complications such as vision loss and loss of limbs due to accelerated atherosclerosis can be prevented or delayed. **Cognitive Level:** Applying **Client Need:** Pharmacological and Parenteral Therapies **Integrated Process:** Teaching and Learning **Content Area:** Pharmacology **Strategy:** The wording of the question indicates that the correct responses are true statements. Read each statement and determine whether it is a true or false statement and use the process of elimination to make your selections, using knowledge of the disease process of diabetes mellitus and information about insulin and its effects on the body. **Reference:** Wilson, B. A., Shannon, M., & Shields, K. (2010). *Pearson nurse's drug guide 2010*. Upper Saddle River, NJ: Pearson Education, pp. 802–813.

10 **Answer: 3** **Rationale:** The priority learning need in treatment of an insulin reaction is that the client understands to take some form of oral glucose, such as orange juice or crackers and peanut butter. The protein prevents a rebound hypoglycemia. This is the most appropriate action because it fixes the problem within a reasonable time frame. The problem can be remedied most of the time without notifying the prescriber so this is a lesser priority. Scheduling serum glucose levels would be routine and not in relation to an insulin reaction; instead the client would monitor finger-stick glucose at home. Ingesting fluid would not contribute to the recovery from drug-induced hypoglycemia. **Cognitive Level:** Analyzing **Client Need:** Pharmacological and Parenteral Therapies **Integrated Process:** Teaching and Learning **Content Area:** Pharmacology **Strategy:** Recall that an insulin reaction is a critical event and the priority action needs to focus on reversing the low blood glucose. With this in mind, easily eliminate each of the incorrect options. **Reference:** LeMone, P., Burke, K., & Bauldoff, G. (2011). *Medical-surgical nursing: Critical thinking in patient care* (5th ed.). Upper Saddle River, NJ: Pearson Education, pp. 1232–1238.

Posttest

1 **Answer: 1** **Rationale:** The expected growth rate with growth hormone therapy is 3 to 5 inches in the first year. Height and weight is measured monthly. Growth hormone is discontinued when optimum adult height is attained, fusion of epiphyseal plates has occurred, or when there is no response to growth hormone. Growth hormone is related to growth of long bones, not fat deposition. **Cognitive Level:** Analyzing **Client Need:** Pharmacological and Parenteral Therapies **Integrated**

Process: Teaching and Learning **Content Area**: Pharmacology **Strategy**: Correlate the action of the drug with the expected outcome. Parents may expect a more rapid rate of growth than is typical. Eliminate 2 options because of the words *daily* and *must*, respectively. Use knowledge of growth hormone to make the final selection. **Reference**: Adams, M. P., & Koch, R. W. (2010). *Pharmacology: Connections to nursing practice.* Upper Saddle River, NJ: Pearson Education, pp. 1106–1112.

2 **Answer: 1** **Rationale**: Insulin contributes to the metabolism of fats, proteins, and carbohydrates. The client should ingest a balanced diet. It is appropriate for the spouse to learn to administer the insulin if the client becomes unable to. Regular exercise can increase peripheral use of glucose. Napping in the afternoon would have no significant impact on insulin administration. **Cognitive Level**: Applying **Client Need**: Pharmacological and Parenteral Therapies **Integrated Process**: Nursing Process: Assessment **Content Area**: Pharmacology **Strategy**: Select the option most closely associated with the function of insulin. **Reference**: LeMone, P., Burke, K., & Bauldoff, G. (2011). *Medical-surgical nursing: Critical thinking in patient care* (5th ed.). Upper Saddle River, NJ: Pearson Education, p. 536.

3 **Answer: 1, 2, 4** **Rationale**: Ginseng lowers glucose levels. Tolbutamide (Orinase) interacting with alcohol can lead to a *disulfiram-like* (Antabuse) reaction causing complaints of headache and flushing of the skin. This is an important teaching point for the client who has a history of alcoholism, even if currently not drinking. Beta blockers reduce the sympathomimetic response to hypoglycemic reactions. Hence, signs and symptoms of hypoglycemia are less likely to occur. Aplastic anemia is a side effect of tolbutamide, not thiazide diuretics. Garlic does not interact with tolbutamide to increase the risk of bleeding. **Cognitive Level**: Analyzing **Client Need**: Pharmacological and Parenteral Therapies **Integrated Process**: Teaching and Learning **Content Area**: Pharmacology **Strategy**: Presume the major focus will be on increasing the risk of hypoglycemia as well as the disulfiram-like (Antabuse) reaction. **Reference**: Wilson, B. A., Shannon, M., & Shields, K. (2011). *Pearson nurse's drug guide 2011.* Upper Saddle River, NJ: Pearson Education, p. 1528.

4 **Answer: 4** **Rationale**: The primary purpose of the cabergoline (Dostinex) is to reduce or eliminate lactation related to hyperprolactinemia. The drug has no effect on calcium levels. Hot flashes are a side effect of the drug. Hypotension is a common side effect. **Cognitive Level**: Analyzing **Client Need**: Pharmacological and Parenteral Therapies **Integrated Process**: Nursing Process: Evaluation **Content Area**: Pharmacology **Strategy**: Specific knowledge of this medication is needed to answer the question. Align the drug's action with the client's health needs and the disease process. **Reference**: Wilson, B. A., Shannon, M., & Shields, K. (2011). *Pearson nurse's drug guide 2011.* Upper Saddle River, NJ: Pearson Education, p. 217.

5 **Answer: 2** **Rationale**: In the presence of adrenal insufficiency, metyrapone (Metopirone) may cause an adrenal crisis by reducing the synthesis of cortisol. The drug is utilized for diagnosis of Cushing disease. Aldosterone is a mineralocorticoid, while metyrapone influences glucocorticoids. Pheochromocytoma is related to excessive secretion of catecholamines and would not cause an adrenal crisis, which is related to decreased glucocorticoid level. Diabetes is more likely to develop with high levels of glucocorticoids. **Cognitive Level**: Applying **Client Need**: Pharmacological and Parenteral Therapies **Integrated Process**: Nursing Process: Diagnosis **Content Area**: Pharmacology **Strategy**: First recall that an adrenal crisis results from insufficient amounts of hormones produced by the adrenal cortex. With this in mind, look for the option that identifies hypofunction of the adrenal gland. Alternatively, determine the relationship between adrenal function and the function of the drug. **Reference**: Adams, M. P., & Koch, R. W. (2010). *Pharmacology: Connections to nursing practice.* Upper Saddle River, NJ: Pearson Education, p. 1171.

6 **Answer:** **Rationale**: Alcohol and caffeine should be avoided during long-term hydrocortisone therapy because they contribute to the development of peptic ulcer disease. Heartburn or indigestion should be reported; they are adverse effects of this medication and may signal peptic ulcer disease. Corticosteroids inhibit the inflammatory and immune response. A slow healing wound should be reported to the health care provider. Replacement steroids should not be abruptly discontinued. If needed, the client should be tapered off the medication to avoid withdrawal symptoms and/or adrenal insufficiency. Replacement corticosteroids may contribute to secondary diabetes. It is unlikely that an improvement of blood glucose or hemoglobin A1C will occur. **Cognitive Level**: Applying **Client Need**: Pharmacological and Parenteral Therapies **Integrated Process**: Teaching and Learning **Content Area**: Pharmacology **Strategy**: The wording of the question indicates that more than one option is correct. Choose the options that contain true statements based on the wording of the question. **Reference**: Adams, M. P., & Koch, R. W. (2010). *Pharmacology: Connections to nursing practice.* Upper Saddle River, NJ: Pearson Education, p. 1168.

7 **Answer: 2** **Rationale**: Desmopressin (DDAVP) is a drug used to treat diabetes insipidus. The manifestations listed are all signs of water intoxication, which could occur as an excessive effect of the medication. Carbamazepine (Tegretol) prolongs the effect of DDAVP and could lead to water retention. The drug has no known effects on the immune system. Hypertension may develop with overhydration, but the headache is related more to the swelling of the brain cells. The client's symptoms are not related to dehydration. **Cognitive Level**: Applying **Client Need**: Pharmacological and Parenteral Therapies **Integrated Process**: Nursing Process: Assessment **Content Area**: Pharmacology

Strategy: Associate the drug with antidiuretic hormone and note that the symptoms related to fluid overload. Use the process of elimination to choose the option that seems most likely to pose a risk of fluid retention. Reference: Wilson, B. A., Shannon, M., & Shields, K. (2011). *Pearson nurse's drug guide 2011*. Upper Saddle River, NJ: Pearson Education, p. 439.

8 **Answer: 1** Rationale: The excessive levels of thyroxine in hyperthyroidism lead to symptoms such as tachycardia, anxiety, and diaphoresis. Propranolol (Inderal) is a beta-adrenergic blocker and is used to treat the sympathetic nervous system responses. Although the disease affects the volume of hair and heat tolerance, propranolol has no direct effect on heat tolerance or scalp hair. Because of the excessive thyroxine secretion, the metabolic process is increased, which results in dyspnea without exertion. The purpose of the propranolol is to reduce the cardiovascular signs and symptoms, not respiratory symptoms. Because propranolol reduces tachycardia and palpitations, the insomnia and restlessness may decrease, but this is not the primary purpose for the administration of the drug. Cognitive Level: Applying Client Need: Pharmacological and Parenteral Therapies Integrated Process: Nursing Process: Evaluation Content Area: Pharmacology Strategy: The critical words in the question are *intended outcomes*. Associate the signs and symptoms of the disease profile along with the actions of propranolol (Inderal) and use the process of elimination to make a selection. Reference: Wilson, B. A., Shannon, M., & Shields, K. (2011). *Pearson nurse's drug guide 2011*. Upper Saddle River, NJ: Pearson Education, pp. 1302–1306.

9 **Answer: 2** Rationale: Because calcium influences cardiac contractility and neural transmission, it can potentiate the actions of digoxin (Lanoxin). The nurse should monitor for severe bradycardia. Hypotension is more likely to occur than hypertension, and tingling around the mouth is more indicative of hypocalcemia. Nausea and vomiting are side effects associated with digoxin, but not diarrhea. Neither is related to a drug interaction between calcium and digoxin. Sloughing of tissue at the site is associated with injection of calcium, but this is not a drug interaction. Cognitive Level: Applying Client Need: Pharmacological and Parenteral Therapies Integrated Process: Nursing Process: Planning Content Area: Pharmacology Strategy: Correlate the potential combined effect of both drugs on the heart. Eliminate 2 options first because they are least related to the heart, and then eliminate a third option because it contains a symptom of hypocalcemia. Reference: Wilson, B. A., Shannon, M., & Shields, K. (2011). *Pearson nurse's drug guide 2011*. Upper Saddle River, NJ: Pearson Education, pp. 471–475.

10 **Answer: 4** Rationale: Ergocalciferol (vitamin D) regulates calcium and phosphorus metabolism and increases blood levels of both elements. Magnesium may reduce calcium absorption. Exercise contributes to bone maintenance. Calcium may reduce the effects of verapamil (Calan). Absorption of calcium is not affected. Cognitive Level: Applying Client Need: Pharmacological and Parenteral Therapies Integrated Process: Nursing Process: Implementation Content Area: Pharmacology Strategy: Determine the relationship between the elements most likely to enhance absorption of calcium. Reference: Wilson, B. A., Shannon, M., & Shields, K. (2011). *Pearson nurse's drug guide 2011*. Upper Saddle River, NJ: Pearson Education, pp. 219–220.

References

Abrams, A. (2009). *Clinical drug therapy: Rationales for nursing practice* (9th ed.). Philadelphia, PA: Lippincott Williams & Wilkins.

Adams, M., Holland, L., & Bostwick, P. (2011). *Pharmacology for nurses: A pathophysiologic approach* (3rd ed.). Upper Saddle River, NJ: Pearson Education.

Adams. M. P., & Urban, C. Q. (2013). *Pharmacology: Connections to nursing practice* (2nd ed.). Upper Saddle River, NJ: Pearson Education.

Aschenbrenner, D., & Venable, S. (2009). *Drug therapy in nursing* (3rd ed.). Philadelphia, PA: Lippincott Williams & Wilkins.

Drug Facts & Comparisons® (Updated monthly). St. Louis, MO: A. Wolters Kluwer.

Karch, A. M. (2010). *Focus on nursing pharmacology* (5th ed.). Philadelphia, PA: Lippincott Williams & Wilkins.

Kee, J. (2009). *Laboratory and diagnostic tests and nursing implications* (8th ed.).

Upper Saddle River, NJ: Pearson Education.

Lehne, R. (2010). *Pharmacology for nursing care* (7th ed.). St. Louis, MO: Mosby.

LeMone, P., Burke, K. M., & Bauldoff, G. (2011). *Medical-surgical nursing: Critical thinking in patient care* (5th ed.). Upper Saddle River, NJ: Pearson Education.

ANSWERS & RATIONALES

Gastrointestinal System Medications

7

Chapter Outline

Gastrointestinal (GI) Stimulants
Medications to Decrease GI
  Tone and Motility
  (Anticholinergics and
  Antispasmodics)
Antidiarrheals

Laxatives
Antiemetics
Histamine H$_2$ Antagonists
Proton Pump Inhibitors
Mucosal Protective Agents
Antacids

Antimicrobials for *Helicobacter
  pylori* Organisms
Medications Used to Dissolve
  Gallstones
Pancreatic Enzyme
  Replacement

Objectives

➤ Describe general goals of therapy when administering
   gastrointestinal system medications.
➤ Describe the use and side effects of antacids.
➤ Identify the actions of various forms of laxatives.
➤ Discuss the effects of H$_2$-receptor antagonists, proton pump
   inhibitors, and mucosal protectants on the gastrointestinal tract.
➤ Describe nursing considerations related to administration
   of antiemetics.
➤ Identify specific food and drug interactions associated with various
   gastrointestinal system medications.
➤ Describe nursing considerations related to administration of
   pancreatic enzyme replacements.
➤ List significant client education points related to gastrointestinal
   system medications.

NCLEX-RN® Test Prep

Use the accompanying online resource,
NursingReviewsandRationales, to test
yourself with hundreds of NCLEX®-style
practice questions.

Review at a Glance

antacid agent that reduces or neutralizes acidity
anticholinergic antagonist to parasympathetic action or other cholinergic
receptors
antispasmodic agent that prevents
or relieves spasms
cathartic agent with purgative action

H$_2$ antagonist antagonist agent
against histamine that decreases gastrin
secretion
Helicobacter pylori bacteria
found in gastric mucosa that produces
urease and is associated commonly with
gastric and duodenal ulcers

laxative agent used to cause a bowel
movement or loosening of the bowels
surfactant a surface-active agent
also known as a wetting agent, tension
depressant, detergent, and emulsifier

PRETEST

1 After a 2-year-old ingested a full bottle of children's aspirin, the parent gives the child 2 doses of ipecac syrup found hidden at the back of the medicine cabinet and then rushes the child to the urgent care clinic. It has been over 40 minutes and the child has not vomited. What should the nurse be prepared to do at this time?

1. Call poison control center.
2. Administer activated charcoal.
3. Offer milk or carbonated soda.
4. Explain that ipecac is no longer sold over the counter.

2 A client with gastroesophageal reflux disease (GERD) is taking metoclopramide (Reglan) as prescribed. What client statement tells the nurse that the medication teaching session was effective?

1. "The purpose of this drug is to increase GI motility."
2. "This drug decreases the tone of the lower esophageal sphincter."
3. "This drug will prevent or stop diarrhea from occurring."
4. "This drug kills the *H. pylori* organism that causes peptic ulcer disease."

3 A client is taking dicyclomine (Antispas) for irritable bowel syndrome (IBS). Which nursing assessment is the best indicator that the client is self-administering the medication properly?

1. Presence of mucus in stool
2. Weighs 10 pounds less than last examination
3. Bowel sounds are hypoactive
4. Nutritional intake within normal ranges

4 A client, who is allergic to aspirin (ASA), has acute diarrhea. The nurse concludes that which antidiarrheal medication should not be given to this client?

1. Attapulgite (Kaopectate)
2. Bismuth subsalicylate (Pepto-Bismol)
3. Diphenoxylate with atropine (Lomotil)
4. Loperamide (Imodium)

5 The nurse determines that further instructions are needed if a client with diarrhea makes which statement?

1. "I need to avoid intake of dairy products."
2. "I should take Kaopectate as directed."
3. "I should call my health care provider if diarrhea lasts more than 2 days."
4. "If the diarrhea persists, I should start taking psyllium hydrophilic (Metamucil)."

6 The nurse concludes that docusate sodium (Colace) is appropriate for use in which of the following clients? Select all that apply.

1. A client preparing for a colonoscopy who needs a bowel prep
2. A postoperative client taking opioid analgesics for pain
3. A client who experienced a myocardial infarction 24 hours ago
4. A client trying to reduce the chances of chronic constipation
5. A client with painful hemorrhoids

7 A healthy adult client has been taking a laxative 3 days per week for 9 months. What primary risk should the nurse address in a teaching plan with this client?

1. Risk of electrolyte imbalance
2. Risk of drug dependence
3. Risk of fluid imbalance
4. Risk for inadequate nutritional status.

8 After noting a new order for loperamide (Imodium) 4 mg PO q6h prn for a 71-year-old client, the nurse should provide which of the following instructions to unlicensed assistive personnel (UAP)?

1. Set up seizure precautions.
2. Set up safety precautions.
3. Measure vital signs every 4 hours.
4. Place a commode at the bedside.

9 After being diagnosed with an open-cratered gastric ulcer, a 19-year-old female client starts crying and refuses to take the prescribed medications. The nurse should complete which of the following activities at this time? Select all that apply.

1. Explain in detail the action of ranitidine (Zantac).
2. Sit with client to allow her to express her feelings.
3. Teach client about ways to prevent future ulcerations.
4. Explain risks associated with not treating the open-crater gastric ulcer.
5. Encourage the client to ingest the dose of misoprostol (Cytotec).

10 Because magnetic resonance imaging (MRI) revealed an open-cratered gastric ulcer, a semi-comatose female client is receiving misoprostol (Cytotec). The nurse, who is a team leader in a nursing home, provides the following instructions to the unlicensed assistants (UAP). Place the activities in the order of priority.

1. Keep a log of client's bowel pattern
2. Report restlessness
3. Place bed protector beneath client
4. Report vaginal spotting
5. Maintain head of bed at 35 degrees

➤ *See pages 248–250 for Answers and Rationales.*

I. GASTROINTESTINAL (GI) STIMULANTS

A. Action and use

1. Decrease reflux by increasing sphincter tone and enhancing acid clearance and decreasing gastric emptying
2. Decrease or prevent nausea and vomiting due to chemotherapy, and to facilitate small bowel intubations
3. Used for delayed gastric emptying caused by diabetic gastroparesis, gastroesophageal reflux disease (GERD), or postoperative nausea and vomiting
4. Stimulate gastric motility without stimulating gastric, biliary, or pancreatic secretion
5. Sensitize tissues to action of acetylcholine and induce release of prolactin
6. Methoscopalamine blocks effect of acetylcholine, relaxing smooth muscles
7. Dexpanthenol minimizes risk of paralytic ileus when used postoperatively

B. Common medications: see Table 7-1

C. Administration considerations

1. Metoclopramide PO should be taken 30 minutes before meals and bedtime
2. Metoclopramide IV should be given 30 minutes prior to chemotherapy for anti-emetic effect

D. Contraindications

1. Hypersensitivity, history of seizure disorders, pheochromocytoma, and Parkinson's disease (metoclopramide)
2. Contraindicated in clients where overstimulation may be dangerous, such as with GI hemorrhage, obstruction, or perforation
3. Contraindicated with allergy to dextran, marked hemostatic defects, congestive heart failure (CHF), and renal failure (dexpanthenol)
4. Use with caution in clients with a history of depression, seizure disorder, or hypertension
5. Lactation: excreted in breast milk, so caution should be used in nursing mothers

Practice to Pass

What GI drug has been withdrawn by the Food and Drug Administration because of adverse effects of QT prolongation?

Table 7-1	Gastrointestinal Stimulants	
Generic (Trade) Name	**Route**	**Uses**
Dexpanthenol [dextro-pantothenyl alcohol] (Ilopan, Panthoderm)	IM, IV, Topical	Prophylactic use immediately after major abdominal surgery to minimize paralytic ileus development, intestinal atony, postoperative or postpartum flatus, resumption of GI motility following paralytic ileus, eczema, dermatosis, diaper rash, chafing
Methoscopolamine bromide (Pamine, Pamine Forte)	PO	Adjunctive therapy in the treatment of peptic ulcer
Metoclopramide (Maxolon, Clopra, Octamide, Reglan)	PO, IM, IV	Relief of acute symptoms or recurrent symptoms of diabetic gastroparesis or GERD, prevention of nausea and vomiting, facilitation of small bowel intubation (single dose), stimulation of gastric emptying and movement of barium, improvement of lactation, relief of nausea or vomiting associated with many etiologies including pregnancy

E. Significant drug interactions
1. Metoclopramide is metabolized by P450 liver enzyme system and should not be taken with inhibitors of this enzyme such as macrolides, antifungals, and some protease inhibitors; may decrease absorption of digoxin
2. Concomitant use of metoclopramide, hyoscyamine, and tricyclic antidepressants may antagonize effects of metoclopramide
3. Levodopa has the opposite effect and may antagonize metoclopramide effect
4. Metoclopramide may increase hypertensive effects of monoamine oxidase (MAO) inhibitors and decrease absorption of digoxin from GI tract
5. Increased toxic and immunosuppressive effects of cyclosporine

F. Significant food interactions: none reported

G. Significant laboratory studies: serum electrolyte levels, falsely elevated glucose level

H. Side effects
1. Drowsiness, diarrhea, restlessness, fatigue
2. Parkinson's-like symptoms
3. Transient hypertension

I. Adverse effects/toxicity
1. Seizures
2. Agranulocytosis
3. Depression with suicide ideations

J. Nursing considerations
1. Monitor for possible hypernatremia and hypokalemia, particularly if client has CHF or liver cirrhosis
2. Extrapyramidal symptoms may occur in young adults and the elderly and with high-dose treatment of metoclopramide
3. Monitor BP carefully when administering metoclopramide IV

K. Client education
1. Report signs and symptoms of side effects
2. Report signs of acute dystonia immediately
3. Do not drive for a few hours after taking metoclopramide
4. Drink adequate amounts of fluids
5. Avoid humid environments with methoscopolamine

II. MEDICATIONS TO DECREASE GI TONE AND MOTILITY (ANTICHOLINERGICS AND ANTISPASMODICS)

A. **Action and use**
   1. **Anticholinergics** antagonize the action of acetylcholine at specific cholinergic receptor sites
   2. **Antispasmodics** are similar and they are believed to relax smooth muscle
   3. Used for treatment of spasms of GI tract such as pylorospasm, ileitis, and irritable bowel syndrome
B. **Common medications (Table 7-2)**
C. **Administration considerations**: give medication 30 to 60 minutes before meals and at bedtime for therapeutic effect
D. **Contraindications**
   1. Narrow-angle glaucoma, obstructive GI disease, paralytic ileus, obstructive uropathy, adhesions between iris and lens, myocardial ischemia, toxic megacolon
   2. Excreted in breast milk, may cause infant toxicity and decreased milk production
   3. Use with caution with renal dysfunction
E. **Significant drug interactions**
   1. Use of another anticholinergic drug may result in increased anticholinergic side effects
   2. Atropine may increase the effect of phenothiazines
   3. Increased effects of atenolol with anticholinergic drugs
   4. Decreased effectiveness of all antipsychotic medications with dicyclomine
   5. Decreased effects of haloperidol and phenothiazines with propantheline bromide
   6. Antacids decrease absorption of anticholinergics
   F. Significant food interactions: none reported
G. **Significant laboratory studies**: serum electrolyte levels
H. **Side effects**
   1. Hypersensitivity
   2. Urticaria, rash, dry mouth, nausea, vomiting, constipation, urinary hesitance and retention
   3. Impotence, blurred vision, worsening of glaucoma
   4. Palpitations, headache, flushing, drowsiness, dizziness, confusion

Table 7-2 Medications to Decrease GI Tone and Motility: Anticholinergics/Antispasmodics

Generic (Trade) Name	Route	Uses
Dicyclomine hydrochloride (Bentyl)	PO	Functional bowel or irritable bowel syndrome
Glycopyrrolate (Robinul, Robinula forte)	PO	Peptic ulcer, reduce salivary, tracheobronchial, and pharyngeal secretions, protect against the peripheral muscarinic effects of cholinergic agents
Hyoscyamine sulfate (L-hyoscyamine)	PO	Irritable bowel syndrome, peptic ulcer disease, spastic or functional disorders, cystitis, neurogenic bladder, parkinsonism, biliary and renal colic, rhinitis, anticholinesterase poisoning, partial heart block associated with vagal activity, and to decrease operative secretions
Methscopolamine bromide	PO	Peptic ulcer disease
Propantheline bromide	PO	Peptic ulcer disease
Tizanidine (Zanflex)	PO	Management of increased muscle tone associated with spasticity

I. **Adverse effects/toxicity**
   1. May cause dilated, nonreactive pupils, visual changes
   2. Tachycardia
   3. Dysphagia, decreased or absent bowel sounds
   4. Hyperthermia, hypertension, increased respiratory rate

J. **Nursing considerations**
   1. An understanding of the factors contributing to the diarrhea is essential in effective treatment
   2. Clients who lose significant potassium with diarrhea are at risk for the development of paralytic ileus and cardiac dysrhythmias
   3. They should also be monitored for metabolic acidosis because of the loss of bicarbonate and impaired renal excretion of acids
   4. Document indications and present medications
   5. Monitor vital signs, urine output, and visual changes
   6. Monitor intake and output (I & O)

K. **Client education**
   1. Avoid exposure to high temperatures because of risk of hyperthermia
   2. Report side effects to health care provider
   3. Dietary and fluid interventions to decrease constipation
   4. Report any additional medications prescribed
   5. Self-monitor I & O
   6. Take drug as prescribed

III. ANTIDIARRHEALS

A. **Action and use**
   1. Slow and/or inhibit GI motility by acting on nerve endings of the intestinal wall, thereby reducing the volume of stools, increasing viscosity and decreasing fluid and electrolyte loss
   2. Used for symptomatic relief of acute nonspecific diarrhea and diarrhea of inflammatory disease

B. **Common medications (Table 7-3)**

Table 7-3 Antidiarrheals		
Generic (Trade) Name	**Route**	**Uses**
Bismuth subsalicylate (Pepto-Bismol)	PO	Indigestion, nausea, diarrhea, control traveler's diarrhea, relieve gas and abdominal cramping, chronic infantile diarrhea, prevention of traveler's diarrhea
Diphenoxylate HCl (Lomotil)	PO	Diarrhea, traveler's diarrhea
Loperamide hydrochloride (Apo-Loperamide, Imodium, Kaopectate, Maalox antidiarrheal capsule)	PO	Acute non-specific diarrhea, chronic diarrhea associated with inflammatory bowel disease, reduction of discharge volume from ileostomy, traveler's diarrhea
Octreotide acetate (Sandostatin)	subQ	Suppression or inhibition of severe diarrhea associated with metastatic carcinoid tumors, profuse watery diarrhea, reduction of growth hormone in clients with acromegaly
Opium (Paregoric)	PO	Management of short bowel syndrome, diarrhea
Rifaximin (Xifaxan)	PO	Clients 12 years and older with traveler's diarrhea caused by noninvasive E. coli

C. **Administration considerations**
   1. Shake suspensions well; chew tablets thoroughly
   2. Stool may appear gray-black (may mask GI bleeding)
   3. Do not give concurrently with other medications
   4. Seek medical care if diarrhea persists for more than 2 days in an adult
   5. Do not use to treat diarrhea in children; seek medical attention
   6. Do not give to clients with *C. difficile*

D. **Contraindications**
   1. Presence of bloody diarrhea, diarrhea associated with pathogens such as *E. coli*, salmonella, shigella or pseudomembranous colitis, or other bacterial toxins
   2. Avoid use if obstructive bowel disease is suspected
   3. Avoid bismuth subsalicylate if allergic to aspirin
   4. Difenoxine/atropine sulfate may cause serious side effects in nursing infants; therefore, should not be used for children under 2 years of age

E. **Significant drug interactions**
   1. Allergies to aspirin or other salicylates since bismuth subsalicylate contains salicylate
   2. Avoid aspirin use as concomitant use with bismuth subsalicylate, which may cause aspirin toxicity
   3. Bismuth may also decrease tetracycline absorption in the GI tract
   4. Diphenoxylate/atropine sulfate and difenoxin/atropine sulfate may increase the sedative effects of barbiturates, narcotics, and alcohol
   5. Concomitant use with MAO inhibitors may increase the risk of hypertensive crisis

F. **Significant food interactions**: none reported

G. **Significant laboratory studies**: diphenoxylate may increase serum amylase levels

H. **Side effects**
   1. Nausea and vomiting
   2. Dry mouth, dizziness, drowsiness, constipation
   3. Temporary darkening of stools and tongue may occur with bismuth salicylate

I. **Adverse effects/toxicity**
   1. Clinical signs and symptoms of overdose include drowsiness, decreased blood pressure (BP), seizures, apnea, blurred vision, dry mouth, and psychosis
   2. Risk of aspirin toxicity with concurrent use of aspirin and bismuth subsalicylate
   3. Other adverse effects include central nervous system (CNS) depression, respiratory depression, hypotonic reflexes, angioedema, anaphylaxis, and paralytic ileus

J. **Nursing considerations**
   1. Note allergies
   2. Document onset, duration, and frequency of symptoms
   3. Document previous therapies used
   4. Note current medications
   5. Identify any causative factors; perform stool analysis if necessary and ordered
   6. Assess for evidence of dehydration or electrolyte imbalance
   7. Monitor vital signs and I & O
   8. Note presence of comorbid conditions
   9. Check abdomen for tenderness, distention, bowel sounds, or masses
   10. Administer bismuth and tetracycline 1 hour apart

K. **Client education**
   1. Withhold solid food for 24 hours with acute diarrhea
   2. Foods that aggravate diarrhea include milk products, fruit and fruit juices, coffee, tea with caffeine, and chocolate
   3. Drink fluids to avoid dehydration and alleviate dry mouth
   4. Follow the BRAT diet—bananas, rice, applesauce, tea/toast—to avoid dehydration if recommended by health care provider (controversial)

Practice to Pass

How long should a client take an over-the-counter (OTC) antidiarrheal medication before consulting the health care provider?

5. Do not exceed prescribed dose
6. Consult health care provider if diarrhea persists over 2 days
7. Use caution in activities requiring alertness if dizziness or drowsiness is present (possible side effects)
8. Report fever, nausea and vomiting, abdominal pain or distention
9. Avoid OTC antacids, dairy products, and other foods that aggravate diarrhea
10. Use good personal hygiene to avoid skin irritation or breakdown because of diarrhea
11. Avoid alcohol ingestion while taking medication
12. Notify health care provider if pregnant or breastfeeding

IV. LAXATIVES

A. Bulk-forming laxatives

1. Action and use
   a. Include nonabsorbable polysaccharide and cellulose derivatives
   b. Bulk-forming **laxatives** absorb water to increase bulk in fecal mass
   c. Peristalsis is stimulated by the increased fecal mass, which decreases bowel transit time
   d. They generally produce a laxative effect within 12 to 14 hours but may require 2 to 3 days for full effect
   e. Are frequently used to prevent straining with defecation in clients who are post–myocardial infarction or have other conditions in which straining at stool could be harmful

2. Common medications (Table 7-4)

3. Administration considerations

   a. Since these agents rely on water to increase their bulk, it is essential that adequate fluids be given for bowel absorption
   b. These agents may also cause intestinal and esophageal obstruction when insufficient liquid is administered with the dose
   c. Each dose should be given with a full glass of liquid (240 mL)
   d. Use sugar-free preparations in clients with phenylketonuria

4. Contraindications
   a. Not recommended for clients with intestinal stenosis, ulceration, or adhesions
   b. Use cautiously in clients with swallowing difficulties to ensure aspiration does not occur
   c. Do not use if fecal impaction is present

5. Significant drug interactions: decreased GI absorption may occur with digitalis, anticoagulants, nitrofurantoin, and salicylates

6. Significant food interactions

   a. Dietary management of constipation can be aided by encouraging the intake of fluid and fiber
   b. Fiber increases stool bulk and water retention in the bowel
   c. A dietary bulk-forming nutrient such as bran is an appropriate adjunctive therapy for constipation
   d. Bran is only partially fermented by bacteria, resulting in increased stool bulk, accelerated transit time, and promotion of normal defecation
   e. Rapid increases in dietary roughage may cause abdominal bloating and flatulence
   f. Adequate fluid intake is also necessary in order to prevent fecal impaction

   g. Generally 240 to 360 mL of fluid with each tablespoon of bran is sufficient
   h. Avoid foods that reduce stool, such as bananas, rice, breads, and cheeses

7. Significant laboratory studies: none reported

Table 7-4 Laxatives

Generic (Trade) Name	Usual Adult Dosage Range	Route
Bulk forming laxatives		
Methylcellulose (Citrucel)	1 tsp (19 grams) in 8 oz of water 1–3 times a day	PO
Calcium polycarbophil (Fibercon)	2 tablets 1–4 times a day	PO
Psyllium (Metamucil)	3–4 grams in 8 oz of liquid 1–3 times a day	PO
Stimulant laxatives		
Casanthranol (Pericolace)	1–2 capsules at HS	PO
Senna (Senokot)	2 tablets at HS	PO
Bisacodyl (Dulcolax)	10–15 mg at HS	PO
	1 suppository	PR
Castor oil (Neoloid, Purgo)	15 to 60 mL	PO
Hyperosmotic laxatives		
Lactulose (Kristalose)	10–20 grams in 4 oz water	PO
Polyethylene glycol (Miralax)	17 grams in 8 oz water daily	PO
Glycerin (Glycerol)	3-gram suppository	Rectal
Stool softeners (surfactants)		
Docusate sodium (Colace)	50–300 mg daily	PO
Docusate potassium (Dialose)	100–300 mg daily	PO
Docusate calcium (Doxidan)	240 mg daily	PO
Saline laxatives		
Magnesium hydroxide (Milk of Magnesia)	30–60 mL at HS	PO
Sodium phosphate (Fleets)	1.25 oz enema	Rectal
	2–3 tablets daily	PO
	1 suppository daily	Rectal

8. Side effects
   a. Abdominal discomfort and/or bloating, flatulence
   b. Nausea and vomiting, diarrhea
9. Adverse effects/toxicity
   a. Rare reports of allergic reactions to karaya such as urticaria, rhinitis, dermatitis, bronchospasm
   b. Esophageal obstruction, swelling, or blockage may occur when insufficient fluid is used in mixing a bulk-forming laxative
10. Nursing considerations
    a. Assess degree of abdominal distention, bowel sounds, and bowel elimination patterns
    b. Assess swallowing ability, adequately mix agents in liquid and encourage additional fluid intake
    c. Monitor for aspiration
    d. If administered via feeding tube, it must be a large bore tube, and medication must be adequately dissolved in liquid and given rapidly with adequate flushing
    e. Add at least 8 oz (240 mL) of water or juice to drug
    f. Separate psyllium administration from digoxin, salicylates, and anticoagulants by 2 hours
    g. Use sugar-free preparations in diabetic clients

11. Client education
    a. These agents require adequate hydration to be effective
    b. Additional fluids and exercise are helpful in aiding bowel elimination
    c. Mix powder preparation with at least 8 oz fluid and drink immediately and follow with another 8 oz of fluid
    d. Bulk-forming laxatives may decrease appetite if taken before meals
    e. Take bulk-forming laxative 2 hours after meals and any oral medications
    f. Use sodium and sugar-free preparations if they are appropriate to individual diet restrictions
    g. Full effect of medication may not occur for 2 to 3 days

B. **Stimulant cathartics**
    1. Action and use
        a. Called stimulants because they stimulate peristalsis via mucosal irritation or intramural nerve plexus activity, which results in increased motility
        b. **Cathartics** are agents with purgative actions
        c. It is proposed that stimulant laxatives modify the permeability of the colonic mucosal cells, which results in intraluminal fluid and electrolyte secretion
        d. Defecation occurs between 6 to 12 hours after oral administration of these agents
        e. Rectal administration of bisacodyl and senna produces catharsis within 15 minutes to 2 hours
    2. Common medications (see Table 7-4 again)
    3. Administration considerations
        a. Bedtime administration of dose promotes a morning bowel movement
        b. Swallow tablet whole; do not crush
        c. Do not take within 1 hour of antacids, or milk
        d. Mix castor oil with 8 oz of water or juice; this drug is usually limited to use for rapid bowel evacuation, such as before radiological procedures
    4. Contraindications
        a. Contraindicated with abdominal pain, nausea and vomiting, symptoms of appendicitis, rectal bleeding, gastroenteritis, intestinal obstruction, fecal impaction
        b. Castor oil may induce premature labor
        c. Use senna cautiously with nursing mothers as senna is excreted in breast milk
    5. Significant drug interactions: antacids and drugs that increase gastric pH may result in GI irritation or cramping
    6. Significant food interactions: do not take within 1 hour of milk
    7. Significant laboratory studies: none reported
    8. Side effects
        a. Nausea and vomiting, abdominal cramps, diarrhea, laxative dependence
        b. Muscle weakness, fluid and electrolyte imbalance
        c. Rectal burning or irritation with suppository use
    9. Adverse effects/toxicity
        a. Hypokalemia, hypocalcemia
        b. Metabolic acidosis or alkalosis
    10. Nursing considerations
        a. Evaluate for nausea and vomiting, abdominal pain, or diarrhea
        b. Evaluate for medication effectiveness
        c. Monitor for fluid and electrolyte imbalances
        d. Administer medication 1 hour before or after ingestion of milk or an antacid
        e. Encourage increased fluids and diet alterations to include increased amounts of high-fiber foods
        f. Evaluate for laxative dependence and offer counseling

Practice to Pass

What substance can be given to counteract the effects of ipecac syrup?

11. Client education

  a. Discourage client from chronic use of laxatives; use beyond 1 week should be avoided

  b. These agents may produce a cathartic colon if used for several years; the colon develops abnormal motor function, and on x-ray resembles ulcerative colitis; usually discontinuation of laxative use restores normal bowel function

  c. Increase fluid intake and diet high in fiber

  d. Report signs and symptoms of side effects immediately

  e. Take medications 1 hour before or after ingestion of milk or an antacid

C. Hyperosmotic cathartics

1. Action and use

  a. They increase osmotic pressure within the intestinal lumen, which results in luminal retention of water, softening the stool

  b. Lactulose is an unabsorbed disaccharide metabolized by colonic bacteria primarily to lactic acid, formic, and acetic acids

  c. It has been proposed that these organic acids may contribute to the osmotic effect

  d. Used for treatment of occasional constipation

  e. Used to reduce ammonia levels (Lactulose)

2. Common medications (see Table 7-4 again)

3. Administration considerations

  a. Glycerin is available only for rectal administration (suppository or enema) for treatment of acute constipation; its laxative effect occurs within 15 to 30 minutes

  b. Lactulose may require 24 to 48 hours for effect; it is also more costly and should be reserved for acute constipation

  c. Dissolve 17 grams Miralax in 8 oz water and use once daily for up to 2 weeks; it may take 2 to 4 days for results to occur

4. Contraindications

  a. Contraindicated in bowel obstruction

  b. Use lactulose cautiously in clients with diabetes mellitus

5. Significant drug interactions: antibiotics may decrease laxative effect by elimination of bacteria needed to digest active form

6. Significant food interactions: none reported

7. Significant laboratory studies: serum electrolyte levels

8. Side effects

  a. Glycerin: rectal irritation and burning, hyperemia of the rectal mucosa

  b. Lactulose and Miralax: flatulence, abdominal cramps and bloating, diarrhea

9. Adverse effects/toxicity: fluid and electrolyte imbalances

10. Nursing considerations

  a. Miralax should always be dissolved in 8 oz of water

  b. Dilute lactulose in water or juice to decrease sweet taste

  c. Monitor frequency and consistency of stools

  d. Monitor for electrolyte imbalances, especially in older adults

11. Client education

  a. Miralax should be dissolved in 8 oz water

  b. Medication may take 2 to 4 days for effect

  c. Contact prescriber if unusual bloating, cramping, or diarrhea occurs

  d. Prolonged use may result in electrolyte imbalance and laxative dependence

  e. Take medication with juice to improve taste

D. Stool softeners (surfactants)

1. Action and use

  a. Used on a scheduled basis for clients who are likely to become constipated, such as with hospitalization, bed rest, postsurgical status, and for those receiving opioid analgesic medications

      b. Stool softeners are often referred to as emollient laxatives

      c. They are anionic **surfactants** that lower the fecal surface tension in vitro by allowing water and lipid penetration

      d. Softening of the feces generally occurs after 1 to 3 days

      e. Some preparations combine a stool softener such as docusate sodium with a stimulant, such as casanthranol to make a single combination product (e.g., Pericolace)

      f. Used for constipation associated with dry, hard stools and to decrease strain of defecation

  2. Common medications (see Table 7-4 again)

  3. Administration considerations

      a. Do not give with mineral oil

      b. Offer fluids after each PO dose

  4. Contraindications

      a. Contraindicated with any hypersensitivity to the drug

      b. Contraindicated with intestinal obstruction, undiagnosed abdominal pain, vomiting or other signs of appendicitis, fecal impaction, or acute abdomen

      c. Docusate sodium should not be used by clients with congestive heart failure (CHF) because of sodium content

  5. Significant drug interactions: may increase absorption of mineral oil

  6. Significant food interactions: none reported

  7. Significant laboratory studies: none reported

  8. Side effects

      a. Mild abdominal cramping, diarrhea

      b. Dependence with long-term use or excessive use

      c. Bitter taste

  9. Adverse effects/toxicity (all rare)

      a. Throat irritation has occurred with docusate sodium solution

      b. Docusate potassium has been associated with hyperkalemia when used in clients who have renal insufficiency or renal failure

  10. Nursing considerations

      a. Monitor frequency and consistency of stools

      b. Monitor for electrolyte imbalances especially in older adults

  11. Client education

      a. Take medication with milk or juice to decrease bitter taste

      b. Increase fluid intake if not contraindicated by another condition such as CHF or renal failure

      c. It may require 1 to 3 days to soften fecal matter

      d. Consult with dietitian regarding dietary changes to increase fiber foods

      e. Avoid prolonged use

E. Lubricants

  1. Action and use

      a. Provide lubrication of feces and hinder water reabsorption into the colon

      b. Used to treat constipation and prepare client for bowel studies or surgery

  2. Common medication

      a. Mineral oil

      b. Usual adult dose is 12.5 to 45 mL at HS PO or 120 mL at HS rectal

  3. Administration considerations

      a. Mineral oil is indigestible, and its absorption is limited considerably in the non-emulsified formulation

      b. Onset of action when taken orally is 6 to 8 hours

4. Contraindications
   a. Abdominal pain, nausea, and vomiting
   b. Signs and symptoms of appendicitis or acute abdomen, and fecal impaction or bowel obstruction
5. Significant drug interactions
   a. Stool softeners increase mineral oil absorption
   b. May impair absorption of fat-soluble vitamins (A, D, E, K), anticoagulants, birth control pills, cardiac glycosides, and sulfonamides
6. Significant food interactions: do not give with food as it may delay gastric empty-ing, separate by 2 hours
7. Significant laboratory studies: none reported
8. Side effects
   a. Nausea and vomiting, diarrhea, abdominal cramps
   b. Decreased absorption of nutrients
   c. Laxative dependence may occur with excessive or long-term use
   d. Anal pruritis, irritation, and hemorrhoids
9. Adverse effects/toxicity: aspiration of the product may cause lipoid pneumonia
10. Nursing considerations
   a. Because of possible aspiration and diminished vitamin absorption, do not administer to young children (younger than 6 years of age), pregnant women, older adults, and debilitated clients
   b. Do not administer the medication at bedtime
   c. Avoid administration of drug to clients lying flat in bed because of risk of aspiration
   d. Do not give within 2 hours of food because of possible decrease in gastric emptying
   e. Cautionary use in older adults because of increased risk of aspiration
   f. Monitor medications and alter administration times to avoid decreased absorp-tion caused by mineral oil
11. Client education
   a. Avoid chronic use; fat-soluble vitamin absorption could be impaired
   b. Do not take mineral oil with stool softeners because of risk of toxic levels
   c. Mineral oil may leak through the anal sphincter; report side effects to health care provider
   d. Do not take medication when lying flat or at bedtime to reduce risk of aspira-tion of oil droplets

F. **Saline laxatives**
1. Action and use
   a. Magnesium, sulfate, phosphate, and citrate salts are used when rapid bowel evacuation is required, as in bowel evacuation in preparation for procedures or surgery
   b. The mechanism of action of these poorly absorbed ions is unclear, but it is believed that they produce an osmotic effect that increases intraluminal volume and stimulates peristalsis
   c. Magnesium may cause cholecystokinin release from the duodenal mucosa promoting increased fluid secretion and motility of the small intestine and colon
   d. Orally administered magnesium and sodium phosphate salts are effective within 30 minutes to 6 hours
   e. Phosphate-containing rectal enemas evacuate the bowel within 2 to 15 minutes
2. Common medications (see Table 7-4 again)

3. Administration considerations
   a. Use magnesium salts cautiously for clients with renal impairment because absorption of magnesium salts may cause hypermagnesemia
   b. Use sodium phosphate salts cautiously for clients with CHF when sodium restriction is necessary
4. Contraindications
   a. Saline agents are not recommended for children under 2 years of age because of the potential for hypocalcemia in this population
   b. Abdominal pain, nausea and vomiting, or other signs and symptoms of appendicitis or acute abdomen
   c. Intestinal obstruction, edema, CHF, megacolon or impaired renal function
5. Significant drug interactions: concomitant use with antacids may inactivate both
6. Significant food interactions: none reported
7. Significant laboratory studies: none reported
8. Side effects: cramping and urgency to defecate
9. Adverse effects/toxicity
   a. Safe when administered for short-term management
   b. They may cause significant fluid and electrolyte imbalances when used for prolonged periods or in certain clients
10. Nursing considerations
    a. Dehydration and electrolyte imbalances may occur from repeated administration without appropriate fluid replacement
    b. Encourage increased fluid intake
    c. Monitor drug effectiveness
11. Client education
    a. Use appropriate dose and avoid frequent or prolonged use due to risk of laxative dependence
    b. Report side effects or lack of effectiveness to health care provider
    c. Increase fluid intake as allowed or tolerated

V. ANTIEMETICS

A. Action and use

1. Emesis is a complex reflex brought about by activation of the vomiting center (a nucleus of neurons located in the medulla oblongata)
2. Certain stimuli activate the vomiting center directly (e.g., gastrointestinal irritation) while other stimuli (e.g., drugs, toxins, radiation) act within the medulla to stimulate the chemoreceptor trigger zone (CTZ); presumably, it is by altering the function of these neuroreceptors that emetogenic compounds and antiemetic drugs produce their effects
3. Receptors involved are influenced by acetylcholine, histamine, serotonin, dopamine, benzodiazepines, and cannabinoids
4. Phenothiazines: suppress emesis by blockade of dopamine receptors in the CTZ
5. Butyrophenones: suppress emesis by blocking dopamine receptors in the CTZ
6. Metoclopramide: inhibits dopamine receptors in CTZ
7. Cannabinoids are approved to treat nausea and vomiting associated with cancer chemotherapy; mechanism of action is unknown
8. Dronabinol is also approved as an appetite stimulant for clients with acquired immunodeficiency syndrome (AIDS)
9. Benzodiazepines: primary effect is suppression of anxiety; most effective for management of cancer chemotherapy–associated nausea and vomiting when combined with metoclopramide and dexamethasone

10. Glucocorticoids: mechanism for suppression of emesis is unknown; they are effective alone and in combination with other antiemetics in the treatment of emesis associated with cancer chemotherapy
11. Antihistamines: anticholinergic effect reducing motion sickness and vomiting
12. Ondansetron: blocks serotonin receptors to reduce nausea
13. Aprepitant: a substance P and neurokinin 1 receptor antagonist that does not affect serotonin

B. **Common medications (Table 7-5)**
C. **Administration considerations**
1. Frequently, antiemetic combinations are more beneficial than single-drug treatment, particularly for cancer chemotherapy management of emesis; this may suggest that there is more than one mechanism triggering the emesis
2. As a rule, prophylactic drugs are generally given by mouth; however, management of active emesis is usually through parenteral or rectal administration of medications

Table 7-5 Antiemetics

Generic (Trade) Name	Route	Uses
Aprepitant (Emend)	PO	Combined with other antiemetics to prevent acute or prolonged nausea and vomiting (N/V) associated with emetogenic cancer chemotherapy, particularly high-dose cisplatin
Buclizine hydrochloride (Bucladin-S)	PO	Control N/V and dizziness associated with motion sickness
Chlorpromazine HCl (Chlopromanyl, Thorazine)	PO, suppository	Control N/V and intractable hiccups
Cyclizine (Marezine)	PO	Control N/V and dizziness associated with motion
Dolasetron mesylate (Anzemet)	PO, IM, IV	Prevent N/V associated with chemotherapy, prevent and treat postoperative N/V
Dronabinol (Delta-9 tetrahydrocannabinol)	PO	N/V associated with cancer chemotherapy in clients who do not respond to other antiemetic medications
Granisetron hydrochloride (Kytril)	IV	Prevent N/V associated with chemotherapy, prevent and treat postoperative N/V
Hydroxyzine hydrochloride (Vistaril)	PO, IM	Treat N/V
Meclizine hydrochloride (Antivert)	PO	Prevent N/V and motion sickness
Metoclopramide (Reglan)	PO, IM, IV	Prophylaxis of postoperative nausea
Ondansetron hydrochloride (Zofran)	PO, IV	Treat N/V associated with chemotherapy or postoperative N/V
Palonosetron hydrochloride (Aloxi)	IV	Prevent N/V associated with chemotherapy
Perphenazine (Apo-Perphenazine, Phenazine, Trilafon)	PO, IM, IV	Severe N/V and intractable hiccups
Prochlorperazine (Compazine)	PO, IM, IV	Severe N/V
Promethazine hydrochloride (Phenergan)	PO, IM, IV	N/V and motion sickness
Scoplamine (Transderm Scop)	Topical	N/V and motion sickness
Thiethylperazine maleate (Torecan)	IM	N/V and vertigo
Trimethobenzamide hydrochloride (Tigan, Trimazide)	PO, suppository, IM, IV	Treat N/V

3. Anticipatory nausea and vomiting should be treated 1 hour before meals or treatment
4. Parenteral preparations should be given deep IM to avoid leakage of the drug into the subcutaneous tissues

D. Contraindications

1. Generally contraindicated with CNS depression and coma
2. Use cautiously in clients with glaucoma, seizures, intestinal obstruction, prostatic hyperplasia, asthma, and cardiac, pulmonary, or hepatic disease
3. Aprepitant is contraindicated with hypersensitivity, lactation, or concurrent use of pimozide
4. Use Aprepitant cautiously with warfarin, vinblastine, vincristine, docetaxel, ironotecen, imatinib, and paclitaxel
5. Dolasetron mesylate is contraindicated with prolonged QT interval or second- or third-degree AV block
6. Dronabinol is contraindicated with allergy to sesame oil, or with use of ritonavir, alcohol, sedatives or hypnotics, psychotomimetics, or tricyclic antidepressants

E. Significant drug interactions

1. Epinephrine including ephedrine, may increase hypotension
2. Avoid use with MAO inhibitors
3. Antihistamines and CNS depressants may increase CNS depression
4. Levodopa may have decreased action
5. Phenytoin may increase toxicity
6. Meclizine may mask signs of ototoxicity with such medications as aminoglycosides, salicylates, and loop diuretics
7. Glucocorticoids cause hyperglycemia
8. Rifampin decreases dolasetron levels

F. Significant food interactions: none reported

G. Significant laboratory studies

1. Monitor BUN and creatinine (kidney function)
2. May mask response of skin testing; discontinue 4 days prior to testing
3. May cause hyperglycemia, false-positive or false-negative pregnancy test, may increase liver enzyme levels
4. Dexamethasone may increase glucose and cholesterol levels, decrease potassium, calcium, and thyroxine levels

H. Side effects

1. Phenothiazines can produce extrapyramidal reactions, anticholinergic effects, hypotension, and sedation; be alert for aspiration
2. Butyrophenones can also produce extrapyramidal reactions, sedation, and hypotension
3. Cannabinoids may cause temporal disintegration, dissociation, depersonalization, and dysphoria

I. Adverse effects/toxicity

1. Cannabinoids are contraindicated for clients with psychiatric disorders
2. Phenothiazines: agranulocytosis, thrombocytopenia

J. Nursing considerations

1. Dronabinol and nabilone have a high potential for abuse
2. Check vital signs regularly for risk of hypotension or tachycardia
3. Observe for side effects and adverse reactions
4. Monitor I & O for urine retention
5. Obtain baseline electrocardiogram with dolasetron
6. Observe for mood changes or involuntary movements
7. Monitor lab values: liver function tests, electrolytes, and renal function (blood urea nitrogen and creatinine)
8. Store dronabinol in refrigerator

9. Ensure client safety
10. Monitor for anticholinergic effects: dry mouth, constipation, or visual changes

K. Client education
1. Avoid activities that require alertness
2. Report adverse effects to health care provider
3. Avoid alcohol and CNS depressant drugs
4. Diabetic clients need to monitor blood glucose
5. Take medications as prescribed
6. Avoid excessive sunlight and ultraviolet light because of risk for photosensitivity
7. Use sugarless hard candy or ice chips to avoid dry mouth
8. Increase fluids and dietary fiber to decrease risk of constipation
9. Take medication 30 to 60 minutes before any activity that causes nausea for best effect

VI. HISTAMINE H₂ ANTAGONISTS

A. Action and use
1. Reduce gastric acid secretion by blocking histamine H_2 in the gastric parietal cells
2. Reduce total pepsin output
3. Histamine **H_2 antagonists** (agents against histamine decreasing gastric secretion) are used to treat duodenal ulcer, gastric ulcer, hypersecretory conditions such as Zollinger-Ellison syndrome, reflux esophagitis
4. Used to prevent stress ulcers in critically ill clients, and as combination therapy to treat *Helicobacter pylori* (bacteria found in gastric mucosa) infection

B. Common medications (Table 7-6)

C. Administration considerations
1. Intravenous (IV) administered drugs should not be mixed with other medications
2. Avoid antacid use within 1 hour of administration
3. May be given as single dose, twice daily, or with meals and at bedtime

D. Contraindications
1. Hypersensitivity to drug
2. Use caution in clients with impaired renal or hepatic function

Table 7-6 **Histamine H_2 Antagonists**

Generic (Trade) Name	Route	Uses
Cimetidine (Tagamet)	PO, IM, IV	Short-term treatment for duodenal ulcer or benign gastric ulcer, pathological hypersecretory condition such as Zollinger-Ellison syndrome, prophylactic of stress-induced ulcers, acute upper GI bleeding in critically ill clients, gastroesophageal reflux disease, heartburn and indigestion
Famotidine (Pepcid)	PO, IV	Short-term treatment for duodenal ulcer or benign gastric ulcer, pathological hypersecretory condition such as Zollinger-Ellison syndrome, prophylactic of stress-induced ulcers, acute upper GI bleeding in critically ill clients, gastroesophageal reflux disease, heartburn and indigestion
Nizatidine (Axid)	PO	Short-term treatment of duodenal ulcer and benign gastric ulcer, gastroesophageal reflux disease, prevention of heartburn and acid indigestion
Ranitidine hydrochloride (Zantac)	PO, IM, IV	Short-term treatment for duodenal ulcer or benign gastric ulcer, pathological hypersecretory condition such as Zollinger-Ellison syndrome, prophylactic of stress-induced ulcers, acute upper GI bleeding in critically ill clients, gastroesophageal reflux disease, heartburn and indigestion, erosive esophagitis

E. **Significant drug interactions**
1. Decreased ketaconazole absorption with famotidine
2. Cimetidine: decreased metabolism of beta-adrenergic blockers, phenytoin, lidocaine, procainamide, quinidine, benzodiazepines, metronidazole, tricyclic antidepressants, oral contraceptives, and warfarin causing increased risk of toxicity
3. Cimetidine alters absorption of ketoconazole, ferrous salts, indomethacin and tetracyclines, and may decrease concentration of digoxin
4. Nizatidine may increase salicylate levels with high doses of aspirin
5. Ranitidine may increase diazepam absorption, increase hypoglycemic effects of glipizide, increase procainamide levels and increase warfarin effect

F. **Significant food interactions**: none reported

G. **Significant laboratory studies**
1. Ranitidine: false-positive urine prolactin
2. Cimetidine: false-negative allergen skin test, increased prolactin, alkaline phosphatase and creatinine levels and may alter gastroccult testing caused by blue dye used in tablets
3. Famotidine may cause false-negative allergen results and may increase liver enzyme levels
4. Nizatidine may cause false-positive urobilinogen

H. **Side effects**
1. Somnolence, diaphoresis, rash, headache, hypotension
2. Taste disorder, diarrhea, constipation, dry mouth
3. Cardiac dysrhythmias
4. Impotence with cimetidine

I. **Adverse effects/toxicity**
1. Rare but may include agranulocytosis, neutropenia, thrombocytopenia, aplastic anemia, and pancytopenia
2. Anaphylaxis

J. **Nursing considerations**
1. Reduced dosages usually required for clients with hepatic or renal impairment
2. Assess medications for possible interactions
3. Evaluate nutritional status and dietary interventions
4. Evaluate need for smoking cessation and alcoholic abuse programs
5. Give cimetidine with meals and at bedtime

K. **Client education**
1. Avoid smoking, which causes gastric stimulation
2. Avoid **antacid** (agent reducing acidity) use within 1 hour of dose
3. Take medications only as directed
4. Once-a-day dosage should be taken at bedtime; if prescribed more than daily, take before meals
5. Avoid gastric irritants such as alcohol, aspirin, or nonsteroidal anti-inflammatory drugs (NSAIDs)
6. Report any side effects to health care provider
7. Cigarette smoking decreases drug effectiveness

Practice to Pass

What information would you share with a pregnant female client with peptic ulcer disease who asks you about taking misoprostol (Cytotec)?

VII. PROTON PUMP INHIBITORS

A. **Action and use**
1. Block acid production by inhibiting the H+ 2 K + ATPase at the secretory surface of the gastric parietal cells, thereby blocking the formation of gastric acid
2. Used for treatment of erosive or ulcerative gastroesophageal reflux disease (GERD) or duodenal ulcers, active benign gastric ulcers, and nonsteroidal anti-inflammatory drug (NSAID)–associated gastric ulcers (short term)

Table 7-7	Proton Pump Inhibitors	
Generic (Trade) Name	Route	Uses
Esomeprazole (Nexium)	PO	GERD, heartburn, erosive esophagitis, duodenal ulcer, duodenal ulcer with *Helicobacter pylori*, gastric ulcer related to nonsteroidal anti-inflammatory drugs (NSAIDs)
Lansoprazole (Prevacid)	PO	Short-term treatment of erosive esophagitis, GERD, duodenal or gastric ulcer, long-term treatment of pathological hypersecretory conditions, maintenance therapy for healing erosive esophagitis and duodenal ulcers
Omeprazole (Losec, Prilosec, Zegerid)	PO	Heartburn, *Helicobacter pylori* with amoxicillin, metronidazole, and clarithromycin, treatment of pathological hypersecretory conditions, benign gastric ulcer, duodenal ulcer, first-line therapy for GERD
Pantoprazole (Pantoloc, Protonix, Protonix IV)	PO, IV	Short-term and long-term treatment of GERD, erosive esophagitis, pathological hypersecretory conditions such as Zollinger-Ellison syndrome, neoplastic conditions, peptic ulcer
Rabeprazole (Aciphex)	PO	*Helicobacter pylori*, pathological hypersecretory conditions such as Zollinger-Ellison syndrome, erosive and ulcerative GERD, daytime and nighttime heartburn

3. Used for healing and reduction in relapse rates of heartburn symptoms in erosive or ulcerative GERD (maintenance)
4. Used for treatment of pathological hypersecretory conditions such as Zollinger-Ellison syndrome (long term)

B. **Common medications (Table 7-7)**

C. **Administration considerations**
1. May give with antacids
2. If unable to swallow capsules, lansoprazole and esomeprazole capsules may be opened and sprinkled on applesauce before taking
3. To give per nasogastric (NG) tube, dilute capsule contents in 40 mL juice
4. Omeprazole, pantoprazole, and rabeprazole must be swallowed whole
5. Pantoprazole IV: should be administered over a period of 15 minutes at a rate not greater than 3 mg/min (7 mL/min)
6. Pantoprazole IV should be administered using the in-line filter provided

D. **Contraindications**: not recommended in children or nursing mothers

E. **Significant drug interactions**
1. Rabeprazole and pantoprazole may alter absorption of gastric pH dependent drugs such as ketoconazole, digoxin, iron preparations, and ampicillin
2. Esomeprazole may affect drugs metabolized by CYP2C19
3. Lansoprazole may alter theophylline levels; give at least 30 minutes before sucralfate
4. Omeprazole may potentiate diazepam, phenytoin, and warfarin
5. Omeprazole should be taken 30 minutes before sucralfate; it may alter absorption of pH dependent medications
6. Hypoglycemia could occur if rabeprazole is combined with itraconazole or gemfibrozil
7. Esomeprazole increases serum levels and increases risk of toxicity of benzodiazepines
8. Esomeprazole interferes with absorption of ketoconazole, iron salts, and digoxin

F. **Significant food interactions**: none reported but administer before meals

G. **Significant laboratory studies**
1. May increase liver enzymes
2. Monitor theophylline levels with lansoprazole (Prevacid)
3. May need to monitor diazepam and phenytoin levels and prothrombin times more frequently with omeprazole (Prilosec)

H. Side effects
1. Headache, diarrhea, constipation, abdominal pain, nausea, flatulence
2. Rash, hyperglycemia, dizziness, pruritis, dry mouth
3. Injection site reaction with pantoprazole

I. Adverse effects/toxicity
1. Pancreatitis, liver necrosis, hepatic failure, toxic epidermal necrolysis
2. Stevens–Johnson syndrome
3. Agranulocytosis, myocardial infarction (MI), shock, cerebral vascular accident (CVA)
4. GI hemorrhage

J. Nursing considerations
1. Dosage should be reduced in severe liver disease
2. Document reason for therapy, duration of symptoms, and drug efficacy
3. Monitor for side effects
4. Monitor laboratory test results including liver function tests, CBC, and measures of renal function (BUN, creatinine)
5. Review any diagnostic findings
6. Assess for pregnancy or lactation
7. Increase water intake to 8 to 10 glasses per day to prevent constipation

K. Client education
1. Be aware of side effects; report diarrhea
2. Take medications as prescribed; do not increase dose
3. Follow prescribed diet and activities to decrease symptoms
4. Medication is generally for short-term therapy; keep health care appointments for treatment of continued signs and symptoms
5. Esomeprazole and omeprazole should be taken before meals
6. Notify health care provider of any difficulty swallowing since omeprazole, pantoprazole, and rabeprazole must be swallowed whole
7. Lansoprazole and esomeprazole capsules may be opened and sprinkled

Practice to Pass

A proton pump inhibitor has been ordered for a client with recent cerebral vascular accident (CVA). What nursing assessment should be performed?

VIII. MUCOSAL PROTECTIVE AGENTS

A. Action and use
1. Misoprostol (Cytotec) inhibits gastric secretion, protects gastric mucosa by increasing bicarbonate and mucus production and decreases pepsin levels
2. Sucralfate (Carafate) protects the site of ulcer from gastric acid by forming an adherent coating with albumin and fibrinogen; it absorbs pepsin decreasing its activity
3. Misoprostol (Cytotec) is used for the prevention of gastric ulcers; investigational use with duodenal ulcers
4. Sucralfate (Carafate) is used for short-term treatment of duodenal ulcers with continued maintenance treatment at lower doses; investigational use for gastric ulcers

B. Common medications (Table 7-8)

Table 7-8 **Mucosal Protective Agents**

Generic (Trade) Name	Route	Uses
Misoprostol (Cytotec)	PO	Prevention of NSAID- or aspirin-induced gastric ulcers, gastric ulcer, duodenal ulcer
Sucralfate (Carafate)	PO	Short-term care for duodenal ulcer given up to 8 weeks, oral and esophageal ulcers related to radiation or chemotherapy, gastric ulcer, reflux and peptic esophagitis, gastritis related to aspirin or NSAID, stress ulcer

C. **Administration considerations**
1. Sucralfate should be taken 1 hour before meals and bedtime or 2 hours after meals
2. Sucralfate should be taken 2 hours after medications and not within 2 hours of antacids
3. Misoprostol should be taken on empty stomach and not within 30 minutes (before or after) food intake

D. **Contraindications**
1. Misoprostol is contraindicated in clients who are allergic to prostaglandins, or who are pregnant or lactating
2. Use cautiously with clients with renal impairment and clients older than 64 years old
3. Safety has not been established for children under 18 years old
4. Misoprostol may cause miscarriage with serious bleeding
5. No known contraindications with sucralfate but safety in children and during lactation is not fully established

E. **Significant drug interactions**
1. Sucralfate: decreased absorption of digoxin, fluoroquinolones, ketoconazole, phenytoin, quinidine, ranitidine, tetracycline, and theophylline; dosing medications 2 hours before sucralfate eliminates the interactions
2. Antacids may decrease binding of sucralfate
3. Misoprostol decreases the availability of aspirin

F. **Significant food interactions**: none reported

G. **Significant laboratory studies**
1. Misoprostol may decrease basal pepsin secretion
2. No laboratory interactions with sucralfate

H. **Side effects**
1. Dizziness, headache, constipation, diarrhea, nausea, vomiting, flatulence, dry mouth, and rash
2. Misoprostol may cause spotting, cramping, dysmenorrhea, menstrual disorders, and postmenopausal bleeding

I. **Adverse effects/toxicity**
1. Angioedema
2. Respiratory difficulty, laryngospasm
3. Seizures

J. **Nursing considerations**
1. Assess GI symptoms
2. Assess for pregnancy via serum test prior to beginning misoprostol and should be negative within first 2 weeks of therapy
3. Monitor concomitant medications
4. Give medications according to prescription
5. Monitor for side effects
6. Assess respiratory status, swallowing, or change in gag reflex

K. **Client education**
1. Avoid gastric irritants such as caffeine, alcohol, smoking, and spicy foods
2. Take medication as prescribed and do not share with others
3. Report side effects to health care provider for possible dosage change
4. Use contraception while on misoprostol
5. Female clients should report any abnormal vaginal bleeding
6. Do not take misoprostol if pregnant; if the client becomes pregnant while taking misoprostol, she should stop taking it
7. Avoid pregnancy at least 1 month or 1 menstrual cycle after stopping medication
8. Increase fluids and fiber to decrease constipation
9. Use antacids properly to decrease interaction
10. Report immediately any difficulty swallowing or breathing

IX. ANTACIDS

A. Action and use
1. Neutralize gastric acid
2. Used for symptomatic relief of hyperacidity associated with GI disorders
3. Used as an antiflatulent to alleviate symptoms of gas and bloating

B. Common medications (Table 7-9)

C. Administration considerations: antacids should be taken at least 2 hours apart from other drugs where a drug interaction may occur

D. Contraindications
1. Safety has not been established for use of antacids by lactating women
2. Magnesium hydroxide is contraindicated in the presence of abdominal pain, nausea, vomiting, diarrhea, severe renal dysfunction, fecal impaction, rectal bleeding, colostomy, and ileostomy
3. Aluminum carbonate antacids: prolonged use of high doses in presence of low serum phosphate
4. Calcium carbonate antacids: hypercalcemia and hypercalciuria, severe renal disease, renal calculi, GI hemorrhage or obstruction, dehydration
5. Dihydroxyaluminum sodium carbonate: aluminum sensitivity, severe renal disease, dehydration, clients on sodium-restricted diets

E. Significant drug interactions
1. Antacids increase the gastric pH, which may decrease the absorption of other drugs, such as digoxin, ciprofloxacin, ofloxacin, norfloxacin, phenytoin, iron supplements, isoniazid, ethambutol, and ketoconazole
2. Antacids may bind with other drugs, therefore decreasing the drug's absorption and effectiveness, such as tetracycline

Table 7-9 Antacids

Generic (Trade) Name	Route	Uses
Aluminum hydroxide (Amphogel)	PO	Relief of gastric acidity, esophageal reflux, hiatal hernia, duodenal ulcer
Aluminum carbonate (Basaljel)	PO	Relief of gastric acidity, esophageal reflux, hiatal hernia, duodenal ulcer
Aluminum phosphate (Phosphajel)	PO	Relief of gastric acidity, esophageal reflux, hiatal hernia, duodenal ulcer
Calcium acetate (PhosLo)	PO	Hyperacidity, acid indigestion, peptic esophagitis, hiatal hernia, control of hyperphosphatemia in chronic renal failure (CRF)
Calcium carbonate (Tums, Dicarbisol)	PO	Hyperacidity, acid indigestion, peptic esophagitis, hiatal hernia, control of hyperphosphatemia in CRF
Calcium citrate (Citracal)	PO	Hyperacidity, acid indigestion, peptic esophagitis, hiatal hernia, control of hyperphosphatemia in CRF
Calcium phosphate (Tricalcium phosphate)	PO	Hyperacidity, acid indigestion, peptic esophagitis, hiatal hernia, control of hyperphosphatemia in CRF
Magnesium hydroxide and aluminum hydroxide (Maalox)	PO	Peptic ulcer, hyperacidity, gastritis, peptic esophagitis, hiatal hernia
Magnesium hydroxide, aluminum hydroxide, and simethicone (Mylanta)	PO	Peptic ulcer, hyperacidity, gastritis, peptic esophagitis, hiatal hernia
Dihydroxyaluminum sodium carbonate (Rolaids)	PO	Peptic ulcer, hyperacidity, gastritis, peptic esophagitis, hiatal hernia

F. **Significant food interactions**: none reported
G. **Significant laboratory studies**: prolonged use of antacids may alter aluminum, calcium, sodium, and phosphate levels
H. **Side Effects**
1. Belching, constipation, flatulence, diarrhea
2. Gastric distention
3. Acid rebound if antacids are given frequently
I. **Adverse effects/toxicity**
1. Hypophosphatemia (anorexia, malaise, tremors, muscle weakness)
2. Aluminum toxicity (dementia) may occur with repeated dosing
3. Hypercalcemia and metabolic alkalosis may occur with antacids containing calcium carbonate
4. May worsen hypertension and heart failure from increased sodium intake with use of those antacids containing sodium carbonate
J. **Nursing considerations**
1. Shake suspension well
2. Flush NG tube with water after administration
3. Observe for signs and symptoms of altered phosphate levels: anorexia, muscle weakness, and malaise
K. **Client education**
1. Increase fluids, fiber, and exercise to avoid constipation
2. Take as directed; do not exceed maximum dose
3. Keep medication out of reach of children
4. Drink sufficient fluids (8–10 glasses/day)
5. Antacids may interact with certain medications; notify health care provider of any prescribed medications; do not take antacids within 45 minutes to 2 hours of other medications or absorption of other drug may be decreased
6. Do not use unless prescribed if diagnosed with kidney disease

X. ANTIMICROBIALS FOR *HELICOBACTER PYLORI* ORGANISMS

A. **Action and use**
1. Antisecretory and antimicrobial action against most strains of *Helicobacter pylori*
2. Used for eradication of *Helicobacter pylori* infection and reduce the risk of duodenal ulcer recurrence
B. **Common medications (Table 7-10)**

Table 7-10 Antimicrobials for *Helicobacter pylori*

Generic (Trade) Name	Usual Adult Dosage Range	Route
Lansoprazole, amoxicillin, clarithromycin (Prevpak)	bid for 10–14 days	PO
Bismuth subsalicylate, metronidazole, tetracycline (Helidac)	qid for 14 days	PO
Omeprazole, clarithromycin (Prilosec/Biaxin)	Omeprazole 40 mg daily and clarithromycin 500 mg tid for 2 weeks then omeprazole 20 mg daily for 2 weeks	PO
Ranitidine bismuth citrate, clarithromycin (Titrec/Biaxin)	Ranitidine bismuth citrate 400 mg bid and clarithromycin 500 mg tid for 2 weeks then ranitidine bismuth citrate 400 mg bid for 2 weeks	PO
Lansoprazole, amoxicillin (Prevacid/Amoxil)	Lansoprazole 30 mg and Amoxil 1 gram tid for 14 days	PO

C. Administration considerations
   1. Swallow all pills whole except bismuth, which should be chewed and not swallowed whole
   2. If dose is missed, continue with normal dosage regimen, do not double dose
D. Contraindications
   1. Allergy to any component of therapy
   2. Avoid coadministration with pimozide or terfenadine because of risk of cardiac dysrhythmias
   3. Pregnant women should not take regimens containing clarithromycin
E. Significant drug interactions
   1. May alter absorption of drugs dependent on gastric pH: ketoconazole, ampicillin, iron, or digoxin
   2. Safety in children is not established
F. Significant food interactions: none reported
G. Significant laboratory studies
   1. Abnormal liver function tests
   2. May increase theophylline levels
   3. May interfere with prothrombin times
   4. May alter serum levels of drugs metabolized by P450 enzyme system
H. Side effects
   1. Rash, nausea, vomiting, diarrhea, abnormal taste, abdominal pain, dyspepsia
   2. Headache, photosensitivity
   3. Transient CNS reactions such as anxiety, behavior changes, tinnitus, and vertigo
I. Adverse effects/toxicity: ventricular dysrhythmias
J. Nursing considerations
   1. Note signs and symptoms, onset, and duration of symptoms
   2. Document allergy status
   3. Determine pregnancy status
   4. Document previous therapies used
   5. Document confirmation of infection
K. Client education
   1. Compliance with drug therapy is important to eliminate infection
   2. Avoid gastric irritants such as smoking, alcohol, and caffeine
   3. Use stress reduction techniques as indicated
   4. Report side effects to prescriber
   5. Report continued symptoms to prescriber
   6. Bismuth-containing preparations may cause darkening of tongue and stool
   7. Review drug packaging as some preparations are prepackaged
   8. Do not double dose if dose is missed
   9. Use additional contraceptive measures as antibiotics can decrease birth control pill effectiveness
   10. Avoid prolonged exposure to sun

XI. MEDICATIONS USED TO DISSOLVE GALLSTONES

A. Action and use
   1. Ursodiol (Actigall) is used to dissolve gallbladder stones smaller than 20 mm; it is absorbed in the small bowel, secreted into hepatic bile ducts and expelled into the duodenum in response to eating; it is a natural-occurring bile acid that inhibits hepatic synthesis and secretion of cholesterol
   2. Chenodiol (Chenex) reduces cholesterol content of gallstones (must have high cholesterol content and not be radiopaque stones)
B. Common medications: Ursodiol (Actigall) and chenodiol (Chenix)
C. Administration considerations: use beyond 24 months has not been established

D. Contraindications
1. Do not use for clients with calcified cholesterol stones, radiopaque stones, or radiolucent bile pigment stones
2. Excretion in breast milk is not known, use with caution
3. Avoid in clients with acute cholecystitis, biliary obstruction, pancreatitis, allergy to bile acids, and chronic liver disease

E. **Significant drug interactions**: antacids and bile acid sequestrants (cholestyramine, colestipol) may interfere with the action of ursodiol by decreasing its absorption

F. **Significant food interactions**: none reported

G. **Significant laboratory studies**: none reported

H. Side effects
1. Nausea, vomiting, abdominal pain, constipation, diarrhea, rash
2. Headache, fatigue, anxiety, sweating
3. Thinning of hair, arthralgia

I. **Adverse effects/toxicity**: diarrhea

J. Nursing considerations
1. If no dissolution of partial stone is observed in 12 months, drug will probably not be effective
2. Gallbladder ultrasound should be done every 6 months the first year of therapy
3. Document indications and length of therapy
4. Determine pregnancy status
5. If infection present, combine with anti-infective agents

K. Client education
1. Avoid antacid use with drug unless prescribed
2. Therapy may take up to 24 months
3. Stones may recur
4. Limit dietary fat
5. Report any side effects to prescriber
6. Discuss contraceptive methods because birth control pills may decrease drug effect
7. Stress importance of follow up visits and diagnostic tests

XII. PANCREATIC ENZYME REPLACEMENT

A. Action and use
1. Replacement of pancreatic enzyme in conditions where there is a deficiency of exocrine pancreatic secretions, such as with cystic fibrosis, chronic pancreatitis, postpancreatectomy, steatorrhea, malabsorption syndrome, or postgastrectomy
2. Helps to digest fat, and absorb fat, proteins, and carbohydrates

B. Common medications (Table 7-11)

C. Administration considerations
1. Swallow tablets or capsules whole, do not crush or chew
2. If swallowing is difficult, open capsules and give contents in applesauce or pudding to swallow without chewing
3. Take medications with meals and snacks

D. Contraindications
1. Hypersensitivity to pork protein or enzymes
2. Contraindicated in acute pancreatitis

E. Significant drug interactions
1. If given with antacids the change in gastric pH may cause the enteric coated capsules to dissolve in the stomach and inactivate the product
2. Pancreatic lipase is inactivated at pH less than 4
3. If antacids allow the enteric coating to dissolve too soon, the drug will be inactivated by the gastric acid

Table 7-11	Pancreatic Enzyme Replacement (Lipase, Amylase, Protease)	
Generic (Trade) Name	**Usual Adult Dosage Range**	**Route**
Pancrelipase (Creon 5)	2–4 capsules with meals and snacks	PO
Pancrelipase (Ku-Zyme)	1–2 capsules with meals and snacks	PO
Pancrelipase (Pancrease)	400 lipase units/kg per meal	PO
Pancrelipase (Viokase)	1–4 tablets with meals	PO

Note: Dosage is adjusted on an individual basis according to extent of enzyme deficiency, dietary fat content, and enzyme activity of individual drug formulation.

4. This drug needs to travel into the less acidic duodenum before breaking down for therapeutic effect; if given with oral iron supplements the enzymes may decrease the effect of the iron

F. **Significant food interactions**: none reported

G. **Significant laboratory studies**: elevated serum uric acid

H. **Side effects**
   1. Nausea
   2. Diarrhea
   3. Abdominal cramps

I. **Adverse effects/toxicity**: hyperuricemia

J. **Nursing considerations**
   1. Monitor for side effects and monitor steatorrhea, as it should diminish with appropriate dose of medication
   2. Assess and monitor to maintain good nutritional status
   3. Document indications for therapy
   4. Document allergies
   5. Assess swallowing ability or difficulty

K. **Client education**
   1. Take before or with meals with plenty of water
   2. Report any side effects to health care provider
   3. Report joint pain and swelling
   4. Review dietary interventions with clients; consult with dietitian for counseling and meal planning

Case Study

A 45-year-old male client comes to the nurse practitioner stating he wakes often at night with coughing and burning he describes as heartburn. He drinks 1–2 alcoholic beverages per evening, usually with distilled liquor, and then wine with dinner. He eats heavy dinners with dessert. He prefers mint ice cream and coffee for dessert. The nurse practitioner prescribes a regimen with omeprazole (Prilosec) every morning and Maalox 30 mL qid.

1. How will you instruct the client about gastro-esophageal reflux disease and its relationship to symptoms?

2. What will you instruct the client about his diet, particularly the evening meal?

3. What medication will be prescribed if the client is diagnosed with *H. pylori?*

4. How will you instruct the client about his medications?

For suggested responses, see page 543.

POSTTEST

1 When the nurse teaches a client about the side effects of anticholinergic medications, what signs or symptoms should be included?

1. Urinary retention, constipation, or dilated pupils
2. Pupillary constriction, bronchoconstriction, or bradycardia
3. Inability to obtain an erection, irregular heart rhythm
4. Increased salivation, dysphagia, confusion, restlessness

2 A pregnant client asks the nurse about laxatives that are safe for use during pregnancy. After explaining that the health care provider should be consulted before using any drug, the nurse should instruct the client to abstain from using which laxative at any time during pregnancy?

1. Bisacodyl (Dulcolax)
2. Mineral oil (generic)
3. Castor oil (Neoloid)
4. Sodium bisphosphonate (Fleets Phospho-Soda)

3 After a family member reported altered mental function in a client with end-stage liver disease, the health care provider prescribed lactulose (Cephulac) 30 mL PO tid. The home health nurse reviews the client's chart for which laboratory test(s) to monitor medication effectiveness?

1. Alanine aminotransferase (ALT) and aspartate aminotransferase (AST)
2. Blood urea nitrogen (BUN) and creatinine
3. Bilirubin and urobilinogen
4. Serum ammonia

4 A client asks, "How does diphenoxylate (Lomotil) help stop diarrhea?" Which of the following is the *best* response by the nurse?

1. "It slows down the motility of the intestine thereby increasing fluid absorption."
2. "Because of the increased sodium in the stool fluid moves into the bloodstream."
3. "It increases the bulk in the intestines resulting decreased peristalsis."
4. "It decreases circulation of blood to the bowels making them less reactive to stimulation."

5 The nurse should consult with the prescriber if oral mineral oil is prescribed for which of the following clients? Select all that apply.

1. Client with dysphagia following a cerebral vascular accident (CVA)
2. Client who has suspected appendicitis
3. Client who has a fecal impaction
4. Client who has infrequent heartburn
5. Client who has steatorrhea

6 The nurse is selecting candidates for a health screening project regarding the abuse of laxatives. The *best* client group includes which of the following?

1. Older adult clients with congestive heart failure (CHF)
2. Clients with irritable bowel syndrome (IBS)
3. Clients with bulimia nervosa or anorexia nervosa
4. Clients who are obese

7 An otherwise healthy client diagnosed with cholecystitis reports to the emergency department with severe pain. The nurse is most likely to administer which of the following drugs with an appropriate order?

1. Codeine sulfate
2. Bethanecol (Urecholine)
3. Dicyclomine (Bentyl)
4. Morphine sulfate (generic)

8 A client has cholelithiasis, but is a poor surgical candidate because of comorbid conditions. The nurse is most likely to teach the client about which of the following medications?

1. Ursodiol (Actigall)
2. Omeprazole (Prilosec)
3. Cimetidine (Tagamet)
4. Ibuprofen (Motrin)

9 A client who has a history of a seizure disorder is newly diagnosed with a gastric ulcer. The client has maintained seizure-free status using phenytoin (Dilantin). The nurse would question a new order for which of the following drugs to treat symptoms caused by the ulcer?

1. Famotidine (Pepcid)
2. Cimetidine (Tagamet)
3. Nizatidine (Axid)
4. Ranitidine (Zantac)

10 A client has a new order to take bisacodyl (Dulcolax). To enhance a rapid medication effect, the nurse instructs the client to take the medication in which way?

1. On an empty stomach
2. With plenty of fluids
3. With meals
4. At bedtime

➤ See pages 250–251 for Answers and Rationales.

ANSWERS & RATIONALES

Pretest

1 **Answer: 2** **Rationale:** The ipecac syrup should have been discarded as it is no longer on the market. Vomiting should occur within 15–30 minutes after ingestion of ipecac. Activated charcoal absorbs ipecac syrup and decreases its effect by inhibiting absorption from the GI tract into the general circulation. If absorbed, ipecac can result in cardiotoxicity. While calling the poison control center may be necessary, it is not the highest priority action to ensure the safety of the client. Milk or carbonated drinks are used when poisons or hazardous chemicals need to be neutralized. The ipecac needs to be removed or bound to prevent absorption. This is an inappropriate time for teaching. **Cognitive Level:** Analyzing **Client Need:** Pharmacological and Parenteral Therapies **Integrated Process:** Nursing Process: Implementation **Content Area:** Pharmacology **Strategy:** Apply knowledge of drug characteristics to the question. The critical thinking question within the test item is, "What is the risk to the client if ipecac remains in the GI tract?" **Reference:** Wilson, B. A., Shannon, M., & Shields, K. (2011). *Pearson nurse's drug guide 2011.* Upper Saddle River, NJ: Pearson Education, pp. 299–300.

2 **Answer: 1** **Rationale:** Metoclopramide is a GI stimulant, increasing motility of the GI tract, shortening gastric emptying time, and thus reducing the risk of the esophagus being exposed to gastric contents. Decreased lower esophageal sphincter (LES) tone will increase the risk of gastric contents being regurgitated upward into the esophagus. Because the drug increases GI motility, it can cause diarrhea rather than combating it. GERD can place clients at increased risk for *H. pylori* bacterial infection; however, anti-infectives would be used to treat this infection. **Cognitive Level:** Applying **Client Need:** Pharmacological and Parenteral Therapies **Integrated Process:** Nursing Process: Evaluation **Content Area:** Pharmacology **Strategy:** First recall the pathophysiology of GERD. Consider that if GERD results in backward flow of gastric contents, it is logical for the drug prescribed to promote forward movement of gastric contents. **Reference:** Wilson, B. A., Shannon, M., & Shields, K. (2011). *Pearson nurse's drug guide 2011.* Upper Saddle River, NJ: Pearson Education, pp. 998–1000.

3 **Answer: 4** **Rationale:** Dicyclomine hydrochloride relieves GI smooth muscle spasm, alleviating the symptoms and leading to a balanced state of nutritional and fluid status. Presence of mucus in the stool is one of the Manning criteria associated with irritable bowel syndrome (IBS). During the recovery phase the weight should be stable with no further weight loss. Bowel sounds should be normal, not hypoactive. **Cognitive Level:** Analyzing **Client Need:** Pharmacological and Parenteral Therapies **Integrated Process:** Nursing Process: Evaluation **Content Area:** Pharmacology **Strategy:** The drug name Antispas is a clue that the drug is an antispasmodic by action. Recall that spasms are a major sign or symptom of irritable bowel syndrome (IBS) and focus on the data that is the most normal as the answer to the question. **Reference:** Wilson, B. A., Shannon, M., & Shields, K. (2011). *Pearson nurse's drug guide 2011.* Upper Saddle River, NJ: Pearson Education, pp. 464–466.

4 **Answer: 2** **Rationale:** Bismuth subsalicylate has a salicylate base and is contraindicated in clients who are allergic to aspirin, also known as acetylsalicylic acid. Attapulgite and loperamide may be given safely to a client allergic to aspirin. Diphenoxylate with atropine contains codeine as well as atropine as ingredients. **Cognitive Level:** Applying **Client Need:** Pharmacological and Parenteral Therapies **Integrated Process:** Nursing Process: Planning **Content Area:** Pharmacology **Strategy:** Associate the word *salicylate* with aspirin and use the process of elimination to pick the medication that contains salicylate in the generic name. **Reference:** Wilson, B. A., Shannon, M., & Shields, K. (2011). *Pearson nurse's drug guide 2011.* Upper Saddle River, NJ: Pearson Education, pp. 183–184.

5 **Answer: 4** **Rationale:** Metamucil is a bulk-forming laxative that could aggravate diarrhea, and this statement indicates that the client has a lack of understanding. The other statements made by the client are true and indicate proper understanding. Dairy products may aggravate diarrhea and it is helpful to avoid these during a bout of diarrhea. Kaopectate is an antidiarrheal agent that is commonly used to manage this health problem, which is usually self-limiting. The client should contact the health care provider if diarrhea persists more than 2 days. **Cognitive Level:** Applying **Client Need:** Pharmacological and Parenteral Therapies **Integrated Process:** Nursing Process: Evaluation **Content Area:** Pharmacology **Strategy:** The critical words in the question are *further instructions*, indicating that the correct option is an incorrect client statement. Associate the primary problem (diarrhea) with the action of Metamucil (accelerated peristalsis). Since this drug would worsen the client's symptoms, this is the incorrect statement and is therefore the answer to the question. **Reference:** Wilson, B. A., Shannon, M., & Shields, K. (2011). *Pearson nurse's drug guide 2011.* Upper Saddle River, NJ: Pearson Education, pp. 1313–1314.

6 **Answer: Rationale:** Docusate sodium (Colace) is appropriate for the postoperative client taking opioid analgesics, the client who had a myocardial infarction 24 hours ago, and the client with painful hemorrhoids. The client preparing for a colonoscopy would likely use a stimulant laxative and the client trying to reduce the chances of chronic constipation would likely use a bulk-forming laxative. **Cognitive Level:** Analyzing **Client Need:** Pharmacological and Parenteral Therapies **Integrated Process:** Nursing Process: Assessment **Content Area:** Pharmacology **Strategy:** Recall the specific drug action of a stool softener and match that to the benefit needed in a client with the conditions listed. Note that the wording of the question indicates that more than one option is correct. **Reference:** Adams, M. P., & Koch, R. W. (2010). *Pharmacology: Connections to nursing practice.* Upper Saddle River, NJ: Pearson Education, pp. 1030–1032.

7 **Answer: 2 Rationale:** Laxatives are included on the list of drugs in which misuse results in addiction. A healthy client who regularly ingests a laxative needs to be taught about laxatives and addiction. A fluid and/or electrolyte imbalance may be present, but the primary focus is to address the cause and not the outcome. Since the client is healthy, one can presume the nutritional status is adequate. **Cognitive Level:** Applying **Client Need:** Pharmacological and Parenteral Therapies **Integrated Process:** Teaching and Learning **Content Area:** Pharmacology **Strategy:** The critical terms are *healthy* and *9 months*. The term *healthy* indicates the laxative is not needed physically, suggesting that there may be a psychosocial concern. Focus on the term *9 months* to apply principles of drug misuse or abuse. **Reference:** Adams, M. P., & Koch, R. W. (2010). *Pharmacology: Connections to nursing practice.* Upper Saddle River, NJ: Pearson Education, pp. 1030–1032.

8 **Answer: 4 Rationale:** Loperamide is indicated for the treatment of diarrhea. If this is a new order, then critical thinking suggests that the diarrhea is relatively new in onset. Placing a commode at the bedside would provide

for proper management of an older adult client with diarrhea. There is no evidence that ingestion of normal dosages of this drug usually causes seizures. There is also no evidence that ingestion of normal dosages of this drug places the client at significant risk for falls or significant changes in vital signs. **Cognitive Level:** Applying **Client Need:** Management of Care **Integrated Process:** Communication and Documentation **Content Area:** Pharmacology **Strategy:** First recognize that the drug in the question is an antidiarrheal agent, and then select the option that addresses meeting bowel elimination needs in an older adult client. **Reference:** Wilson, B. A., Shannon, M., & Shields, K. (2011). *Pearson nurse's drug guide 2011.* Upper Saddle River, NJ: Pearson Education, pp. 910–911.

9 **Answer: 2, 4, 5 Rationale:** Discussion of feelings with another person helps the client manage emotional reactions. The nurse does not know why the client is crying. Although the client is emotionally upset, the nurse is obligated to inform the client of the risks associated with refusing medication. Although the client does need to know that ranitidine (Zantac) is an H_2-receptor blocker that reduces gastric acid production, resulting in less exposure of the open crater to irritants, the client does not appear to be ready for teaching. Because it seals the open crater and protects it from gastric contents, misoprostol (Cytotec) is commonly used in open-crater gastric ulcers. The nurse should encourage the client to take the medication to reduce risk of perforation. **Cognitive Level:** Analyzing **Client Need:** Pharmacological and Parenteral Therapies **Integrated Process:** Communication and Documentation **Content Area:** Pharmacology **Strategy:** Discriminate between risks to the client and client needs. Think about the conditions that would assure client rights and guarantee quality nursing care. **Reference:** Wilson, B. A., Shannon, M., & Shields, K. (2011). *Pearson nurse's drug guide 2011.* Upper Saddle River, NJ: Pearson Education, pp. 1024–1025.

10 **Answer: 4, 2, 3, 5, 1 Rationale:** Misoprostol is administered for open-cratered gastric ulcers. The nurse may want to elevate the head of the bed because of the high risk of aspiration of blood. Maintaining an airway and breathing are high in priority. One side effect is abdominal pain, and increased restlessness could indicate the client is experiencing pain, making this second in priority. Ingestion of misoprostol (Cytotec) can result in diarrhea. To prevent skin breakdown, placing a bed protector beneath the buttocks as the third action will help the skin to remain clean and dry. A log would help determine the bowel pattern and would be done fourth as it is a routine care activity. One side effect of the drug is spotting. This problem lacks the immediacy of aspiration, pain, and maintaining skin integrity, and would be done last if it occurs. **Cognitive Level:** Analyzing **Client Need:** Pharmacological and Parenteral Therapies **Integrated Process:** Nursing Process: Planning **Content Area:** Pharmacology **Strategy:** Make decisions about the priorities by determining what will place the client most at risk, followed by routine care activities and then items that may not occur at all. **Reference:** Wilson, B. A., Shannon, M., & Shields, K. (2011). *Pearson nurse's drug guide 2011.* Upper Saddle River, NJ: Pearson Education, pp. 1024–1025.

Posttest

1 **Answer: 1** **Rationale:** Anticholinergic effects include drying of mucous membranes, dilated pupils, and decreased motility of the GI tract, which may result in constipation. Pupillary constriction, bronchoconstriction, and bradycardia are the opposite of anticholinergic outcomes. The parasympathetic system participates in establishing an erection, hence, blockers would result in erectile dysfunction, and the drugs increase the heart rate. Because dry mouth is an anticholinergic effect, excessive salivation is incorrect. **Cognitive Level:** Applying **Client Need:** Pharmacological and Parenteral Therapies **Integrated Process:** Teaching and Learning **Content Area:** Pharmacology **Strategy:** Recall that when there is more than one part to an option, all parts must be correct for that option to be correct. Next, recall that side effects are exaggerations of parasympathetic function to help you choose correctly. **Reference:** Adams, M. P., & Koch, R. W. (2010). *Pharmacology: Connections to nursing practice.* Upper Saddle River, NJ: Pearson Education, pp. 214–217.

2 **Answer: 3** **Rationale:** Because it may induce premature labor, castor oil (Neoloid) is a Pregnancy Category X preparation. Bisacodyl (Dulcolax) is Pregnancy Category C, while mineral oil and sodium bisphosphonate (Fleets Phospho-Soda) are listed as unknown. It is recommended that the client utilize preventive methods such as adequate dietary fiber and at least 8 glasses of fluid per day. **Cognitive Level:** Applying **Client Need:** Pharmacological and Parenteral Therapies **Integrated Process:** Teaching and Learning **Content Area:** Pharmacology **Strategy:** Correlate the characteristics of the laxative with the risks to the fetus. Specific knowledge is needed to answer this question. **Reference:** Adams, M. P., & Koch, R. W. (2010). *Pharmacology: Connections to nursing practice.* Upper Saddle River, NJ: Pearson Education, pp. 1030–1032.

3 **Answer: 4** **Rationale:** Elevated serum ammonia levels are commonly associated with hepatic encephalopathy. AST and ALT are liver enzymes indicating liver impairment. The enzyme level does not have a direct relationship to the cause of the impaired mental function. BUN and creatinine levels provide evidence of renal function. Bilirubin is elevated and urobilinogen may be normal or decreased in liver disease. Neither test would provide information regarding the hepatic encephalopathy. **Cognitive Level:** Applying **Client Need:** Pharmacological and Parenteral Therapies **Integrated Process:** Nursing Process: Assessment **Content Area:** Pharmacology **Strategy:** Correlate the altered mental function with the elevated ammonia levels. Next, recall that this medication helps to reduce ammonia levels in clients with severe liver disease. **Reference:** Wilson, B. A., Shannon, M., & Shields, K. (2011). *Pearson nurse's drug guide 2011.* Upper Saddle River, NJ: Pearson Education, pp. 725–726.

4 **Answer: 1** **Rationale:** Diphenoxylate (Lomotil) inhibits nerve endings that cause the intestinal movement. Decreasing the velocity increases opportunity for absorption of fluid resulting in increased viscosity of the stools. The drug is a narcotic with a structure similar to meperidine (Demerol) and has no effect on the shifts of sodium Increased bulk would increase peristalsis. The drug primarily affects the nervous system and not the circulatory system **Cognitive Level:** Analyzing **Client Need:** Pharmacological and Parenteral Therapies **Integrated Process:** Teaching and Learning **Content Area:** Pharmacology **Strategy:** The core issue of the question is specific information about the drug action of diphenoxylate (Lomotil). Associate "low" mobility (motil) with Lomotil. **Reference:** Wilson, B. A., Shannon, M., & Shields, K. (2011). *Pearson nurse's drug guide 2011.* Upper Saddle River, NJ: Pearson Education, pp. 493–494.

5 **Answer: 1, 2, 3, 5** **Rationale:** Mineral oil should not be administered to clients with swallowing problems due to increased risk of aspiration leading to lipoid pneumonia. If a drug that may increase peristalsis is introduced it may intensify the signs or symptoms or blur the clinical picture in a client with appendicitis. The client with fecal impaction needs to be disimpacted and may require enemas. Steatorrhea causes excessive stimulation of peristalsis because of the excessive fat content in the stool. There is no contraindication to giving this medication to a client with occasional heartburn, since this is likely due to food intolerance. **Cognitive Level:** Applying **Client Need:** Pharmacological and Parenteral Therapies **Integrated Process:** Nursing Process: Planning **Content Area:** Pharmacology **Strategy:** Correlate the clinical profile of the diseases or alterations with the actions of the drug. **Reference:** Adams, M. P., & Koch, R. W. (2010). *Pharmacology: Connections to nursing practice.* Upper Saddle River, NJ: Pearson Education, pp. 1030–1031.

6 **Answer: 3** **Rationale:** Clients with eating disorders such as anorexia nervosa or bulimia nervosa are most likely to abuse laxatives. Older adults often believe having a stool every day is healthy and they are also a group that may excessively use laxatives, but they are not as at risk as clients who have eating disorders. Clients with irritable bowel syndrome (IBS) are not likely to disturb the GI tract with drugs that could further irritate the tissue. Clients who are obese are more likely to be inactive and ingest diets high in fat and cholesterol. **Cognitive Level:** Analyzing **Client Need:** Pharmacological and Parenteral Therapies **Integrated Process:** Nursing Process: Assessment **Content Area:** Pharmacology **Strategy:** First eliminate 2 options because they are least likely to abuse laxatives overall. Next associate the characteristic of laxative abuse with the group most likely to demonstrate compulsive behaviors, which helps you to choose correctly between the clients who are older adults and those with eating disorders. **Reference:** Adams, M. P., & Koch, R. W. (2010). *Pharmacology: Connections to nursing practice.* Upper Saddle River, NJ: Pearson Education, pp. 1030–1032.

7 **Answer: 4** **Rationale**: Morphine sulfate (generic) is the drug of choice of the options listed because it is an opioid analgesic that is strong enough to relieve the pain, and it does not intensify biliary spasms, although this was a widely held notion in the past. Codeine sulfate is not utilized because it is a weaker opioid analgesic, although morphine sulfate is commonly administered. Bethanecol (Urecholine) is a cholinergic drug that results in increased smooth muscle tone and motility. Dicyclomine (Bentyl) is an antispasmodic that could decrease the biliary spasms, but is not an analgesic. The pain is also related to the inflammatory process. **Cognitive Level**: Applying **Client Need**: Pharmacological and Parenteral Therapies **Integrated Process**: Nursing Process: Planning **Content Area**: Pharmacology **Strategy**: The core issue of the question is which drug will relieve severe pain in a client with cholecystitis. Eliminate 2 options because they are not opioid analgesics. Choose between the remaining 2 options because 1 is stronger. Correlate the best remedy in relation to the total disease profile. **Reference**: Wilson, B. A., Shannon, M., & Shields, K. (2011). *Pearson nurse's drug guide 2011*. Upper Saddle River, NJ: Pearson Education, pp. 436–438.

8 **Answer: 1** **Rationale**: Ursodiol (Actigall) is a naturally occurring bile acid used to dissolve gallstones. It is believed to suppress hepatic synthesis and secretion of cholesterol as well as intestinal absorption. Omeprazole (Prilosec) is a proton pump inhibitor that reduces gastric acid production. Cimetidine (Tagamet) is an H_2 antagonist that reduces gastric acid production, but is not designed to treat cholelithiasis. Ibuprofen (Motrin) is a nonsteroidal anti-inflammatory drug (NSAID) and may be needed should the client develop a fever secondary to the process of inflammation. **Cognitive Level**: Applying **Client Need**: Pharmacological and Parenteral Therapies **Integrated Process**: Nursing Process: Planning **Content Area**: Pharmacology **Strategy**: The wording of the question suggests that the correct answer will be a drug that will treat the gallstones since surgery is not an option. Determine the actions of each of the drugs listed and then correlate the disease process with the action of the drug. **Reference**: LeMone, P., Burke, K., & Bauldoff, G. (2011). *Medical-surgical nursing: Critical thinking in patient care* (5th ed.). Upper Saddle River, NJ: Pearson Education, p. 723.

9 **Answer: 2** **Rationale**: All of the drugs listed are histamine 2 (H_2)-receptor blockers that inhibit the secretion of gastric acid. Cimetidine (Tagamet) interacts with a large number of drugs. Because it decreases the hepatic metabolism of phenytoin, they should not be administered concurrently. Famotidine (Pepcid) has no known drug interactions with phenytoin. Nizatidine (Axid) does not interfere with phenytoin therapy and ranitidine reduces the absorption of several antibiotics. **Cognitive Level**: Applying **Client Need**: Pharmacological and Parenteral Therapies **Integrated Process**: Nursing Process: Planning **Content Area**: Pharmacology **Strategy**: Review each of the drugs in the options and determine the one that has the highest risk of negative interaction with the anti-epileptic drug. **Reference**: Wilson, B. A., Shannon, M., & Shields, K. (2011). *Pearson nurse's drug guide 2011*. Upper Saddle River, NJ: Pearson Education, pp. 1463–1465.

10 **Answer: 1** **Rationale**: Taking bisacodyl (Dulcolax) on an empty stomach will result in a more rapid effect. Drinking plenty of fluids is a good general measure to reduce the risk of constipation. Taking the medication with a meal will delay absorption. If taking at bedtime, the client will have a bowel movement in the morning. **Cognitive Level**: Applying **Client Need**: Pharmacological and Parenteral Therapies **Integrated Process**: Nursing Process: Implementation **Content Area**: Pharmacology **Strategy**: Note that 2 options are opposites, making it more likely that 1 of them is correct. Consider that food will slow down or delay drug action to help choose the option citing to take the medication on an empty stomach. **Reference**: Wilson, B. A., Shannon, M., & Shields, K. (2011). *Pearson nurse's drug guide 2011*. Upper Saddle River, NJ: Pearson Education, pp. 179–180.

References

Abrams, A. (2009). *Clinical drug therapy: Rationales for nursing practice* (9th ed.). Philadelphia, PA: Lippincott Williams & Wilkins.

Adams, M., Holland, L., & Bostwick, P. (2011). *Pharmacology for nurses: A pathophysiologic approach* (3rd ed.). Upper Saddle River, NJ: Pearson Education.

Adams. M. P, & Urban, C. Q. (2013). *Pharmacology: Connections to nursing practice* (2nd ed.). Upper Saddle River, NJ: Pearson Education.

Aschenbrenner, D., & Venable, S. (2012). *Drug therapy in nursing* (4th ed.). Philadelphia, PA: Lippincott Williams & Wilkins.

Drug Facts & Comparisons® (updated monthly). St. Louis, MO: A. Wolters Kluwer.

Karch, A. M. (2010). *Focus on nursing pharmacology* (5th ed.). Philadelphia, PA: Lippincott Williams & Wilkins.

Kee, J. (2009). *Laboratory and diagnostic tests and nursing implications* (8th ed.). Upper Saddle River, NJ: Prentice Hall.

Lehne, R. (2010). *Pharmacology for nursing care* (7th ed.). St. Louis, MO: Mosby, Inc.

LeMone, P., Burke, K. M., & Bauldoff, G. (2011). *Medical-surgical nursing: Critical thinking in client care* (5th ed.). Upper Saddle River, NJ: Pearson Education.

8 Immune System Medications

Chapter Outline

NCLEX-RN® Test Prep

Use the accompanying online resource, NursingReviewsandRationales, to test yourself with hundreds of NCLEX®-style practice questions.

Objectives

➤ Describe the general goals of therapy when administering immune system medications.
➤ Identify the primary uses, interactions, major side effects, and adverse or toxic effects of the most commonly prescribed immunostimulant and immunosuppressant medications.
➤ Describe the recommended childhood immunization schedule.
➤ Identify side effects and adverse effects associated with the administration of immunizations.
➤ List contraindications associated with the administration of vaccines.
➤ Explain the nursing considerations related to the administration of medications commonly used to treat multiple sclerosis (MS), myasthenia gravis, rheumatoid arthritis, and systemic lupus erythematosus.
➤ List the significant client education points related to immune system medications.

Review at a Glance

active immunity immunity acquired by having a disease or by injection of infectious organisms

antigen a substance that produces formation of antibodies

cellular immunity host immunity that has been enhanced with increases in white blood cells and both helper and suppressor T-cell function

colony-stimulating factors factors that stimulate glycoproteins to produce blood cells, thus stimulating immunity and bone marrow development

glycoprotein compounds of carbohydrates and proteins that, when produced, increase blood cell production

immunosuppression ability to suppress body's response to an antigen

immune sera an injection that provides passive immunity following exposure to certain communicable diseases

neutropenia abnormally low neutrophil count

vaccine injections of living attenuated organisms or dead organisms that assist a human host to develop protection from a communicable disease

PRETEST

1 A client is scheduled to receive filgrastim (Neupogen) 5 mcg/kg/day. The nurse considers that the dose should be withheld and the prescriber notified if which assessment data is noted?

1. Hematocrit 37%, hemoglobin 12 grams/dL
2. Mental depression
3. Bone pain
4. Neutrophils 8,000/mm^3

2 A client being cared for at home is taking sargramostim (Leukine). The charge nurse at the home health agency instructs the unlicensed assistive personnel (UAP) to report which most important drug side effect(s) if noted?

1. Early morning oral temperature of 99 (tympanic membrane)
2. Pericardial and pleural friction rub
3. Dyspnea on exertion and dependent edema
4. Mental depression and fatigue

3 A 61-year-old female client has severe rheumatoid arthritis that is being managed with leflunomide (Arava) and infliximab (Remicade). After the client reported having an elevated temperature of 99.8°F, the nurse concludes that this may be related to which of the following?

1. Development of viral or bacterial infection
2. Joint inflammation
3. Probable dehydration
4. Vaginal yeast infection

4 After the intramuscular administration of immune globulin (BayGam), the nurse should provide which instructions to the client? Select all that apply.

1. Apply ice pack to injection site.
2. Postpone receiving live vaccine for at least 3 months.
3. Use protective measures for the next 2 months until immunity develops.
4. Notify nurse if chills and fever develop.
5. Urinary output is likely to decrease.

5 A client with a seizure disorder is taking an antiepileptic medication along with cyclosporine (Sandimmune). Which of the following nursing interventions will the nurse include in the plan of care? Select all that apply.

1. Consult with the prescriber regarding the need to increase the cyclosporine dosage.
2. Evaluate for symptoms of elevated blood pressure.
3. Consult with the prescriber regarding the need to lower the antiepileptic dosage.
4. Routinely monitor blood glucose levels for hyperglycemia.
5. Monitor the client for seizures.

6 Two days after receiving oprelvekin (Neumega), the client, whose regular prescriptions include oral furosemide (Lasix) 20 mg daily and oral digoxin (Lanoxin) 0.25 mg daily, calls the home health agency and reports onset of dyspnea and peripheral edema. What are the best instructions for the nurse to give to the client at this time? Select all that apply.

1. "Do not drink anything by mouth until evaluated by the health care provider."
2. "Call 911 or emergency medical services (EMS) to obtain immediate assistance."
3. "Take your prescribed diuretics and weigh yourself tomorrow morning."
4. "Lie down with your head elevated 45–90 degrees."
5. "Take an extra dose of your Lasix and digoxin now."

7 The nurse would place highest priority on which nursing diagnosis and associated nursing intervention when working with a client who is receiving cyclosporine (Sandimmune)?

1. Risk for Ineffective Tissue Perfusion: monitor for high blood pressure.
2. Acute Pain: administer analgesic as prescribed.
3. Deficient Fluid Volume: encourage fluids.
4. Altered Neurological Status: set up safety precautions.

8 Several clients were exposed to hepatitis A. The nurse should question a prescription for immune serum globulin (ISG) by the intramuscular (IM) route that is written for a client with which of the following?

1. Diabetes insipidus
2. Exposure to rubeola
3. Exposure to hepatitis B
4. Platelet count less than 100,000/mm^3

9 A new parent asks the obstetrics nurse for information about immunizations for their infant. Which information should be included in client teaching? Select all that apply.

1. "Immunizations to prevent contagious diseases are required by law."
2. "Infants tend to be more susceptible to contagious diseases."
3. "Immunizations are safe without side effects."
4. "The injections are inexpensive or free at the health department."
5. "Immunity to disease develops immediately after the first immunization, so you may consider not having booster vaccines."

10 A client being treated for myasthenia gravis presents to the emergency department with severe ataxia and tremors. The nurse immediately prepares to administer which of the following medications per protocol order?

1. Edrophonium (Tensilon)
2. Ambenonium (Mytelase)
3. Neostigmine (Prostigmine)
4. Atropine (generic)

➤ *See pages 276–278 for Answers and Rationales.*

I. IMMUNOMODULATORS

A. Description

1. Immunomodulators alter the body's immune system actions
2. They can either suppress or enhance a client's immune response
3. Depending on the desired immune response, the client is given either an immune stimulant or an **immunosuppressant**, a drug that suppresses the body's response to an **antigen** (a substance that triggers antibody formation)

B. Immunostimulants

1. **Colony-stimulating factors (CSFs)**
   a. Action and use
      1) Colony-stimulating factors are **glycoproteins** that increase production of blood cells that enhance an individual's **cellular immunity** (host immunity that has been enhanced with increases in white blood cells and both helper and suppressor T-cell functions) by increasing number of lymphocytes and inhibiting tumor growth
      2) They increase development of leukocytes, which is adversely affected by chemotherapy agents used after bone marrow transplantation or to treat cancer
      3) These medications reduce **neutropenia** (abnormally low neutrophil count) and decrease incidence of infection; they assist in mobilization of stem cells allowing for stem cell collection
   b. Common medications (Table 8-1)
   c. Administration considerations
      1) Sargramostim (Leukine) (GM-CSF)
         a) Multiple results—including increasing number of neutrophils, eosinophils, and monocytes—and increasing bactericidal activity of other immune cells
         b) Commonly used for clients with acute lymphocytic leukemia or Hodgkin disease; typically started when the absolute neutrophil count (ANC) is less than 500 cells/mm^3

Table 8-1	**Common Immunostimulant Medications**	
Generic (Trade) Name	Route	Uses
Sargramostin (CSF-GM) (Leukine)	IV or subQ	Treatment of neutropenia following bone marrow transplant Myeloid reconstitution after autologous bone marrow transplantation Accelerate myeloid recovery in non-Hodgkin lymphoma and acute lymphoblastic leukemia Mobilize hematopoietic progenitor cells for collection by leukopheresis
Filgrastim (Neupogen)	IV or subQ	Reduce incidence of infections in client with nonmyeloid malignancies receiving myelosuppressive anticancer drugs Reduce time for neutrophil recovery following chemotherapy, severe chronic neutropenia Orphan drug use—myelodysplastic syndrome, aplastic anemia
Pegfilgrastim (Neulasta)	subQ	Reduce time for neutrophil recovery following chemotherapy

2) Filgrastim (Neupogen)

   a) Has 2 actions: increases bone marrow production of neutrophils and enhances function of existing neutrophils

   b) Is generally given by subcutaneous administration, although it may be given IV

   c) With each further chemotherapy administration, dose of Neupogen should be increased by 5 mcg/kg; with bone marrow transplantation or collection of stem cells, increase dose by 10 mcg/kg/day; dose of Neupogen with severe chronic neutropenia 5 to 6 mcg/kg, 1 to 2 times per day

 d. Contraindications

   1) Sargramostim (Leukine): pregnancy, hypersensitivity to yeast products or *E. coli* products, leukemic myeloblasts in the bone marrow; use cautiously with hepatic or renal insufficiency and lactation

   2) Filgrastim (Neupogen) and pegfilgrastim (Neulasta): pregnancy (Category C) and hypersensitivity to *E. coli* products (*E. coli* is used to produce this drug)

   e. Significant drug interactions

   1) Lithium increases the effectiveness of CSFs

   2) Do not administer either before or after 24 hours after chemotherapy because the drugs produce opposing effects

   f. Significant food interactions: none reported

   g. Significant lab studies

 1) Baseline and routine complete blood count (CBC) with differential and platelet count; report neutrophil count of greater than $10,000/\text{mm}^3$ to prescriber

   2) Assess creatinine, blood urea nitrogen (BUN), liver enzymes before and after administration

   h. Side effects

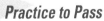 **1)** Bone pain, especially to bones with large amounts of bone marrow; usually managed with nonopioid analgesics

   2) Splenomegaly occurs in up to 30% of clients with long-term therapy

   3) Supraventricular dysrhythmia, tachycardia, myocardial infarction (MI) (with high leukocyte counts)

   4) Nausea, vomiting, anorexia, constipation, diarrhea

   i. Adverse effects/toxicity

   1) General

      a) MI, gastrointestinal (GI) hemorrhage, thrombus formation, and stroke (generally from high leukocyte counts)

      b) Adult respiratory distress syndrome (ARDS), pleural effusion

   2) Sargramostim (Leukine)

      a) Plan to withhold medication if ANC rises above 10,000 cells/mm^3

      b) Respiratory distress occurring during first IV infusion administration: signs include shortness of breath, hypotension, and tachycardia

Practice to Pass

What 3 assessments for hypersensitivity reaction are necessary for a client with hypersensitivity to *E. coli* products?

3) Filgrastim (Neupogen) and pegfilgrastim (Neulasta): report neutrophil count of 20,000/mm^3 to health care provider

j. Nursing considerations

1) Assess CBC and platelet count before administration and 2 times per week during medication administration

2) Assess renal and hepatic function

3) Assess for excessive myeloid blasts in bone marrow

4) Do not administer during pregnancy, and cautiously with lactation

5) Client is at an increased risk for infection due to low WBC counts; evaluate for symptoms such as fever, chills, rash, or nonhealing areas; teach to avoid exposure to infection

6) Leukocytosis may occur as a result of the medication; evaluate for elevated WBCs during therapy

k. Client education

1) Report pain in joints and bones

2) Maintain good hygiene and avoid exposure to crowds because of susceptibility to infection

3) Teach to report even mild symptoms of infection such as fever, sore throat, chills, and rash

4) Teach symptoms of allergic response, though this risk is low for this class of medications

2. Cell-stimulating medications

a. Action and use

1) Interferons

a) Biologic response modifiers with antiviral, anti-inflammatory, and antineoplastic activity

b) Slow spread of viral infections by stimulating activities of leukocytes, phagocytes, and T-cells

c) Used in clients with acquired immunodeficiency syndrome–related Kaposi's sarcoma, chronic hepatitis B or C, chronic myelogenous leukemia, and multiple sclerosis (MS)

d) Interferon alfa-2b (intron A) suppresses growth of cancer cells and nonspecifically inhibits viral replication

e) Interferon beta-1a and beta-1b are effective in treating MS (these medications will be discussed later in the chapter)

2) Interleukins

a) Biologic response modifiers that prevent thrombocytopenia and stimulate platelet production; they also possess an antitumor action and promote inflammation

b) Cause T-cell replication, which results in lymphokine-activated killer cells, which destroy only cancer cells and maintain normal cells

c) Aldesleukin (Proleukin) is used to treat metastatic renal carcinoma and prevents severe thrombocytopenia; also approved for other carcinomas listed in Table 8-2

b. Common medications (Table 8-2)

c. Administration considerations

1) Interferons: interferon alfa-2b (Intron A)

a) Given IV, IM, or subcutaneously

b) Initially causes flulike symptoms and resulting lack of appetite that usually lessens with therapy

c) May cause thrombocytopenia, which may be treated with oprelvekin (Neumega), a platelet-enhancing medication

d) May cause elevated liver enzymes

Practice to Pass

What assessment related to laboratory values should the nurse make when administering colony-stimulating factors?

Table 8-2	Common Cell-Stimulating Medications	
Generic (Trade) Names	**Route**	**Uses**
Aldesleukin (Proleukin)	IV	Treatment of metastatic renal cell carcinoma; breast, ovarian, colon, brain, head and neck, and lung carcinoma; lymphoma Considered an orphan drug when used for adult metastatic melanoma
Anakinra (Kineret)	SubQ	Reduce signs and symptoms of severe, acute rheumatoid arthritis in clients over age 17 who have not responded to methotrexate therapy, or sulfasalazine, hydrochloroquine, gold, pencillamine, leflunomide, azathioprine
Denileukin diftitox (Ontak)	IV	Treatment of cutaneous T-cell lymphoma in which cells excrete CD25 component of Interleukin 2 receptor

      2) Aldesleukin (Proleukin)
         a) Because of drug's ability to cause serious effects in every body system, it is given in a hospital that has an intensive care unit with medical specialists available
         b) Is administered in multiple brief IV infusions because of short half-life
         c) Treatment of overdose: dexamethasone
      3) Denileukin diftitox (Ontak); acute hypersensitivity reactions can occur within hours of infusion; severity can be reduced with use of acetaminophen (Tylenol), diphenhydramine (Benadryl), nonsteroidal anti-inflammatory drugs (NSAIDs), or corticosteroids
   d. Contraindications
      1) Interferons: interferon alfa-2b (Intron A):
         a) Autoimmune hepatitis or hepatic decompensation
         b) Neonates and infants: contains benzyl alcohol, which may cause neurologic complications
         c) Use caution in patients with liver impairment or herpes zoster, or who have recent exposure to chickenpox
      2) Interleukins: aldesleukin
         a) Multiple contraindications; clients with significant cardiac, nervous system, pulmonary, renal, or hepatic problems should not use this drug
         b) May worsen patients with autoimmune diseases including diabetes mellitus and rheumatoid arthritis (RA)
   e. Significant drug interactions (interleukins)
      1) Potential interaction with almost any drug, causing additive effects or organ damage
      2) Because of increased bleeding risk, use caution with aspirin, NSAIDs, and platelet inhibitors
      3) Avoid vaccines during and for 3 months after therapy
   f. Significant food interactions: disulfiram-type reactions can occur if levasimole is combined with alcohol
   g. Significant laboratory studies
      1) Interferons: interferon alfa-2b (Intron A): monitor platelet function and liver enzymes
      2) Interleukins: baseline CBC, electrolytes, renal, and liver panel (renal and hepatic impairment is likely during therapy)
   h. Side effects
      1) Interferons: interferon alfa-2b (Intron A)
         a) Monitor platelet count, as Intron A may cause thrombocytopenia

            b) Most common effects are flulike symptoms, which include fever, chills, weight loss, and fatigue that generally improves over time

            c) Possible depression and suicidal ideation, even after discontinuation of drug

        2) Aldesleukin: cardiac dysrhythmias, fluid retention, lethargy, and myalgia

  i. Adverse effects/toxicity

        1) Interferons: hepatotoxicity-medication may cause elevation in liver enzymes, resulting in need to discontinue drug

        2) Interleukins

            a) Capillary leak syndrome, which can cause death

            b) Severe hypotension, causing organ damage due to decreased blood supply

            c) Aldesleukin: dexamethasone treats many symptoms of toxicity

  j. Nursing considerations

        1) Interferons: interferon alfa-2b (intron A)

            a) Monitor body weight due to lack of appetite

            b) Evaluate for symptoms of thrombocytopenia

            c) Monitor cardiac function especially in older adults, who are at increased risk for cardiotoxicity

        2) Interleukins

            a) Assess for renal and hepatic impairment

            b) Perform thorough comprehensive assessment before administering initial dose to assess for presence or history of diseases

            c) Maintain fluid and electrolyte balance particularly to prevent encephalopathy and mental status changes

            d) Assess for neutropenia or thrombocytopenia

        3) Provide optimal hygiene practices

        4) Monitor for weight gain

  k. Client education

        1) Interferons: interferon alfa-2b (Intron A)

            a) Avoid exposure to infection such as crowded places or public transportation

            b) Notify health care provider immediately for symptoms of infection such as rash, sore throat, or diarrhea

            c) Report signs of depression, lethargy, or excessive sleeping immediately

        2) Interleukins

            a) Plan for fatigue and flulike symptoms by prevention of over-scheduling, and taking acetaminophen before and after injections

            b) Report symptoms of bleeding or infection to health care provider

            c) Report symptoms of depression, kidney, or liver failure immediately

C. Immunosuppressants

  1. Action and use

    a. Immunosuppressants are medications used to inhibit inflammatory response and block immune response to an antigen

    b. These medications inhibit T-cell function and also block production of antibodies by B cells

    c. They are used to prevent rejection of transplanted organs

    d. Immunosuppressants may include antibodies, cytotoxic agents and antimetabolites, calcineurin inhibitors, and kinase inhibitors

        1) Antimetabolites class: inhibits aspects of lymphocyte replication and includes some drugs that treat cancer

        2) Calcineurin inhibitors: disrupt T-cell function by binding to intracellular messenger calcineurin; often used in treatments for psoriasis

        3) Antibodies: these medications are antibodies against T cells or T-cell receptors (note suffix *–ab* in these medication names)

2. Common medications (Table 8-3)
3. Administration considerations
   a. Antimetabolites: use caution when clients have viral or bacterial infections or other immune problem
      1) Mycophenolate (CellCept)
         a) Usually given intravenously initially then changed to oral dosing
         b) Primarily used for renal transplant clients; often used concurrently with corticosteroids and cyclosporine
      2) Azathioprine (Imuran)
         a) Given usually to suppress kidney transplant rejection; however, may be used with severe RA
         b) Oral administration or intravenous
   b. Calcineurin inhibitors: administered intravenously
      1) Cyclosporine (Sandimmune): tends to be less toxic than other immunosuppressants; used to prevent transplant rejection
      2) Tacrolimus (Prograf): is administered 6 hours after transplant

Table 8-3   Common Immunosuppressant Medications

Generic (Trade) Name	Route	Actions	Uses
Alefacept (Amevive)	IV	Interferes with lymphocyte activation and reduces CD4+ and CD8+ T-lymphocyte counts	Treatment of chronic psoriasis
Azathioprine (Imuran)	PO	Inhibits DNA synthesis leading to DNA damage and chromosome breakage	Immunosuppressant therapy following kidney transplant, severe refractory rheumatoid arthritis
Basiliximab (Simulect)	IV	Immunosuppressant agent produced by recombinant DNA technology	Prophylaxis of acute rejection in renal transplant clients; used in combination with cyclosporine and corticosteroids
Daclizumab (Zenapax)	IV	Immunosuppressant monoclonal antibody	Prophylaxis of acute rejection in renal transplant clients; used in combination with cyclosporine and corticosteroids
Cyclosporine (Sandimmune)	PO, IV	Inhibits T-helper and T-suppressor cells, lymphokine production, and release of interleukin-2 and T-cell growth factor	Prophylaxis to prevent kidney, liver, and heart transplant rejection; treatment of chronic rejection in clients who have received immunosuppressive agents, rheumatoid arthritis, recalcitrant plaque psoriasis
Muromonab-CD3 (Orthoclone OKT3)	IV	Murine monoclonal antibody to the antigen in human T cells; immunosuppressant that enables T cells	Acute allograft rejection in renal transplant clients; treatment of steroid-resistant acute allograft rejection in cardiac and hepatic transplant recipients
Mycophenolate (CellCept)	PO, IV	Inhibits T-lymphocyte activation	Prophylaxis of organ rejection in clients receiving allogenic renal, hepatic, and heart transplants; unlabeled use: refractory uveitis
Sirolimus (Rapamune)	PO	Inhibits T-lymphocyte activation and proliferation	Prophylaxis for kidney transplant rejection; used with corticosteroids and cyclosporine; unlabeled use: psoriasis treatment
Tacrolimus (Protopic, Prograf)	PO	Inhibits T-lymphocyte activation	Prophylaxis for liver or renal organ rejection, moderate to severe atopic dermatitis; unlabeled use: prophylaxis in bone marrow, cardiac, pancreas, pancreatic island cell, small bowel transplants, autoimmune disease, recalcitrant psoriasis

   c. Antibodies such as basiliximab (Simulect), daclizumab (Zenapax), muromonab CD3 (Orthoclone OKT3):
      1) Primarily used post-transplant
      2) Avoid vaccinations for at least 2 weeks following last dose of drugs
   4. Contraindications
      a. Allergy to drug
      b. Pregnancy or lactation
      c. Use cautiously with renal or hepatic impairment and with exposure to viral infections
   5. Significant drug interactions
      a. General
         1) Increased risk of hepatic or renal toxicity in clients taking other renal or hepatotoxic medications
         2) There are multiple medication interactions that may increase or decrease effectiveness of medications; see product literature
      b. Calcineurin inhibitors
         1) Cyclosporine: antiepileptic medications decrease cyclosporine levels; angiotensin-converting enzyme (ACE) inhibitors, NSAIDs increase cyclosporine levels
         2) Tacrolimus: increased risk of toxicity with metoclopramide, nicardipine, cimetidine, clarithromycin
   6. Significant food interactions: increased serum levels of calcineurin inhibitors are associated with administration of cyclosporine and grapefruit juice or grapefruit by 50–200%
   7. Significant laboratory studies
      a. Aspartate aminotransferase (AST) and alanine aminotransferase (ALT)
      b. BUN and creatinine
      c. CBC and platelet count
      d. Blood glucose and potassium levels (may cause hyperkalemia and hyperglycemia)
   8. Side effects
      a. Antimetabolites: nausea, vomiting, bone marrow suppression
      b. Calcineurin inhibitors: hypertension and reduction in renal output
      c. Antibodies: local site reactions and influenza-like symptoms
      d. General effects: increased risk for infection
      e. Hypertension
      f. Bone marrow suppression
   9. Adverse effects/toxicity
      a. Antimetabolites: leukopenia, thrombocytopenia, anemia
      b. Azathioprine (Imuran): drug has high potential for toxicity, causing decreased leukocyte or platelet count
      c. Calcineurin inhibitors: nephrotoxicity and hepatotoxicity
      d. Antibodies: anaphylaxis, infections
   10. Nursing considerations
      a. Assess for signs and symptoms of infection and opportunistic infections
      b. Provide supportive care for flulike symptoms
      c. Review drug interactions, as there are multiple drug interactions for all of these drug classes that may either increase or decrease drug effectiveness
      d. Assess nutritional status
      e Encourage well-balanced meals with small frequent feedings
      f. Avoid use of live vaccines
      g. Maintain blood studies as ordered such as CBC, platelet count, and renal and hepatic function tests

Practice to Pass

What learning objectives are appropriate for the nurse to develop for a client who will be receiving immunosuppressant agents?

11. Client education
    a. Need for lab studies, prevention of infection, and all aspects of medication administration including action, side effects, and nursing implications; also report signs of infection

    b. Birth control methods should be utilized until after discontinuation of drug therapy

II. IMMUNIZATIONS

A. Vaccines

1. Action and use
   a. **Vaccines** are injectable or oral suspensions containing live or weakened micro-organisms that when injected produce antibodies to fight against a disease
   b. **Active immunity** results from introduction of a specific protein antigen by way of a vaccine; body responds by developing antibodies to confer a long-lasting immunity to that organism
   c. Vaccines are used to prevent diseases that may have high mortality and morbidity
2. Common medications (Figure 8-1 and Table 8-4)
3. Administration considerations
   a. Live vaccines should be administered at least 1 month apart
   b. Hepatitis A is a 2-dose series for clients at risk
   c. Hepatitis B: initial dose followed by second dose 1 month later, and a third dose 6 months after initial dose
   d. Measles, mumps, and rubella; total amount of reconstituted vial is adminis-tered subQ
4. Contraindications

   a. Vaccines should not be administered during a moderate to severe febrile illness, pregnancy, cancer, leukemia, and while on immunosuppressive drug therapy

   b. Do not administer for 3 months after blood products have been administered
   c. Do not administer influenza vaccine to clients who are hypersensitive to chicken or egg products
5. Significant drug interactions: immunosuppressive drug therapy
6. Significant food interactions: none reported
7. Significant laboratory studies: monitor antibody titer levels
8. Side effects

   a. Pain, swelling, or redness at injection site
   b. Flulike symptoms
   c. Hypersensitivity (rarely noted)
9. Adverse effects/toxicity: rarely clients may experience a hypersensitivity reaction
10. Nursing considerations
    a. Determine administration guidelines and timing of immunization administration
    b. Adhere to individual vaccine storage recommendations to ensure vaccine potency
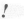
    c. Assess client for acute infection prior to administration
    d. Maintain documentation of immunization administration and client reaction to administration; provide client or caretaker with a record of immunizations administered
    e. Administer all vaccines for which client is eligible at different sites, using different syringes
    f. Observe client for manifestations of adverse reactions and have epinephrine available in case of hypersensitivity reactions
    g. Provide acetaminophen (Tylenol) after administration as needed
    h. Apply heat to injection site as needed for comfort

Vaccine ▼ Age ▶	Birth	1 month	2 months	4 months	6 months	9 months	12 months	15 months	18 months	19–23 months	2–3 years	4–6 years	
Hepatitis B[1]	Hep B	HepB					HepB						Range of recommended ages for all children
Rotavirus[2]			RV	RV	RV[2]								
Diphtheria, tetanus, pertussis[3]			DTaP	DTaP	DTaP		see footnote[3]	DTaP				DTaP	
Haemophilus influenzae type b[4]			Hib	Hib	Hib[4]		Hib						Range of recommended ages for certain high-risk groups
Pneumococcal[5]			PCV	PCV	PCV		PCV					PPSV	
Inactivated poliovirus[6]			IPV	IPV			IPV					IPV	
Influenza[7]							Influenza (Yearly)						
Measles, mumps, rubella[8]							MMR		see footnote[8]			MMR	Range of recommended ages for all children and certain high-risk groups
Varicella[9]							Varicella		see footnote[9]			Varicella	
Hepatitis A[10]							Dose 1[10]				HepA Series		
Meningococcal[11]							MCV4 — see footnote[11]						

This schedule includes recommendations in effect as of December 23, 2011. Any dose not administered at the recommended age should be administered at a subsequent visit, when indicated and feasible. The use of a combination vaccine generally is preferred over separate injections of its equivalent component vaccines. Vaccination providers should consult the relevant Advisory Committee on Immunization Practices (ACIP) statement for detailed recommendations, available online at http://www.cdc.gov/vaccines/pubs/acip-list.htm. Clinically significant adverse events that follow vaccination should be reported to the Vaccine Adverse Event Reporting System (VAERS) online (http://www.vaers.hhs.gov) or by telephone (800-822-7967).

Figure 8-1a

Recommended Childhood and Adolescent Immunization Schedule—United States, 2012

Source: Department of Health and Human Services, Recommended Immunization Schedule for Persons Aged 0–6 Years. www.cdc.gov/vaccines/recs/schedules/downloads/child/0-6yrs-schedule-pr.pdf. Information provided by Centers for Disease Control and Prevention (CDC), Atlanta, GA 30333.

Vaccine ▼ Age ▶	7–10 years	11–12 years	13–18 years	
Tetanus, diphtheria, pertussis[1]	1 dose (if indicated)	1 dose	1 dose (if indicated)	Range of recommended ages for all children
Human papillomavirus[2]	see footnote[2]	3 doses	Complete 3-dose series	
Meningococcal[3]	See footnote[3]	Dose 1	Booster at 16 years old	
Influenza[4]		Influenza (yearly)		Range of recommended ages for catch-up immunization
Pneumococcal[5]		See footnote[5]		
Hepatitis A[6]		Complete 2-dose series		
Hepatitis B[7]		Complete 3-dose series		
Inactivated poliovirus[8]		Complete 3-dose series		Range of recommended ages for certain high-risk groups
Measles, mumps, rubella[9]		Complete 2-dose series		
Varicella[10]		Complete 2-dose series		

This schedule includes recommendations in effect as of December 23, 2011. Any dose not administered at the recommended age should be administered at a subsequent visit, when indicated and feasible. The use of a combination vaccine generally is preferred over separate injections of its equivalent component vaccines. Vaccination providers should consult the relevant Advisory Committee on Immunization Practices (ACIP) statement for detailed recommendations, available online at http://www.cdc.gov/vaccines/pubs/acip-list.htm. Clinically significant adverse events that follow vaccination should be reported to the Vaccine Adverse Event Reporting System (VAERS) online (http://www.vaers.hhs.gov) or by telephone (800-822-7967).

Figure 8-1b

Recommended Childhood and Adolescent Immunization Schedule—United States, 2012

Source: Department of Health and Human Services, Recommended Immunization Schedule for Persons Aged 7–18 Years. www.cdc.gov/vaccines/recs/schedules/downloads/child/7-18yrs-schedule-pr.pdf. Information provided by Centers for Disease Control and Prevention (CDC), Atlanta, GA 30333.

!

Practice to Pass

What client education should be implemented during a hepatitis A outbreak?

11. Client education
   a. Discuss with client and family risk of contracting vaccine-preventable illnesses as well as signs and symptoms
   b. Instruct on treatment of flulike symptoms using acetaminophen or NSAIDs such as ibuprofen
   c. Instruct on importance of keeping a record of immunizations and being up to date in immunization administration
   d. Provide a copy of the Current Vaccine Information Statement for each vaccine administered; these are available from the Centers for Disease Control

Vaccine	Minimum Age for Dose 1	Minimum Interval Between Doses			
		Dose 1 to dose 2	Dose 2 to dose 3	Dose 3 to dose 4	Dose 4 to dose 5
**Persons aged 4 months through 6 years**					
Hepatitis B	Birth	4 weeks	8 weeks and at least 16 weeks after first dose; minimum age for the final dose is 24 weeks		
Rotavirus[1]	6 weeks	4 weeks	4 weeks[1]		
Diphtheria, tetanus, pertussis[2]	6 weeks	4 weeks	4 weeks	6 months	6 months[2]
Haemophilus influenzae type b[3]	6 weeks	4 weeks if first dose administered at younger than age 12 months 8 weeks (as final dose) if first dose administered at age 12–14 months No further doses needed if first dose administered at age 15 months or older	4 weeks[3] if current age is younger than 12 months 8 weeks (as final dose)[3] if current age is 12 months or older and first dose administered at younger than age 12 months and second dose administered at younger than 15 months No further doses needed if previous dose administered at age 15 months or older	8 weeks (as final dose) This dose only necessary for children aged 12 months through 59 months who received 3 doses before age 12 months	
Pneumococcal[4]	6 weeks	4 weeks if first dose administered at younger than age 12 months 8 weeks (as final dose for healthy children) if first dose administered at age 12 months or older or current age 24 through 59 months No further doses needed for healthy children if first dose administered at age 24 months or older	4 weeks if current age is younger than 12 months 8 weeks (as final dose for healthy children) if current age is 12 months or older No further doses needed for healthy children if previous dose administered at age 24 months or older	8 weeks (as final dose) This dose only necessary for children aged 12 months through 59 months who received 3 doses before age 12 months or for children at high risk who received 3 doses at any age	
Inactivated poliovirus[5]	6 weeks	4 weeks	4 weeks	6 months[5] minimum age 4 years for final dose	
Meningococcal[6]	9 months	8 weeks[6]			
Measles, mumps, rubella[7]	12 months	4 weeks			
Varicella[8]	12 months	3 months			
Hepatitis A	12 months	6 months			
**Persons aged 7 through 18 years**					
Tetanus, diphtheria/ tetanus, diphtheria, pertussis[9]	7 years[9]	4 weeks	4 weeks if first dose administered at younger than age 12 months 6 months if first dose administered at 12 months or older	6 months if first dose administered at younger than age 12 months	
Human papillomavirus[10]	9 years	Routine dosing intervals are recommended[10]			
Hepatitis A	12 months	6 months			
Hepatitis B	Birth	4 weeks	8 weeks (and at least 16 weeks after first dose)		
Inactivated poliovirus[5]	6 weeks	4 weeks	4 weeks[5]	6 months[5]	
Meningococcal[6]	9 months	8 weeks[6]			
Measles, mumps, rubella[7]	12 months	4 weeks			
Varicella[8]	12 months	3 months if person is younger than age 13 years 4 weeks if person is aged 13 years or older			

1. **Rotavirus (RV) vaccines (RV-1 [Rotarix] and RV-5 [Rota Teq]).**
   - The maximum age for the first dose in the series is 14 weeks, 6 days; and 8 months, 0 days for the final dose in the series. Vaccination should not be initiated for infants aged 15 weeks, 0 days or older.
   - If RV-1 was administered for the first and second doses, a third dose is not indicated.
2. **Diphtheria and tetanus toxoids and acellular pertussis (DTaP) vaccine.**
   - The fifth dose is not necessary if the fourth dose was administered at age 4 years or older.
3. ***Haemophilus influenzae* type b (Hib) conjugate vaccine.**
   - Hib vaccine should be considered for unvaccinated persons aged 5 years or older who have sickle cell disease, leukemia, human immunodeficiency virus (HIV) infection, or anatomic/functional asplenia.
   - If the first 2 doses were PRP-OMP (PedvaxHIB or Comvax) and were administered at age 11 months or younger, the third (and final) dose should be administered at age 12 through 15 months and at least 8 weeks after the second dose.
   - If the first dose was administered at age 7 through 11 months, administer the second dose at least 4 weeks later and a final dose at age 12 through 15 months.
4. **Pneumococcal vaccines.** (Minimum age: 6 weeks for pneumococcal conjugate vaccine [PCV]; 2 years for pneumococcal polysaccharide vaccine [PPSV])
   - For children aged 24 through 71 months with underlying medical conditions, administer 1 dose of PCV if 3 doses of PCV were received previously, or administer 2 doses of PCV at least 8 weeks apart if fewer than 3 doses of PCV were received previously.
   - A single dose of PCV may be administered to certain children aged 6 through 18 years with underlying medical conditions. See age-specific schedules for details.
   - Administer PPSV to children aged 2 years or older with certain underlying medical conditions. See *MMWR* 2010:59(No. RR-11), available at http://www.cdc.gov/mmwr/pdf/rr/rr5911.pdf.

5. **Inactivated poliovirus vaccine (IPV).**
   - A fourth dose is not necessary if the third dose was administered at age 4 years or older and at least 6 months after the previous dose.
   - In the first 6 months of life, minimum age and minimum intervals are only recommended if the person is at risk for imminent exposure to circulating poliovirus (i.e., travel to a polio-endemic region or during an outbreak).
   - IPV is not routinely recommended for U.S. residents aged 18 years or older.
6. **Meningococcal conjugate vaccines, quadrivalent (MCV4).** (Minimum age: 9 months for Menactra [MCV4-D], 2 years for Menveo [MCV4-CRM])
   - See Figure 1 ("Recommended immunization schedule for persons aged 0 through 6 years") and Figure 2 ("Recommended immunization schedule for persons aged 7 through 18 years") for further guidance.
7. **Measles, mumps, and rubella (MMR) vaccine.**
   - Administer the second dose routinely at age 4 through 6 years.
8. **Varicella (VAR) vaccine.**
   - Administer the second dose routinely at age 4 through 6 years. If the second dose was administered at least 4 weeks after the first dose, it can be accepted as valid.
9. **Tetanus and diphtheria toxoids (Td) and tetanus and diphtheria toxoids and acellular pertussis (Tdap) vaccines.**
   - For children aged 7 through 10 years who are not fully immunized with the childhood DTaP vaccine series, Tdap vaccine should be substituted for a single dose of Td vaccine in the catch-up series; if additional doses are needed, use Td vaccine. For these children, an adolescent Tdap vaccine dose should not be given.
   - An inadvertent dose of DTaP vaccine administered to children aged 7 through 10 years can count as part of the catch-up series. This dose can count as the adolescent Tdap dose, or the child can later receive a Tdap booster dose at age 11–12 years.
10. **Human papillomavirus (HPV) vaccines (HPV4 [Gardasil] and HPV2 [Cervarix]).**
    - Administer the vaccine series to females (either HPV2 or HPV4) and males (HPV4) at age 13 through 18 years if patient is not previously vaccinated.
    - Use recommended routine dosing intervals for vaccine series catch-up; see Figure 2 ("Recommended immunization schedule for persons aged 7 through 18 years").

Clinically significant adverse events that follow vaccination should be reported to the Vaccine Adverse Event Reporting System (VAERS) online (http://www.vaers.hhs.gov) or by telephone (800-822-7967). Suspected cases of vaccine-preventable diseases should be reported to the state or local health department. Additional information, including precautions and contraindications for vaccination, is available from CDC online (http://www.cdc.gov/vaccines) or by telephone (800-CDC-INFO [800-232-4636]).

Figure 8-1c

Recommended Childhood and Adolescent Immunization Schedule—United States, 2012

Source: Department of Health and Human Services, Recommended Immunization Schedule for Persons Aged 4 Months–18 Years Who Start Late or Are More Than 1 Month Behind. www.cdc.gov/vaccines/recs/schedules/downloads/child/catchup-schedule-pr.pdf. Information provided by Centers for Disease Control and Prevention (CDC), Atlanta, GA 30333.

Table 8-4	Immunizations and Common Immune Sera			
Generic (Trade) Name	**Route**	**Actions**	**Uses**	
BCG (TICE BCG) haemophilus B conjugate vaccine and hepatitis B surface antigen	Percutaneously	Prevention of tuberculosis with high-risk exposure Immunization against haemophilus B and hepatitis B	Prevention of tuberculosis, haemophilus B, and hepatitis B	
Cytomegalovirus immune globulin	IV	Attenuation of cytomegalovirus	Cytomegalovirus related to kidney transplant	
Diphtheria and tetanus toxoids, combined (Dt, Td) diphtheria and tetanus toxoids and acellular pertussis vaccine absorbed (DTaP)	IM	Stimulates active immunity against diphtheria, tetanus, and pertussis	Prevention of diphtheria, tetanus, and pertussis	
Diphtheria and tetanus toxoids and whole cell pertussis vaccine with haemophilus B conjugate vaccine DTwp-HIB (Tetraimmune)	IM	Stimulates active immunity against diphtheria, tetanus, pertussis, and haemophilus B	Prevention of diphtheria, tetanus, pertussis, and haemophilus B Administered to children 2 months to 5 years	
Diphtheria and tetanus toxoid	IM	Stimulates active immunity against diphtheria and tetanus	Prevention of diphtheria and tetanus	
Hepatitis A vaccine (Havrix, Vaqta)	IM	Simulates immunity against hepatitis A	Prevention of hepatitis A infection	
Hepatitis B vaccine (Energix-B, Recombivax-HB)	IM	Stimulates immunity against hepatitis B	Prevention of hepatitis B infection	
Influenza virus vaccine (FluShield, Fluogen, Fluzone)	IM	Stimulates active immunity to influenza virus antigens	Prevention of influenza virus	
Influenza virus vaccine (FluMist)	Intranasal 2 mL	Stimulates active immunity to influenza virus antigens	Prevention of influenza virus	
Japanese encephalitis (JE-VAX)	subQ	Stimulate active immunity from Japanese encephalitis	Immunization of persons older than age 1 year who reside in or travel to endemic areas Prevention of Japanese encephalitis	
Measles (Attenuvax)	subQ	Stimulate active immunity to measles	Immunization of persons older than age 1 year who reside or travel to endemic regions	
Measles, mumps, and rubella (MMR-II)	subQ	Stimulate active immunity to measles, mumps, and rubella	Immunization of persons greater than 15 months of age	
Measles and rubella, live (MR vax II)	subQ	Stimulate active immunity to measles and rubella	Immunization of children age 1 year and older	
Meningococcal polysaccharide vaccine (Menomune-A/C/Y/W-135)	subQ	Stimulates immunity to meningococcal infections	Immunization against meningococcal infections in endemic regions	
Mumps virus vaccine live (Mumpsvax)	subQ	Stimulate active immunity to mumps	Immunization against mumps in persons age 1 year and older	
Palivizumab (Synagis)	IM	Monoclonal antibody that interferes with the ability of respiratory syncytial virus to replicate in and infect cells	It prevents RSV in high-risk pediatric clients	
Pneumococcal vaccine polyvalent (Pneumovax 23)	subQ or IM	Stimulates active immunity to pneumococcal infection	Immunization against pneumococcal infections	

Table 8-4	Immunizations and Common Immune Sera (Continued)			
Generic (Trade) Name	**Route**	**Actions**	**Uses**	
Pneumococcal 7-valent conjugate vaccine (Prevnar)	IM	Stimulates active immunity to pneumococcal infection	Assists prevention of invasive pneumococcal disease in infants and children	
Poliovirus vaccine: inactivated (IPOL)	subQ	Stimulate active immunity to polio	Immunization against polio in children and adults	
Respiratory syncytial virus immune globulin (RS-VIG, RespiGam)	IV	Passive transfer of antibodies from healthy adults	Polyclonal human hyperimmune globulin	
Rubella virus vaccine: live (Meruvax II)	subQ	Stimulates active immunity to rubella virus	Immunization for children older than age 1 year and adults Do not administer to clients who are pregnant or hypersensitive to neomycin	
Rubella and mumps vaccine: Live (Biavax II)	subQ	Stimulates immunity to rubella and mumps	Immunization of children older than age 1 year and adults	
Smallpox vaccine	One drop of live virus in 2–3 prepared punctures on upper arm	Stimulates active immunity to smallpox	Active immunization against smallpox disease Currently not administered as a regular childhood immunization	
Typhoid vaccine	subQ	Stimulates active immunity to typhoid fever	Immunization against typhoid fever	
Varicella virus vaccine	subQ	Stimulates active immunity against chickenpox	Immunization in adults and children over age 12 months	
Yellow fever vaccine (YF-Vax)	subQ	Simulates active immunity to yellow fever	Immunization of travelers to endemic areas	

      e. Adults should be immunized against tetanus every 10 years

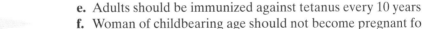

      f. Woman of childbearing age should not become pregnant for 3 months after receiving a rubella immunization

B. Immune sera

    1. Action and use

      a. Immune sera provide passive immunity to a disease

      b. They can be used prophylactically to prevent disease following exposure

    2. Common medications (Table 8-4)

    3. Administration considerations (Table 8-4)

    4. Contraindications: hypersensitivity to immune sera and use cautiously with thrombocytopenia and disorders affecting coagulation

    5. Significant drug interactions: none reported

    6. Significant food interactions: none reported

    7. Significant laboratory studies: none reported

    8. Side effects

      a. Allergic reaction

      b. Flulike symptoms

      c. Irritation at injection site

    9. Adverse effects/toxicity: anaphylaxis

   10. Nursing considerations

      a. Monitor for signs and symptoms of hypersensitivity reaction following administration

Table 8-5	Common Antitoxin Medications	
Generic/Trade Names	**Route**	**Uses**
Rabies immune globulin	IM	Postexposure prevention of rabies
Antirabies serum, equine	IM or to bite wound	Horse serum used if human rabies immune globulin is unavailable
Botulism antitoxin	See drug insert	Obtained from horses immunized against *Clostridium botulinum*; used to treat botulism

      b. Provide comfort for flulike symptoms
      c. Apply heat to irritated injection site
      d. Do not administer to clients with a history of coagulation disorders
      e. Document the medication administered, dosage, date, and response to medication
  11. Client education
      a. Treatment of flulike symptoms (client and family)
      b. Signs and symptoms of anaphylaxis and to seek emergency care if noted (client and family)
      c. There is no evidence to support linkage of immunization such as MMR to autism
      d. Provide documentation to the client and family on the medication administered

C. Antitoxins
  1. Action and use: these are antibodies provided in immune sera for specific toxins that are released from invading pathogens
  2. Common medications (Table 8-5)
  3. Administration considerations: antirabies serum can be applied to animal bite wound
  4. Contraindications: hypersensitivity to antitoxin or horse serum, malignancy, and use cautiously with pregnancy
  5. Significant drug interactions: immunosuppressive drug therapy
  6. Significant food interactions: none reported
  7. Significant laboratory studies: none reported
  8. Side effects: irritation and pain at injection site
  9. Adverse effects/toxicity: hypersensitivity to medication and severe pain at injection site
  10. Nursing considerations
      a. Monitor client response to medication
      b. Assess vital signs before and after administration
      c. Cleanse wound in case of animal bite
      d. Document client's response to medication

      e Test sensitivity to horse serum and have epinephrine available
      f. Assess for neurologic response to botulism antitoxin
  11. Client education
      a. Intended effects of medication
      b. Adverse effects of medication
      c. Wound care of client's animal bite

III. MEDICATIONS TO TREAT MULTIPLE SCLEROSIS MS

A. Action and use
  1. The goal of medication therapy for MS is to decrease inflammation, suppress immune system to prevent nerve tissue destruction, and to reduce fatigue and ataxia

2. A wide variety of medications are used to treat MS, including beta-adrenergic blockers, corticosteroids, anti-inflammatory agents, and interferon
3. Medications to treat MS slow disease progression and assist in decreasing severity of attacks
4. Immunomodulators administered include interferon beta-1a (Avonex), interferon beta-1b (Betaseron), and glatiramer acetate (Copaxone, Copolymer-1)
   a. Interferons reduce T-cell proliferation
   b. Glatiramer acetate (Copaxone, Colpolymer-1) modifies immune process, which is responsible for pathogenesis of MS
5. The following adrenocorticosteroid agents are used to sustain remission and treat exacerbations: adrenocorticotropic hormone (ACTH) (Acthar), prednisone (Deltasone, Metcorten, and Orasone), and methylprednisolone (Medrol and Solumedrol)
6. The following muscle relaxants are given to relieve spasticity associated with MS baclofen (Lioresal), dantrolene (Dantrium), and diazepam (Valium)
7. Immunosuppressants such as azathioprine (Imuran) and cyclophosphamide (Cytoxan), an antineoplastic drug, are given to slow progression of disease
B. **Common medications (Table 8-6)**
C. **Administration considerations:**
   1. Typically, medications are started as soon as a diagnosis of MS is made and should be continued indefinitely only if toxicity occurs or no benefit is noted
   2. Beta-1b (Betaseron) should be discontinued in 6 months if disease does not enter remission

Table 8-6 **Common Medications to Treat Multiple Sclerosis**

Generic (Trade) Name	Route	Actions	Uses
Azathioprine (Imuran)	PO	Decreases severity of symptoms and disease progression	Administered for autoimmune component of disease
Interferon Beta-1a (Avonex) (Rebif)	IM (Avonex) subQ (Rebif)	Blocks replication of viruses and stimulates host immunoregulatory activities	Treatment of relapsing forms of MS Slows accumulation of physical disability; treatment of initial MS attack if brain scan abnormalities show characteristics of MS
Interferon Beta-1b (Betaseron)	subQ	Interferons are produced by human leukocytes in response to viral infections and other stimuli; blocks replication of viruses, thus stimulating host immunoregulatory activities	Reduction in frequency of clinical exacerbations in relapsing and remitting MS
Cyclophosphamide (Cytoxan)	IV, PO	Reduces rate of progression of disease by interfering with replication of susceptible cells	Reduction in rate and progression of MS symptoms
Glatiramer acetate (Copaxone)	subQ	Prevents destruction of brain and nerve tissue	Reduction in frequency and relapse of relapsing and remitting MS
Mitoxantrone hydrochloride (Novantrone)	IV	Cytotoxic cell cycle nonspecific, which is DNA reactive and causes death of both proliferating and nonproliferating cells	Antineoplastic agent used to treat chronic progressive relapsing, or worsening relapsing remitting MS

D. Contraindications

1. These medications should be administered cautiously in presence of hepatic or renal insufficiency and when client has been diagnosed with a neoplasm
2. Contraindicated in pregnancy, lactation, and hypersensitivity to drug

E. Significant drug interactions

1. Do not administer these medications with hepatotoxic or nephrotoxic medications

F. Significant food interactions: do not administer these medications with grapefruit juice or grapefruit; effectiveness of medication will be reduced if this occurs

G. Significant laboratory studies

1. AST/ALT
2. Blood glucose
3. BUN and creatinine
4. Calcium, phosphorus, uric acid
5. CBC and platelet count

H. Side effects

1. Azathioprine (Imuran): an increased risk of infection and renal or hepatic insufficiency; leukopenia and thrombocytopenia have also been noted
2. Inteferons: anorexia, nausea, vomiting, dizziness, and flulike symptoms
3. Glatiramer acetate (Copaxone): anxiety, diarrhea, flulike symptoms, hypertonia, and pain at injection site; may cause a reaction resembling myocardial ischemia

I. Adverse effects/toxicity

1. Medications used to treat symptoms of MS have been noted to increase pulmonary edema leading to chest pain and shortness of breath
2. Medications, depending on action, may either stimulate immune response or suppress some aspects of immune function

J. Nursing considerations

1. Assess client for signs and symptoms of pulmonary edema, chest pain, shortness of breath, GI symptoms, or other adverse effects
2. Assess laboratory tests as ordered by prescriber
3. Monitor blood pressure (BP), pulse, and cardiac output
4. Provide comfort measures when client experiences flulike symptoms
5. Assess injection sites for inflammation and pain

K. Client education

1. Side effects of medication and need for periodic laboratory studies; report side and adverse effects to prescriber
2. Drink 2 liters fluid daily and with cyclophosphamide, observe urine for blood
3. Need for supportive care of flulike symptoms, including adequate fluid intake, rest, and use of acetaminophen for relief of pain and fever
4. How to recognize signs and symptoms of pulmonary edema and to report them
5. Avoid pregnancy while taking cytotoxic medications

Practice to Pass

What nursing interventions should be implemented to relieve the flulike symptoms that are side effects during administration of medications to treat multiple sclerosis?

IV. MEDICATIONS TO TREAT MYASTHENIA GRAVIS

A. Action and use

1. The goal of anticholinesterase medications is to treat symptoms of myasthenia gravis (MG)
2. These medications increase concentration of acetylcholine at neuromuscular junction
3. They are used to increase nerve impulses and their strength

B. Common medications (Table 8-7)

C. Administration considerations

1. Edrophonium (Tensilon): is for diagnostic purposes only; administer IV slowly while observing client response; response will often be immediate

Table 8-7	Common Medications to Treat Myasthenia Gravis		
Generic (Trade) Name	**Route**	**Actions**	**Uses**
Ambenonium (Mytelase)	PO	Increases concentration of acetylcholine (Ach) at sites of cholinergic transmission; prolongs and inhibits enzyme acetylcholinesterase causing parasympathomimetic effects, facilitating transmission at skeletal neuromuscular junction	Provide symptomatic control of myasthenia gravis
Edrophonium (Enlon, Reversol, Tensilon)	IV, IM	Increases concentration of Ach at sites of cholinergic transmission; prolongs and exaggerates effects of Ach by inhibiting enzyme anticholinesterase, facilitating transmission at skeletal neuromuscular junction	Diagnosis and treatment of myasthenia gravis
Neostigmine (Prostigmine)	IM, subQ, PO	Increases concentration of Ach at cholinergic transmission sites and prolongs effect of Ach at skeletal neuromuscular junction	Symptomatic control of myasthenia gravis
Pyridostigmine (Reganol, Mestinol)	PO	Increases concentration of Ach at sites of cholinergic transmission and prolongs effects of Ach by inhibiting acetylcholinesterase, facilitating transmission at skeletal neuromuscular junction	Treatment of myasthenia gravis

2. Neostigmine (Prostigmine): can be administered subQ during an acute exacerbation of MG

3. Pyridostigmine (Reganol, Mestinon): a timed-release preparation can be administered at bedtime; can also be administered IM during acute exacerbation

4. Corticosteroids or immunosuppressants may be added to plan of care during exacerbation or over time if medications become ineffective

D. **Contraindications**
   1. Pregnancy and lactation
   2. Bradycardia, intestinal or urinary obstruction, peritonitis
   3. Hypersensitivity to drug
   4. Use cautiously in clients with asthma, heart disease, Parkinson's disease, and seizure disorders

E. **Significant drug interactions**
   1. Combination of MG medications and NSAIDs poses a threat of GI bleeding because of increase in GI secretions
   2. Decreased effects of neostigmine occur with ambenonium and corticosteroids

F. **Significant food interactions**: none reported

G. **Significant laboratory studies**
   1. ALT/AST
   2. BUN and creatinine

H. **Side effects**
   1. Bradycardia, hypotension, or cardiac arrest
   2. Increased gastric secretions or diarrhea
   3. Increased urinary urgency
   4. Involuntary incontinence of stool
   5. Nausea and vomiting

I. **Adverse effects/toxicity**
   1. Severe cholinergic reaction includes excessive salivation, sphincter relaxation, diarrhea, and vomiting
   2. During administration of edrophonium (Tensilon), observe for cholinergic reaction and have atropine available as an antidote

J. Nursing considerations

1. Assess respiratory and general muscle strength including swallowing and heart rate prior to administration
2. Administer doses with meals to enhance absorption and decrease GI irritation
3. Administer doses on time to prevent difficulty with respirations and swallowing caused by under-medication or late medication administration
4. Administer IV preparations slowly to prevent cholinergic reaction
5. Have atropine available to counteract cholinergic reaction but also be aware that atropine may mask parasympathetic effects of anticholinesterase overdose
6. Assess client's response to the medication and ability to perform activities of daily living (ADLs)

K. Client education

1. All aspects of medication administration
2. How to coordinate medication administration with ADLs
3. Overmedication will result in cholinergic reaction
4. Assessment of apical pulse
5. Side effects of medications
6. Take medications with food to decrease GI irritation
7. Report muscle weakness promptly to prescriber

V. MEDICATIONS TO TREAT RHEUMATOID ARTHRITIS

A. Action and use

1. Management of RA in early stages is accomplished with use of NSAIDs and disease-modifying antirheumatic drugs (DMARDs)
2. These medications decrease the erythrocyte sedimentation rate, thus reducing inflammation, stiffness, swelling, and pain
3. DMARDs include the newest RA treatments using biologic therapies
   a. Medications including etanercept (Enbrel) and infliximab (Remicade) are tumor necrosis factor (TNF) antagonists, which decrease inflammation and modulate cellular immune responses
   b. Adalimumab (Humira) works in clients with polyarthritis to decrease inflammation

B. Common medications (Table 8-8)

C. Administration considerations

1. DMARDs: a client may take multiple DMARDs and analgesics; it may take several months to achieve therapeutic effects
   a. Hydroxychloroquine (Plaquenil): often used in conjunction with corticosteroid therapy
   b. Methotrexate (Rheumatrex): an antimetabolite primarily used for severe RA intravenously
   c. Biologic therapies: administer only one medication of this type; examples include etanercept (Enbrel) and adalimumab (Humira): for treatment of moderate to severe RA, administered subQ
   d. Gold salts and medications such as penicillamine (Depen) may be used but are more toxic than other DMARDs

D. Contraindications

1. Never administer medications to clients who have a known allergy to animal products
2. Contraindicated with pregnancy, lactation, liver disease, or renal disease
3. Use cautiously in clients with immunosuppression or malignancy

E. Significant drug interactions

1. Do not administer these drugs with any agents known to be hepatotoxic
2. Use caution when administering anakinra with etanercept (tumor necrosis factor blocker) because of increased risk for neutropenia and resulting risk for severe infection

Table 8-8	Common Medications to Treat Rheumatoid Arthritis (RA)			
Generic (Trade) Names	**Route**	**Actions**	**Uses**
Anakinra (Kineret)	subQ	Blocks activity of interleukin-1 by competitively inhibiting interleukin-1 activity from binding to interleukin-1 type receptors	Slow progression of structural damage in moderate-to-severe active RA following one failure with DMARDs
Auranofin (Ridaura)	PO	Inhibits phagocytosis and activities of lysosomal enzymes, thus decreasing rheumatoid factor and immunoglobulins	Manage RA in adults with active classic or definite RA who lack sufficient treatment with NSAIDs
Aurothioglucose (Solganol)	IM	Suppresses and prevents arthritis and synovitis, taken up by macrophages with inhibition of phagocytosis	Treats adult and juvenile RA; most effective early in disease
Etanercept (Enbrel)	subQ	Genetically engineered TNF receptors from Chinese hamsters' ovary cells; assist autoimmune response by deactivating free-floating TNF released by active leukocytes	Inhibits progression of structural damage to improve physical function with moderate to severe RA; assists in delaying structural damage associated with RA
Hylan G-F 20 (Synvisc)	Intraarticular	Lubricating hylan from chicken combs enhances lubrication of knee joint	Relief of arthritic knee pain in clients unresponsive to conventional treatment
Leflunomide (Arava)	PO	Inhibits enzyme dihydroorotate dehydrogenase (DHODH) (active in RA) to assist in relieving inflammation and blocking structural damage caused by autoimmune process	Relieve symptoms and slow progression of RA
Methotrexate (Rheumatrex)	PO	Inhibits folic acid reductase, which inhibits DNA synthesis and cellular replication; selectively affects most rapidly dividing cells	Management of severe RA
Penicillamine (Depen)	PO	Lowers IgM rheumatoid factor, reducing cystine excretion by disulfide interchange with cystine, making the substance more soluble than cystine that is readily excreted	Treatment of severe active RA in clients who have had failure in other treatments
Sodium hyaluronate (Hyalgan)	Intraarticular	Lubricating hylan injected into the knee joint to provide cushioning; it is a hyaluronic acid derivative	Treatment of pain in arthritis in clients who failed to respond to conservative therapy and analgesics

  3. Methotrexate (Rheumatrex): multiple solution incompatibilities
  4. Do not administer biologic modifiers with vaccinations
  5. Biologic modifiers may be used with other DMARDs, but are generally contraindicated with each other due to similar mechanism of action
  6. Etanercept combined with NSAIDs leads to fatal reactions
F. Significant food interactions
  1. Methotrexate results may be decreased with increased caffeine intake
  2. Echinacea increases liver toxicity
G. Significant laboratory studies
  1. Liver function tests
  2. BUN and creatinine
  3. CBC and platelet count

H. Side effects
1. Alopecia
2. Stomatitis, colitis, and diarrhea
3. Dizziness
4. Itching and rash
5. Plaquenil: can cause unusual pigmentation of skin (to a blue-black color)

I. Adverse effects/toxicity
1. Black furry tongue (from superinfection)
2. Hepatotoxicity, pericarditis
3. Pulmonary edema
4. Thrombosis, Stevens–Johnson syndrome, and death
5. Increased eosinophil count or decreased neutrophils, total WBC count, or platelet count

J. Nursing considerations
1. Avoid use of antacids for at least 2 hours after dose administration
2. Assess for bone marrow suppression, pulmonary fibrosis, and GI ulceration or bleeding with methotrexate
3. Protect from exposure to sunlight
4. Assess for side effects to medication
5. Check for proteinuria and hematuria before giving initial dose and during therapy with gold drugs
6. Assess for signs of infection with all DMARDs
7. Stop medications if signs of severe infection develop

K. Client education
1. Use measures to protect self from infection when taking etanercept or anakinra
2. Use good oral hygiene to protect from stomatitis
3. If taking gold preparations, report signs of gold toxicity, including metallic taste and pruritus
4. Monitor for and report bruising, petechiae, bleeding gums, or blood in stool
5. Monitor blood glucose and report elevations
6. Take medications as directed and be aware of side effects, action, use, and contraindications
7. Use contraceptive measures to protect against pregnancy with cytotoxic drugs such as methotrexate

VI. MEDICATIONS TO TREAT SYSTEMIC LUPUS ERYTHEMATOSUS

A. Action and use
1. Cytotoxic drugs or purine analogs are used along with NSAIDs and corticosteroids to treat symptoms of systemic lupus erythematosus (SLE)
2. They provide immunosuppressive action to treat autoimmune diseases
3. Cytotoxic and antineoplastic drugs are used as immunosuppressive agents to decrease cell proliferation in immune system; administered concurrently with corticosteroid therapy

B. Common medications (Table 8-9)
C. Administration considerations (Table 8-9)
D. Contraindications
1. Do not administer with agents that are known to be hepatotoxic
2. Do not administer during pregnancy or lactation

E. Significant drug interactions: if azathioprine (Imuran) is administered with allopurinol (Zyloprim), the azathioprine dose should be reduced

F. Significant food interactions: do not administer azathioprine with grapefruit juice

Table 8-9 Common Medications to Treat Systemic Lupus Erythematosus (SLE)

Generic (Trade) Name	Route	Actions	Uses
Azathioprine (Imuran)	PO	Suppresses cell-mediated hypersensitivity and alters antibody production	Administered for autoimmune component of disease
Cyclophosphamide (Cytoxan)	PO, IV	Lymphocytes are sensitive to drug effects in immunosuppression	Treatment of SLE
Cyclosporine (Sandimmune)	PO	Inhibits T-helper and T-suppressor cells, lymphokine production, and release of interleukin-2 and T-cell growth factor	Prophylaxis against kidney, liver, and heart transplantation; treatment of chronic rejection in clients who have received immunosuppressants; RA, recalcitrant plaque psoriasis, and SLE
Methotrexate (Rheumatrex)	PO	Inhibits folic acid reductase, which inhibits DNA synthesis and cellular replication in rapidly dividing cells	Management of SLE

G. **Significant laboratory studies**
   1. Liver and renal function tests
   2. Blood glucose
   3. CBC and platelet count
   4. Calcium, phosphorus, and uric acid
H. **Side effects**
   1. Alopecia
   2. Stomatitis, diarrhea, and colitis
   3. Dizziness
   4. Itching or rash
   5. Leukopenia or thrombocytopenia
I. **Adverse effects/toxicity**
   1. Black furry tongue
   2. Hepatotoxicity
   3. Pericarditis
   4. Pulmonary edema
   5. Stevens–Johnson Syndrome
   6. Death
J. **Nursing considerations**
   1. Assess for side effects of medications
   2. Assess for pulmonary edema and shortness of breath
   3. Assess laboratory tests as ordered by provider
K. **Client education**
   1. How to protect self from infection
   2. Need for proper oral hygiene to protect from stomatitis
   3. How to self-monitor blood glucose level and report elevations
   4. Be aware of all aspects of medication therapy, including side effects, actions, use, and contraindications
   5. How to recognize pulmonary edema and to report to provider

Case Study

A 15-year-old girl is diagnosed with untreatable liver failure and esophageal varices with hemorrhage, and her name is placed on the national transplant list. Two weeks later, she received a liver transplant. Both before and after surgery she stated she was anxious and depressed. Three weeks after surgery she was discharged on these medications:

- *Tacrolimus (Prograf) 3 mg PO bid*
- *Magnesium oxide 1 tablet PO bid*
- *Azathioprine (Imuran) 50 mg 2 ½ tablets PO every other day*
- *Esomeprazole (Nexium) 1 tablet PO bid*
- *Milk of magnesia 30 mL PO every other day*

One week after discharge, she fainted and experienced extreme abdominal pain. She was readmitted with signs of liver transplant rejection. A liver biopsy was performed and surgery was done to repair a closing portal vein. An order for methylprednisolone (SoluMedrol) 125 mg IVP every 8 hours was added to her medication list. Laboratory studies obtained included AST/ALT, CBC with

platelets, chemistry profile, arterial blood gases, and serum bilirubin.

1. What are the priority nursing diagnoses for this client both preoperatively and postoperatively?

2. Prior to the administration of the previously listed medications, what diagnostic studies and assessments should the nurse make?

3. What should be included in a teaching plan for this client and her family?

4. What nursing interventions should be implemented prior to discharge following the portal vein repair?

5. What is the rationale for the administration of SoluMedrol following the portal vein repair?

For suggested responses, see page 543.

POSTTEST

① The client asks how filgrastim (Neupogen) will help with the management of cancer. The nurse should provide which response?

1. "Filgrastim (Neupogen) will reduce your fatigue level."
2. "Filgrastim (Neupogen) will increase your ability to resist infection."
3. "Filgrastim (Neupogen) reduces the nausea and vomiting that accompanies chemotherapy."
4. "Filgrastim (Neupogen) will protect your heart during chemotherapy administration."

② Following an autologous bone marrow transplant, a client is receiving sargramostim (Leukine). The nurse is most likely to give *priority* to the assessment of which of the following?

1. Bone pain, myalgia, or arthralgia
2. Hypotension, tachycardia, or cardiac rhythm changes
3. Nausea, vomiting, and diarrhea
4. Myalgia, weight gain, and increased uric acid levels

③ Because a client with rheumatoid arthritis (RA) developed insulin-dependent diabetes mellitus, the nurse gives priority to which of the following assessments?

1. Client response to corticosteroids
2. Ability to fill syringes and give injections
3. Ability to exercise
4. Eating a balanced diet

4 A client is receiving cortisone after receiving a liver transplant. Several months later, what assessment data is of greatest concern to the home health nurse?

1. Ability to perform activities of daily living (ADLs)
2. Psychological response to receiving another person's body part
3. Eye examination results of intraocular pressure (IOP) and lens density
4. Presence of fine tremors and gingival hyperplasia

5 Prior to the administration of chemotherapy to a client with cancer, a nurse is *most likely* to administer which of the following medications?

1. Epoetin alfa (Epogen)
2. Granisetron hydrochloride (Kytril)
3. Dexamethasone (Decadron)
4. Vinblastine sulfate (Velban)

6 A client with a renal transplant is receiving tacrolimus (Prograf). The nurse reviews the results of which of the following laboratory tests prior to drug administration?

1. LDH (lactic dehydrogenase) and CPK (creatinine phosphokinase)
2. Serum uric acid and serum protein
3. Serum calcium levels and serum albumin levels
4. Serum AST (aspartate aminotransferase) and ALT (alanine aminotransferase)

7 A client with multiple sclerosis (MS) has been prescribed interferon alfa-2b (Intron-A). Which intervention should the nurse include in the plan of care?

1. Request a prescription to treat clinical depression.
2. Instruct the client to change body positions slowly.
3. Encourage the client to seek grief counseling.
4. Encourage routine hydration with water.

8 An infant girl with a tympanic membrane temperature of 101°F is scheduled to receive the second diphtheria, pertussis, and tetanus (DPT) vaccine along with the inactivated poliovirus vaccine (IPV). The nurse should take which action?

1. Withhold vaccines and reschedule her visit when she is not febrile.
2. Administer injection and instruct mother to administer an antipyretic when she gets home.
3. Administer acetaminophen orally and give immunizations.
4. Obtain titers on needed immunizations and withhold them until results are obtained.

9 A client with multiple sclerosis who receives cyclophosphamide (Cytoxan) and digoxin (Lanoxin) reports nausea to the outpatient clinic nurse. The nurse would place highest priority on which of the following actions?

1. Evaluate the cyclophosphamide (Cytoxan) level.
2. Administer an oral antiemetic daily.
3. Provide six small, frequent meals.
4. Evaluate the digoxin level.

10 When a nurse discovers that a renal transplant recipient eats grapefruit for breakfast and is taking cyclosporine (Sandimmune) as an immunosuppressant drug, the nurse should provide which instructions? Select all that apply.

1. "This combination is likely to cause epigastric burning."
2. "Grapefruit and cyclosporine have interactions that affect the drug dosage."
3. "Take loperamide (Imodium) for diarrhea if it occurs."
4. "Be sure to watch for signs and symptoms of organ rejection."
5. "This combination could cause confusion or kidney failure."

➤ *See pages 278–279 for Answers and Rationales.*

POSTTEST

ANSWERS & RATIONALES

Pretest

1 **Answer: 4** **Rationale:** Filgrastim (Neupogen) is a colony-stimulating factor. The goal of the therapy is to increase the neutrophil count to a normal level. The range is 5,000–8,000/mm^3. Thus, if the count returns to high normal level, it may be appropriate to withhold the dose and confirm future orders. Although the drug can cause anemia, the hemoglobin and hematocrit are within normal limits. There is no evidence that mental depression is caused by this drug. Because of the nature of the drug, the depression would probably be treated and the medication continued. Because of the risks to the client, the drug would be continued and the bone pain would be managed with opioid analgesics. **Cognitive Level:** Applying **Client Need:** Pharmacological and Parenteral Therapies **Integrated Process:** Nursing Process: Planning **Content Area:** Pharmacology **Strategy:** The critical words are *withholding the dose*. Consider the action of the drug to reason that the correct answer must either identify the intended outcome or a severe adverse effect. With this in mind, recall that the drug is intended to stimulate white blood cell production, and note the normal value to choose it as the correct option. **Reference:** Wilson, B. A., Shannon, M. T., & Shields, K. M. (2012). *Pearson nurse's drug guide 2012.* Upper Saddle River, NJ: Pearson Education, pp. 634–636. Adams, M., & Koch, R. (2010). *Pharmacology: Connections to nursing practice.* Upper Saddle River, NJ: Pearson Education, p. 673.

2 **Answer: 3** **Rationale:** Pericarditis, a side effect of this drug, can result in heart failure. Signs and symptoms include dyspnea on exertion and dependent edema. Unlicensed assistive personnel (UAP) are capable of noting this data while performing or assisting with activities of daily living. A slight temperature elevation accompanies pericarditis but is not representative of impaired cardiac function. Assessments of pericardial and pleural friction rub are beyond the skill level of support staff. Mental depression and fatigue need to be reported but the dyspnea and the edema take priority over these elements. **Cognitive Level:** Analyzing **Client Need:** Pharmacological and Parenteral Therapies **Integrated Process:** Communication and Documentation **Content Area:** Pharmacology **Strategy:** Use the syllable *gram* in the word *sargramostim* to recall the increase in heart size associated with congestive heart failure. Next recall the scope of practice of unlicensed assistive personnel (UAP) to select the most important abnormal data that is within their scope to collect. **Reference:** Wilson, B. A., Shannon, M. T., & Shields, K. M. (2012). *Pearson nurse's drug guide 2012.* Upper Saddle River, NJ: Pearson Education, pp. 1367–1369. Adams, M., & Koch, R.

(2010). *Pharmacology: Connections to nursing practice.* Upper Saddle River, NJ: Pearson Education, p. 674.

3 **Answer: 1** **Rationale:** Immunosuppression and biologic response modifier drugs are used to treat severe rheumatoid arthritis. These medications increase the client's susceptibility to infection. Fever without an infectious process is also a side effect. It is not likely that the elevation in body temperature is due to joint inflammation; an increased temperature from joint inflammation is more likely to be localized. Dehydration is possible but not as likely as the increased susceptibility to infection. Antibiotics are more likely to lead to vaginal yeast infections because of overgrowth of normal flora as a side effect of treatment. **Cognitive Level:** Analyzing **Client Need:** Pharmacological and Parenteral Therapies **Integrated Process:** Nursing Process: Assessment **Content Area:** Pharmacology **Strategy:** Recall that arthritis is an inflammatory process. Consider that these drugs reduce the inflammatory response resulting in a reduced ability to fight pathogens and increasing the client's susceptibility to infection. **Reference:** Wilson, B. A., Shannon, M. T., & Shields, K. M. (2012). *Pearson nurse's drug guide 2012.* Upper Saddle River, NJ: Pearson Education, p. 781. Adams, M., & Koch, R. (2010). *Pharmacology: Connections to nursing practice.* Upper Saddle River, NJ: Pearson Education, pp. 670–674.

4 **Answer: 1, 2, 3, 4** **Rationale:** Significant pain and tenderness is likely to occur at the injection site. The drug may interfere with the development of antibodies following administration of live viruses so vaccinations should be postponed for at least 3 months. Immunity occurs several weeks after administration so the client should use measures to protect against infection in the interim. Fever and chills are indicative of hypersensitivity. Because of the diuretic effect of maltose (a preservative), urinary output may increase rather than decrease. **Cognitive Level:** Analyzing **Client Need:** Pharmacological and Parenteral Therapies **Integrated Process:** Teaching and Learning **Content Area:** Pharmacology **Strategy:** Correlate drug characteristics with the purpose of the prescription. **Reference:** Wilson, B. A., Shannon, M. T., & Shields, K. M. (2012). *Pearson nurse's drug guide 2012.* Upper Saddle River, NJ: Pearson Education, pp. 771–772.

5 **Answer: 1, 2** **Rationale:** Because concurrent administration of antiepileptic medications and cyclosporine (Sandimmune) will cause decreased therapeutic levels of the cyclosporine, an increase in the cyclosporine dosage needs to be made to ensure the appropriate therapeutic effect. The client is more likely to experience hypertension than hypotension. The antiepileptic medication will need to be administered at the proper dosage level that controls the seizures. Monitoring for seizures is an assessment, not an intervention, and it places the client at risk for ineffective immunosuppressant therapy. Cyclosporine does not generally interfere with antiepileptic medication levels. **Cognitive Level:** Analyzing **Client Need:** Pharmacological and Parenteral Therapies **Integrated Process:** Nursing Process: Implementation **Content Area:** Pharmacology **Strategy:** Use knowledge of the relationship between antiepileptics and cyclosporine (Sandimmune) to choose correctly. **Reference:** Wilson, B. A., Shannon, M. T., & Shields, K. M. (2012). *Pearson nurse's drug guide 2012.* Upper Saddle River, NJ: Pearson Education, p. 387–389. Adams, M., & Koch, R. (2010). *Pharmacology: Connections to nursing practice.* Upper Saddle River, NJ: Pearson Education, p. 743.

6 **Answer: 1, 2, 4** **Rationale:** Fluid retention, cardiac dysrhythmias, and dyspnea are side effects of oprelvekin (Neumega). The nature of the signs and symptoms warrant immediate attention. Hence, calling for immediate assistance is the best match. Although the client needs to be NPO until health care assistance is available, this instruction does nothing to relieve the hypoxia or address the immediacy of the client's needs. Lying down with the head elevated will reduce the oxygen demand, but does nothing to resolve the problem. Although the diuretic would likely help with fluid volume overload, delaying medical attention will put the client at greater risk. An extra dose of digoxin (Lanoxin) could lower the heart rate or cause toxicity. Thus, the client needs to be evaluated by a health care provider before taking medications. **Cognitive Level:** Analyzing **Client Need:** Pharmacological and Parenteral Therapies **Integrated Process:** Communication and Documentation **Content Area:** Pharmacology **Strategy:** Apply knowledge of drug side effects with client's clinical profile and use principles of priority setting (airway, breathing, and circulation) to choose the best instruction for the client. **Reference:** Wilson, B. A., Shannon, M. T., & Shields, K. M. (2012). *Pearson nurse's drug guide 2012.* Upper Saddle River, NJ: Pearson Education, pp. 1111–1112. Adams, M., Holland, L., & Bostwick, P. (2011). *Pharmacology for nurses: A pathophysiologic approach* (3rd ed.). Upper Saddle River, NJ: Pearson Education, pp. 391, 397, 452–457.

7 **Answer: 1** **Rationale:** A side effect of cyclosporine (Sandimmune) is hypertension that places the client at risk for ineffective tissue perfusion to the kidneys, brain, and heart. Chest pain and leg cramps are occasionally associated with cyclosporine. Nephrotoxicity is associated with the drug, but hypervolemia is more likely. Tremors are a side effect of the drug, but this does not override the significance of uncontrolled hypertension. **Cognitive Level:** Applying **Client Need:** Pharmacological and Parenteral Therapies **Integrated Process:** Nursing Process: Implementation **Content Area:** Pharmacology **Strategy:** Specific drug knowledge is needed to answer the question. If needed, use the ABCs—airway, breathing, and circulation—to choose correctly. **Reference:** Adams, M., & Koch, R.

(2010). *Pharmacology: Connections to nursing practice.* Upper Saddle River, NJ: Pearson Education, p. 743.

8 **Answer: 4** **Rationale:** Intramuscular immune serum globulin should not be administered to clients with a history of coagulation disorders (platelet count of less than 100,000/mm^3). It can be administered to clients with diabetes insipidus, but should be avoided in clients with diabetes mellitus. It is administered to clients exposed to rubeola and hepatitis B to provide passive immunity. **Cognitive Level:** Applying **Client Need:** Pharmacological and Parenteral Therapies **Integrated Process:** Nursing Process: Planning **Content Area:** Pharmacology **Strategy:** Think of immunoglobulin therapy and hypocoagulation as repelling each other. Choose the option that represents this connection in thinking. **Reference:** Abrams, A., Pennington, S., Lammon, C., & Goldsmith, T. (2009). *Clinical drug therapy: Rationales for nursing practice* (9th ed.). Philadelphia, PA: Lippincott Williams & Wilkins, pp. 617–620.

9 **Answer: 1, 2, 4** **Rationale:** Because of the reduced immunity, children are more prone to many contagious diseases. Without the immunizations, control of contagious illnesses would cause a high rate of mortality and morbidity in children as well as spreading to others. Although immunizations are mandatory, the new parent is probably more concerned about the new baby; however, the client does need to understand the importance of immunizations. All of the immunizations commonly have minor side effects. Information about cost may allay fears that the parent cannot afford the immunization, thus increasing compliance. Immunity begins with the first vaccine, but the child does not have full immunity until all doses are given. **Cognitive Level:** Applying **Client Need:** Pharmacological and Parenteral Therapies **Integrated Process:** Communication and Documentation **Content Area:** Pharmacology **Strategy:** When determining the appropriate response, consider the client and intended recipient along with the purpose of the immunizations. **Reference:** Abrams, A., Pennington, S., Lammon, C., & Goldsmith, T. (2009). *Clinical drug therapy: Rationales for nursing practice* (9th ed.). Philadelphia, PA: Lippincott Williams & Wilkins, pp. 625–635. Karch, A. M. (2010). *Focus on nursing pharmacology* (5th ed.). Philadelphia, PA: Lippincott Williams & Wilkins, pp. 291–294.

10 **Answer: 4** **Rationale:** In myasthenia gravis, fewer receptors for acetylcholine are available, resulting in a lack of muscular contraction. Because they maximize the available receptors, cholinesterase inhibitors are the drugs of choice. Side effects of this category include dysrhythmic muscular contractions. Atropine (an anticholinergic medication) counteracts the cholinergic reaction of the medication. Edrophonium (Tensilon) is a cholinesterase inhibitor. It prevents the destruction of acetylcholine, improving muscular contractions. If muscular contractions improve, it is determined that a diagnosis of myasthenia gravis exists. Edrophonium, neostigmine (Prostigmine), and ambenonium (Mytelase) are in the same category and would increase symptoms. **Cognitive Level:** Applying **Client Need:** Pharmacological and Parenteral Therapies **Integrated Process:** Nursing Process: Planning **Content Area:** Pharmacology **Strategy:** Consider from the symptoms described that the client may be experiencing excessive drug effects, after recalling that the symptoms of the disease include muscle weakness. From there, choose the medication that is the antidote to the prescribed medication. **Reference:** Abrams, A., Pennington, S., Lammon, C., & Goldsmith, T. (2009). *Clinical drug therapy: Rationales for nursing practice* (9th ed.). Philadelphia, PA: Lippincott Williams & Wilkins, pp. 313–317.

Posttest

1 **Answer: 2** **Rationale:** Filgrastim (Neupogen) increases the number of neutrophils whose function is to act against invading microorganisms. The drug may cause anemia, which may compound the feelings of fatigue rather than reduce them. The drug may cause nausea and vomiting rather than reduce it. It may cause changes in the electrocardiogram and is not cardioprotective. **Cognitive Level:** Applying **Client Need:** Pharmacological and Parenteral Therapies **Integrated Process:** Teaching and Learning **Content Area:** Pharmacology **Strategy:** Associate the syllable *fil* in *filgrastim* with filling the gap in the neutrophil count caused by chemotherapy. Recall the function of neutrophils to then choose the correct option. **Reference:** Wilson, B. A., Shannon, M. T., & Shields, K. M. (2012). *Pearson nurse's drug guide 2012.* Upper Saddle River, NJ: Pearson Education, pp. 634–636.

2 **Answer: 2** **Rationale:** Hypotension, tachycardia, and thrombocytopenia are major side effects of sargramostim (Leukine). They take priority because they affect circulation. The other options indicate signs or symptoms that are side effects of the drug but they do not have priority over those that affect circulatory status. Bone pain, myalgia, and arthralgia are common side effects. Nausea, vomiting, and diarrhea are side effects that should be managed, but would *not* receive priority over cardiovascular changes. Myalgia, weight gain, and increased uric acid levels are side effects of the drug that would also be secondary priorities. **Cognitive Level:** Applying **Client Need:** Pharmacological and Parenteral Therapies **Integrated Process:** Nursing Process: Assessment **Content Area:** Pharmacology **Strategy:** Associate the drug with musculoskeletal and cardiac complications. Then prioritize using the ABCs (airway, breathing, and circulation). **Reference:** Adams, M., & Koch, R. (2010). *Pharmacology: Connections to nursing practice*. Upper Saddle River, NJ: Pearson Education., p. 674. Wilson, B. A., Shannon, M. T., & Shields, K. M. (2012). *Pearson nurse's drug guide 2012.* Upper Saddle River, NJ: Pearson Education, pp. 1367–1369.

3 **Answer: 2** **Rationale:** The diagnosis of rheumatoid arthritis (RA) may limit fine motor movements of the hands that are needed for self-administration of insulin, and this client may need further assistance from family or other caregivers. Corticosteroids may increase the glucose level, but making sure the insulin is injected takes priority. Exercise is known to increase the utilization of glucose, resulting in a decreased level of glucose in the central circulating volume; however, the primary focus of insulin-dependent diabejtes management is injection of insulin. Eating a balanced diet has similar importance to exercise in the management of diabetes, but ability to manage medication therapy takes priority because the client depends on exogenous insulin injection. **Cognitive Level:** Analyzing **Client Need:** Pharmacological and Parenteral Therapies **Integrated Process:** Nursing Process: Assessment **Content Area:** Pharmacology **Strategy:** With diabetes, consider health maintenance needs. With rheumatoid arthritis (RA), determine the possible psychomotor interference with the ability to manage the disease and use this rationale to focus on ability to manage medication therapy. **Reference:** Aschenbrenner, D., & Venable, S. (2009). *Drug therapy in nursing* (3rd ed.). Philadelphia, PA: Lippincott Williams & Wilkins, pp. 428–442, 1059–1070.

4 **Answer: 3** **Rationale:** Long-term use of corticosteroids to prevent organ rejection can result in the development of cataracts and glaucoma. While fatigue and weakness prevented normal activities before the transplant, the client's ability to manage personal needs increases after the transplant. Clients often experience mental depression following the transplant. While psychosocial needs are important as well, the nurse should give the potential loss of sight priority. Overgrowth of gums and fine tremors are minor side effects of the drug. **Cognitive Level:** Applying **Client Need:** Pharmacological and Parenteral Therapies **Integrated Process:** Nursing Process: Assessment **Content Area:** Pharmacology **Strategy:** The time line in the question refers to long-term intended and adverse effects associated with the use of cortisone. Use specific knowledge about the drug to make a selection. **Reference:** Aschenbrenner, D., & Venable, S. (2009). *Drug therapy in nursing* (3rd ed.). Philadelphia, PA: Lippincott Williams & Wilkins, pp. 669–689.

5 **Answer: 2** **Rationale:** Granisetron hydrochloride (Kytril) is a serotonin-blocker that is effective against emetogenic chemotherapy agents. Administration before infusing chemotherapy prevents the onset of nausea and vomiting commonly associated with this drug category. Epoetin alfa (Epogen) is administered *after* chemotherapy to treat anemia. Glucocorticoids are used as adjuncts to chemotherapy rather than prior to administration. Vinblastine sulfate (Velban) is a vinca alkaloid, a type of chemotherapy. **Cognitive Level:** Applying **Client Need:** Pharmacological and Parenteral Therapies **Integrated Process:** Nursing Process: Planning **Content Area:** Pharmacology **Strategy:** Note that the critical words in the question are *prior to*. Next determine the categories of the drugs in the various options and recall that medications that end in *setron* are antiemetics. Finally, associate the use of this drug with chemotherapy-induced nausea and vomiting. **Reference:** Wilson, B. A., Shannon, M. T., & Shields, K. M. (2012). *Pearson nurse's drug guide 2012.* Upper Saddle River, NJ: Pearson Education, pp. 714–716.

6 **Answer: 4** **Rationale:** AST (aspartate aminotransferase) and ALT (alanine aminotransferase), which are liver enzymes, are relevant since tacrolimus (Prograf) and other immunosuppressant drugs are hepatotoxic. LDH (lactic dehydrogenase) is found in many tissues and is not specifically used for determining liver damage. CPK (creatinine phosphokinase) is utilized in the diagnosis of cardiac, neurologic, and muscle damage. The drug does not significantly affect these tissues. Changes in uric acid levels are related to gout. Serum protein is used more commonly for the diagnosis of lymphoma or myeloma. Serum calcium levels are more likely to be elevated with decreased parathyroid function or with decreased bone resorption. Because of the long half-life (12–18 days) of albumin, it is not an effective test for determining whether or not the drug should be administered. **Cognitive Level:** Applying **Client Need:** Pharmacological and Parenteral Therapies **Integrated Process:** Nursing Process: Assessment **Content Area:** Pharmacology **Strategy:** The core issue of the question is knowledge that this medication is hepatotoxic. With this in mind, select the laboratory tests that best reflect liver function. **Reference:** Wilson, B. A., Shannon, M. T., & Shields, K. M. (2012). *Pearson nurse's drug guide 2012.* Upper Saddle River, NJ: Pearson Education, pp. 1437–1439.

7 **Answer: 4** **Rationale:** Interferon alfa-2a is a biological response modifier used in treatment of multiple illnesses, including multiple sclerosis (MS). A history of depression or suicidal tendencies may prevent the use of the drug; however, an antidepressant would not generally need to be requested from the health care provider. Dizziness, hypotension, and tachycardia are not common side effects of interferon. The need for grief counseling would not be related to administration of this drug. Hydration status should be monitored by the nurse, particularly in the initial stage of treatment, due to the elimination of the drug in the kidneys in order to prevent toxicity. **Cognitive Level:** Applying **Client Need:** Pharmacological and Parenteral Therapies **Integrated Process:** Nursing Process: Implementation **Content Area:** Pharmacology **Strategy:** Specific drug knowledge is needed to answer this question. Associate need for hydration with this medication. **Reference:** Wilson, B. A., Shannon, M. T., & Shields, K. M. (2012). *Pearson nurse's drug guide 2012.* Upper Saddle River, NJ: Pearson Education, pp. 793–795.

8 **Answer: 1** **Rationale:** Since fever is a side effect of the vaccine, the immunization should be withheld. It would be difficult to separate a response to the immunization from a febrile disease. Diagnosis of the problem should

be made before treatment is initiated. Administering an antipyretic is more appropriate for prevention of a fever after the vaccine is administered. The fever remains of unknown origin and further diagnosis is needed. Titers should be performed after immunization or actually having the disease. **Cognitive Level:** Applying **Client Need:** Pharmacological and Parenteral Therapies **Integrated Process:** Nursing Process: Implementation **Content Area:** Pharmacology **Strategy:** Recall that immunization stimulates the immune process, which could make it difficult to interpret the significance of fever. Use general nursing knowledge of vaccines and the immune response to make a selection. **Reference:** Adams, M., & Koch, R. (2010). *Pharmacology: Connections to nursing practice.* Upper Saddle River, NJ: Pearson Education, pp. 757–758.

9 **Answer: 4** **Rationale:** Cyclophosphamide (Cytoxan) combined with digoxin (Lanoxin) may result in digoxin toxicity, so the health care team must continually assess for signs and symptoms of toxicity. Nausea is an early sign of digoxin toxicity. Nausea and vomiting are also side effects of cyclophosphamide, but because cyclophosphamide may increase the risk of digoxin toxicity, the best response is to explore the digoxin level first. The nurse should administer an antiemetic but not orally. Nausea needs to be relieved before eating. **Cognitive Level:** Applying **Client Need:** Pharmacological and Parenteral Therapies **Integrated Process:** Nursing Process: Assessment **Content Area:** Pharmacology **Strategy:** As an early strategy for many questions, consider the possibility of drug toxicity when symptoms are reported. Next associate the symptom of nausea with digoxin (Lanoxin) toxicity to answer this particular question. **Reference:** Adams, M., & Koch, R. (2010). *Pharmacology: Connections to nursing practice.* Upper Saddle River, NJ: Pearson Education, p. 967.

10 **Answer: 2, 5** **Rationale:** The combination of grapefruit and cyclosporine (Sandimmune) will result in an increased serum cyclosporine level. The most common adverse effects include nephrotoxicity and neurotoxicity. Epigastric burning may be related to the ingestion of the fruit, but is not related to the combination with the drug. Diarrhea is not a consequence of this combination. Since the combination is more likely to increase the cyclosporine levels, organ rejection is not likely. **Cognitive Level:** Applying **Client Need:** Pharmacological and Parenteral Therapies **Integrated Process:** Communication and Documentation **Content Area:** Pharmacology **Strategy:** Consider that a question that focuses on a food and a drug or on 2 or more drugs usually aims at testing knowledge of the interactions between them. With this in mind, eliminate 2 options first and then use drug knowledge to choose between the remaining 2. **Reference:** Wilson, B. A., Shannon, M. T., & Shields, K. M. (2012). *Pearson nurse's drug guide 2012.* Upper Saddle River, NJ: Pearson Education, pp. 387–389. Adams, M., & Koch, R. (2010). *Pharmacology: Connections to nursing practice.* Upper Saddle River, NJ: Pearson Education, p. 743.

References

Abrams, A. (2009). *Clinical drug therapy: Rationales for nursing practice* (9th ed.). Philadelphia, PA: Lippincott Williams & Wilkins.

Adams, M., Holland, L., & Bostwick, P. (2011). *Pharmacology for nurses: A pathophysiologic approach* (3rd ed.). Upper Saddle River, NJ: Pearson Education.

Adams, M., & Urban, C. (2013). *Pharmacology: Connections to nursing practice* (2nd ed.). Upper Saddle River, NJ: Pearson Education.

Aschenbrenner, D., & Venable, S. (2009). *Drug therapy in nursing* (3rd ed.). Philadelphia, PA: Lippincott Williams & Wilkins.

Drug Facts & Comparisons® (Updated monthly). St. Louis, MO: A. Wolters Kluwer.

Karch, A. M. (2010). *Focus on nursing pharmacology* (5th ed.). Philadelphia, PA: Lippincott Williams & Wilkins.

Kee, J. (2010). *Laboratory and diagnostic tests and nursing implications* (8th ed.). Upper Saddle River, NJ: Pearson Education.

Lehne, R. (2010). *Pharmacology for nursing care* (7th ed.). St. Louis, MO: Mosby.

LeMone, P., Burke, K., & Bauldoff, G. (2011). *Medical–surgical nursing: Critical thinking in patient care* (5th ed.). Upper Saddle River, NJ: Pearson Education.

Wilson, B. A., Shannon, M. T., Shields, K. M. (2012). *Pearson nurse's drug guide 2012.* Upper Saddle River, NJ: Pearson Education.

Integumentary System Medications

9

Chapter Outline

General Agents
Protective Agents
Antipruritics

Anti-Infectives
Corticosteroids
Keratolytics

Acne Medications
Burn Medications
Debriding Medications

Objectives

➤ Describe the principles related to skin absorption.
➤ Identify the general properties of topical dermatological medications.
➤ Describe the actions, purposes, and safe use of dermatological medications.
➤ Discuss the nursing considerations when administering medications for the integumentary system.
➤ Describe the general goals of therapy when administering integumentary medications.
➤ List the significant client education points related to integumentary medications.

NCLEX-RN® Test Prep

Use the accompanying online resource, NursingReviewsandRationales, to test yourself with hundreds of NCLEX®-style practice questions.

Review at a Glance

acne most common chronic skin disease of adolescents and young adults that affects hair follicles and sebaceous glands; characterized by noninflammatory and inflammatory lesions that often involve face, chest, and back

antiseptics chemical agents that inhibit growth of microorganisms but do not necessarily kill them

creams emulsions of oil in water; more complex preparations than ointments

emollients occlusive agents that make skin soft and pliable by increasing hydration of stratum corneum

herpes simplex an acute viral disease marked by groups of vesicles on skin, often on borders of lips or nares or on genitals

lotions liquid suspensions or dispersions intended for external use

ointments water-in-oil emulsions; semisolid preparations of medicinal substances in a base, such as petrolatum or lanolin

papules small, circumscribed, superficial, solid elevations of skin

pediculosis parasitic infestation caused by lice; may involve hair, body, or pubic area

powder finely divided solid drug or mixture of drugs

pruritus intense itching that is relieved fully by controlling the causative primary illness

psoriasis a chronic, genetically influenced skin disorder characterized by periodic exacerbation of erythematous papules and plaques covered by prominent, thick silvery-white scales

scabies parasitic infestation caused by a mite

tinea pedis a superficial fungal infection of skin of feet; also known as athlete's foot

PRETEST

1 A client newly diagnosed with psoriasis has been prescribed betamethasone (Diprolene) as treatment for the disorder. What statement made by the client indicates further information is needed about this medication?

1. "This drug will also help cure my acne."
2. "I should report an elevated temperature if it occurs."
3. "After applying the medication, I should either leave the skin exposed or cover it lightly."
4. "It should only be applied to the affected skin area."

2 The nurse teaches the parents to apply as ordered which of the following topical applications to the skin of a child with impetigo?

1. Ketoconazole (Nizoral)
2. Mupirocin (Bactroban)
3. Capsaicin (Capsin)
4. Acyclovir (Zovirax) ointment

3 A client is diagnosed with atopic dermatitis. The nurse should expect that which classes of drugs will be prescribed either alone or in combination? Select all that apply.

1. Antihistamines
2. Analgesics
3. Antimicrobials
4. Topical anesthetics
5. Antifungals

4 A participant in a skin care research project asks the nurse educator to justify the recommendation of a sunscreen. Which response by the nurse provides the best rationale?

1. "Sunscreens neutralize the sun's rays."
2. "Sunscreens are waterproof and thus block the sun's rays."
3. "Sunscreens absorb the sun's rays and distribute the heat to other body parts."
4. "Sunscreens prevent sunburn by absorbing and reflecting the sun's rays."

5 An adult client with a pediculosis infestation has an order for an efficient and effective drug to treat the condition. The nurse anticipates writing out which information as an instruction to the client about application methods?

1. Chlorhexidine (Hibiclens): Apply with sterile gloves
2. Lindane (Kwell): Leave in place for 12–24 hours
3. Collagenase (Santyl): Apply with fingertips
4. Terbinafine (Lamisal): Apply a thin layer

6 Permethrin (Elimite Cream) is prescribed for an adult client, and the nurse needs to provide the client with instructions for use. Place the directions in proper sequence that the nurse will provide to the client.

1. Comb hair using a fine-toothed comb.
2. Shampoo hair.
3. Apply Permethrin (Elimite Cream) cream to hair and work through to scalp.
4. Let sit for 10 minutes.
5. Wash hair to remove drug.

7 The nurse teaches the client that which medication is one of the most effective drugs of choice for the treatment of acne?

1. Mafenide (Sulfamylon)
2. Benzoyl peroxide
3. Chlorhexidine (Hibiclens)
4. Cryotherapy

8 The school nurse explains to a group of adolescents at a school health fair that which of the following medications is considered the most effective anti-acne agent?

1. Tetracycline
2. Penicillin G
3. Clindamycin (Cleocin T)
4. Isotretinoin (Accutane)

9 After administering silver sulfadiazine (Silvadene) to a client with burns, the nurse determines the effectiveness of the medication by performing which client assessment?

1. Measure body temperature.
2. Weigh client daily
3. Review serum potassium levels.
4. Assess separation of eschar.

10 During the first 24 hours, the nurse manages one of the most common complications associated with burn injury by administering which medications as prescribed for the client?

1. Famotidine (Pepcid) 20 mg IV q12h
2. Calcium-based antacids after meals
3. Furosemide (Lasix) 20 mg IV bid
4. Crotamiton (Eurax) cream, once daily for 2 days

➤ *See pages 304–306 for Answers and Rationales.*

PRETEST

I. GENERAL AGENTS

A. Soaps

1. Action and use
   a. Deodorant soaps are relatively harsh soaps that contain triclosan or triclocarban as topical antibacterial agents and are useful in decreasing body odor, preventing bacterial spread, and assisting in treatment of cutaneous infections
   b. True soaps mechanically remove bacteria and are effective at removing all sebum and environmental dirt
   c. Synthetic detergent bars are generally milder and compose a group of products known as beauty bars
   d. Allergic sensitization can occur to fragrances, dyes, antibacterial agents, or other additives in soaps
   e. Cleansing ingredients in shampoos are detergents that have different abilities to cleanse and lather
   f. Medicated shampoos may be used for dandruff, seborrheic dermatitis, or **psoriasis** (a chronic skin disorder characterized by periodic exacerbations of erythematous papules and plaques covered by prominent, thick silvery-white scales)

2. Common preparations (see Box 9-1)
3. Nursing considerations
   a. Assess any skin symptom, beginning with a history
   b. Monitor for local adverse effects/irritation from use of selected soap(s) and/or shampoo(s)
   c. Read product literature carefully because some shampoos are not recommended for small children

Box 9-1	Soaps	Shampoos
Soaps and Shampoos	**Deodorant Soaps: Harsh** Dial Lever 2000 Safeguard **True Soaps** Ivory **Synthetic Detergent Soaps: Mild** Dove Oil of Olay Neutrogena Tone	**Unmedicated** Too numerous to list **Medicated** Head & Shoulders Intensive Treatment Dandruff Shampoo (selenium sulfide 1%) and other related products Selsun Blue Dandruff Shampoo and other related products

4. Client education
   a. Soaps can be irritating to people with dry skin, especially in winter with low humidity
   b. Apply a moisturizing preparation after bathing if dry skin is a problem
   c. How to properly use any prescribed shampoo

B. **Cleansers**
   1. Action and use
      a. Cleansers are used for preoperative cleansing of skin
      b. Cleansers may be used for treatment of wounds or abrasions
      c. May also be bacteriostatic or bactericidal depending on agent
   2. Common preparations (see Table 9-1)
   3. Nursing considerations
      a. Assess any skin symptom, beginning with a history
      b. Monitor for local irritation and/or drying as an adverse effect of these topical preparations
   4. Client education
      a. Proper use of any prescribed cleanser
      b. If wounds or abrasions are present, explain inflammatory process and wound healing process

C. **Lotions**
   1. Action and use
      a. **Lotions** historically were "shake lotions" or suspensions of a **powder** (finely divided solid drug or mixture of drugs) in water
      b. With a shake lotion, as water in the lotion evaporates, a coating of powder is left on skin, producing a drying effect
      c. Today other types of liquid emulsions of thin, uniform consistency are also referred to as lotions
   2. Common preparation: Calamine lotion (Calamox, Resinol, Clamatum); it is a preparation of calamine, zinc oxide, glycerin bentonite magma, calcium hydroxide, and others
   3. Nursing considerations
      a. Shake the lotion before application to place powder in suspension
      b. Monitor for local and systemic adverse effects of topical preparation

Table 9-1 **Cleansers**

Agent	Use
Povidone-iodine (Betadine, others)	Bactericidal
Iodine (Iodine Topical, Iodine Tincture)	Cleansing action
Benzalkonium chloride (Benza, Zephiran)	Bacteriostatic; can support growth of certain pseudomonas species; is inactivated by soap; do not cover with an occlusive dressing
Alcohol	Bactericidal; is not as effective as povidone-iodine
Hydrogen peroxide	Germicidal; has mechanical effectiveness; do not use after epithelium is formed because it will continue to debride newly growing cells
Chlorhexidine gluconate (Hibiclens, others)	Cleansing action
Hexachlorophene (Phisohex, Septisol)	Cleansing action
Oxychlorosene sodium (Clorpactin XCB, Clorpactin WCS-90)	Cleansing action
Sodium hypochlorite (Dakin's)	Cleansing action

4. Client education
   a. Proper use of any prescribed lotion (supervise initial use if appropriate to ensure correct application)
   b. Some preparations of calamine lotion also contain diphenhydramine (Benadryl), which can cause drowsiness; use these products cautiously until effect of these agents is known

D. Emollients
   1. Action and use
      a. **Emollients** are occlusive agents that make skin soft and pliable by increasing hydration of stratum corneum and by filling gaps in stratum corneum created by dry, contracted skin cells
      b. Include silicone oils, propylene glycol, isopropyl palmitate, and octyl stearate
      c. Can also function as skin protectants if they soothe symptom of **pruritus** (intense itching) due to exposed, traumatized nerve endings
      d. Moisturizers are intended to mimic function of sebum on skin; function is based on mechanisms of occlusion and humectancy
      e. The occlusion function employs petrolatum, lanolin, cocoa butter, or mineral oil to prevent evaporation of water from skin
      f. The humectancy function employs substances that attract moisture to skin, (e.g., glycerin, sorbitol, propylene glycol)
   2. Common preparations (see Box 9-2)
   3. Nursing considerations
      a. Assess any skin symptom, beginning with a history
      b. Unless otherwise directed by product instructions, apply to skin after bathing while skin is slightly moist
   4. Client education
      a. Explain to clients what contents to look for in over-the-counter (OTC) moisturizers that will indicate product is of high quality
      b. Proper use of any prescribed emollient

E. Protectants
   1. Action and use
      a. Several preparations are designed to protect skin from wetness
      b. Help prevent and treat diaper rash, prickly heat, and/or chafing
   2. Common preparations (see Box 9-3)
   3. Nursing considerations
      a. Assess any skin symptom, beginning with a history
      b. Monitor skin for desired effect

Box 9-2	Aquaphor	Lac-Hydrin cream
Emollients	Cetaphil lotion	Lac-Hydrin lotion 12% (prescription only)
	Curel moisturizing lotion	Lubriderm dry skin lotion
	Dermasil lotion	Lubriderm sensitive lotion
	Eucerin crème or lotion	Lubriderm Bath & Shower Oil
	Eucerin Plus crème	Moisturel lotion
	Eucerin Plus lotion	Neutrogena emulsion
	Eucerin Light lotion	Penecare lotion
	Keri lotion	White petrolatum

Box 9-3	A and D Ointment (lanolin, petrolatum, others)
Protectants	A and D Medicated Diaper Rash Ointment (white petrolatum, zinc oxide, cod liver oil, light mineral oil, others)
	Balmex Ointment (zinc oxide, balsam Peru, beeswax, mineral oil, others)
	Caldesene Medicated Powder or Ointment (powder: calcium undecylenate; ointment: white petrolatum, zinc oxide, others)
	Clocream Skin Protectant Cream (each ounce contains vitamins A and D equivalent to 1 ounce of cod liver oil, many others)
	Desitin Cornstarch Baby Powder (zinc oxide 10% with cornstarch, others)
	Desitin Ointment (zinc oxide 40% with cod liver oil in a petrolatum-lanolin base, others)

   4. Client education
      a. Powders should be kept away from face to avoid inhalation
      b. Some preparations should not be used on broken skin
      c. If diaper rash or skin irritation worsens or does not improve within 7 days of beginning self-care, consult health care provider

Practice to Pass

A 6-month-old infant has diaper rash. What would you include in a teaching plan for the mother?

F. Therapeutic baths
   1. Action and use
      a. General rule: balneotherapy describes a bath or soak for treatment of large affected skin areas
      b. Baths remove crusts, scales, and/or old medications
      c. Assist in the relief of itching and acute dermatoses
      d. Medications can be placed in water
      e. Bath temperature should be 37.7° to 46°C
      f. Client should be placed in bath for 20–30 minutes
      g. Tub should be filled one-third to one-half full
   2. Common preparations (Table 9-2)
   3. Nursing considerations
      a. Assess condition of skin including excoriation, drainage, odor, color, and temperature
      b. Assess for pain prior to bathing
      c. Assess range of motion and client safety, particularly in presence of oils
      d. Apply clean gloves to assist client during bath
      e. Fill tub one-third to one-half full
      f. With use of medicated tars, bathroom should be well ventilated due to volatile fumes
      g. Assess skin for achievement of therapeutic effects
      h. Minimize fluctuation in bath and room temperatures during bath

Table 9-2 **Common Additives to Therapeutic Baths**

Therapeutic Bath Solution	Use
Water	Provides wet dressing effect
Saline	Treats wide disseminated lesions
Colloidal (Aveeno, oatmeal)	Decreases itching, antipruritic
Sodium bicarbonate	Provides soothing soak, which cools skin, usually a rash
Medicated tars	Psoriasis and eczema
Bath oil	Emollient action and antipruritic for acute generalized eczema
Starch	Soothes skin

4. Client education
   a. Safety measures with the use of bath oils and how to prevent falls
   b. Blot skin to dry it after bath
   c. Intended effects of bath
   d. Wear light clothing after bath

G. Soaks and wet dressings
1. Action and use
   a. General rule: acute lesions that are oozing, weeping, and crusting respond best to medication in aqueous, drying preparations
   b. General rule: scaling chronic lesions respond best to medication in moisturizing, lubricating preparations

   c. Open soaks are applied for 20 minutes, 3 times a day
   d. Closed soaks use a water-impermeable substance (occlusion) over a wet soak; this method causes heat retention, which is excellent for debridement but may lead to maceration; are applied for 1 to 2 hours, 2–3 times a day
   e. Continuous closed soaks are left in place for 24 hours to treat thick crusts; it is important to rewet dressing 4–5 times a day
2. Common preparations (Table 9-3)
3. Nursing considerations
   a. Assess any skin symptom, beginning with a history
   b. Monitor for achievement of intended effects
4. Client education
   a. In a health care institution, carry out prescribed soak procedure
   b. Teach procedure to clients for type of soak recommended or prescribed if scheduled for discharge

H. Rubs and liniments
1. Action and use: these are OTC preparations for temporary relief of minor aches and pains of muscles and joints associated with strains, bruises, sprains, sports injuries, simple backache, and arthritis
2. Common preparations (see Box 9-4)
3. Nursing considerations
   a. Assess symptom for which agent is to be used
   b. Monitor for achievement of intended effects
4. Client education
   a. Clean skin of all other **ointments** (water-in-oil emulsions), **creams** (more complex preparations of oil in water than ointments), sprays, or liniments before applying the product
   b. Apply to affected areas no more than 3–4 times daily
   c. Some products have specific directions (i.e., BenGay should not be used with heating pad or tight bandage)

Table 9-3 Soaks and Wet Dressings

Agent	Use
Burow's Solution (Domeboro, others): 5% aluminum acetate solution, 1 Domeboro tablet or packet to 1 pint of tap water	Acts as astringent to decrease exudation by precipitation of protein
Acetic Acid 0.1–1% solution: ½-cup white vinegar to 1 quart water	May be helpful for wounds infected with *Pseudomonas* organisms
Potassium permanganate: 1:4,000–1:16,000 solution	Formerly considered to be useful for fungal infections, but use has decreased because of staining property
Salt solution: 1 tbsp. salt to 1 quart of water	Wetting action

Box 9-4	**Aspercreme External Analgesic Rub with Aloe**
Rubs and Liniments	Available as crème, lotion
	Contains trolamine salicylate, aloe vera gel, many others

BenGay External Analgesic Products
Ointment, cream, arthritis formula cream
Contains menthol in alcohol base gel, methyl salicylate, camphor, others

Sportscream External Analgesic Rub
Available as crème, lotion
Contains trolamine salicylate, acetyl alcohol, others

Therapeutic Mineral Ice, Pain Relieving Gel, Icy Hot
Contain menthol, others

Capsaicin (Capsin)
Active ingredient from cayenne peppers

Practice to Pass

A client has osteoarthritis of both knees and does not want to take pills several times a day. Explain specific suggestions you could give to this client regarding a topical agent.

I. **Powders**

1. Action and use: hygroscopic agents that absorb and retain moisture and assist in reducing friction between bedding and skin
2. Common preparations: bentonite, cornstarch, talc, and zinc oxide
3. Nursing considerations
   a. Assess skin for breakdown or signs of reduced friction
   b. Keep skin clean and dry
4. Client education
   a. General skin care and proper application of powder
   b. Importance of changing position to reduce pressure and avoiding friction during repositioning

II. **PROTECTIVE AGENTS**

A. **Description**
   1. This section is limited to discussion of sunscreen preparations and protective dressings
   2. For other preparations that can be defined as offering protection, see previous section on *Protectants*

B. **Sunscreen preparations**
   1. Actions and use
      a. These are important because they can prevent skin cancer
      b. Chemical sunscreens absorb ultraviolet radiation in the spectrum of ultraviolet light (UVL) most responsible for sunburns
      c. Chemical absorbers formulated against ultraviolet B rays (UVB) include cinnamates, *p*-aminobenzoic acid (PABA) and PABA esters, or salicylates
      d. Chemical absorbers formulated against ultraviolet A rays (UVA) include benzophenones
      e. Physical sunscreens reflect or scatter light to prevent skin penetration
      f. Physical sunscreens contains ingredients such as titanium dioxide, zinc oxide, talc
      g. Effectiveness of a sunscreen is indicated by its sun protection factor (SPF), which is the ratio between exposures to ultraviolet wavelengths and development of skin erythema; an SPF of 6 means product offers 6 times the protection as the use of no sunscreen

    h. Sunscreens range from 12 to 80 SPF

    i. A water-resistant sunscreen should continue to function after 40 minutes in water

    j. A waterproof sunscreen withstands 80 minutes in water

2. Common preparations (see Table 9-4)

3. Nursing considerations: assess skin for degree of burn if not used effectively

4. Client education

    a. Follow product directions and avoid contact between product and eyes

    b. Apply sunscreen if outdoors between 10 a.m. and 3 p.m. daily

    c. Use products with SPF of 15 or greater

    d. Reapply sunscreen every 2 hours or per product directions when swimming or if sweating

    e. Choose sunscreen according to need (see Table 9-5)

C. Protective dressings

1. Action and use

    a. Includes occlusive biosynthetic dressings for certain wound therapies

    b. As an example, DuoDERM as a hydrocolloid dressing hydrates wound surface; wound fluid interacts with wafer of the preparation and melts it, forming a moist, jelly-like substance that keeps wound moist and promotes healing

2. Common dressings (see Table 9-6)

3. Nursing considerations

    a. Assess any skin wound, beginning with a history

    b. Inspect dressing at least daily for leaks, dislodgment, wrinkling, or odor

    c. Change dressing when it becomes dislodged, leaks, or develops an odor

    d. If wound has substantial drainage, dressing might need to be changed every 24–48 hours, but generally is left in place for 3–7 days

    e. When changing dressing, leave residue that is difficult to remove; it will wear off in time; attempts to remove can irritate surrounding skin

4. Client education: proper use of any prescribed occlusive biosynthetic dressing

Practice to Pass

Your cousin, who is fair-skinned, is planning to visit Florida for the first time. She has never seen the ocean and "can't wait to go to the beach." What would you discuss with her before she leaves?

Table 9-4 **Common Sunscreen Preparations**

Brand Name	SPF	Active Ingredients
Coppertone Broad Spectrum Lotion	25	Avobenzone, benzophenones, cinnamates
DuraScreen	15	Benzophenones, cinnamates
Johnson's Baby Sunblock Lotion	30	Benzophenones, cinnamates, salicylates
Neutrogena Sunblock	30	Cinnamates, menthyl anthranilate, octocrylene
Shade UVA/UVB	15, 25, 30, 45	Avobenzone benzophenones, cinnamates
Sundown Sport	15	Titanium dioxide, zinc oxide
Total Eclipse Lotion	15	Benzophenones, salicylates, PABA
Water Babies UVA/UVB	12, 25, 30, 45	Benzophenones, cinnamates, octocrylene

Table 9-5 **Required Skin Protection and SPF**

Required Skin Protection	Recommended SPF
Minimal	2–11 SPF
Moderate	12–29 SPF
High	30 or above

Table 9-6	Common Protective Wound Dressings					
Dressing	**Transmits Oxygen**	**Transmits Water Vapor**	**Excludes Bacteria**	**Absorbs Fluids**	**Transparent**	**Adhesive**
Bioclusive	+	+	2	2	+	+
DuoDERM	2	2	+	+	2	+
Geliperm	+	+	+	+	+	+
Intrasite	2	2	+	+	2	+
Op-site	+	+	+	2	+	+
Replicare	2	2	+	2	2	+
Tegasorb	2	2	+	+	2	+
Tegaderm	+	+	?	2	+	+
Vigilon	+	2	2	+	+	2
Zenoderm	+	+	+	+	+	+

+ = has the stated action

2 = does not have the stated action

? = may or may not have the stated action

III. ANTIPRURITICS

A. Description
1. Antipruritics stop the intense itching known as pruritis
2. Pruritus causes more clients to visit health care provider than any other dermatological symptom
3. Pruritus has a multitude of causes and treatment needs to be tailored to specific cause
4. Types of pruritis include winter pruritus, senior pruritus, lichen simplex chronicus, external otitis, pruritus ani (e.g., pinworm infestation in children), and genital pruritus

B. Action and use
1. Antipruritic medication therapy for some types of pruritis might include topical corticosteroids to decrease inflammation and/or methods to promote skin hydration
2. Antipruritic therapy may also necessitate use of a systemic antihistamine
3. Antipruritic lotions contain a powder in water and should be shaken well; powder has active ingredients that treat the affected area; apply to affected area every 3–4 hours or as recommended

C. Common medications (see Box 9-5)

D. Nursing considerations
1. Take a history of this systemic symptom and any associated skin symptoms
2. Monitor for local and systemic adverse effects of any topical preparation
3. Monitor for anticholinergic adverse reactions if systemic antihistamines of the anticholinergic type are used

E. Client education
1. General bathing should be limited to once or twice a week and only mild soaps should be used; any soap chosen should be used sparingly
2. Negative effects of scratching and the need to interrupt any itch-and-scratch cycle
3. Maintain cool environment, especially in the bedroom for sleep

Box 9-5	**Lotion or cream**	**Systemic H₁ Blockers or Combination**

Box 9-5

Antipruritic Agents

Lotion or cream
Aveeno Anti-itch Lotion or Cream

Aveeno Moisturizing Lotion or Cream

Eucerin Crème or Lotion

Sarna Topical Lotion (camphor, menthol, and phenol)

Zonalon Cream

Calamine Lotion

Hydrating baths
Aveeno (colloidal oatmeal)

Aveeno Oil (e.g., colloidal oatmeal, mineral oil, glyceryl stearate)

Systemic H₁ Blockers or Combination
Hydroxyzine hydrochloride (Atarax)

Hydroxyzine pamoate (Vistaril)

Chlorpheniramine (Chlor-Trimeton)

Cyproheptadine hydrochloride (Periactin)

Unsafe
Benzocaine and other "-caine" derivatives

Antihistamines such as astemizole (Hismanal)

IV. ANTI-INFECTIVES

A. Antibacterials
1. Action and use
   a. Common causative organisms of skin infections are *streptococcus pyogenes* and *staphylococcus aureus*
   b. Certain topical antibiotics are used to inhibit growth of *Propionibacterium acnes* and reduce inflammatory lesions of acne
   c. Topical antibacterial therapy may be useful for prophylaxis of infections in wounds and injuries
2. Common medications (see Table 9-7)
3. Nursing considerations
   a. Assess any skin symptom, beginning with a history
   b. Assess for hypersensitivity to any ingredient in product to be used; this would constitute a contraindication for use
   c. Monitor for skin irritation and any signs of superinfection

Table 9-7 Antibacterial and Antiviral Agents

Generic (Trade) Name	Usual Adult Dosage	Action	Uses
Bacitracin (Baciguent Topical)	Apply to affected area 5 times per day. If needed, apply a sterile dressing.	Inhibits cell wall synthesis	Primarily used to treat staphylococci in minor skin abrasions or treat superficial skin infections
Bacitracin, Polymixin B, Neosporin (Mycitracin Topical, others)	Apply to affected area 3 times per day. If needed, apply a sterile dressing.	Inhibits cell wall synthesis and 30S ribosome	Primarily used to treat *Bacillus subtilis, Streptomyces fradiae*, and secondarily infected skin problems
Chloramphenicol (Chloromycetin)	Used infrequently due to dose-related bone marrow suppression; used only when necessary. Sensitization from topical use may prevent effective treatment in serious infections.	Inhibits cell wall replication	*Streptococcus venezuelae*
Clindamycin phosphate (Cleocin T, others)	Apply thinly to an affected area bid. Vaginal application: one applicator intravaginally at hour of sleep for 7 days.	Inhibits protein synthesis, causing cell death	Treat acne vulgaris and bacterial vaginosis

Table 9-7 Antibacterial and Antiviral Agents (Continued)

Generic (Trade) Name	Usual Adult Dosage	Action	Uses
Erythromycin and benzoyl peroxide (Benzamycin)	Acne: Apply to affected areas morning and evening Dermatologic ointment: Apply to affected area 1–5 times per day	Bacteriostatic or bactericidal, binding to cell membrane, changing protein function and causing cell death	Treat acne vulgaris, prophylaxis against infection in minor abrasions, and susceptible skin organisms
Gentamicin sulfate (Garamycin, others)	Apply to affected areas tid or qid and cover with a sterile dressing if needed	Inhibits protein synthesis in susceptible gram-negative bacteria; disrupts cell membrane and causes cell death	Treat minor skin abrasions and superficial infections of skin
Meclocycline sulfosalicylate (Meclan Topical)	Apply to affected areas in the a.m. and hour of sleep	Suppresses growth of *Propionibacterium acnes*; synthetic derivative of oxytetracycline	Suppresses growth of *Propionibacterium acnes*
Metronidazole (MetroGel, MetroCream)	Apply a thin layer to inflammatory papules, pustules, and erythema of rosacea bid for 3–9 weeks Vaginal: *nonpregnant women only*—1 applicator 1–2 times per day for 5 days	Inhibits DNA synthesis in anaerobes causing cell death	Treatment of inflammatory papules, pustules, and erythema of rosacea Treatment of *Gardnerella vaginalis*
Mupirocin (Bactroban)	Apply small, thin layer to affected area tid	Inhibits bacterial protein synthesis by binding to bacterial transfer-RNA	Treat impetigo due to *S. aureus*, beta-hemolytic streptococcus, and *streptococcus pyogenes*
Neomycin (Mycifradin Sulfate Topical)	Apply to affected area 1–3 times per day	Aminoglycoside antibiotic obtained from *Streptomyces fradiae*	Treat short-term eye, ear, and skin infections
Tetracycline (Achromycin Topical, others)	Apply to cleansed area bid	Broad-spectrum antibiotic derived from *Streptomyces aurofaciens*	Treat superficial skin infections
Acyclovir (Zovirax)	0.5-inch ribbon to affected area, rub in gently 6 times per day	Inhibits viral DNA replication	Recurrent herpes labialis
Docusanol (Abreva)	Apply 5 times per day for 10 days	Inhibits viral DNA replication	Recurrent herpes labialis
Imiquimod (Aldara)	Apply a thin layer to warts, rub in gently 3 times per week at hour of sleep for 16 weeks, remove imiquimod with soap and water	Inhibits viral DNA replication	Treat external genital and perianal warts; typical nonhyperkeratotic actinic keratoses on face or scalp; basal cell carcinoma in immunocompromised clients
Penciclovir (Denavir)	Apply a thin layer to affected area every 2 hours while awake for 4 days	Inhibits viral DNA replication	Treat cold sores in healthy clients; herpes labialis in lips and face

4. Client education
   a. Wash hands before using any topical antibacterial agent and cleanse area to be treated
   b. May wear gloves
   c. Generally topical agents should be applied sparingly and gently to affected area
   d. With some, a dressing should be applied and with some it should not; follow prescriber instructions

      e. Report worsening of condition, lack of healing, or development of a rash around lesion

      f. Protect skin from sunlight if using gentamicin sulfate (risk of photosensitization)

B. Antivirals

  1. Action and use

      a. Used to treat cutaneous **herpes simplex** (an acute viral disease marked by groups of vesicles on skin, often on borders of lips, nares, or on genitals) primarily

      b. May also be used to treat herpes zoster

      c. With some infections an oral agent may be needed instead of a topical agent

  2. Common medication: acyclovir 5% ointment (Zovirax); see also Table 9-7

  3. Nursing considerations

      a. Assess skin symptoms, beginning with a history

      b. Monitor for local adverse effects of topical product, such as mild pain, burning, stinging; report these to prescriber

  4. Client education

      a. Wash hands before using topical antiviral drug

      b. Use gloves or finger cot when applying product to avoid autoinnoculation of other body sites

      c. Apply as soon as symptoms of herpes lesions begin

      d. Apply sparingly and gently to affected area

      e. Wear loose clothing and keep area clean and dry

      f. Avoid sexual intercourse when visible skin lesions are present

C. Antifungals

  1. Action and use

      a. Clients with limited disease and infection limited to glabrous (smooth, hairless) skin can be treated with topical antifungal agents

      b. Clients with extensive disease and infection of hair and nails are best treated with systemic therapy

      c. Advantages of topical use over systemic use: absence of serious adverse reactions, absence of drug interactions, over-the-counter availability of some preparations, ability to localize treatment to affected sites, no need to monitor laboratory tests

      d. New drugs have caused decrease in use of keratolytics and **antiseptics** (chemical agents that inhibit growth of microorganisms but do not necessarily kill them) used in the past

  2. Common medications

      a. Topical agents (see Table 9-8)

      b. Oral agents include fluconazole (Diflucan), griseofulvin (Fulvicin, Grispeg), itraconazole (Sporanox), ketoconazole (Nizoral), and terbinafine (Lamisil)

Table 9-8 **Topical Antifungals**

Generic (Trade) Name	Usual Adult Dose	Action	Uses
Amphoteracin B	Apply liberally to lesions bid to qid for 2–4 weeks	Fungal cell death	Treat mucocutaneous and cutaneous *Candida* infections
Butenafine hydrochloride (Mentax)	Apply to affected area once a day for 4 weeks	Inhibits sterol synthesis	Treat interdigital pedia, tinea corporis, ringworm, tinea cruris
Butoconazole nitrate (Gynazole-I)	Apply intravaginally in a single dose	Alters fungal cell membrane permeability, preventing cellular replication	Treat vulvovaginal candidiasis

Table 9-8 Topical Antifungals (Continued)

Generic (Trade) Name	Usual Adult Dose	Action	Uses
Ciclopirox olamine (Loprox, Penlac Nail Lacquer)	Apply directly to finger- and toenails Tinea: Massage cream into affected area and surrounding skin bid in a.m. and p.m. Onychomycosis: Paint affected nail under nail surface and nail bed once daily at bedtime (after 7 days remove lacquer with alcohol; trim away unattached nail)	Synthetic broad-spectrum antifungal agent; inhibits transport of amino acids within fungal cell; interferes with synthesis of RNA, DNA, and fungal protein	Treat onychomycosis of fingernails and toenails
Clotrimazole (Lotrimin, others)	Apply a thin layer to affected areas bid in a.m. and p.m. Intravaginal: 1 applicator at bedtime for 7 days or one 500 mg vaginal tablet at bedtime as one-time dose	Alters fungal cell membrane permeability, preventing cell replication	Treat tinea pedis, tinea cruris, tinea corporis, tinea versicolor, vulvovaginal and oropharyngeal candidiasis
Econazole nitrate (Spectazole, Econostatin)	Apply to affected areas bid for tinea cruris, tinea corporis, tinea pedis, and cutaneous candidiasis Apply sufficient amount to affected areas once daily for tinea versicolor	Fungicidal for certain microorganisms	Active against many dermaphytes Treatment of tinea pedis, tinea cruris, tinea corporis, cutaneous candidiasis
Genetian violet	Apply to areas bid; do not apply to active lesions	Absorbed into skin; should not come in contact with active lesions; alters cellular permeability	Treat topical mycosis
Ketoconazole (Nizoral)	Apply 1–2 times per day to affected areas and surrounding skin	Interferes with synthesis of ergosterol, increasing cell membrane permeability and inhibiting fungal growth	Treat tinea corporis, tinea cruris, and tinea versicolor
Naftifine hydrochloride (Naftin)	Apply cream once daily; apply gel twice daily; cream or gel may be used up to 4 weeks	Interferes with synthesis of ergosterol (principal sterol in fungus cell membrane)	Treat *C. albicans*, *Epidermophyton floccosum*, *Microsporum canis*, *M. audouinii, M. gypseum*, *Trichophyton rubrum*, *T. mentagrophytes, T. tonsurans*
Oxiconazole (Oxistat)	Apply once daily to affected area at hour of sleep	Alters fungi cell membrane, resulting in increased permeability	Treat tinea pedis, tinea cruris, and tinea corporis
Sertaconazole nitrate (Ertaczo)	Apply daily up to 1 month	Inhibits CYP-dependent synthesis of ergosterol; alters cell wall permeability and results in cell death	Tinea pedis caused by *Trichophyton mentagrophytes*, *T. rubrum*, or *Epidermophyton floccosum*
Terbinafine (Lamisil, Lamisil DermaGel)	Apply 1–2 times per day to affected and surrounding areas for 1–7 weeks	Inhibits sterol biosynthesis in fungi and results in cell death	Tinea pedis, tinea cruris, and tinea corporis due to *Epidermophyton floccosum*, *Trichophyton mentagrophyte*, or *T. rubrum*
Tolnaftate (Absorbine, others)	Apply 0.5–1 cm of cream bid or 3 drops of solution bid; powder may be applied prophylactically	Distorts hyphae and stunts mycelial growth on susceptible fungi	Tinia pedis, tinea corporis, tinea capitis, tinea unguium

3. Nursing considerations
   a. Assess any skin symptom, beginning with a history
   b. Assess for predisposing factors, such as trauma, general health, suppressed immune status, hygiene practices and exposure to infectious agent
   c. Monitor for local adverse effects of topical preparations, which often include irritation, burning, or stinging depending on specific product used
   d. Do not apply gentian violet to active lesions
   e. Monitor for skin sensitization, noted by increased redness, swelling, weeping, or any burning or itching that were not present before treatment began
   f. Systemic effects of topical products are negligible, since absorption rates generally are only 3–6%
   g. Ensure affected area is cultured before starting topical amphoteracin treatment
4. Client education
   a. Use products as directed for full course of therapy (may be prolonged); apply liberally to clean and dry skin
   b. Leave exposed to air; do not apply protective dressing unless specifically ordered
   c. To prevent such fungal infections as **tinea pedis** (a superficial fungal infection of skin of feet; athlete's foot)
      1) Wear shower shoes or thongs in public or communal showers and locker rooms
      2) Wear footwear of natural fibers (leather shoes, cotton or wool socks)
      3) Avoid going barefoot
      4) Change socks daily
   d. To avoid other fungal infections, practice adequate hygiene
      1) Keep affected areas clean, dry, and well ventilated (loose clothing)
      2) Use powders to keep skin dry and prevent maceration; these may or may not contain antifungal ingredients

D. Antiparasitics
1. Action and use
   a. Used to treat parasitic infestations such as **scabies** (caused by *Sarcoptes scabiei* mite) or **pediculosis** (caused by lice); may involve hair (tinea capitis), body (tinea corporis), or pubic area (tinea pubis)
   b. Recurrence of scabies is generally related to reinfection in incomplete treatment rather than resistance of mite
   c. Crotamiton can be used in clients with scabies and pediculosis capitis who are ragweed sensitive
2. Common medications (see Table 9-9)
3. Nursing considerations
   a. Assess any skin symptom, beginning with a history
   b. Although client may bathe, ensure skin is cool and dry before application of scabicide to prevent systemic absorption
   c. Monitor for local adverse effects, including irritation, pruritis, burning, or stinging

Practice to Pass

A mother has an 8-year-old daughter who has come home from school with a note from the school nurse that says head lice have been noted on 2 children in her classroom. What would you include in a teaching plan for the mother?

Table 9-9 Antiparasitics

Agent	Uses
Crotamiton (Eurax cream, lotion)	Scabies
Malathion (Ovide lotion)	Pediculosis capitis and their ova
Permethrin (Elimite cream, Nix liquid)	Pediculosis capitis, scabies
Pyrethrin, piperonyl butoxide (liquid, Rid shampoo)	Pediculosis capitis, pediculosis corporis, pediculosis pubis
Lindane (Kwell cream, lotion, shampoo)	Pediculosis capitis, pediculosis pubis, scabies

      d. Monitor for systemic effect of dizziness with lindane because it affects nervous system; avoid use in infants, children, older adults, and clients with known seizure disorders because of risk of seizures

  4. Client education

      a. After bathing, ensure skin is dry and cool before applying scabicide to reduce risk of seizures from systemic absorption

      b. For scabies

        1) Apply thin layer to dry skin from neck down and rub in thoroughly over entire body

        2) Permethrin and lindane: leave on 8 to 12 hours, remove thoroughly with washing

        3) Crotamiton: apply again after 24 hours, remove with washing 48 hours after initial application

      c. For pediculosis capitis

        1) Lindane lotion: apply lotion to dry hair, rub in thoroughly, leave on for 12 hours, then remove thoroughly

        2) Lindane shampoo: apply shampoo to dry hair, lather with small amount water, work into hair for 4 minutes, rinse thoroughly

        3) Second treatment in 7–10 days may be needed with malathion, RID

V. CORTICOSTEROIDS

A. Description

  1. Topical corticosteroids are commonly used with skin disorders

  2. Systemic corticosteroids may also be used with skin disorders

B. Action and use

  1. Corticosteroids enter cell and bind to cytoplasmic receptors to produce an anti-inflammatory, antipruritic, and antiproliferative effect

  2. Indicated for relief of inflammatory and pruritic manifestations and for minor skin irritations, rashes, and itching

  3. Clinical effectiveness of corticosteroids relates to four properties

      a. Vasoconstriction; decreases erythema

      b. Antiproliferative effects; inhibits DNA synthesis and mitosis

      c. Immunosuppression; mechanism poorly understood

      d. Anti-inflammatory effects; inhibits formation of prostaglandins

  4. Responsiveness of diseases to topical corticosteroids varies: highly responsive diseases include psoriasis, atopic dermatitis in children, seborrheic dermatitis, intertrigo

  5. Penetration of preparation varies according to skin site

  6. Using these products on thin skin, on older adult or pediatric clients, or under occlusion will increase incidence of adverse reactions

  7. Adverse effects more common since introduction of higher potency preparations

  8. Local adverse reactions include atrophy, hypopigmentation, striae

  9. Topical corticosteroids can cause systemic adverse reactions, including suppression of hypothalamic–pituitary–adrenal axis; occurs most frequently in clients using topical corticosteroids that are covered with an occlusive dressing or in clients with liver failure

  10. Low-potency agents are best used for diffuse eruptions, those involving face or occluded areas such as axilla or groin, and chronic dermatoses

  11. Medium-potency agents are appropriate for acute flare-ups of chronic dermatoses and acute self-limited eruptions where they can be used for periods of 14–21 days

  12. High-potency agents best used for acute localized eruptions for a short time of 7–14 days

13. High-potency agents should be avoided on areas susceptible to increased penetration and adverse reactions, such as face, intertriginous areas, perineum
14. A twice-a-day application is usually sufficient; more frequent application does not appear to improve response
15. Abrupt discontinuation of mid- or high-potency corticosteroids may result in rebound flare-up of disorder

C. **Common medications (see Table 9-10)**
D. **Nursing considerations**
1. Assess any skin symptom, beginning with a history
2. Apply sparingly and gently in a thin film to affected area, usually 2–3 times per day
3. At times, the preparation should be rubbed in thoroughly
4. Do not use occlusive dressings or tight-fitting diapers, which may increase systemic absorption
5. Do not apply to open skin lesions
6. Avoid direct contact to eyes

Table 9-10	Topical Corticosteroids	
Potency Class	**Generic Name**	**Brand Name**
Lowest potency	Alclometasone 0.05% cream, ointment	Aclovate
	Desonide 0.05% cream, ointment, lotion	Desowen, Tridesilon
	Dexamethasone 0.04% aerosol	Decaspray
	Hydrocortisone 1% cream	Ala-Cort, others
	Hydrocortisone 1% lotion	Acticort 100, others
	Hydrocortisone 1% ointment, hydrocortisone 2.5% cream, ointment	Cortizone-10, Hycort, others
	Methylprednisolone acetate 0.25% ointment	Medrol
	Methylprednisolone acetate 1% ointment	Medrol
Low potency	Betamethasone valerate 0.025% cream	Valisone
	Clocortolone 0.1% cream	Cloderm
	Fluocinolone acetonide 0.01% cream, solution	Synalar
	Flurandrenolide 0.025% cream, ointment	Cordran
	Hydrocortisone valerate 0.2% cream	Westcort
	Triamcinolone acetonide 0.025% cream, ointment	Kenalog
Intermediate potency	Betamethasone benzoate 0.025% cream, gel, lotion	Uticort
	Betamethasone valerate 0.1% cream, ointment, lotion	Valisone
	Desoximetasone 0.05% cream, ointment	Topicort LP
	Fluocinolone acetonide 0.025% cream	Cutivate
	Halcinonide 0.025% cream, ointment	Halog
	Mometasone furoate 0.1% cream, ointment, lotion	Elocon
	Triamcinolone acetonide 0.1% cream, ointment	Kenalog
High potency	Amcinonide 0.1% cream, ointment	Cyclocort
	Betamethasone dipropionate 0.05% cream, ointment, lotion	Diprosone
	Desoximetasone 0.25% cream, ointment	Topicort
	Flucinolone 0.2% cream	Synalar HP
	Flucinolone 0.05% cream, ointment	Lidex
	Halcinonide 0.1% cream, ointment, solution	Halog
	Triamcinolone acetonide 0.5% cream, ointment	Kenalog
Very high potency	Augmented betamethasone dipropionate 0.05% ointment	Diprolene
	Clobetasol propionate 0.05% cream, ointment	Temovate
	Diflorasone 0.05% gel, ointment	Fluorone, others
	Halobetasol propionate 0.05% cream, ointment	Ultravate

! 7. Monitor for local adverse skin effects, which include acneiform skin lesions, dryness, itching, burning, allergic contact dermatitis, hypopigmentation, overgrowth of bacteria/fungi/viruses (secondary infection), skin atrophy, or striae

! 8. Monitor for systemic adverse effects, which are more likely to include hirsutism (usually of face), moon facies, alopecia (scalp), and immunosuppression

! 9. These drugs, especially those of higher potency, should be tapered and not discontinued abruptly

! **E. Client education**

1. Use exactly as directed; do not overuse
2. Do not apply to open wounds or weeping areas
3. Before using, wash and dry area gently
4. Report worsening of condition, signs of infection, or lack of healing

VI. KERATOLYTICS

A. Description
1. These agents reduce thickness of hyperkeratotic stratum corneum
2. They reduce keratinocyte adhesion (remove or soften horny layer of skin)

B. Action and use
1. Used to treat disorders of keratinization (e.g., forms of ichthyosis that generally have genetic component)
2. Some are used to treat certain warts
3. They are available in different concentrations
4. Concentration necessary for keratolytic action differs among available agents

C. Common medications (see Table 9-11)

D. Nursing considerations
1. Assess any skin symptom, beginning with a history
2. Monitor for local adverse effects of topical preparations
3. Warts will become blanched and necrotic in 24–48 hours
4. Assess neurological function; polyneuropathy may appear in 2 weeks and persist up to 9 months

E. Client education
1. Purpose of agent, use, side effects, symptoms of toxicity, and anticipated length of treatment
2. Use as directed; method will vary somewhat depending on condition for which it is used
3. Do not breastfeed while using podofilox
4. Have sex partner examined for warts as applicable

Practice to Pass

The client has two plantar warts on the ball of his left foot. What would you include in a plan of action for the client?

Table 9-11 Keratolytics			
Generic (Trade) Name	**Usual Adult Dosage**	**Action**	**Uses**
Podophyllum resin (Podoben, Podofin) and Podofilox	10% solution; repeat 1–2 times per week for up to 4 applications Verruca vulgaris 0.5% solution every 12 hours for up to 4 weeks	Cytotoxic and keratolytic agent with caustic action; directly affects epithelial cell metabolism	Benign growths of external genitalia and perianal warts, papillomas, and fibroids
Salicylic acid (Panscol ointment, others)	20% ointment	Softens scales of outer horny layer of skin	Corns, warts, conditions of scalp, acne, and dermatitis

VII. ACNE MEDICATIONS

A. Description

1. Generally a staged approach is used
2. Mild **acne** (noninflammatory and inflammatory lesions that most commonly involve face, chest, back), consisting of some comedones or few inflammatory lesions, is treated by topical therapy with agents such as salicylic acid, azelaic acid, benzoyl peroxide, and topical antibiotics
3. Moderate acne consisting of *comedones* (blackheads) and **papules** (small, circumscribed, superficial, solid elevations of skin) can be managed by gradually increasing strength of topical tretinoin
4. Severe acne consisting of inflammatory papules and nodulocystic disease requires systemic antibiotics and isotretinoin (Accutane)

B. Action and use

1. Choice of vehicle for topical preparation depends on whether client has dry or oily skin
2. Local adverse reactions to some topical preparations include erythema, burning or stinging, excessive dryness, and increased susceptibility to sunburn
3. Most clients will develop tolerance to local side effects within 3–4 weeks

C. Common medications (see Tables 9-12 and 9-13)

Table 9-12 Topical Acne Medications

Generic/Trade Name	Usual Adult Dosage	Action	Uses
Adapalene (Differin)	Apply a thin layer at hour of sleep after washing	Retinoid-like compound; modulates cellular differentiation; produces anti-inflammatory action	Acne vulgaris
Benzoyl peroxide (Benzac, Benzagel)	Wash affected areas and apply gel preparation	Antibacterial, keratolytic activity	Acne vulgaris
Azelaic acid (Azelex, Finacea 20%)	Wash and dry skin and apply a thin layer of medication to affected areas twice a day	Antibacterial, keratolytic that competitively inhibits tyrosinase; inhibits comedone formation	Acne vulgaris
Clindamycin (Evoclin, Clindesse)	1% foam applied once daily to affected areas after washing	Antibacterial	Acne vulgaris
Clindamycin and Benzoyl Peroxide (Benzaclin)	Apply gel to affected areas twice daily after washing	Antibacterial and keratolytic activity	Acne vulgaris
Sodium sulfacetamide	Apply a thin layer twice daily to affected areas after washing with mild soap and water	Antibacterial	Acne vulgaris
Tazarotene (Tazorac)	Apply thin layer every evening after washing	Retinoid	Acne vulgaris
Tetracycline (Achromycin, others)	Apply thin layer to cleansed area twice a day	Suppresses growth of *Propionibacterium acnes* in sebaceous follicles, reducing free fatty acid content in sebum	Acne vulgaris
Tretinoin cream (Avita) 0.25%	Apply thin layer once daily	Retinoid	Acne vulgaris
Tretinoin (Retin-A)	Apply to cover once daily after cleansing	Retinoic acid derivative; increases mitotic activity and turnover of follicular epithelial cells; loosens keratin debris; promotes drainage of preexisting comedones; inhibits new comedone formation; maximal result in 6 weeks	Acne vulgaris

Table 9-13 Oral Medications for Acne Vulgaris

Generic (Trade) Name	Usual Adult Dose	Action	Uses
Isotretinoin (Accutane)	0.5–1 mg/kg/day in 2 divided doses	Regulation of cell differentiation and proliferation of altered lipid composition (highly toxic vitamin A)	Severe recalcitrant cystic acne unresponsive to conventional therapy
Tetracycline (Achromycin, Monodox, Sumycin, Doryx, Vibramycin)	500–1,000 mg bid to qid	Anti-acne action by suppressing growth of *Propionibacterium acnes* in sebaceous follicles, reducing free fatty acid content in sebum	Acne vulgaris

D. Nursing considerations
1. Assess skin lesions as baseline and periodically to evaluate effectiveness of therapy
2. Monitor for local adverse effects of topical preparations, such as excessive drying, erythema, and hypersensitivity
3. Monitor for systemic adverse effects as particular to individual product
4. Do not apply adapalene with salicylic acid

5. Do not administer tetracycline to woman who is pregnant or attempting pregnancy

E. Client education
1. Purpose, use, side effects, and anticipated length of treatment
2. Treatment is designed to control, not cure; therefore, periodic breakouts (especially premenstrual flares) may still occur
3. With topical preparation, wash and dry skin; massage thin film gently into affected areas twice daily
4. Discontinue use and notify prescriber if severe irritation occurs
5. Avoid getting product into eyes, mouth, and mucous membranes; wash hands after use

6. With certain preparations, minimize exposure to sun and UV light; drying of skin may also lead to photosensitivity

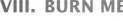
7. Accutane is a teratogen; females of child-bearing age must strictly avoid becoming pregnant; they should have negative pregnancy test within 2 weeks before starting therapy and monthly during therapy
8. There is no connection between acne and diet

VIII. BURN MEDICATIONS

A. Description of burn therapy
1. Clients who have partial-thickness burns of more than 5–10% of body, full-thickness burns, burns associated with electrical current, or burns of ears, eyes, face, hands, feet, and perineum should be referred to a hospital prepared to handle burn clients
2. Remaining clients who have superficial-thickness burns and partial-thickness burns of less than 5% of body should receive wound care and close follow-up
3. Goals of therapy are to decrease inflammation, prevent infection, relieve pain, and promote healing

B. Actions and use: topical agents are used to prevent infection in burn wounds, which could rapidly lead to sepsis

C. Common medications (see Table 9-14)

D. Adverse effects
1. Mafenide (sulfamylon): pain, burning, or staining at application sites for 20–30 minutes after application; clients with impaired renal function: high blood level of agent may lead to metabolic acidosis; watch for respiratory alkalosis as an indicator

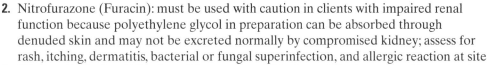

Table 9-14 Burn Medications			
Generic (Trade) Name	Usual Adult Dose	Action	Uses
Mafenide (sulfamylon)	Apply to clean, debrided wound 1–2 times per day with sterile gloves	Bacteriostatic against Pseudomonas aeruginosa and Clostridia	Continue applications after whirlpool baths until healing occurs
Nitrofurazone (Furacin)	Apply to burn directly or place medication on gauze daily	Inhibits aerobic and anaerobic cycles in bacterial carbohydrate metabolism	Adjunct treatment of bacterial infection in partial and full-thickness burns; prevention of infection at skin graft sites
Silver sulfadiazine (Silvadene, Thermazene, SSD Cream)	Apply 1–2 times per day to clean debrided wounds; thickness of layer should be 1/16 in.	Silver released from preparation is toxic to bacteria; silver prevents replication of *S. aureus*, *E. coli*, *Klebsiella*, others	Applications of silver sulfiadazine to burn sites

2. Nitrofurazone (Furacin): must be used with caution in clients with impaired renal function because polyethylene glycol in preparation can be absorbed through denuded skin and may not be excreted normally by compromised kidney; assess for rash, itching, dermatitis, bacterial or fungal superinfection, and allergic reaction at site

3. Silver sulfadiazine (Silvadene, Thermazene, SSD Cream): leukopenia, skin necrosis, erythema multiforme, skin discoloration, rashes; up to 10% may be absorbed; hazardous to use in clients with G6PD deficiency

E. **Nursing considerations**

1. Agents are applied under sterile conditions once or twice daily to a thickness of approximately 1/16 in. to a clean and debrided wound

2. If hospitalized, client may undergo hydrotherapy (bathing in whirlpool) to aid debridement prior to application

3. Client should be premedicated with analgesic, whenever possible, half-hour prior to burn wound cleansing; provide emotional support during dressing changes and/or hydrotherapy

4. Wound may be covered or left open

5. Monitor for adverse effects as outlined in Table 9-14

6. Watch for signs of infection and WBC count in clients receiving silver sulfadiazine because of leukopenic effect

F. **Client education**

1. Purpose, use, side effects, and anticipated length of treatment

2. Use as directed if using preparation as an out-patient

IX. DEBRIDING MEDICATIONS

A. **Description**

1. Debriding agents are used to remove dirt, damaged tissue, and cellular debris from a wound to prevent infection and to promote healing

2. Their effectiveness in removing necrotic tissue, clotted blood, purulent exudates, or fibrinous accumulations has been questioned

B. **Action and use**

1. Appear most effective when wound base has collagen that must be removed before epithelialization can proceed

2. Specific indications may vary (e.g., collagenase is indicated for stage 3 and 4 pressure ulcers)

C. **Common medications (see Table 9-15)**

Table 9-15	Debriding Preparations	
Agent	**Action**	**Notes**
Collagenase (Santyl)	Digests collagen; active at pH 6–8, takes 10–14 days	Active at pH 6–8, such enzymes tend to be inactivated by extremes of pH; also inactivated by hydrogen peroxide, heavy metals like silver, detergents, and by iodine, nitrofurazone, and hexachlorophene
Sutilains (Travase)	Digests necrotic soft tissues by proteolytic action	See above
Fibrinolysin and deoxyribonuclease (Elase)	Deoxyribonuclease attacks DNA; fibrinolysin attacks fibrin of blood clots and fibrinous exudates	Hypersensitivity reactions can occur; serious adverse reactions reported when using ointment preparation containing chloramphenicol
Papain and urea (Panafil White)	Ointment source is papaya	Chlorophyll derivatives control wound odor
Papain, urea, chlorophyllin copper complex (Panafil)	Source is papaya	See above
Trypsin, Balsam Peru, castor oil (Granulex)	Source of trypsin is bovine pancreas	Balsam Peru is capillary bed stimulant used to improve circulation; castor oil used to reduce premature epithelial cornification

D. Nursing considerations
  1. Assess skin problem before use
  2. Monitor progress in wound healing
E. Client education
  1. Explain purpose, use, and side effects of medications
  2. Assess client's understanding about anticipated length of treatment

Case Study

A 16-year-old male has severe acne vulgaris, which is nonresponsive to conventional treatment with Benzaclin and Tetracycline orally. The dermatologist begins isotretinoin (Accutane) 35 mg PO bid. The client weighs 70 kg and is 6 feet tall. He is to continue using Benzaclin twice daily.

1. What is the action of Benzaclin?

2. What is the action of isotretinoin?

3. Is this the proper dosage for isotretinoin to be administered to this young man?

4. What client education should be provided to the client and his family?

For suggested responses, see pages 543–544.

POSTTEST

1 Because a client diagnosed with psoriasis vulgaris is using a prescribed topical corticosteroid, what activity should the nurse perform?

1. Protect the unaffected skin from staining.
2. Heat cream before applying.
3. Provide continuous occlusive therapy.
4. Apply warm, moist dressings over occlusive dressing.

2 After 5-fluorouracil (Adrucil) cream is prescribed for a client diagnosed with basal cell carcinoma, what client teaching should the nurse perform?

1. The drug will cause increasing tenderness as lesions ooze and erode.
2. The drug will cause the lesion to become dry, shrink, and fall off.
3. The drug will decrease the sensitivity of the lesion.
4. Vigorously massage the lesion after application.

3 The nurse teaches the client how to manage an infestation of scabies with crotamiton (Eurax) by providing which of the following directions?

1. Rotate the container gently before using. Do not shake.
2. Vigorously massage the solution into the skin.
3. Comb the hair with a fine-toothed comb every day for 7 days.
4. Apply the product to inflamed areas first.

4 The nurse is most likely to utilize a DuoDerm dressing for which of the following clients assigned to the nurse's care for the shift?

1. Client who has a necrotic wound with a thick layer of eschar attached
2. Client who has a new, partial-thickness burned area
3. Client who has a wound that needs debriding
4. Client who has an uninfected venous stasis ulcer

5 After a health care provider prescribed minocycline (Minocin) for a client with acne, the nurse explains to the client that which of the following is a disadvantage of this preparation?

1. Suppression of sebum production
2. Lupus-like syndrome and pigmentation changes
3. Open pores promoting excessive production of accumulated sebum
4. Occurrence of spontaneous abortions

6 A nurse is administering a very high-potency topical corticosteroid clobetasol (Temovate 0.05%) to certain assigned clients. Which of the following clients is most at risk for systemic absorption?

1. 35-year-old with psoriasis
2. 72-year-old with eczema
3. 59-year-old with seborrhea
4. 38-year-old with contact dermatitis

7 A nurse is discussing treatment options for a client with acne vulgaris. The nurse should explain to the client that anti-acne medications work in which of the following ways? Select all that apply.

1. Inhibiting viral replication
2. Inhibiting sebaceous gland overactivity
3. Reducing bacterial colonization
4. Preventing follicles from becoming plugged with keratin
5. Reducing inflammation of lesions

8 After listening to the nurse explain the use of isotretinoin (Accutane) to a 19-year-old female client, the client demonstrates understanding of the most important point by making which statement at the end of the teaching session?

1. Apply thick layer of isotretinoin twice a day.
2. Increase exposure to sun for added benefit.
3. Have pregnancy test prior to beginning therapy and use contraception.
4. Keep lips moist and lubricated to prevent inflammation.

POSTTEST

9 The client with a burn injury reports a stinging and burning sensation when topical mafenide acetate (Sulfamylon) is applied. The nurse should perform which of the following?

1. Withhold medication and notify the prescriber.
2. Remove that dose of the medication.
3. Pre-medicate client with moderate analgesic before applying.
4. Chill preparation before applying.

10 A nurse working in a burn center frequently applies topical burn medications to burn wounds. The nurse should anticipate that which medications may be prescribed topically for a newly admitted client with burns? Select all that apply.

1. Mafenide (Sulfamylon)
2. Sulfisoxazole (Gantrinsin)
3. Silver sulfadiazine (Silvadene)
4. Nitrofurazone (Furacin)
5. Trimethoprim

➤ *See pages 306–307 for Answers and Rationales.*

ANSWERS & RATIONALES

Pretest

1 Answer: 1 Rationale: Betamethasone (Diprolene) is a corticosteroid that is used in the treatment of psoriasis. The client needs to know that acne can occur as a side effect of this medication rather than curing it. The other options indicate correct understanding by the client. The client should report temperature in case symptoms of infection are masked; only the affected skin area should be treated and the site should be left exposed or covered only lightly with a dressing. Cognitive Level: Analyzing Client Need: Pharmacological and Parenteral Therapies Integrated Process: Teaching and Learning Content Area: Pharmacology Strategy: The critical words in the question are *further information is needed*. This indicates that the correct option is an incorrect statement on the part of the client. Recognize this medication as a glucocorticoid and then recall common adverse effects to choose correctly. Reference: Wilson, B. A., Shannon, M., & Shields, K.(2011). *Pearson nurse's drug guide 2011*. Upper Saddle River, NJ: Pearson Education, p. 1639.

2 Answer: 2 Rationale: Mupirocin (Bactroban) is a topical antimicrobial agent effective against impetigo caused by *Staphylococcus aureus*, beta-hemolytic streptococci, and *Streptococcus pyogenes*. Ketoconazole (Nizoral) is an antifungal agent. Capsaicin (Capsin) is a topical analgesic made from hot peppers. Acyclovir (Zovirax) is an antiviral agent. Cognitive Level: Applying Client Need: Pharmacological and Parenteral Therapies Integrated Process: Teaching and Learning Content Area: Pharmacology Strategy: First recognize that the disease is of bacterial origin. Then associate the drug names with the type of microorganism against which they are effective. Use the process of elimination to choose the

antibacterial drug. Reference: Wilson, B. A., Shannon, M., & Shields, K.(2011). *Pearson nurse's drug guide 2011*. Upper Saddle River, NJ: Pearson Education, p. 1655.

3 Answer: 1, 2 Rationale: Pharmacotherapy of dermatitis is symptomatic and involves lotions and ointments to control itching and skin flaking. Antihistamines may be used to control inflammation and reduce itching, and analgesics or topical anesthetic may be prescribed for pain relief. Cognitive Level: Applying Client Need: Pharmacological and Parenteral Therapies Integrated Process: Nursing Process: Planning Content Area: Pharmacology Strategy: Note that the question is asking for identification of what types of drugs may be used to treat atopic dermatitis. Note that the wording of the question indicates that more than one option will be correct. Reference: Adams, M. P. & Koch, R. W. (2010). *Pharmacology: Connections to nursing practice*. Upper Saddle River, NJ: Pearson, p. 1325.

4 Answer: 4 Rationale: The sunscreens frequently recommended are zinc oxide and titanium ointments that include PABA (p-aminobenzoic acid). The sun protective factor (SPF) means that if an individual normally burns in 10 minutes, an SPF 15 would mean sunburn would occur within $10 \times 15 = 150$ minutes. No chemical changes occur between the skin and the sun's rays. The waterproof characteristic limits or prevents washing away when the skin is exposed to moisture. Heat absorbed by the skin can be distributed to other body parts, but have no relationship to sunscreens. Cognitive Level: Applying Client Need: Pharmacological and Parenteral Therapies Integrated Process: Teaching and Learning Content Area: Pharmacology Strategy: The core issue of the question is an understanding of the basis of how sunscreens act and the ability to phrase this information in a way that is accurate and understandable to a client. Use basic nursing knowledge and the process of elimination to make a selection. **Reference:** Adams, M. P., & Koch, R. W. (2010). *Pharmacology: Connections to nursing practice*. Upper Saddle River, NJ: Pearson Education, p. 1331.

5 **Answer: 2** **Rationale:** Lindane (Kwell) is the drug of choice because it is well absorbed by the nervous system of the parasite (lice), resulting in death. It should be left in place for at least 12–24 hours. Chlorhexidine (Hibiclens) is a skin, dental, and wound cleanser. Sterile gloves may be needed for cleansing wounds but not to treat an infestation. Collagenase (Santyl) is an enzyme used in skin debriding and should not be touched with the fingers. Terbinafine (Lamisal) is an oral or nasal antifungal agent for tinea infections. **Cognitive Level:** Applying **Client Need:** Pharmacological and Parenteral Therapies **Integrated Process:** Teaching and Learning **Content Area:** Pharmacology **Strategy:** The critical term is *efficient and effective*. Associate the nature of the parasite with the drug and the application method. **Reference:** Adams, M. P., & Koch, R. W. (2010). *Pharmacology: Connections to nursing practice*. Upper Saddle River, NJ: Pearson Education, p. 1318.

6 **Answer: 5, 1, 2, 3, 4** **Rationale:** Shampooing the hair prior to application removes oils and cosmetic preparations and leads to increased drug penetration. To be effective the drug needs to be in contact with all infested areas so it is important to saturate the hair and scalp. Once applied, the recommended exposure time is 10 minutes. (Some residue may remain for 8 hours but normal exposure is 10 minutes.) The hair should be washed again to remove the drug after the recommended exposure time is completed. Combing with a fine-toothed comb removes dead lice once the treatment is complete. **Cognitive Level:** Analyzing **Client Need:** Pharmacological and Parenteral Therapies **Integrated Process:** Teaching and Learning **Content Area:** Pharmacology **Strategy:** Note the critical phrase *to sequence the events*, and from there visualize the process of a therapeutic shampoo to place the options in order. **Reference:** Wilson, B. A., Shannon, M., & Shields, K. (2011). *Pearson nurse's drug guide 2011*. Upper Saddle River, NJ: Pearson Education, pp. 896–897.

7 **Answer: 2** **Rationale:** Benzoyl peroxide inhibits growth of *Propionibacterium acnes* (a gram-positive microorganism). It is effective against inflammatory and noninflammatory acne. The microbe is less likely to develop antibiotic resistance to this agent and it is available in a variety of concentrations. Mafenide (Sulfamylon) is effective against gram-positive and gram-negative microorganisms, but the adverse risks are too significant for the treatment of acne. Chlorhexidine (Hibiclens) is used for the treatment of gingivitis. Cryotherapy is a treatment used for various types of warts. The goal is to destroy the skin cells containing the virus. **Cognitive Level:** Applying **Client**

Need: Pharmacological and Parenteral Therapies **Integrated Process:** Teaching and Learning **Content Area:** Pharmacology **Strategy:** Specific knowledge of these agents is needed to answer the question. Associate the drug actions with client needs and the offending microbe, and use the process of elimination to make a selection. **Reference:** Wilson, B. A., Shannon, M., & Shields, K. (2011). *Pearson nurse's drug guide 2011*. Upper Saddle River, NJ: Pearson Education, p. 1553.

8 **Answer: 4** **Rationale:** Isotretinoin (Accutane), an oral agent, is effective against acne because it reduces the size of the sebaceous glands and decreases gland cell differentiation and proliferation, as well as lipid composition of sebum on the skin surface. The other products are also used for acne, but are topical preparations and are less effective. Tetracycline suppresses the growth of *P. acne* but lacks the other significant actions. There is no evidence that penicillin or clindamycin (Cleocin T) act against *P. acne*. **Cognitive Level:** Applying **Client Need:** Pharmacological and Parenteral Therapies **Integrated Process:** Teaching and Learning **Content Area:** Pharmacology **Strategy:** Specific knowledge of the various anti-acne products is needed to answer this question. Review these quickly now if this question was difficult. **Reference:** Wilson, B. A., Shannon, M., & Shields, K.(2011). *Pearson nurse's drug guide 2011*. Upper Saddle River, NJ: Pearson Education, p. 1653.

9 **Answer: 1** **Rationale:** Infection is one of the primary complications associated with the burned client. Silver sulfadiazine (Silvadene) reduces bacterial growth and if treatment is successful, not only will the burned area heal but the client will not experience infection signaled by fever. The drug will not prevent fluid loss through burned tissue. Hypokalemia can occur, but silver sulfadiazine has no direct influence on its prevention or management. Appropriate separation of eschar should be noted as an appropriate assessment if an enzyme such as collagenase was used. **Cognitive Level:** Applying **Client Need:** Pharmacological and Parenteral Therapies **Integrated Process:** Nursing Process: Assessment **Content Area:** Pharmacology **Strategy:** Since burns damage the primary defense or barrier to invasion of microbes, it is logical to address elements associated with infection first. **Reference:** Wilson, B. A., Shannon, M., & Shields, K. (2011). *Pearson nurse's drug guide 2011*. Upper Saddle River, NJ: Pearson Education, pp. 1401–1403.

10 **Answer: 1** **Rationale:** Curling's ulcer may develop within 24 hours after a severe burn related to decreased blood flow and mucosal damage. For this reason, histamine 2-receptor antagonists such as famotidine (Pepcid) are ordered to reduce secretion of gastric acid. Clients with severe burns are usually NPO. A diuretic such as furosemide (Lasix) increases urinary output at the expense of reducing central circulating volume that results in decreased cardiac output. Crotamiton (Eurax), an antiparasitic used to treat scabies, is not indicated for use with the burned client. **Cognitive Level:** Applying **Client Need:** Pharmacological and Parenteral Therapies **Integrated Process:** Nursing Process: Implementation **Content Area:** Pharmacology **Strategy:** Consider that burn injury is a major stressor. Next recall that the body's response to stress includes shunting of blood away from the gastrointestinal (GI) tract, ultimately leading to GI bleeding. Then choose the drug that will reduce secretion of stomach acid. **Reference:** Wilson, B. A., Shannon, M., & Shields, K. (2011). *Pearson nurse's drug guide 2011.* Upper Saddle River, NJ: Pearson Education, pp. 1198–1199.

Posttest

1 **Answer: 1** **Rationale** Application of warm, moist dressings enhances drug's penetration of the skin. Tar preparations are more prone to staining. Subjecting the medication to a change in temperature may reduce its effectiveness. More than 12 hours of occlusive therapy can increase the risk of systemic absorption. **Cognitive Level:** Applying **Client Need:** Physiological Integrity **Nursing/Integrated Concepts:** Nursing Process: Implementation **Content Area:** Pharmacology **Strategy:** Consider that a critical concern with administration of topical medications is their ability to penetrate the skin. With this in mind, determine the best method for maximizing absorption. **Reference:** Adams, M. P., & Koch, R. W. (2010). *Pharmacology: Connections to nursing practice.* Upper Saddle River, NJ: Pearson Education, pp. 32–34.

2 **Answer: 1** **Rationale:** Clients should be warned about the unsightly appearance of the lesion and that tenderness at the site is to be expected. Sloughing will occur before crusting and dryness occurs. Lesion will be sore and inflamed rather than have decreased sensitivity. Massage may promote systemic absorption and is not recommended. **Cognitive Level:** Applying **Client Need:** Pharmacological and Parenteral Therapies **Integrated Process:** Teaching and Learning **Content Area:** Pharmacology **Strategy:** Because of the depth of the lesion, associate sloughing with the drug. **Reference:** Adams, M. P., & Koch, R. W. (2010). *Pharmacology: Connections to nursing practice.* Upper Saddle River, NJ: Pearson Education, pp. 973–975.

3 **Answer: 3** **Rationale:** Since some parasites may become resistant to the medications, the hair shaft should be checked regularly for at least a week. The container should be shaken well before use. Vigorous massage will result in systemic absorption. Applying drug to the inflamed areas can result in systemic absorption. **Cognitive Level:** Applying **Client Need:** Pharmacological and Parenteral Therapies **Integrated Process:** Nursing Process: Implementation **Content Area:** Pharmacology **Strategy:** Determine the best method for maximizing the drug's effectiveness. The option that provides for this will be

the answer to the question. **Reference:** Adams, M. P., & Koch, R. W. (2010). *Pharmacology: Connections to nursing practice.* Upper Saddle River, NJ: Pearson Education, p. 1318–1320.

4 **Answer: 4** **Rationale:** DuoDerm is a hydrophilic dressing indicated for noninfected ulcers with moderate drainage. The thick eschar at the wound edges should be removed before applying DuoDerm. DuoDerm is designed for draining wounds. Fibrinolysin and desoxyribonuclease (Elase) debride wounds by digesting the fibrin or blood clots inside the wound. **Cognitive Level:** Applying **Client Need:** Pharmacological and Parenteral Therapies **Integrated Process:** Nursing Process: Planning **Content Area:** Pharmacology **Strategy:** Specific knowledge of the purposes of various wound care products is needed to answer the question. Eliminate 2 options first because they are similar. Next, recall that this is a protective agent that absorbs drainage to help choose the correct option. **Reference:** Smith, S. F., Duell, D. J., & Marin, B. C. (2011). *Clinical nursing skills: Basic to advanced skills* (8th ed.). Upper Saddle River, New Jersey: Pearson Education, p. 926.

5 **Answer: 2** **Rationale:** Minocycline (Minocin) can lead to development of a lupus-like syndrome and also may cause increased pigmentation changes. It reduces the acne process by reducing the infectious processes. It is an antibiotic and has no effect on the patency of pores. There is no evidence that the drug leads to spontaneous abortions. **Cognitive Level:** Applying **Client Need:** Pharmacological and Parenteral Therapies **Integrated Process:** Teaching and Learning **Content Area:** Pharmacology **Strategy:** Associate the drug with "major" eruptions and increased pigmentation. **Reference:** Wilson, B. A., Shannon, M., & Shields, K. (2011). *Pearson nurse's drug guide 2011.* Upper Saddle River, NJ: Pearson Education, p. 1668.

6 **Answer: 2** **Rationale:** Excessive absorption is more likely to occur in the older adult because the skin is thinner and more permeable. Excessive absorption is not likely in younger clients, such as those that are 35 years old, 59 years old, and 38 years old. **Cognitive Level:** Applying **Client Need:** Pharmacological and Parenteral Therapies **Integrated Process:** Nursing Process: Planning **Content Area:** Pharmacology **Strategy:** Recall the age-related changes in the skin. Align absorption rates with the client's age. **Reference:** Wilson, B. A., Shannon, M., & Shields, K. (2011). *Pearson nurse's drug guide 2011.* Upper Saddle River, NJ: Pearson Education, 1454–1456.

7 **Answer: 2, 3** **Rationale:** Anti-acne medications inhibit sebaceous gland overactivity, reduce bacterial colonization, prevent follicles from becoming plugged with keratin, and reduce inflammation of lesions. They do not inhibit viral replication, as acne is caused by bacteria, not viruses. **Cognitive Level:** Applying **Client Need:** Pharmacological and Parenteral Therapies **Integrated Process:** Nursing Process: Implementation

Content Area: Pharmacology **Strategy:** Recall the pathophysiology of acne vulgaris and then choose the pharmacological options that address this correctly. **Reference:** Adams, M. P. & Koch, R. W. (2010). *Pharmacology: Connections to nursing practice.* Upper Saddle River, NJ: Pearson, pp. 1319–1321.

8 **Answer: 3** **Rationale:** Isotretinoin, an oral preparation, is a known teratogen that may result in spontaneous abortion and/or major fetal abnormalities such as hydrocephalus. Prevention of pregnancy is mandatory during isotretinoin therapy. The drug is not topical. Clients should avoid sun exposure to prevent risk of developing skin cancer. Inflammation of the lips is a side effect of isotretinoin, but this concern does not override the significance of the risk to the fetus. **Cognitive Level:** Applying **Client Need:** Pharmacological and Parenteral Therapies **Integrated Process:** Teaching and Learning **Content Area:** Pharmacology **Strategy:** Associate the drug with birth defects. Select the option that most represents the knowledge needed to adequately manage isotretinoin therapy. **Reference:** Wilson, B. A., Shannon, M., & Shields, K. (2011). *Pearson nurse's drug guide 2011.* Upper Saddle River, NJ: Pearson Education, p. 1661.

9 **Answer: 3** **Rationale:** Mafenide acetate (Sulfamylon) is a water-soluble cream that is used to treat burns. It may cause a severe stinging or burning sensation for 20 minutes after it is applied. A moderate analgesic may provide some comfort. The prescriber needs to be notified if an analgesic has not been prescribed. Attempting to remove the medication could increase the pain sensation. If the medication is the best application to treat or prevent infection, the focus should be on helping the client manage the discomfort. The temperature of the medication is not the causative factor. Cold application may stimulate a greater sensation of discomfort. **Cognitive Level:** Applying **Client Need:** Pharmacological and Parenteral Therapies **Integrated Process:** Nursing Process: Implementation **Content Area:** Pharmacology **Strategy:** Associate the medication with severe drug-induced pain and use the process of elimination to select the option that matches this concern. **Reference:** Wilson, B. A., Shannon, M., & Shields, K. (2011). *Pearson nurse's drug guide 2011.* Upper Saddle River, NJ: Pearson Education, pp. 931–932.

10 **Answer: 1, 3, 4** **Rationale:** Mafenide (Sulfamylon), silver sulfadiazine (Silvadene), and nitrofurazone (Furacin) may be ordered topically for burn treatment. Sulfisoxazole (Gantrinsin) is a short-acting, oral sulfonamide that is taken by mouth for various infections but is not used to treat burns. Trimethoprim is used to treat urinary tract infections and otitis media, not burn wounds. **Cognitive Level:** Applying **Client Need:** Pharmacological and Parenteral Therapies **Integrated Process:** Nursing Process: Implementation **Content Area:** Pharmacology **Strategy:** Note that the question is asking for identification of which topical drugs may be used to treat burn injury. Note that the wording of the question indicates that more than one option will be correct. **Reference:** Adams, M. P. & Koch, R. W. (2010). *Pharmacology: Connections to nursing practice.* Upper Saddle River, NJ: Pearson Education, p. 844.

References
Abrams, A. (2009). *Clinical drug therapy: Rationales for nursing practice* (9th ed.). Philadelphia: Lippincott Williams & Wilkins.

Adams, M., Holland, L., & Bostwick, P. (2011). *Pharmacology for nurses: A pathophysiologic approach* (3rd ed.). Upper Saddle River, NJ: Pearson Education.

Adams, M., & Urban, C. (2013). *Pharmacology: Connections to nursing practice* (2nd ed.). Upper Saddle River, NJ: Pearson Education.

Aschenbrenner, D., & Venable, S. (2012). *Drug therapy in nursing* (4th ed.). Philadelphia: Lippincott Williams & Wilkins.

Drug Facts & Comparisons® (updated monthly). St. Louis, MO: A. Wolters Kluwer.

Karch, A. M. (2010). *Focus on nursing pharmacology* (5th ed.). Philadelphia: Lippincott Williams & Wilkins.

Kee, J. (2009). *Laboratory and diagnostic tests and nursing implications* (8th ed.). Upper Saddle River, NJ: Prentice Hall.

Lehne, R. (2010). *Pharmacology for nursing care* (7th ed.). St. Louis, MO: Mosby, Inc.

LeMone, P., Burke, K. M., & Bauldoff, G. (2011). *Medical-surgical nursing: Critical thinking in patient care* (5th ed.). Upper Saddle River, NJ: Pearson Education.

Wilson, B. A., Shannon, M. T., & Shields, K. M. (2012). *Pearson nurse's drug guide 2012.* Upper Saddle River, NJ: Pearson Education.

ANSWERS & RATIONALES

Neurological and Musculoskeletal System Medications

Chapter Outline

NCLEX-RN® Test Prep

Use the accompanying online resource, NursingReviewsandRationales, to test yourself with hundreds of NCLEX®-style practice questions.

Objectives

➤ Describe general goals of therapy when administering neurological and musculoskeletal system medications.
➤ Identify significant nursing considerations related to administering opioid analgesics.
➤ Explain side effects and adverse effects of acetylsalicylic acid (aspirin), acetaminophen (Tylenol), and nonsteroidal anti-inflammatory drugs (NSAIDs).
➤ Identify major antiepileptic medication classifications.
➤ Describe significant client education points related to the administration of antiepileptics.
➤ Explain nursing considerations related to the administration of central nervous system (CNS) stimulants.
➤ Explain nursing considerations related to the administration of medications commonly used to treat Parkinson's disease, Alzheimer's disease, narcolepsy, and attention deficit/hyperactivity disorder.
➤ Identify primary uses, interactions, major side effects and adverse or toxic effects of the most commonly prescribed musculoskeletal relaxants.
➤ List significant client education points related to neurological and musculoskeletal system medications.

Review at a Glance

attention deficit/hyperactivity disorder also called ADHD; a condition in which a person demonstrates inattention, impulsivity, and possibly hyperactivity in a persistent pattern for more than a 6-month period
anorexia loss of appetite

diplopia double vision
epilepsy a chronic disorder characterized by recurring seizures in which there is a disturbance in some type of behavior (i.e., motor, sensory, autonomic, consciousness, or mentation)

gamma-aminobutyric acid (GABA) an excitatory neurotransmitter that is one of the amino acids
gingival hyperplasia increased growth of gum tissue; an adverse effect of antiepileptics, especially phenytoin (Dilantin)

hepatotoxicity a state in which liver damage has occurred; symptoms include dark urine, clay-colored stools, yellowing of skin, sclera, itching, abdominal pain, fever, and diarrhea

intracranial pressure pressure inside skull; when increased may cause serious to disastrous sequelae

level of consciousness state of awareness that includes orientation (arousal and wakefulness) and cognition (sum of cerebral mental functions)

narcolepsy inability to stay awake during the day, regardless of amount of sleep or stimulation

nystagmus involuntary oscillation of eyes

paresthesias abnormal sensations, whether spontaneous or evoked

psychomotor seizures a term referring to complex partial (focal) seizures that cause client to lose consciousness or black out for a few seconds; characteristic behavior may include lip smacking, patting, and picking at clothes

reticular activating system a diffuse system that extends from lower brain stem to cerebral cortex; controls sleep–wakefulness cycle, consciousness, focused attention, and sensory perceptions

spasms involuntary contractions of large muscle groups (arms, legs, neck)

spasticity increased resistance to passive movement, often more pronounced at extremes of range of motion and followed by a sudden or gradual release of resistance

status epilepticus a true neurological emergency in which a seizure

lasts more than 4 minutes or seizures are so frequently repeated or prolonged that they created a lasting condition (more than 30 minutes)

Stevens–Johnson syndrome an acute inflammatory disorder of the skin and mucous membranes (toxic epidermal necrolysis)

tonic–clonic seizures formerly grand mal seizures; tonic phase begins with a sudden loss of consciousness and a major tonic contraction (stiffening of body and extremities) that lasts for about 1 minute; clonic phase is characterized by violent, rhythmic, muscular contractions and hyperventilation that lasts from 30 seconds to a minute; postictal phase is a deep sleep followed by a period of confusion and lethargy that can last minutes to hours

PRETEST

❶ Methylphenidate (Ritalin) is newly prescribed for a client with narcolepsy. The nurse reports which priority health history component to the prescriber?

1. Congestive heart failure (CHF)
2. Diabetes mellitus
3. Irritable bowel syndrome
4. Anemia

❷ A medication regimen has controlled the seizures of an adult client for several days and includes the medication phenytoin (Dilantin). Prior to discharge, the nurse should place highest priority on including which information in the teaching plan? Select all that apply.

1. Many seizure disorders will eventually stop on their own.
2. Adherence to medication therapy is essential to avoid recurrence of seizures.
3. Side effects may include confusion and headache.
4. The client cannot drive a vehicle permanently.
5. Lab work for drug levels will need to be done routinely.

❸ The nurse should include which instruction to a client taking ergotamine tartrate (Gynergen) for treatment of cluster headaches?

1. "Take the medication every 4 hours."
2. "Take the medication with plenty of water."
3. "You will feel energetic and warm after taking the medication."
4. "Lie down in a darkened room after taking the medication."

❹ Because a client with a spinal cord injury has developed spasticity, the nurse prepares to teach the client about which newly prescribed medication?

1. Dexamethasone (Decadron)
2. Dantrolene (Dantrium)
3. Donepezil (Aricept)
4. Dobutamine (Dobutrex)

5 An opioid analgesic has been administered to a client postoperatively. The nurse would make which priority follow-up assessments? Select all that apply.

1. Respiratory rate and level of consciousness
2. Blood pressure and heart rate
3. Interactions with foods and other prescribed drugs
4. History of drug abuse and pain management history
5. Pain level

6 The nurse would include which precaution when teaching a client with liver disease about the use of over-the-counter (OTC) acetaminophen, aspirin, or nonsteroidal anti-inflammatory drugs (NSAIDs)?

1. "Take your temperature before taking one of these drugs."
2. "Consult your health care provider before taking one of these medications."
3. "You should have your cholesterol level measured before using these medications."
4. "Taper the discontinuance of any of these medications over a 3-day period."

7 Because phenytoin (Dilantin) was ordered stat for a client who was just admitted to the nursing unit from the emergency department, which assessments are of highest priority for the nurse to perform?

1. Hydration status and emotional response to seizures
2. Blood urea nitrogen, creatinine, and urine output
3. Seizure activity, mental status, and respiratory status
4. Electrolytes, serum osmolality, and leg edema

8 A client with chronic depression has a new medication order for phenelzine (Nardil). The nurse calls the prescriber to clarify the order if the client is already taking which of the following drugs? Select all that apply.

1. Propranolol (Inderal)
2. Meperidine (Demerol)
3. Glucagon (GlucaGen)
4. Carbamazepine (Tegretol)
5. Dicyclomine (Bentyl)

9 The nurse would include in a teaching plan for a client diagnosed with seizure disorder that which of the following drug groups can potentiate the effects of the prescribed carbamazepine (Tegretol)?

1. Nonsteroidal anti-inflammatory drugs (NSAIDs)
2. Anorexiants and amphetamines
3. Anticholinergics
4. Hydantoins and benzodiazepines

10 The client with a spinal cord injury is taking dantrolene (Dantrium) for spasticity. The nurse instructs the client to notify the health care provider immediately if which adverse effects occur? Select all that apply.

1. Persistent diarrhea
2. Change in blood or urine glucose levels
3. Abdominal pain, scleral jaundice
4. Painful urination and urinary frequency
5. Change in hearing or smell

➤ *See pages 341–342 for Answers and Rationales.*

I. ANALGESICS

A. Opioids

1. Action and use
   a. Symptomatic relief of severe acute and chronic pain
   b. Most commonly used in postoperative settings and to treat pain caused by malignancy
   c. Produce effects by binding to opioid receptors throughout central nervous system (CNS) and peripheral tissues
   d. Considered controlled substances by FDA
   e. Classified by their ability to stimulate or block opioid receptors or by the severity of pain for which they are used

f. Onset of action is immediate if given by intravenous (IV) route and rapid if given by intramuscular (IM) route, subcutaneously (subQ), or by mouth (PO)

g. Peak action is from 1–2 hours and duration up to 12 hours depending on formulation

h. These agents cross the blood–brain and placental barriers and also into breast milk

2. Common medications (Table 10-1)

3. Administration considerations

    a. Check respiratory rate prior to administration due to CNS depressant effects

    b. May increase **intracranial pressure** (ICP, pressure inside skull); never administer an opioid to a client with a traumatic brain injury because it could mask symptoms of deteriorating level of consciousness (LOC)

    c. Opioids may be given short-term for acute pain, or on a long-term basis for chronic pain; tolerance should not be confused with addiction in clients requiring long-term pain management therapy

    d. Clients with severe heart, liver or kidney disease, respiratory or seizure disorders should be closely monitored

    e. Initial therapy begins with decreased dosages for older adults or debilitated clients

    f. Double check dosages for neonates, infants, and children with prescriber or pharmacist

    g. Use caution if given to clients more prone to addiction because of possibility of dependence; however, do not withhold if client is experiencing pain

    h. Determine client's pattern of use if long term; be aware that some opioids, such as Oxycontin, are used as street drugs

4. Contraindications

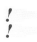

    a. Hypersensitivity reactions occur frequently

    b. Check for sensitivity prior to administration

    c. Do not use with clients who have acute bronchial asthma or upper airway obstruction, increased ICP, seizure disorders, pancreatitis, acute ulcerative colitis, or severe liver or kidney insufficiency; traumatic brain injury

Table 10-1   **Common Opioid Analgesics**

Type	Generic (Trade) Name	Route
Pure agonists (No ceiling effect, increase in analgesia by increase in dose)	Codeine (Paveral)	IM, PO
	Hydrocodone bitartrate (Vicodin)	PO, subQ
	Oxycodone (Oxycontin)	PO
	Propoxyphene (Darvon)	PO
	Morphine sulfate (Duramorph)	PO, IV
	Fentanyl citrate (Sublimaze Duragesic)	IM, trans-dermal patch
	Oxymorphone (Numorphan)	subQ, IM, IV
	Hydromorphone hydrochloride (Dilaudid)	PO, IM, IV, subQ
	Meperidine (Demerol)	PO, IM, IV, subQ
	Methadone hydrochloride (Dolophine)	PO, IM, subQ
	Levorphanal tartrate (Levo-Dromoran)	PO, subQ
Mixed agonists–antagonists (Have ceiling effect)	Pentazocine hydrochloride (Talwin)	PO, IM, IV, subQ
	Butorphanol tartrate (Stadol)	IM, IV
	Dezocine (Dalgan)	IM, IV
	Nalbuphine hydrochloride (Nubain)	subQ, IM, IV

5. Significant drug interactions
   a. Barbiturates, other narcotics, hypnotics, antipsychotics, or alcohol can increase CNS depression when combined with opiates
   b. Combined use with monoamine oxidase (MAO) inhibitors may precipitate hypertensive crisis
   c. Analgesia may be inhibited if used with phenothiazines
6. Significant food interactions: alcohol may have additive effect
7. Significant laboratory studies: monitor liver and kidney function to determine ability to excrete medication and metabolites
8. Side effects
   a. Nausea and vomiting (N/V), **anorexia** or loss of appetite
   b. Sedation, light-headedness, dizziness
   c. Constipation, GI cramps, urinary retention, oliguria
   d. Pruritus (these effects decrease over time)
9. Adverse effects/toxicity
   a. Respiratory depression, respiratory arrest
   b. Circulatory depression
   c. Increased ICP
10. Nursing considerations
    a. Assess pain for type, intensity, and location of prior to administration (use pain scale)
    b. Assess for respiratory rate, depth, and rhythm; if less than 12 breaths/min withhold medication and notify prescriber
    c. Assess for CNS changes including **level of consciousness** (LOC), which is the state of awareness, as well as dizziness, drowsiness, hallucinations, and pupil size
    d. Assess client for allergic reactions such as rash or urticaria
    e. Administer opiate for pain and antiemetic for N/V
    f. Evaluate the therapeutic response and maintain comfort
    g. Monitor vital signs regularly
    h. Assess older adults frequently because of possible slower biotransformation and sensitivity to CNS drugs
    i. Note that there are multiple formulations and strengths of most opioids; double-check orders and medication before administration
11. Client education
    a. Avoid alcohol and other CNS depressants while using opioids
    b. Do not take over-the-counter (OTC) medications without approval by prescriber
    c. Avoid ambulation, smoking, driving, or other activities without assistance after administration of medication until drug response is known
    d. Report any CNS changes, allergic reactions, or shortness of breath
    e. Long-term use can lead to withdrawal symptoms with termination of use, including N/V, cramps, fever, faintness, and anorexia; this is considered dependence, not addiction

B. **Opioid antagonists**
   1. Actions and use
      a. Include naloxone (Narcan) and naltrexone (ReVia)
      b. Compete with opioids at opiate receptor sites, blocking effects of opioids
      c. Used to reverse respiratory depression and sedation induced by overdose of opioids, pentazocine, and propoxyphene
      d. Onset of effect 1–2 minutes, duration 45 minutes
   2. Side effects
      a. Reversal of analgesia
      b. Increased blood pressure (BP)

Practice to Pass

You are caring for a client with a patient-controlled analgesia (PCA) pump that has morphine sulfate as the medication. The client has been out of surgery for 1½ hours. He reports that his hands itch and he has a rash. What would you do first?

    c. Tremors, hyperventilation, drowsiness, nervousness, rapid pulse

    d. Hyperpnea and N/V

3. Adverse effects/toxicity

    a. Hypotension

    b. Ventricular tachycardia and fibrillation

    c. Seizures

    d. Hepatitis

    e. Pulmonary edema

4. Nursing considerations

    a. Assess vital signs every 3–5 minutes

    b. Assess arterial blood gases (ABGs)

    c. Assess cardiac status: tachycardia, hypertension

    d. Monitor electrocardiogram (ECG)

    e. Assess respiratory function (rate, rhythm) and LOC

    f. Administer only with resuscitative equipment nearby

    g. Evaluate therapeutic response, LOC, and need for reversal of respiratory depression

    h. In clients with physical dependence on narcotics, administration of naloxone may precipitate symptoms of withdrawal

C. Nonopioids

  1. Acetylsalicylic acid (Aspirin)

    a. Action and use

      1) Is a salicylate medication

      2) Inhibits prostaglandins involved in production of inflammation, pain and fever

      3) Blocks pain impulses in CNS

      4) Antipyretic action results from vasodilation of peripheral vessels

      5) Powerfully inhibits platelet aggregation

      6) Relieves mild to moderate pain, including pain caused by rheumatoid arthritis, osteoarthritis, acute rheumatic fever, systemic lupus erythematosus (SLE), bursitis, transient ischemic attacks (TIA), post–myocardial infarction (MI), prophylaxis of MI, stroke, and angina

    b. Administration considerations

      1) Dosage varies depending on age of client and condition being treated

      2) Gastric irritation may be decreased by administering with full glass of water, milk, food, or antacid

      3) Pills can be crushed or chewed, but do not crush enteric-coated preparations

      4) Give 30 minutes prior to or 2 hours following meals

      5) Administer at least 30 minutes prior to physical therapy or planned activity to minimize discomfort

    c. Contraindications

      1) History of hypersensitivity to salicylates, or other nonsteroidal anti-inflammatory drugs (NSAIDs), GI bleeding, bleeding disorders

      2) Contraindicated in children younger than 12 years old because of risk of Reye syndrome, children or teenagers with chicken pox or flulike symptoms, pregnancy 3rd trimester, lactation

      3) Contraindicated with vitamin K deficiency, peptic ulcer disease, anemia, renal or hepatic dysfunction

    d. Significant drug interactions

      1) Decreased effects of aspirin (ASA) with antacids (high-dose), and urinary alkalizers

      2) Increased bleeding with anticoagulants and alcohol

      3) Increased GI bleeding when taken concurrently with corticosteroids

    4) Increased effects of warfarin, insulin, thrombolytic agents, penicillins, phenytoin, valproic acid, oral hypoglycemics, and sulfonamides

    5) Increased salicylate levels (leads to toxicity) with ammonium chloride, urinary acidifiers, and nizatidine

    6) Decreased effects of probenecid, spironolactone, sulfinpyrazone, sulfonamides, NSAIDs, beta blockers

  e. Significant food interactions: increased risk of bleeding with horse chestnut, kelpware, dong quai, feverfew, red clover, and ginger; caffeine may increase absorption of aspirin

  f. Significant laboratory studies

    1) Increases coagulation studies, liver function studies, serum uric acid, amylase, CO_2, and urinary protein

    2) Decreases serum potassium, cholesterol, and T_3 and T_4 concentrations

    3) Interference with urine catecholamines, pregnancy test, and urine glucose tests (Clinistix, Tes-Tape)

  g. Side effects

    1) Increased prothrombin time (PT), activated partial thromboplastin time (APTT), bleeding time

    2) Stimulation, drowsiness, dizziness, confusion, headache, hallucinations

    3) Diarrhea, heartburn, anorexia, and N/V

    4) Rash, urticaria, bruising

    5) Tinnitus

  h. Adverse effects/toxicity

    1) Hematologic: thrombocytopenia, agranulocytosis, leukopenia, neutropenia, and hemolytic anemia

    2) Seizures, coma

    3) GI bleeding, hepatitis

    4) Reye syndrome (children), characterized by encephalopathy and fatty liver degeneration

  i. Nursing considerations

    1) Assess for allergy to salicylates prior to administration

    2) Assess liver function tests, renal function tests (BUN, creatinine), and blood studies including complete blood count (CBC), hematocrit (Hct), hemoglobin (Hgb), PT if on long-term therapy

    3) Assess for **hepatotoxicity** (state of liver damage): dark urine, clay-colored stools, yellowing of skin, sclera, itching

    4) Abdominal pain, fever, diarrhea, especially if on long-term therapy

    5) Evaluate for therapeutic responses such as decreased pain, inflammation, and fever

    6) Assess for aspirin toxicity when administered with ammonium chloride

  j. Client education

    1) Report any symptoms of hepatotoxicity or renal toxicity

    2) Report visual changes, tinnitus, allergic reactions, and bleeding

    3) Take medication with 8 oz water, milk, or food, and sit upright for 30 minutes following dose

    4) Do not exceed recommended dose; acute salicylate poisoning may result

    5) Do not combine with other OTC medications that also contain ASA

    6) Therapeutic response can take up to 2 weeks

    7) Avoid alcohol ingestion to decrease chance of GI bleeding

    8) This medication should not be given to children or teens with flulike or chickenpox symptoms (risk of Reye syndrome)

    9) May need to be discontinued 7–10 days prior to surgery to reduce risk for excessive bleeding

2. Acetaminophen (Tylenol)
    a. Action and use
        1) May block pain impulses peripherally that occur in response to inhibition of prostaglandin synthesis
        2) Possesses weak anti-inflammatory properties
        3) Antipyretic action results from inhibition of prostaglandins in the CNS resulting in peripheral vasodilation, sweating, and dissipation of heat
        4) Used for mild to moderate pain or fever, especially when ASA or NSAIDs are not tolerated
    b. Administration considerations
        1) Usual dose is 325 to 600 mg q4–6h PO or by rectum (PR); maximum dose is 4 grams per day
        2) Oral forms may be crushed or given as whole or chewable tablets
        3) May give with food or milk to increase gastric tolerance
        4) Co-administration with high-carbohydrate meal may significantly retard absorption rate
        5) Intravenous use: only one formulation available (Ofirmev); administered via a 15-minute infusion for mild to moderate post-surgical pain management
    c. Contraindications
        1) Hypersensitivity to acetaminophen or phenacetin
        2) In children younger than 3 years unless directed by prescriber
        3) Repeated administration to clients with anemia or hepatic diseases, including alcoholism, malnutrition, or thrombocytopenia
    d. Significant drug interactions
        1) Decreased effect and increased hepatotoxicity with barbiturates, alcohol, carbamazepine, hydantoins, rifampin, sulfinpyrazone
        2) Cholestyramine decreases absorption
        3) Hypoprothrombinemia may occur when used concurrently with warfarin
        4) Bone marrow suppression may occur with zidovudine
    e. Significant food interactions: caffeine enhances analgesic effect; alcohol increases risk of liver damage
    f. Significant laboratory studies: interference with Chemstrip G, Dextrostix, Visidex II (false increases in urinary glucose), 5-HIAA (false increases), blood glucose (false decreases), serum uric acid (false increases)
    g. Side effects: rash; otherwise negligible with recommended dosage
    h. Adverse effects/toxicity
        1) Anaphylaxis
        2) Hematology: leukopenia, neutropenia, hemolytic anemia, thrombocytopenia, pancytopenia
        3) GI: hepatotoxicity with hepatic necrosis
        4) Angioedema
        5) Toxicity: cyanosis, anemia, neutropenia, jaundice, pancytopenia, CNS stimulation, delirium followed by vascular collapse, seizures, coma, and death
    i. Nursing considerations
        1) Assess liver function tests, BUN and creatinine, and CBC and PT if on long-term therapy
        2) May cause hepatotoxicity at doses greater than 4 grams/day with chronic use; recommendations for older adults are no more than 3 grams/day
        3) Assess client for chronic poisoning; signs including rapid, weak pulse, dyspnea, cold, clammy extremities; report them immediately to prescriber
        4) Assess for hepatotoxicity: dark urine, clay-colored stools, yellowing of skin, sclera, itching, abdominal pain, fever, diarrhea, especially if on long-term therapy

5) Be prepared to administer acetylcysteine (Mucomyst) as antidote for acetaminophen poisoning

6) Evaluate client for therapeutic response, such as decreased pain or fever

j. Client education

1) Do not exceed recommended dose; acute poisoning with liver damage may result

2) Be aware of acute toxicity symptoms such as N/V, abdominal pain; notify prescriber of these immediately

3) Do not combine with other OTC medications that also contain acetaminophen

4) Recognize signs of chronic overdose such as bleeding, bruising, malaise, fever, and sore throat

5) Notify prescriber of pain or fever lasting longer than 3 days

3. Nonsteroidal anti-inflammatory drugs (NSAIDs)

a. Action and use

1) Inhibit cyclooxygenase and decrease prostaglandins and thromboxane

2) They are used to treat mild to moderate pain, osteoarthritis, rheumatoid arthritis, and dysmenorrhea

b. Common medications (Table 10-2)

Table 10-2 **Common Nonsteroidal Anti-Inflammatory Agents**

Medication	Route	Significant Drug Interactions
Celecoxib (Celebrex)	PO	↑ effect of anticoagulants ↓ effect of ASA, ACE inhibitors, diuretics ↑ adverse reactions of glucocorticoids, NSAIDs, ASA ↑ toxicity: lithium, antineoplastics
Diclofenac sodium (Voltaren, others)	PO	↓ effect of beta blockers, diuretics ↑ effect of anticoagulants, digoxin; increases toxicity of phenytoin, lithium, cyclosporine, methotrexate, ASA Hyperkalemia with potassium-sparing diuretics
Etodolac (Lodine)	PO	↓ effect of beta blockers, diuretics, antacids ↑ effect of anticoagulants, digoxin ↑ toxicity of phenytoin, lithium, cyclosporine, methotrexate, ASA
Fenoprofen (Nalfon)	PO	Phenobarbital ↓ effect of fenoprofen ↓ effect of diuretics ↑ effects of oral anticoagulants and sulfonylureas ↑ GI toxicity with ASA ↑ GI reactions with corticosteroids, alcohol (ETOH)
Flurbiprofen (Ansaid, Ocufen)	PO	↑ effects of oral anticoagulants, heparin, phenytoin, sulfonylureas, and sulfonamides ↑ effect of flurbiprofen: phenytoin, sulfonylureas, sulfonamides
Ibuprofen (Advil)	PO	↓ effect of diuretics effect of antihypertensives, thiazides, furosemide ↑ reactions: corticosteroids, ASA ↑ toxicity: digoxin, lithium, oral anticoagulants, cyclosporine
Indomethacin (Indocin)	PO	↓ effect of antihypertensives ↑ effect of digoxin, penicillamine, phenytoin ↑ toxicity: lithium, methotrexate, cyclosporine, aminoglycosides, ASA, corticosteroids, triamterene, ETOH ↑ risk of bleeding with anticoagulants

Table 10-2	Common Nonsteroidal Anti-Inflammatory Agents (Continued)	
Medication	**Route**	**Significant Drug Interactions**
Ketoprofen (Orudis, Oruvail)	PO	↑ toxicity: lithium, methotrexate, cyclosporine, phenytoin, alcohol ↑ risk of bleeding: warfarin ↑ effects of ketoprofen, ASA, probenecid ↑ GI reactions: corticosteroids, ASA ↓ effect of diuretics, antihypertensives
Ketorolac (Toradol, others)	IV, IM, PO	↑ toxicity: lithium, methotrexate ↑ risk of bleeding: anticoagulants, salicylates ↑ renal impairment: ACE inhibitors ↓ effect of diuretics, antihypertensives
Mefenemic acid (Ponstel)	PO	↑ toxicity: lithium, sulfonylureas, sulfonamides, phenytoin, warfarin ↑ risk of bleeding: anticoagulants, heparin
Nabumetone (Relafen)	PO	↓ effect of diuretics, antihypertensives ↑ risk of bleeding: anticoagulants, thrombolytics, valproic acid, cefamandole, cefotetan, cefoperazone ↑ risk of hematologic reactions: antineoplastics, radiation ↑ GI reactions: salicylates, NSAIDs, ETOH, potassium, corticosteroids
Naproxen (Naprosyn, others)	PO	↑ toxicity: methotrexate, oral anticoagulants, sulfonylureas, probenecid, lithium ↓ effect of diuretics, antihypertensives ↑ GI reactions: ASA, ETOH, corticosteroids Possible renal impairment: ACE inhibitors ↑ risk of bleeding: oral anticoagulants, heparin
Oxyprozin (Daypro)	PO	↓ effect of antihypertensives, diuretics ↑ risk of adverse effects with corticosteroids
Piroxicam (Feldene)	PO	↑ toxicity: cyclosporine, methotrexate, lithium, alcohol, oral anticoagulants, ASA, corticosteroids ↓ effects of antihypertensives, diuretics Hypoglycemia: oral antidiabetics ↑ risk of bleeding: oral anticoagulants, heparin ↑ GI reactions: ASA, ETOH
Sulindac (Clinoril)	PO	↑ risk of bleeding: oral anticoagulants ↑ nephrotoxicity: cyclosporine ↓ sulindac effect with use of diflunisal—**do not use together** ↑ toxicity: methotrexate, sulfonamides, sulfonylureas, probenecid, lithium ↑ GI reactions: ASA, NSAIDs

   c. Administration considerations
     1) Gastric irritation may be decreased by administering with full glass of water, milk, or food
     2) Pills can be crushed or chewed; capsules should not be crushed, dissolved, or chewed
     3) Give 30 minutes before or 2 hours after meals for best absorption
     4) Administer at least 30 minutes prior to physical therapy or planned activity to minimize discomfort
   d. Contraindications
     1) Hypersensitivity
     2) Contraindicated with asthma, severe renal or hepatic disease, GI bleeding, bleeding disorders, peptic ulcer disease, or anemia

    e. Significant drug interactions: see Table 10-2 for specific interactions for each medication

    f. Significant food interactions: food may increase absorption of NSAIDs; increased risk of bleeding with dong quai, feverfew, garlic, ginger, horse chestnut, and red clover; increased risk of photosensitivity with St. John's wort

    g. Significant laboratory studies
       1) Liver function tests
       2) Serum uric acid
       3) Urinary bilirubin, urinalysis, BUN, creatinine
       4) Bleeding time, PT, CBC

    h. Side effects
       1) Nausea, abdominal pain, anorexia
       2) Dizziness, drowsiness

    i. Adverse effects/toxicity
       1) FDA has recommended that NSAID product manufacturers include a boxed warning, highlighting possible increased risk of cardiovascular events and serious risk for GI bleeding associated with their use
       2) Nephrotoxicity including dysuria, hematuria, oliguria, azotemia
       3) Blood dyscrasias, cholestatic hepatitis

    j. Nursing considerations
       1) Assess lab tests for renal, hepatic, and hematologic function before treatment begins and periodically thereafter
       2) Audiometric and ophthalmic exam may be done before, during, and after treatment
       3) Assess for ear and eye problems; blurred vision and tinnitus may indicate toxicity
       4) Evaluate for therapeutic response including decreased pain, stiffness in joints, decreased swelling in joints, ability to move more easily
       5) Client may need to refrain from administration for several days before surgery to reduce risk of operative bleeding

    k. Client education
       1) Take drug with food or fluids to reduce GI irritation
       2) Report blurred vision, ringing, roaring in ears, which may indicate toxicity
       3) Avoid driving or other hazardous activities if dizziness and drowsiness occur, especially in older adults
       4) Report changes in urine pattern, increased weight, edema, increased pain in joints, fever, or blood in urine indicating nephrotoxicity
       5) Therapeutic effects may take up to 1 month, depending on formulation

D. Medications to treat headaches

    1. Action and use: serotonin-selective drugs (known as -*triptans*) relieve pain and inflammation associated with migraine headaches; aimed at prevention with prophylactic therapy and acute symptomatic treatment during an attack

    a. Migraine headaches
       1) Acute therapy directed toward abolishing or limiting headache as it begins
       2) Ergot preparations are alpha-adrenergic agonists or antagonists that cause vasoconstriction or vasodilation, depending on state of vessel; they also block uptake of serotonin by platelets that can cause precipitous decline of serotonin leading to migraine attack
       3) Prophylaxis medications are beta-adrenergic blockers, serotonin antagonists, and antiepileptics

    b. Tension-type headaches
       1) Therapy is directed toward rapid treatment of pain
       2) Prevention and reduction of occurrence is also a goal

   3) Mild analgesics and muscle relaxants are first-line agents; antidepressants may be used with counseling; ASA, acetaminophen, ibuprofen are used for pain; amitriptyline (Elavil) is helpful for muscle contraction pain
 c. Cluster headaches
   1) Treatment is directed at elimination of triggers
   2) Preventative therapies used may include high-dose calcium channel blockers, lithium, methysergide, or corticosteroids
2. Common medications (Table 10-3)
3. Administration considerations
 a. For abortive treatment medications, taking early in headache is imperative
 b. Dose that was effective for last headache should be starting dosage for this headache
4. Contraindications
 a. Hypersensitivity to ergot alkaloids, pregnancy, cardiac disease, hypertension, sepsis, or severe pruritus
 b. Triptans: contraindicated in clients with history of acute myocardial infarction (MI), uncontrolled hypertension, and cerebrovascular diseases such as stroke
5. Significant drug interactions
 a. Beta blockers and calcium channel blockers are additive in effects with these medications
 b. Ergot toxicity can occur if ergot is given with erythromycin or other macrolides
 c. Serotonin-selective drugs have many interactions; see product literature
 d. Triptans should be given cautiously if ergotamine has been taken within the previous 24 hours
6. Significant food interactions: none reported
7. Significant laboratory studies: see specific medications
8. Side effects: see Table 10-3
9. Adverse effects/toxicity: see Table 10-3
10. Nursing considerations
 a. Assess for medication-specific side effects as well as efficacy of treatment
 b. Planning for care must begin with careful history, including treatments that have been effective in past

Table 10-3   **Medications Used to Treat Headaches**

Medication	Route	Therapeutic Indications	Adverse Effects
Ergots			
Ergotamine tartrate (Ergostat)	PO	Abort headache unresponsive to nonnarcotic treatment; cluster headaches	Nausea, vomiting, weakness, numbness, tingling of fingers and toes; possible throat or nasal irritation, altered taste; delirium, seizures, cerebral hemorrhage, intermittent claudication
Dihydroergotamine (Migranal, others)	IM, IV, intranasal	Parenteral treatment for established headache	
Serotonin receptor agonists			
Sumatriptan (Imitrex)	subQ, PO, intranasal	Migraine or cluster headaches	Dizziness, vertigo, fatigue, anxiety, warming sensation, coronary artery vasospasm, dysrhythmias, transient myocardial ischemia, myocardial infarction, cardiac arrest
Almotriptan (Axert)	PO	Acute migraine headache with or without aura	
Eletriptan (Relpax)	PO		
Frovatriptan (Frova)	PO		
Naratriptan (Amerge)	PO		
Rizatriptan (Maxalt)	PO, SL		
Zolmitriptan (Zomig)	PO, SL intranasal		

c. Provide a quiet and low-light environment for client to relax

d. Obtain an accurate dietary history from client to determine if a relationship exists between onset of headache and certain foods

e. Avoid prolonged use of medication

f. When administering triptans, do not break oral disintegrating tablets

g. Beware of ergotamine rebound or an increase in frequency and duration of headache

11. Client education

a. How to identify type of headache: migraine, cluster, or tension

b. Identify triggers for headaches and how to ameliorate them

c. Keep a headache diary

d. Stress reduction, stress management and lifestyle changes, including diet, to minimize headaches

e. Do not eat, drink, or smoke while tablet is dissolving (if using sublingual tablet)

f. Avoid exposure to cold weather for a prolonged period; cold may increase adverse reactions to drug

g. Do not increase dose without consulting prescriber

h. Use comfort measures during attack, such as lying in darkened, quiet room with cold compresses applied to head

II. ANTIEPILEPTICS

A. Hydantoins

1. Action and use

a. Suppress sodium influx across neuronal cell membranes

b. Inhibit spread of seizure activity in motor cortex

c. Used in general **tonic–clonic seizures** (grand mal seizures), **status epilepticus** (seizures that last longer than 4 minutes), and **psychomotor seizures** (complex focal seizures)

2. Common medications (Table 10-4)

3. Administration considerations

a. Fosphenytoin should only be given IV for status epilepticus in emergency department or critical care area; respiratory rate, BP, and ECG should be monitored

b. Do not interchange chewable phenytoin products with capsules

c. Phenytoin readily binds with protein so should not be given with gastric feedings, which inhibit uptake

d. Phenytoin metabolism varies greatly among people, and thus drug levels should be monitored and maintained at 10–20 mcg/mL

e. Carbamazepine given via NG tube should be mixed with D_5W or NS and flush with at least 100 mL solution afterwards

f. Give ethosuximide, diazepam, and carbamazepine with food or milk to reduce GI symptoms

4. Contraindications

a. Hypersensitivity

b. Contraindicated with psychiatric condition, pregnancy, bradycardia, SA and AV node block, Stokes–Adams syndrome, hepatic failure

5. Significant drug interactions: see Table 10-4

6. Significant food interactions: phenytoin absorption is decreased by enteral nutrition products; withhold feedings 30–60 minutes before and after medication administration or per institutional policy and procedure manual; folic acid, calcium, and vitamin D absorption may be decreased by phenytoin

7. Significant laboratory studies: therapeutic phenytoin level of 10–20 mcg/mL

Table 10-4	Antiepileptics		
Generic (Trade) Name	**Route**	**Therapeutic Indications**	**Drug-to-Drug Interactions**
Hydantoins			
Fosphenytoin (Cerebyx)	PO	Grand mal seizures, complex partial seizures, status epilepticus	Many drugs may either ↑ or ↓ fosphenytoin levels: see product literature Tricyclic antidepressants lower the seizure threshold
Phenytoin (Dilantin)	PO, IV	Grand mal, psychomotor, tonic–clonic, nonepileptic seizures, seizures following head injury, prevention of seizures during and after surgery	Antiepileptics may ↑ or ↓ phenytoin levels Phenytoin may ↓ absorption and ↑ metabolism of oral anticoagulants Phenytoin ↑ metabolism of oral contraceptives and corticosteroids Amiodarone, chloramphenicol, omeprazole, and ticlopidine ↑ phenytoin levels Antituberculosis agents ↓ phenytoin levels Gingko may ↓ antiepileptic effectiveness
Iminostilbenes			
Carbamazepine (Tegretol)	PO	Partial or generalized tonic–clonic seizures	Many drug interactions, see product literature
Oxcarbazepine (Trileptal)			
Barbiturates			
Mephobarbital (Mebaral)	PO	Grand mal, petit mal seizures; used in combination with other antiepileptics to manage delirium tremens	↓ metabolism of anticoagulants and corticosteroids ↓ effectiveness with digoxin Griseofulvin ↓ mephobarbital absorption Kava kava and valerian may potentiate sedation
Phenobarbital (Luminal)	PO, IV	Grand mal, partial seizures, status epilepticus	
Succinimides			
Ethosuximide (Zarontin)	PO	Petit mal and myoclonic seizures	↓ ethosuximide levels with carbamazepine ↑ ethosuximide levels with isoniazid Phenobarbital and ethosuximide levels may be altered with ↑ seizure frequency Gingko may ↓ antiseizure effectiveness
Methsuxmide (Celontin)	PO	Petit mal seizures when refractory to other drugs	Lamotrigine concentrations may be ↓ ↓ serum levels along with therapeutic effects of primidone
Benzodiazepines (Anxiolytics)			
Clonazepam (Klonopin)	PO	Myoclonus, status epilepticus, petit mal seizures refractory to succinimides or valproic acid	↑ effect with cimetidine, disulfiram, omeprazole, hormonal contraceptives ↓ effectiveness with theophylline ↑ digoxin level and toxicity
Clorazepate (Tranxene)	PO	Adjunctive therapy for partial seizures	↑ effect with cimetidine, disulfiram, omeprazole, hormonal contraceptives ↓ effectiveness with theophylline ↑ digoxin level and toxicity
Diazepam (Valium, Diastat)	IV, PR	Adjunct therapy for status epilepticus Severe recurrent seizures	↑ effect with cimetidine, disulfiram, omeprazole, hormonal contraceptives ↓ effectiveness with theophylline, ranitidine
Lorazepam (Ativan)	IV	Status epilepticus	↑ CNS depression with barbiturates and opioids ↓ effectiveness with theophylline Risk of toxicity with probenecid, valproate Kava kava ↑ sedation effect

Table 10-4	Antiepileptics		
Generic (Trade) Name	**Route**	**Therapeutic Indications**	**Drug-to-Drug Interactions**
Others			
Ezogabine (Potiga)	PO	Adjunct treatment of partial-onset seizures (adults)	↓ serum levels with carbamazepine or phenytoin ↑ serum digoxin concentration
Felbamate (Felbatol)	PO	Partial and secondary seizures	Use limited to clients with poor control on other antiseizure medications
Gabapentin (Neurontin)	PO	Adjunctive therapy for partial seizures	↓ serum levels when administered with antacids
Lamotrigine (Lamictal)	PO	Partial seizures and adjunctive antiseizure therapy	↓ serum levels with acetaminophen, carbamazepine, phenobarbital, phenytoin, primidone, and hormonal contraceptives ↑ serum levels with folate Oil of primrose may lower seizure threshold
Levetiracetam (Keppra)	PO	Complex partial seizures	↓ sedation when combined with antihistamines, benzodiazepines, opioids, tricyclic antidepressants Do not administer with carbamazepine, clozapine, and drugs that cause leucopenia or neutropenia
Magnesium sulfate	IM, IV infusion	Seizures related to toxemia	Neuromuscular relaxants such as tubocurarine, atracurium, pancuronium, and vecuronium
Pregbalin (Lyrica)	PO	Adjunct therapy partial onset seizures in adults	↑ CNS depression when given with other CNS depressants Fewer drug–drug interactions than many antiepileptic drugs
Tiagabine hydrochloride (Gabitril)	PO	Adjunctive therapy for partial seizures	↑ serum levels with carbamazepine, phenytoin, and primidone Possible interaction with valproate CNS depressants can ↑ sedation
Topiramate (Topamax)	PO	Partial seizures, generalized tonic–clonic seizures	↑ serum levels when given with drugs that inhibit cytochrome such as fluoxetine
Valproate (Valproic acid, divalproex) Sodium (Depakene, Depakote)	PO	Grand mal seizures, petit mal seizures, psychomotor seizures, myoclonic seizures	↑ sedation with CNS depressants ↑ serum levels with salicylates, cimetidine, chlorpromazine, erythromycin, felbamate ↑ effects (more rapid drug metabolism) with carbamazepine, phenobarbital and phenytoin
Zonisamide (Zonegran)	PO	Adjunctive therapy for partial seizures	Should not be administered with sulfonamides Rapid elimination of zonisamide with carbamazepine, phenytoin, phenobarbital, primidone

8. Side effects
    a. Drowsiness, dizziness, insomnia, **paresthesias** (abnormal sensations), depression, suicidal tendencies, aggression, headache, confusion, slurred speech
    b. Hypotension
    c. **Nystagmus** (involuntary oscillation of eye), **diplopia** (double vision), blurred vision
    d. Constipation, N/V, anorexia, weight loss, hepatitis, jaundice, **gingival hyperplasia** (increased growth of gum tissue)
    e. Urine discoloration
    f. Rash, lupus erythematosus, hirsutism
    g. Hypocalcemia

9. Adverse effects/toxicity
    a. Ventricular fibrillation
    b. Hepatitis or nephritis
    c. Agranulocytosis, leukopenia, aplastic anemia, thrombocytopenia, megaloblastic anemia
    d. Lupus erythematosus, **Stevens–Johnson syndrome** (an acute inflammatory disorder of the skin)
    e. Toxicity: bone marrow suppression, N/V, ataxia, diplopia, cardiovascular collapse, slurred speech, confusion

10. Nursing considerations
    a. Assess for seizure activity including type, location, duration, and character; provide seizure precautions
    b. Rapid administration of phenytoin can cause cardiac arrest; be sure to use infusion pump
    c. Assess for mental status, mood, sensorium, affect, and memory (short and long term)
    d. Assess for respiratory depression, rate, depth, and character of respirations
    e. Assess for blood dyscrasias, fever, sore throat, bruising, rash, and jaundice
    f. Evaluate client for therapeutic responses such as decreases in severity of seizures and decreased ventricular dysrhythmias
    g. Administer dose with food to reduce risk of GI upset

11. Client education
    a. Medication regimen including name, dose, schedule, side effects, and possible adverse effects
    b. Urine may turn pink
    c. Do not discontinue medication abruptly or without consulting prescriber; emphasize that abrupt discontinuation may precipitate seizures
    d. Brush teeth with soft toothbrush and do proper flossing to prevent gingival hyperplasia; more frequent visits to dentist may be needed
    e. Carry MedicAlert identification stating medication use
    f. Avoid heavy use of alcohol as it may decrease effectiveness of medication
    g. Do not change brands of medication once seizure activity has stabilized; bio-availability differs among formulations
    h. Hydantoins decrease effectiveness of oral contraceptives; phenytoin has terato-genic effects

B. Barbiturates

1. Action and use
    a. Decrease impulse transmission to cerebral cortex
    b. Are used in all forms of **epilepsy**, a chronic disorder characterized by recurring seizures
2. Common medications (Table 10-4)
3. Administration considerations
    a. Administer IM injection into large muscle mass to prevent tissue sloughing
    b. Use less than 5 mL/site
    c. When ordered IV, give slowly (after dilution) at a rate of 65 mg or less per minute
    d. Give oral dose on empty stomach to increase absorption
4. Contraindications: hypersensitivity, pregnancy, porphyria, and liver disease
5. Significant drug interactions: see Table 10-4
6. Significant food interactions: none reported
7. Significant laboratory studies
    a. Increases serum phosphatase
    b. Affects bromsulphalein retention test which enhances hepatic uptake and excretion of dye

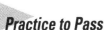

Practice to Pass

Your client is receiving continuous gastric feeding and receiving phenytoin (Dilantin) IV for seizures. The physician decides to change the phenytoin to oral suspension to be administered via the feeding tube. What precautions must you take to ensure that the client's level of antiepileptic does not diminish due to the change in administration method?

8. Side effects
   a. Paradoxical excitement (older adults), drowsiness, lethargy, hangover headache, flushing, hallucinations
   b. Possible confusion, depression, or irritability in children or older adults with high doses
   c. N/V, diarrhea, constipation
   d. Rash, urticaria, local pain, swelling, necrosis
9. Adverse effects/toxicity
   a. Coma
   b. Stevens–Johnson syndrome, angioedema, thrombophlebitis
10. Nursing considerations
   a. Assess for mental status changes such as mood, sensorium, affect, and memory (long and short term)
   b. Assess for respiratory status or depression including rate, rhythm, and depth
   c. Assess for blood dyscrasias, fever, sore throat, bruising, rash, and jaundice
   d. Assess for seizure activity including type, duration, and precipitating factors
   e. Blood studies and liver function tests are done routinely during long-term treatment
   f. Evaluate client for therapeutic responses such as decreased seizures or increased sedation
11. Client education
   a. Medication regimen including name, dose, schedule, side effects, and possible adverse effects
   b. Avoid other CNS depressants including alcohol
   c. Do not discontinue medication abruptly or without consulting prescriber
   d. Avoid hazardous activities until stabilized on drug; drowsiness may occur
   e. Carry MedicAlert bracelet stating medication use
   f. Therapeutic effects may not be seen for 2 to 3 weeks

C. Succinimides

1. Action and use
   a. Suppress calcium influx into neurons, increasing electrical threshold and decreasing ability to generate an action potential
   b. Inhibit spike, wave formation in absence seizures (petit mal), decrease amplitude, frequency, duration, and spread of discharges in minor motor seizures
   c. Used in absence seizures, partial seizures, and tonic–clonic seizures
2. Common medications (Table 10-4)
3. Administration considerations: give with food or milk to decrease GI symptoms
4. Contraindications: hypersensitivity
5. Significant drug interactions: see Table 10-4
6. Significant food interactions: none reported
7. Significant laboratory studies: increased liver function tests and false-positive direct Coomb's test
8. Side effects
   a. Drowsiness, dizziness, fatigue, euphoria, lethargy
   b. Anorexia, N/V, heartburn
   c. Pink urine
   d. Urticaria, pruritic erythema
   e. Myopia, blurred vision
9. Adverse effects/toxicity
   a. Agranulocytosis, aplastic anemia, thrombocytopenia, leukocytosis, eosinophilia, pancytopenia
   b. Stevens–Johnson syndrome
   c. Toxicity: bone marrow depression, N/V, ataxia, diplopia, and cardiovascular collapse

10. Nursing considerations

    a. Assess for mental status changes including mood, sensorium, affect, and behavioral changes
    b. Monitor renal studies including urinalysis, BUN, and creatinine
    c. Monitor blood studies including CBC, Hct, Hgb, reticulocyte counts every week for 4 weeks
    d. Monitor hepatic studies including AST, ALT, and bilirubin
    e. Assess for eye problems; may need regular ophthalmic exams
    f. Assess for allergic reactions such as red, raised rash or exfoliative dermatitis
    g. Assess for blood dyscrasias, fever, sore throat, bruising, rash, or jaundice
    h. Monitor weight weekly; report any signs of anorexia or weight loss

11. Client education

    a. Carry ID card or MedicAlert bracelet with medication, client's name, prescriber's name, and phone number
    b. Avoid driving and other activities that require alertness
    c. Avoid alcohol ingestion and other CNS depressants as they may increase sedation
    d. Do not discontinue medication abruptly or without consulting prescriber
    e. Continue regular dental checkups to identify gingival hyperplasia
    f. Emphasize importance of contraception, as drug therapy is a risk to fetus

D. Benzodiazepines

1. Action and use

    a. Enhance inhibitory neurotransmitter **gamma-aminobutyric acid (GABA)** to decrease anxiety and as an adjunct for seizure activity
    b. Relief of delirium tremens

2. Common medications (Table 10-4)

3. Administration considerations

    a. Give with food or milk to reduce GI symptoms
    b. IV injection should be given into large vein
    c. Administer IV medication at a rate of 5 mg or less per minute

4. Contraindications

    a. Hypersensitivity
    b. Contraindicated in acute narrow-angle glaucoma or psychosis
    c. Contraindicated in children younger than 6 months
    d. Do not give to clients with liver disease (clonazepam), or during lactation (diazepam)

5. Significant drug interactions: see Table 10-4

6. Significant food interactions: none reported

7. Significant laboratory studies: increases AST and ALT, serum bilirubin levels, and 17-OHCS and decreases radioactive iodine uptake

8. Side effects

    a. Dizziness, drowsiness, confusion, headache, fatigue
    b. Orthostatic hypotension
    c. Blurred vision
    d. Constipation, dry mouth
    e. Rash, itching

9. Adverse effects/toxicity

    a. Neutropenia
    b. Respiratory depression
    c. ECG changes, tachycardia

10. Nursing considerations

    a. Assess BP (lying, standing), pulse; if systolic BP drops 20 mmHg, withhold drug, notify prescriber because of orthostatic hypotension

      b. Assess hepatic and renal function, high density lipoprotein, alkaline phosphatase

      c. Assess for mental status changes including mood, sensorium, affect, memory (long and short term)

      d. Assess respiratory status for depression including rate, rhythm, and depth

      e. Assess seizure activity including type, duration, and precipitating factors

      f. Evaluate client for therapeutic responses such as reduced or absent seizure activity, anxiety

11. Client education

      a. Medication regimen including name, dose, schedule, side effects, and possible adverse effects

      b. Avoid other CNS depressants, including alcohol

      c. Do not discontinue medication abruptly or without consulting prescriber

      d. Avoid hazardous activities until stabilized on drug; drowsiness may occur

      e. Use barrier contraceptives while taking benzodiazepines

E. Other antiepileptics

1. Carbamazepine (Tegretol)

      a. Action and use

            1) Inhibits nerve impulses by limiting influx of sodium ions across cell membrane in motor cortex

            2) Used in tonic–clonic, complex-partial, and mixed seizures

      b. Given by oral or enteral (GI tube) route

      c. Administration considerations

            1) Give oral forms with food or milk to reduce GI symptoms

            2) Chewable pills must be chewed or crushed, should not be swallowed whole

            3) Prolonged administration produces physical dependence; withdrawal symptoms will occur if stopped suddenly

      d. Contraindications

            1) Hypersensitivity to carbamazepine or tricyclic antidepressants

            2) Contraindicated with bone marrow depression and concomitant use of MAOIs

      e. Significant drug interactions: see Table 10-4

      f. Significant food interactions: increased peak concentrations of carbamazepine with grapefruit

      g. Significant laboratory studies: increases false negatives for pregnancy tests

      h. Side effects

            1) Increased PT

            2) Syndrome of inappropriate antidiuretic hormone (SIADH), mostly with older adults

            3) Drowsiness, dizziness, confusion

            4) Constipation, diarrhea, N/V

            5) Rash, urticaria

            6) Tinnitus, dry mouth, blurred vision, nystagmus

            7) Hypotension

            8) Fever, dyspnea, pneumonitis

            9) Urinary frequency or retention, increased BUN

      i. Adverse effects/toxicity

            1) Thrombocytopenia, agranulocytosis, leukocytosis, neutropenia, aplastic anemia, eosinophilia

            2) Paralysis, worsening of seizures

            3) Hepatitis

            4) Stevens–Johnson syndrome

            5) Hypertension, CHF, dysrhythmias, AV block

            6) CNS toxicity with lithium

            7) Fatal reaction with MAOIs

j. Nursing considerations

    1) Assess for seizure activity including type, duration, and precipitating factors

    2) Monitor blood, hepatic, and renal studies including red blood cell (RBC) count, Hct, Hgb, reticulocyte count, AST, ALT, bilirubin, urinalysis, BUN, creatinine

    3) Assess mental status including mood, sensorium, affect, and memory (long and short term)

    4) Assess for eye problems; may need regular ophthalmic exams

    5) Assess for allergic reactions including purpura or red, raised rash

    6) Assess for blood dyscrasias, fever, sore throat, bruising, rash, or jaundice

    7) Evaluate client for therapeutic response such as decreased or absent seizure activity

k. Client education

    1) Medication regimen including name, dose, schedule, side effects, and possible adverse effects

    2) Avoid other CNS depressants including alcohol

    3) Do not discontinue medication abruptly or without consulting prescriber

    4) Avoid hazardous activities until stabilized on drug; drowsiness may occur

    5) Carry MedicAlert ID with name, drug, prescriber's name, phone number

    6) Urine may turn pink to brown

2. Valproates

  a. Action and use

    1) Increases levels of GABA in brain, which decreases seizure activity

    2) Use in simple (petit mal), complex (petit mal) absence, or mixed seizures; manic episodes associate with bipolar disorder and migraine headaches

  b. Given by oral or enteral (GI tube) route

  c. Administration considerations

    1) Do not crush tablets or capsules; take them whole

    2) Elixir forms should be given alone; do not dilute with carbonated beverage

    3) May give with food or milk to decrease GI symptoms

  d. Contraindications

    1) Hypersensitivity

    2) Contraindicated during pregnancy and with hepatic disease

  e. Significant drug interactions: see Table 10-4

  f. Significant food interactions: none reported

  g. Significant laboratory studies

    1) Increase the risk of false positive for ketones

    2) Interfere with thyroid function tests

  h. Side effects

    1) Sedation, drowsiness

    2) Constipation, diarrhea, heartburn, N/V

    3) Rash

  i. Adverse effects/toxicity

    1) Thrombocytopenia, leukopenia, lymphocytosis

    2) Hepatic failure, pancreatitis, toxic hepatitis

    3) Rare but fatal adverse effects include elevated ammonia levels with encephalopathy and liver toxicity

  j. Nursing considerations

    1) Assess for seizure activity including type, duration, and precipitating factors

    2) Monitor blood, hepatic and renal studies including RBCs, Hct, Hgb, serum folate, PT, platelets, vitamin D, reticulocyte count, AST, ALT, bilirubin, urine analysis, BUN, creatinine

    3) Assess mental status such as mood, sensorium, affect, and memory (long and short term)

          4) Assess respiratory status/depression including rate, rhythm, and depth

          5) Evaluate for therapeutic response, such as decreased seizure activity

      k. Client education

          1) Medication regimen including name, dose, schedule, side effects, and possible adverse effects

          2) Avoid other CNS depressants including alcohol

          3) Do not discontinue medication abruptly or without consulting prescriber

          4) Avoid hazardous activities until stabilized on drug; drowsiness may occur

          5) Carry MedicAlert ID with name, drug, prescriber's name, and phone number

          6) Physical dependency may result from extended use

          7) Report visual disturbances, rash, diarrhea, light-colored stools, jaundice, or protracted vomiting to provider

III. CENTRAL NERVOUS SYSTEM (CNS) STIMULANTS

    A. Anorexiants

      1. Action and use

        a. Act similar to amphetamines, as indirect sympathomimetic amines with alpha- and beta-adrenergic activity

        b. May have moderate appetite suppressant properties but have short-lived effects and have increased potential for tolerance

      2. Common medication (Table 10-5)

Table 10-5 **Central Nervous System (Adrenergic) Stimulants**

Generic (Trade) Name	Route	Significant Drug Interactions
Anorexiants		
Diethylpropion (Proprion)	PO	↑ BP effects: furazolidone ↑ effects of alcohol, other CNS depressants
Amphetamines		
Amphetamine sulfate (Adderall)	PO	↓ elimination of amphetamine: acetazolamide, sodium bicarbonate ($NaHCO_3$) ↑ elimination of amphetamine: ammonium chloride, ascorbic acid ↓ effects of guanethidine, guanadrel Hypertensive crisis and intracranial hemorrhage may occur if given within 14 days of MAOIs or selegiline ↓ effectiveness of amphetamine: tricyclic antidepressants ↑ BP effects: furazolidone ↑ effects of alcohol, other CNS depressants
Methylphenidate hydrochloride (Ritalin)	PO	Hypertensive crisis: MAOIs within 14 days, or vasopressor ↑ sympathomimetic effect: decongestants, vasoconstrictors ↓ effects of warfarin, tricyclics, antiepileptics
Dextroamphetamine sulfate (Dexadrine)	PO	Hypertensive crisis: MAOIs within 14 days Delayed absorption: barbiturates, phenytoin ↑ effect of dextroamphetamine: acetazolamide, antacids, $NaHCO_3$ ↑ CNS effect: haloperidol, tricyclics, phenothiazines ↓ effect of dextroamphetamine: ascorbic acid, ammonium chloride ↓ effect of adrenergic blockers, antidiabetics
Pemoline (Cylert)	PO	↑ CNS effect: other CNS stimulants
Selective Norepinephrine Reuptake Inhibitor		
Atomoxetine (Strattera)	PO	↑ serum levels when combined with CYP2D6 inhibitors (paroxetine, fluoxetine, quinidine) Withhold MAOIs for 2 weeks before starting atomoxetine

3. Administration considerations
   a. Anorexiant effects of diethylpropion are temporary
   b. Do not abruptly discontinue medication
   c. Should be given on empty stomach; additional dose may be given mid-evening to control nighttime hunger
4. Contraindications
   a. Hypersensitivity
   b. Contraindicated with angle-closure glaucoma, advanced cardiac disease, hyperthyroidism, agitated states, history of drug abuse, and children under 12 years of age
5. Significant drug interactions: see Table 10-5
6. Significant food interactions: none reported
7. Significant laboratory studies: none reported
8. Side effects
   a. Restlessness, insomnia
   b. Palpitations
   c. Dysmenorrhea
9. Adverse effects/toxicity
   a. Decrease in seizure threshold in epilepsy
   b. Tachycardia
10. Nursing considerations
    a. Assess BP and pulse during treatment
    b. Evaluate client for therapeutic response such as decrease in weight over time
    c. Implement psychosocial interventions
11. Client education
    a. Discuss all medications currently taken (including OTC) with provider
    b. Take medications exactly as prescribed; do not use during pregnancy-alert prescriber
    c. Avoid driving or other hazardous activities until reaction to medication is determined
    d. Report palpitations, weight loss, dry mouth, and difficulty swallowing

B. Amphetamines
1. Action and use
   a. Increase release of norepinephrine and dopamine in cerebral cortex to **reticular activating system**, a diffuse system that extends from lower brain stem to cerebral cortex
   b. Used in treating narcolepsy, **attention deficit/hyperactivity disorder (ADHD)**
2. Common medications (Table 10-5)
3. Administration considerations
   a. Give first dose on awakening and give last dose not closer than 6 hours to bedtime
   b. Administer on empty stomach 30 to 60 minutes prior to meal
4. Contraindications
   a. Hypersensitivity
   b. Contraindicated with hyperthyroidism, hypertension, glaucoma, severe arteriosclerosis, drug abuse, cardiovascular disease, anxiety, or lactation
5. Significant drug interactions: see Table 10-5
6. Significant food interactions: none reported
7. Significant laboratory studies: serum thyroxine (T_4) with high amphetamine doses
8. Side effects
   a. Hyperactivity, insomnia, restlessness, talkativeness
   b. Dry mouth, N/V
   c. Impotence, change in libido
   d. Palpitations, tachycardia

Practice to Pass

A female client has started taking an anorexiant as prescribed by her physician for weight reduction. If she has multiple medical diagnoses, what types of medications might need to be adjusted because of the addition of the anorexiant?

9. Adverse effects/toxicity: same as previously described
10. Nursing considerations
    a. Assess vital signs, especially BP, since may reverse antihypertensive medication action
    b. Monitor CBC, urinalysis, and in diabetics, monitor blood glucose levels; changes in insulin may be required
    c. Assess mental status for mood, sensorium, and affect; stimulation, insomnia, or aggressiveness may occur
    d. Assess for withdrawal symptoms including headache, N/V, muscle pain, weakness
    e. Evaluate client for therapeutic responses such as decreased activity in ADHD or absence of sleeping during day in **narcolepsy**
11. Client education
    a. Medication regimen including name, dose, schedule, side effects, and possible adverse drug effects; if a dose is missed, do not double dose
    b. Avoid or decrease caffeine consumption (coffee, tea, cola, chocolate), which may increase irritability or stimulation
    c. Avoid OTC preparations unless approved by prescriber and avoid alcohol consumption
    d. Do not discontinue medication abruptly or without consulting prescriber
    e. Importance of rest
    f. Seizure threshold is decreased in clients with seizure disorders

C. **Nonstimulant medication to treat ADHD**
1. Action and use: selective norepinephrine reuptake inhibitor (SNRI) increases concentration of norepinephrine in prefrontal cortex
2. Common medication: atomoxetine (Strattera)
3. Administration considerations: daily dose is usually weight-based in children and adolescents
4. Contraindications
    a. Hypersensitivity
    b. Concurrent use of MAOIs or MAOI use within last 2 weeks
    c. Serious cardiac or liver disease
    d. Major depressive disorder or presence of suicidal ideation
    e. Efficacy in children under 6 years of age or in older adults is not established
5. Significant drug interactions: see Table 10-5
6. Significant food interactions: increased stimulation and amine effect with caffeine
7. Significant laboratory studies: none reported
8. Side effects
    a. Hyperactivity, insomnia, restlessness, and talkativeness
    b. Dry mouth
    c. Palpitations and tachycardia
    d. Rash
    e. Nausea, vomiting, decreased appetite and weight loss
    f. Sexual dysfunction
9. Adverse effects/toxicity
    a. Suicidal ideation
    b. Dysrhythmias and palpitations
    c. Severe liver injury
10. Nursing considerations
    a. Assess vital signs, especially BP, since increased BP may occur
    b. Assess for mental status changes including mood, sensorium, and affect; stimulation, insomnia, and aggressiveness may occur
    c. Assess client for changes in appetite, sleep, speech patterns

d. Assess client for suicidal ideation

    e. Evaluate client for therapeutic responses such as decreased activity in ADHD

11. Client education

    a. Medication regimen including name, dose, schedule, side effects, and possible adverse effects

    b. Avoid or decrease caffeine consumption (coffee, tea, cola, chocolate), which may increase irritability or stimulation

    c. Avoid OTC preparations unless approved by prescriber and avoid alcohol consumption

    d. Do not discontinue medication abruptly or without consulting prescriber

IV. MEDICATIONS TO TREAT PARKINSON'S DISEASE

A. Anticholinergics

1. Action and use

    a. Block or compete at central acetylcholine receptor sites in autonomic nervous system

    b. Used to decrease involuntary movements and rigidity in parkinsonism

2. Common medications (Table 10-6)

3. Administration considerations

    a. Parenteral dose of trihexyphenidyl is given with client in recumbent position to prevent postural hypotension

    b. Oral form of trihexyphenidyl is given with or after food to prevent GI upset; may give with fluids other than water

    c. Parenteral dose of benztropine is given slowly; keep client under observation at least 1 hour after administering dose and monitor vital signs

    d. Monitor dosage of medication very carefully; even slight overdose can lead to toxicity

4. Contraindications: clients with narrow-angle glaucoma, myasthenia gravis, or GI obstruction should not use

5. Significant drug interactions: see Table 10-6

6. Significant food interactions: none reported

7. Significant laboratory studies: none reported

8. Side effects

    a. Dry mouth, constipation

    b. Urinary retention or hesitancy

    c. Headache or dizziness

9. Adverse effects/toxicity: paralytic ileus

10. Nursing considerations

    a. Monitor I & O; retention may cause decreased urinary output

    b. Assess client for urinary hesitancy and retention; palpate bladder if retention occurs

    c. Assess client for constipation; increase fluids, bulk, and exercise to counteract constipation; assess bowel sounds to rule out paralytic ileus

    d. Assess mental status for affect, mood, CNS depression, worsening of mental symptoms during early therapy

    e. If tolerance occurs during long-term therapy, dose may need to be increased or changed

    f. Protect client from heat

    g. Evaluate for therapeutic responses such as decreased tremors, secretions, absence of N/V

Table 10-6	Medications Used to Treat Parkinson's Disease			

Generic (Trade) Name	Route	Uses	Drug-to-Drug Interactions
Dopaminergic			
Carbidopa-levodopa (Sinemet, Sinemet CR) Levodopa (Dopar, Larodopa)	PO	Parkinson's disease	Antacids may ↑ absorption of levodopa components Antihypertensives may have ↑ hypotensive effects Iron salts ↓ bioavailability MAOIs ↑ risk of severe hypertension Papaverine, phenytoin, phenothiazines and antipsychotics may ↓ antiparkinsonism effects Kava may ↓ dopamine action
Selegiline (Eldepryl)	PO	Parkinson's disease	Adrenergics ↑ pressor response Use cautiously with citalopram, fluoxetine, fluvoxamine, nefazodone, paroxetine, sertraline, venlafaxine Do not administer selegiline for at least 2 weeks after stopping MAOIs Meperidine may cause stupor and rigidity Cacao tree may have vasopressor effects Ginseng may ↑ adverse reactions
Rasagiline (Azilect)	PO	Parkinson's disease	Use with dextromethorphan can cause episodes of psychosis Potentiates levodopa ↑ plasma levels of opioids including meperidine and methadone
Dopamine Agonists			
Apomorphine (Apokyn)	PO	Parkinson's disease	May ↑ CNS depression with other CNS depressants; hypotension and unconsciousness with granisetron and similar drugs; multiple other drug interactions
Bromocriptine (Parlodel)	PO	Parkinson's disease, acromegaly, hyperprolactinemia	Antihypertensives will ↓ BP significantly Ergot alkaloids, estrogens, hormonal contraceptives interfere with bromocriptine Erythomycin ↑ bromocriptine Haloperidol, loxapine, MAOIs, methyldopa, metoclopramide, phenothiazines, reserpine interfere with bromocriptine Levodopa produces additive effects
Pramipexole (Mirapex)	PO	Parkinson's disease	Butyrophenones, metoclopramide, phenothiazines, thiothixenes ↓ pramipexole levels Cimetidine, diltiazem, quinidine, quinine, ranitidine, triamterene, and verapamil ↓ pramipexole clearance Levodopa ↑ adverse effects Black horehound produces ↑ dopaminergic effect
Ropinirole hydrochloride (Requip)	PO	Parkinson's disease	CNS depressants ↑ CNS effects Dopamine antagonists ↓ ropinirole effects Estrogens ↓ ropinirole clearance Erythromycin, fluvoxamine, diltiazem, tacrine ↓ ropinirole clearance
Anticholinergic Agents			
Atropine sulfate	PO, IM, IV	Hypersalivation and irregular movements related to Parkinson's disease	↑ anticholinergic effect with phenothiazines, antidepressants, MAOIs, amantadine ↑ effects of atenolol
Benztropine mesylate (Cogentin)	PO		Amantadine, phenothiazines, tricyclic anti-depressants ↑ anticholinergic effects, intolerance to heat and hyperthermia Cholinesterase inhibitors ↓ efficacy of cholinesterase inhibitors
Diphenhydramine (Benadryl)	PO, IM, IV		CNS medications will ↑ sedation MAOIs ↑ anticholinergic effects

Table 10-6 Medications Used to Treat Parkinson's Disease (Continued)

Generic (Trade) Name	Route	Uses	Drug-to-Drug Interactions
Glycopyrrolate (Robinul)	PO	Hypersalivation and irregular movements related to Parkinson's disease, peptic ulcer disease, and irritable bowel syndrome	↓ effect with antipsychotic agents ↑ anticholinergic effect with tricyclic antidepressants and amantadine ↑ effect of atenolol and digoxin
Hyoscyamine sulfate (Cystospaz, others)	PO, SL		↑ effect with other anticholinergic agents, amantadine, haloperidol, phenothiazines, MAOIs, tricyclic antidepressants, and antihistamines ↓ absorption when given with antacids
Propantheline bromide (generic)	PO		↓ effectiveness with antipsychotic medications, particularly haloperidol ↓ effectiveness with phenothiazines
Scopolamine hydrobromide	PO, subQ, IM, IV		↓ effectiveness with antipsychotic medications, particularly haloperidol ↓ effectiveness with phenothiazines
Trihexyphenidyl (generic)	PO		↓ therapeutic effects of chlorpromazine, haloperidol, phenothiazines MAOIs potentiate drug effects ↑ bioavailability of digoxin
Antiviral			
Amantadine hydrochloride (Symmetrel)	PO	Parkinson's disease and drug-induced extrapyramidal reactions	↑ atropine-like side effects when administered with anticholinergic agents ↑ effects of amantadine when administered with hydrochlorothiazide and triamterene

11. Client education
    a. Void before taking dose of anticholinergic to reduce urinary retention
    b. Avoid driving or other hazardous activities; drowsiness may occur
    c. Avoid OTC medications such as cough and cold preparations with alcohol, and antihistamines unless prescribed by provider; separate antacid use from anticholinergics by 2–4 hours

B. **Medications affecting dopamine level in brain**
    1. Action and use
        a. These medications include amantadine, levodopa, dopamine agonists and MAO type B inhibitors
        b. Amantadine (an antiviral) promotes synthesis and release of dopamine
        c. L-dopa is the immediate natural precursor of dopamine
        d. Dopamine agonists (DA) directly stimulate specific subclasses of dopamine receptors
        e. MAO type B inhibitors (MAOBI) increase dopamine activity by an incompletely understood mechanism
        f. DAs and MAOBIs are used to enhance effects of L-dopa
        g. All are used to increase available dopamine; parkinsonism symptoms are decreased by having more dopamine available to body
    2. Common medications (Table 10-6)
    3. Administration considerations
        a. Administer medication after meals for better absorption and to decrease GI symptoms
        b. Absorption of levodopa and selegiline is decreased with high-protein meals; administer after a low-protein food or snack

Practice to Pass

A client with Parkinson's disease is admitted to the nursing unit after a surgical procedure. What type of medication would you be careful not to administer because he or she takes selegiline, an MAOBI?

4. Contraindications
   a. Hypersensitivity
   b. Narrow-angle glaucoma
   c. Undiagnosed skin lesions
5. Significant drug interactions: see Table 10-6
6. Significant food interactions
   a. Decreased levodopa and selegiline absorption with high-protein foods
   b. With selegiline and rasagiline, tyramine-containing foods may increase hypertensive reactions
7. Significant laboratory studies
   a. Bromocriptine: increases growth hormone, AST, ALT, potassium, BUN, uric acid, alkaline phosphatase
   b. Selegiline results in false positive of urine ketones and glucose; also results in false negative of urine glucose
8. Side effects
   a. N/V, dry mouth, and constipation
   b. Dizziness, headache, and depression
   c. Cough
   d. Cardiac dysrhythmias and orthostatic hypotension
   e. Sleep disturbance, "on–off" phenomenon
9. Adverse effects/toxicity
   a. Amantadine: seizures, CHF, leukopenia
   b. Levodopa: hemolytic anemia, leukopenia, agranulocytosis
   c. DAs: seizures, shock
   d. MAOBIs: tachycardia or sinus bradycardia
   e. Levodopa toxicity: disturbed sleep patterns, hallucinations, personality changes, increased twitching, grimacing, tongue protrusion
10. Nursing considerations
   a. Assess BP and respirations
   b. Assess mental status for affect, mood, behavioral changes, and depression; complete a suicide assessment
   c. Monitor for involuntary movement, akinesia, tremors, staggering gait, muscle rigidity, and drooling
   d. Evaluate for therapeutic responses such as a decrease in akathisia and increased mood
11. Client education
   a. Change positions slowly to prevent orthostatic hypotension
   b. Report side effects such as twitching and eye spasm; may indicate overdose
   c. Use drugs exactly as prescribed; never discontinue them abruptly since this may precipitate parkinsonian crisis
   d. Avoid alcohol use
   e. Do not take foods high in protein with dose
   f. Quit smoking if taking ropinirole because drug clearance is increased (less effectiveness)

V. MEDICATIONS TO TREAT ALZHEIMER'S DISEASE

A. Action and use
   1. Cholinesterase inhibitors elevate acetylcholine concentrations in cerebral cortex
   2. They accomplish this by slowing degradation of acetylcholine released in cholinergic neurons
B. Common medications (Table 10-7)

Table 10-7	Medications Used to Treat Alzheimer's Disease			
Generic (Trade) Name	**Route**	**Uses**	**Drug-to-Drug Interactions**	
Donepezil (Aricept)	PO	Mild to moderate Alzheimer's disease	↓ effects of anticholinergic drugs Bethanechol, succinylcholine produces additive effects Carbamazepine, dexamethasone, phenytoin, Phenobarbital, and rifampin ↑ elimination of donepezil Cholinomimetics, cholinesterase inhibitors produce a synergistic effect Jaborandi tree and pill-bearing spurge may cause toxic effects of donepezil	
Ergoloid mesylate (Hydergine)	PO	Senile dementia of Alzheimer's disease	No clinical significant interactions noted	
Rivastigmine tartrate (Exelon)	PO	Mild to moderate Alzheimer's disease	↓ effects of anticholinergic drugs Bethanechol, succinylcholine, and neuromuscular blockers have synergistic effects Smoking ↑ rivastigmine clearance	
Tacrine (Cognex)	PO	Improves memory loss related to Alzheimer's disease	Decreased activity of anticholinergics ↑ tacrine levels with cimetidine ↑ elimination half-life with theophylline Synergistic effects with succinylcholine, cholinesterase inhibitors, cholinergic agonists	
Memantine hydrochloride (Namenda)	PO	Mild to severe Alzheimer's disease	Cimetidine, hydrochlorothiazide, quinidine, ranitidine, triamterene alter drug levels Amantadine, dextromethorphan, ketamine, can interact and should be used cautiously ↑ effect and possible toxicity of memantine if administered with drugs that alkalinize urine (i.e., carbonic anhydrase inhibitors and sodium bicarbonate)	
Galantamine hydrobromide (Razadyne)	PO	Mild to moderate dementia of Alzheimer's disease	Cimetidine, ketoconazole, paroxetine, erythromycin, succinylcholine, bethanechol can produce galantamine toxicity	

C. Administration considerations

1. Administer medication between meals; may be given with meal to reduce GI symptoms
2. Use rivastigmine cautiously with NSAIDs because of increased risk for bleeding
3. Dosage adjusted to response no more frequently than every 6 weeks

D. Contraindications

1. Hypersensitivity to drug
2. Development of jaundice when taking drug

E. Significant drug interactions: see Table 10-7

F. Significant food interactions: none reported

G. Significant laboratory studies: none reported

H. Side effects

1. Insomnia, headache, dizziness, confusion, ataxia, anxiety, depression, hostility, and abnormal thinking
2. N/V, diarrhea, abdominal pain, and constipation
3. Urinary frequency and incontinence
4. Rash
5. Rhinitis or cough

I. **Adverse effects/toxicity**
1. Seizures
2. Hepatotoxicity
3. Urinary tract infection (UTI)
4. Atrial fibrillation

J. **Nursing considerations**
1. Assess BP for hypotension or hypertension
2. Assess mental status for affect, mood, behavioral changes, depression, hallucinations, and confusion; complete a suicide assessment
3. Assess GI status for N/V, anorexia, constipation, or abdominal pain
4. Assess client for urinary frequency and incontinence
5. Monitor liver function tests frequently
6. Evaluate client for therapeutic responses such as decrease in confusion, improved mood

K. **Client (and/or caregiver) education**
1. Use drug exactly as prescribed, at regular intervals, preferably between meals, may be taken with food to decrease GI upset
2. Report side effects such as twitching, N/V, sweating; they might indicate overdose
3. Notify provider of N/V, diarrhea (dose increase or beginning treatment) or rash
4. Do not increase or abruptly decrease dose; serious consequences may result
5. Drug is not a cure; it only relieves symptoms
6. Stop smoking
7. Use of sodium bicarbonate to treat GI upset can produce toxic levels of memantine
8. Change position slowly to avoid orthostatic hypotension

VI. CENTRALLY ACTING SKELETAL MUSCLE RELAXANTS

A. **Medications for spasticity**
1. Action and use
   a. Decrease synaptic responses at neurotransmitters to decrease frequency, severity of spasms
   b. Used to reduce **spasticity** (increased resistance to passive movement) after spinal cord injuries, stroke, and in cerebral palsy and multiple sclerosis (MS)
2. Common medications (Table 10-8)
3. Administration considerations: see Table 10-8
4. Contraindications
   a. Hypersensitivity to medication
   b. Contraindicated in compromised pulmonary function, active hepatic disease, impaired myocardial function
5. Significant drug interactions: see Table 10-8
6. Significant food interactions: none reported
7. Significant laboratory studies: baclofen increases AST, alkaline phosphatase, and blood glucose levels
8. Side effects: dizziness, weakness, fatigue, drowsiness, disorientation, N/V
9. Adverse effects/toxicity
   a. Seizures
   b. Eosinophilia, hepatic injury
10. Nursing considerations
   a. Monitor BP, weight, blood glucose level, and hepatic function
   b. Assess client for increased seizure activity; drugs decrease seizure threshold
   c. Monitor I & O, check for urinary frequency, retention, or hesitancy
   d. Monitor electroencephalogram (EEG) in epileptic clients due to poor seizure control

Table 10-8 Skeletal Muscle Relaxants

Generic (Trade) Name	Route	Therapeutic Indications	Drug-to-Drug Interactions
Baclofen (Lioresal)	PO	Spasticity in MS and spinal cord injuries	Administration with CNS ↑ depressants ↑ CNS depression MAOIs, tricyclic antidepressants elicit respiratory depression and hypotension
Carisoprodol (Soma)	PO	Relieve pain and discomfort from musculoskeletal disorders	CNS depressants may ↑ CNS depression
Cyclobenzaprine (Flexeril)	PO	Relieve pain and discomfort from musculoskeletal disorders	CNS depressants may ↑ CNS depression Anticholinergic agents ↑ anticholinergic activity MAOIs may exacerbate CNS depression
Dantrolene hydrochloride (Dantrium)	PO	Spasticity of neuromuscular disorders, malignant hyperthermia, metabolic acidosis, hypercarbia	CNS depressants ↑ CNS depression Estrogens ↑ risk of hepatotoxicity Verapamil IV causes cardiovascular collapse when administered to anesthetized clients
Diazepam (Valium)	PO	Relieve pain and discomfort from musculoskeletal disorders Management of anxiety Acute alcohol withdrawal Treatment of tetanus Antiepileptic	↑ CNS depression with alcohol, omeprazole ↑ effect of diazepam if combined with cimetidine, disulfiram, hormonal contraceptives ↓ effectiveness with theophylline and ranitidine
Metaxalone (Skelaxin)	PO	Relieve pain and discomfort from musculoskeletal disorders	Cimetidine, furosemide, cationic drugs such as digoxin, amiloride, vancomycin will ↑ risk of hypoglycemia ↑ risk of lactic acidosis with glucocorticoids and ethanol ↑ risk of hypoglycemia with juniper berries, ginseng, garlic, fenugreek, coriander, dandelion root, celery
Methocarbamol (Robaxin)	PO	Relieve pain and discomfort from musculoskeletal disorders; spasms from black widow spider bite	↑ theophylline clearance ↓ effectiveness in hyperthyroidism ↑ anticoagulant effects Possible toxicity with digitalis glycoside, metoprolol, propranolol
Orphenadrine citrate (Norflex)	PO	Relieve pain and discomfort from musculoskeletal disorders	↑ anticholinergic activity with anticholinergic medications ↑ CNS depression with CNS depressants, particularly phenothiazine Tardive dyskinesia with phenothiazines and haloperidol
Tizanidine (Zanaflex)	PO	Spasticity in clients with MS, spinal cord injury, or brain trauma	↑ depression with alcohol, baclofen, and CNS depressants ↑ effect with hormonal contraceptives Do not use alpha-2 adrenergics

    e. Assess client for allergic reactions, fever, rash, or respiratory distress

    f. Monitor client for severe weakness or numbness in extremities

    g. Monitor client for CNS depression, dizziness, drowsiness, or psychiatric symptoms

    h. Monitor hepatic function (AST, ALT) and renal function (BUN, creatinine, CBC)

    i. Report unusual bleeding

    j. Large doses of relaxants may lead to dependency

    k. Evaluate client for therapeutic responses such as decrease in pain and spasticity

  11. Client education

    a. Do not discontinue medication quickly; hallucinations, spasticity, tachycardia will occur; it should be tapered off gradually by prescriber

     b. Notify prescriber of abdominal pain, jaundiced sclera, clay-colored stools, or change in color of urine (hepatotoxicity)

     c. Do not take alcohol or other CNS depressants

     d. Avoid using OTC medications, cough preparations, or antihistamines, unless recommended by prescriber

     e. Do not break, crush, or chew capsules

B. Medications used for spasms

  1. Action and use

     a. Depress multisynaptic pathways in the spinal cord, causing skeletal muscle relaxation and/or sedation

     b. Used for adjunct relief of **spasms** (involuntary contractions of large muscles) and pain in musculoskeletal conditions

  2. Common medications (Table 10-8)

  3. Administration considerations: see Table 10-8

  4. Contraindications

     a. Hypersensitivity

     b. Contraindicated in children under age of 12, intermittent porphyria, acute recovery phase of MI, heart block, CHF, or thyroid disease

  5. Significant drug interactions: see Table 10-8

  6. Significant food interactions: none reported

  7. Significant laboratory studies: methocarbamol results in false increased levels of VMA, urinary 5-HIAA

  8. Side effects: dizziness, weakness, drowsiness, nausea

  9. Adverse effects/toxicity

     a. Erythema multiforme

     b. Angioedema, anaphylaxis

     c. Dysrhythmias

     d. Seizures

 10. Nursing considerations

     a. Blood studies including CBC, WBC with differentials

     b. During and after injection, assess for CNS effects, rash, conjunctivitis, and nasal congestion

     c. Liver studies including AST, ALT, alkaline phosphatase

     d. EEG in clients with seizures

     e. Assess for allergic reactions including idiosyncratic reaction, anaphylaxis, rash, fever, or respiratory distress

     f. Assess client for severe weakness or numbness in extremities

     g. Assess for CNS depression, dizziness, drowsiness, and psychiatric symptoms

     h. Monitor client for psychological dependency, increased need for drug, and increased pain

     i. Evaluate client for therapeutic responses such as decreased pain, spasm, and spasticity

 11. Client education

     a. Do not discontinue medication abruptly; insomnia, nausea, headache, spasticity, tachycardia will occur

     b. Do not take with alcohol or other CNS depressants

     c. Avoid using OTC medications, cough preparations, antihistamines, unless recommended by provider

     d. Avoid hazardous activities if drowsiness or dizziness occurs

VII. ANTIANXIETY, SEDATIVE, AND HYPNOTICS (REFER TO CHAPTER 11)

Case Study

T. P., a 48-year-old male client, is admitted to the emergency department (ED) after having a seizure while attending church. You are the admitting nurse in the ED. The client has a history of a seizure disorder. He is arousable but lethargic.

1. What questions will you ask the client or the family upon arrival?

2. What initial assessments will you make?

3. What are the priorities of care for the client while he is in the ED?

4. What education points are of highest priority prior to discharge home?

5. Give examples of medications or foods that could interfere with T. P.'s prescribed seizure medications, phenytoin (Dilantin), and phenobarbital (Luminal).

For suggested responses, see page 544.

For suggested responses, see page 544.

POSTTEST

① Because a health care provider prescribed levodopa (Dopar) for a client newly diagnosed with Parkinson's disease, the nurse should place a high priority on teaching the client which information prior to discharge?

1. Side effects include cushingoid symptoms such as moon face and weight gain.
2. Postpone vaccinations during levodopa therapy.
3. Report any ulcerations or sores in the mouth to provider immediately.
4. Avoid taking medication with high-protein foods.

② Which of the following statements made by the client indicates an understanding of client teaching regarding antiepileptic drug therapy?

1. "After taking the medication, I should lie down."
2. "I must be sure to have my cholesterol levels checked regularly."
3. "I need to take this medication regularly to avoid the recurrence of seizures."
4. "I probably will not need this medication very long."

③ The nurse concludes that which statement made by the client with migraine headaches refers to the activity most likely to reduce or eliminate the headaches?

1. "I will be keeping a diary of my headaches so that I can see if there is a pattern."
2. "I will be able to stop my exercise program since it has not helped my headaches."
3. "I will take the pain medication every 4 hours."
4. "Because I have chronic migraine headaches, I have started taking the bus."

④ The provider prescribed methylphenidate (Ritalin) for a client diagnosed with attention deficit/hyperactivity disorder (ADHD). The nurse would question the order if the client has which contraindication?

1. Age less than 12 years
2. History of anemia
3. History of seizures
4. History of Tourette syndrome

5 A health care provider has written a prescription for sibutramine hydrochloride monohydrate (Meridia) for a fashion model who is returning to work after giving birth. The clinic nurse would question the order if the client's current medication list includes which of the following drugs?

1. Naproxen (Naprosyn)
2. Amoxicillin (Amoxil)
3. Captopril (Capoten)
4. Cimetidine (Tagamet)

6 A client has begun taking an anticholinergic medication. The nurse should make it a priority to assess for which unintended manifestations?

1. Tachycardia and hypertension
2. Urinary retention, hesitancy, and constipation
3. Pain resembling the pattern associated with cholecystitis
4. Pain resembling renal colic

7 A client is receiving both selegiline (Eldepryl) and meperidine (Demerol). What instructions should the nurse provide to the unlicensed assistive personnel (UAP)?

1. Set up infection control precautions.
2. Use automatic blood pressure to measure client's blood pressure (BP).
3. Assist client with activities of daily living.
4. Place a "no visitors" sign on the door.

8 The health care provider has prescribed cyclobenzaprine (Flexeril) for a 16-year-old football player who sustained a back injury during the first game of the season. The pediatric office nurse provides which instruction to the client and his parents?

1. Client should avoid prolonged walking while taking the medication.
2. Client should use sunscreen and protective clothing while taking the medication.
3. Client may need to take the drug for the rest of the football season.
4. Client should report edema of the tongue immediately.

9 A 71-year-old nursing home resident has been taking phenytoin (Dilantin) 100 mg PO tid for some time. The nurse carries out which most important health promotion measure as ordered?

1. Administer calcium supplements as well as vitamin D.
2. Wear dark glasses when exposed to the sun.
3. Give medication with food to prevent nausea.
4. Instruct client to massage gums every morning after brushing the teeth.

10 After the health care provider prescribes naproxen (Naprosyn) for a client with rheumatoid arthritis, the nurse explains to the client that maximum relief may take up to how many weeks to occur? Provide a numeric answer.

_____ weeks

➤ *See pages 343–344 for Answers and Rationales.*

ANSWERS & RATIONALES

Pretest

1 **Answer: 1** **Rationale:** Methylphenidate (Ritalin) is a central nervous system stimulant that results in the release of norepinephrine and dopamine, which can lead to hypertension and life-threatening dysrhythmias in the client with chronic heart failure. Methylphenidate can increase the metabolic rate, which could increase the serum glucose level, but this is not significant enough to prohibit its use in a client with diabetes mellitus. The drug can cause anorexia, nausea, and abdominal pain, which could be troublesome for the client with irritable bowel syndrome, but again the risks are not as great as in congestive heart failure (CHF). The drug can result in myelosuppression, so a history of anemia should be monitored, but again this is not as great a risk as CHF. **Cognitive Level:** Analyzing **Client Need:** Pharmacological and Parenteral Therapies **Integrated Process:** Nursing Process: Implementation **Content Area:** Pharmacology **Strategy:** Specific knowledge about how the drug acts is needed to answer the question. Nonetheless, if you know that the drug is a stimulant, you can reason that the drug action may be harmful to a client with heart disease, particularly congestive heart failure (CHF). **Reference:** Wilson, B. A., Shannon, M. T., & Shields, K. M. (2012). *Pearson nurse's drug guide 2012.* Upper Saddle River, NJ: Pearson Education, pp. 976–978.

2 **Answer: 2, 3, 5** **Rationale:** For seizure control, medication must be taken to maintain therapeutic blood levels, even if there is no seizure activity. Seizures affecting adults usually do not resolve spontaneously in the absence of treatment. The most frequent adverse effects of phenytoin (Dilantin) present as central nervous system symptoms. In most states driving is permitted after a client is seizure free for 6 to 12 months. Obtaining a therapeutic blood level between 10 and 20 mcg/mL may take time, particularly initially. **Cognitive Level:** Applying **Client Need:** Pharmacological and Parenteral Therapies **Integrated Process:** Teaching and Learning **Content Area:** Pharmacology **Strategy:** The critical words are *controlled* and *recurrence*. Note that 2 options are essentially providing opposite information, making it more likely that one of them is correct. Use knowledge of the principles of antiepileptic therapy to choose correctly. **Reference:** Aschenbrenner, D., & Venable, S. (2009). *Drug therapy in nursing* (3rd ed.). Philadelphia, PA: Lippincott Williams & Wilkins, pp. 330–342.

3 **Answer: 4** **Rationale:** Cluster headaches are aggravated by light. Darkening the room reduces this noxious environmental stimulus, thereby promoting maximum therapeutic effects. Ergotamine tartrate (Gynergen) should be given orally 1–2 mg followed by 1–2 mg every 30 minutes until the headache abates or until the maximum dose of 6 mg/24 hours. It is unnecessary to drink large amounts of fluids. Tachycardia can be a side effect of this drug, but increased warmth and energy are not associated with this medication. **Cognitive Level:** Applying **Client Need:** Pharmacological and Parenteral Therapies **Integrated Process:** Communication and Documentation **Content Area:** Pharmacology **Strategy:** Associate the disease characteristics with management of cluster headaches and promotion of drug effectiveness. **Reference:** Wilson, B. A., Shannon, M. T., & Shields, K. M. (2012). *Pearson nurse's drug guide 2012.* Upper Saddle River, NJ: Pearson Education, pp. 562–564.

4 **Answer: 2** **Rationale:** Dantrolene (Dantrium) is a central-acting skeletal muscle relaxant known to be effective in managing spasticity after spinal cord injury. Dexamethasone (Decadron), a corticosteroid, decreases inflammation. Spinal cord-related spasms are not caused by inflammation. Donepezil (Aricept), a cholinesterase inhibitor, slows progression of Alzheimer's disease in clients. Dobutamine (Dobutrex), a beta-adrenergic agonist, acts primarily on cardiac tissue. **Cognitive Level:** Analyzing **Client Need:** Pharmacological and Parenteral Therapies **Integrated Process:** Teaching and Learning **Content Area:** Pharmacology **Strategy:** Recall that spasticity is a condition affecting muscles. Associate the drug category (central-acting muscle relaxant) with the client need, which is to inhibit the spasm of muscles. **Reference:** Wilson, B. A., Shannon, M. T., & Shields, K. M. (2012). *Pearson nurse's drug guide 2012.* Upper Saddle River, NJ: Pearson Education, pp. 403–405, 434–437, 485–487, 494–495.

5 **Answer: 1, 2, 5** **Rationale:** The primary purpose of administering opioid analgesics is pain relief. Side effects placing the client at greatest risk are respiratory depression and reduced level of consciousness (LOC). Blood pressure and heart rate could decrease because of diminished sympathetic nervous system stimulation following effective pain relief. Concerns about drug interactions are preadministration concerns also, and should be investigated before the dose is administered. History of drug abuse and past experiences with pain management are preadministration concerns. **Cognitive Level:** Applying **Client Need:** Pharmacological and Parenteral Therapies **Integrated Process:** Nursing Process: Evaluation **Content Area:** Pharmacology **Strategy:** Link the drug category, purpose, action, and primary side effect to nursing practice. **Reference:** Aschenbrenner, D., & Venable, S. (2009). *Drug therapy in nursing* (3rd ed.). Philadelphia, PA: Lippincott Williams & Wilkins, pp. 378–384.

6 **Answer: 2** **Rationale:** A client with liver disease may be at risk for toxicity with acetaminophen, or at increased risk of bleeding if taking aspirin or NSAIDs. Unless temperature elevation is the reason for the prescription, it does not need to be measured. Tachycardia can occur if the drugs are combined with various cold remedies. There is no evidence that changes in cholesterol levels influence administration of these drugs. These drugs may be abruptly withdrawn and do not need to be tapered. **Cognitive Level:** Applying **Client Need:** Pharmacological and Parenteral Therapies **Integrated Process:** Teaching and Learning **Content Area:** Pharmacology **Strategy:** The core issue of the question is the level of risk to a client with liver disease in taking medications. Recall that the liver plays a key role in the biotransformation of many drugs. Use this information and the process of elimination to consider that the client should consult the health care provider before taking these medications. **Reference:** Aschenbrenner, D., & Venable, S. (2009). *Drug therapy in nursing* (3rd ed.). Philadelphia, PA: Lippincott Williams & Wilkins, pp. 377–380.

7 **Answer: 3** **Rationale:** Since the medication was ordered stat, one can conclude the seizure disorder is unstable. The assessments of greatest assistance to the nurse include seizure activity, changes in mental status, and current respiratory status. To prevent toxicity, hydration needs to be attended to later along with the client's emotional needs. Although renal failure can be a side effect of the drug, impaired airway, changes in mental status, and the nature of seizure activity need to be managed first. Although altered electrolyte status and leg edema may need attention if they occur, management of the seizure activity takes priority first. **Cognitive Level:** Applying **Client Need:** Pharmacological and Parenteral Therapies **Integrated Process:** Nursing Process: Planning **Content Area:** Pharmacology **Strategy:** The critical word is *stat*, suggesting that the client's status is unstable. Recognize that phenytoin (Dilantin) is an antiepileptic to choose the option that includes seizure activity. **Reference:** Aschenbrenner, D., & Venable, S. (2009). *Drug therapy in nursing* (3rd ed.). Philadelphia, PA: Lippincott Williams & Wilkins, pp. 330–342.

8 **Answer: 1, 2, 4** **Rationale:** Both propranolol (Inderal), a beta blocker, and monoamine oxidase inhibitors (MAOIs) such as phenelzine have hypotensive effects and should not be administered concurrently. Hyperpyrexia may occur if meperidine (Demerol) and MAOIs are administered concurrently. Because carbamazepine (Tegretol) can significantly compound the depressant and anticholinergic effects of MAOIs, it should *not* be administered within 14 days of taking MAOIs. The outcome of the interactions of the 2 drugs is potentially fatal. Glucagon (GlucaGen) increases glucogenesis, while MAOIs potentiate hypoglycemic activity of oral hypoglycemics, thus offsetting each other's effects. Dicyclomine (Bentyl) is a parasympatholytic resulting in antispasmodic activity, while MAOIs are more likely to compound sympathomimetic activity. **Cognitive Level:** Analyzing **Client Need:** Pharmacological and Parenteral Therapies **Integrated Process:** Teaching and Learning **Content Area:** Pharmacology **Strategy:** Apply knowledge of

the normal effect of monoamine oxidase inhibitors (MAOIs) on neurotransmitters such as norepinephrine, serotonin, and dopamine to the actions of the specific drugs. **Reference:** Wilson, B. A., Shannon, M. T., & Shields, K. M. (2012). *Pearson nurse's drug guide 2012.* Upper Saddle River, NJ: Pearson Education, pp. 457–458, 1192–1195. Aschenbrenner, D., & Venable, S. (2009). *Drug therapy in nursing* (3rd ed.). Philadelphia, PA: Lippincott Williams & Wilkins, pp. 298–299.

9 **Answer: 2** **Rationale:** Amphetamines and anorexiants increase the secretion of norepinephrine, resulting in a decrease in the seizure threshold. Seizures are often associated with the excessive release of acetylcholine. When these drug groups are used concurrently with antiepileptics, the seizure control is more efficient. A reduction in red blood cells may be compounded if given concurrently with nonsteroidal anti-inflammatory drugs (NSAIDs). Since anticholinergics may cause tremors and cerebral dystonia, they would be contraindicated in a client with a seizure disorder. Because of a potential increase in metabolism, administration with other antiepileptics may result in decreased serum levels. **Cognitive Level:** Applying **Client Need:** Pharmacological and Parenteral Therapies **Integrated Process:** Nursing Process: Planning **Content Area:** Pharmacology **Strategy:** The critical word in the question is *potentiate*. This tells you that the correct option is a drug or group of drugs that enhances the antiepileptic effect of carbamazepine (Tegretol). Use specific drug knowledge and the process of elimination to answer the question. **Reference:** Aschenbrenner, D., & Venable, S. (2009). *Drug therapy in nursing* (3rd ed.). Philadelphia, PA: Lippincott Williams & Wilkins, pp. 242, 332–334, 346–347. Wilson, B. A., Shannon, M. T., & Shields, K. M. (2012). *Pearson nurse's drug guide 2012.* Upper Saddle River, NJ: Pearson Education, pp. 234–236, 1043–1044. Adams, M., & Koch, R. (2010). *Pharmacology: Connections to nursing practice.* Upper Saddle River, NJ: Pearson Education, pp. 1090–1091.

10 **Answer: 1, 3, 4** **Rationale:** Dantrolene (Dantrium) is a skeletal muscle relaxant. Hepatotoxicity is an adverse reaction for dantrolene, which may be manifested by abdominal pain and scleral jaundice. Diarrhea is a common side effect, but persistent diarrhea may cause dehydration. Hepatic necrosis may result in changes in the serum glucose levels, but other signs are more indicative of this serious impairment. Painful urination and urinary frequency may occur and should be reported. Changes in hearing or smell are not common side effects of dantrolene. **Cognitive Level:** Applying **Client Need:** Pharmacological and Parenteral Therapies **Integrated Process:** Teaching and Learning **Content Area:** Pharmacology **Strategy:** Apply knowledge of primary side effects of the drug. **Reference:** Wilson, B. A., Shannon, M. T., & Shields, K. M. (2012). *Pearson nurse's drug guide 2012.* Upper Saddle River, NJ: Pearson Education, pp. 403–405.

ANSWERS & RATIONALES

Posttest

1 **Answer: 4** Rationale: High-protein foods significantly decrease absorption of levodopa. For this reason, clients are taught to take it with a low-protein food. Cushingoid symptoms are associated with ingesting cortisone derivatives. There is no need to avoid vaccinations. GI disturbances associated with the drug include anorexia and nausea and vomiting but not mouth ulcerations. **Cognitive Level:** Analyzing **Client Need:** Pharmacological and Parenteral Therapies **Integrated Process:** Teaching and Learning **Content Area:** Pharmacology **Strategy:** Associate levodopa with "leave off the protein." **Reference:** Wilson, B. A., Shannon, M. T., & Shields, K. M. (2012). *Pearson nurse's drug guide 2012.* Upper Saddle River, NJ: Pearson Education, pp. 236–239.

2 **Answer: 3** Rationale: Doses must be taken regularly to maintain therapeutic blood levels, even without seizure activity. The side effects of antiepileptic drugs vary widely. A mild drowsiness can occur with some of them, but it should not be significant enough to require lying down. There is no evidence of an impact on serum cholesterol levels. Most common side effects involve the central nervous system and the hematologic system. Antiepileptic therapy is prescribed for long-term or lifelong use. **Cognitive Level:** Applying **Client Need:** Pharmacological and Parenteral Therapies **Integrated Process:** Nursing Process: Evaluation **Content Area:** Pharmacology **Strategy:** Apply knowledge of the relationships between therapeutic dose levels and seizure activity. **Reference:** Aschenbrenner, D., & Venable, S. (2009). *Drug therapy in nursing* (3rd ed.). Philadelphia, PA: Lippincott Williams & Wilkins, pp. 330–342.

3 **Answer: 1** Rationale: There is evidence that certain lifestyle patterns contribute to development of migraine headaches, which cannot be completely controlled by medications. If the client can identify the triggering factors, the nurse and the client can collaborate and design a plan of care that will reduce or eliminate the headaches. The client should continue to exercise for general health and stress management. The client should take the pain medication when pain is experienced, but frequent ongoing self-administration could result in tolerance. Unless the client is continually impaired, driving is permitted. **Cognitive Level:** Applying **Client Need:** Pharmacological and Parenteral Therapies **Integrated Process:** Nursing Process: Evaluation **Content Area:** Pharmacology **Strategy:** Correlate the management of migraine headaches with "not by medicine alone." **Reference:** Aschenbrenner, D., & Venable, S. (2009). *Drug therapy in nursing* (3rd ed.). Philadelphia, PA: Lippincott Williams & Wilkins, pp. 419–422.

4 **Answer: 4** Rationale: Since methylphenidate (Ritalin) is a stimulant, a history of Tourette syndrome is a contraindication for its use. There are other medications that could be used for treatment of attention deficit/hyperactivity disorder (ADHD), such as pemoline (Cylert) or dextroamphetamine (Dexedrine). Methylphenidate has a calming effect on pediatric clients and is appropriate for use with this age group. Aplastic anemia is a side effect of Cylert. Because it is a stimulant, the use of methylphenidate in clients with a seizure disorder should be done so with caution. **Cognitive Level:** Applying **Client Need:** Pharmacological and Parenteral Therapies **Integrated Process:** Nursing Process: Assessment **Content Area:** Pharmacology **Strategy:** First recall that this medication is a stimulant, and then consider each option in terms of which item would be a contraindication to use of a stimulant. **Reference:** Wilson, B. A., Shannon, M. T., & Shields, K. M. (2012). *Pearson nurse's drug guide 2012.* Upper Saddle River, NJ: Pearson Education, pp. 976–978. Aschenbrenner, D., & Venable, S. (2009). *Drug therapy in nursing* (3rd ed.). Philadelphia, PA: pp. 356–358.

5 **Answer: 3** Rationale: Captopril (Capoten) is an angiotensin converting enzyme (ACE) inhibitor, which is a potent antihypertensive. Sibutramine hydrochloride monohydrate (Meridia) may increase the blood pressure. Nonsteroidal anti-inflammatory drugs (NSAIDs) such as naproxen (Naprosyn), the antibiotic amoxicillin (Amoxil), and the histamine antagonist cimetidine (Tagamet) have no known significant overlapping characteristics with sibutramine. **Cognitive Level:** Applying **Client Need:** Pharmacological and Parenteral Therapies **Integrated Process:** Nursing Process: Implementation **Content Area:** Pharmacology **Strategy:** Recall that most anorexiants increase metabolism, which would increase the basal metabolic rate (BMR). Then consider that an increased BMR would increase physiological processes such as blood pressure. **Reference:** Adams, M., & Koch, R. (2010). *Pharmacology: Connections to nursing practice.* Upper Saddle River, NJ: Pearson Education, pp. 1090–1091.

6 **Answer: 2** Rationale: Anticholinergic medications block the action of acetylcholine, resulting in decreased stimulation in the GI and urinary tract systems. This leads to urinary and bowel problems such as urinary retention, hesitancy, and constipation. Anticholinergic drugs stimulate the parasympathetic system and tachycardia and hypertension indicate sympathetic system stimulation. Cholinergic agonists, not anticholinergics, cause biliary contractions. Renal colic is also more commonly associated with cholinergic agonists rather than anticholinergics. **Cognitive Level:** Applying **Client Need:** Pharmacological and Parenteral Therapies **Integrated Process:** Nursing Process: Assessment **Content Area:** Pharmacology **Strategy:** Correlate the nature of the drug category with the signs and symptoms. Specific knowledge of this drug category is needed to answer this question. **Reference:** Aschenbrenner, D., & Venable, S. (2009). *Drug therapy in nursing* (3rd ed.). Philadelphia, PA: Lippincott Williams & Wilkins, pp. 242–252.

7 **Answer: 2** Rationale: Selegiline (Eldepryl) is a monoamine oxidase inhibitor (MAOI). Concurrent administration of meperidine (Demerol), an opioid analgesic, and selegiline can lead to a life-threatening hypertensive crisis, so the blood pressure will require careful monitoring. Selegiline primarily affects the dopamine levels in the brain and has no effect on the immune system. The client will need to refrain from all activity until it is determined that there is no risk of a hypertensive crisis. Decreased stimulation will be needed if it is determined that the client's blood pressure has become significantly elevated. **Cognitive Level:** Applying **Client Need:** Pharmacological and Parenteral Therapies **Integrated Process:** Nursing Process: Planning **Content Area:** Pharmacology **Strategy:** Associate monoamine oxidase inhibitors (MAOIs) with a hypertensive crisis as the greatest risk to the client. **Reference:** Aschenbrenner, D., & Venable, S. (2009). *Drug therapy in nursing* (3rd ed.). Philadelphia, PA: Lippincott Williams & Wilkins, p. 252. Wilson, B. A., Shannon, M. T., & Shields, K. M. (2012). *Pearson nurse's drug guide 2012.* Upper Saddle River, NJ: Pearson Education, pp. 940–942.

8 **Answer: 4** **Rationale:** Cyclobenzaprine (Flexeril) can cause edema of the tongue, which can place the client at risk for airway obstruction. Because the medication can cause drowsiness, the client should avoid driving and other activities that could lead to injury while taking the medication; however, walking should be safe. The side effects affecting the skin include pruritus and skin rash. The drug is recommended for short-term rather than long-term treatment. **Cognitive Level:** Applying **Client Need:** Pharmacological and Parenteral Therapies **Integrated Process:** Teaching and Learning **Content Area:** Pharmacology **Strategy:** Whenever a new medication is prescribed, an important element of client teaching is the risk of adverse effects. With this in mind, evaluate each option for the worst consequence to choose it as the answer to the question. **Reference:** Wilson, B. A., Shannon, M. T., & Shields, K. M. (2012). *Pearson nurse's drug guide 2012.* Upper Saddle River, NJ: Pearson Education, pp. 380–381.

9 **Answer: 1** **Rationale:** Prolonged phenytoin (Dilantin) therapy may result in osteoporosis, especially in clients with limited sun exposure and who are more at risk of the disease. Since osteoporosis is a chronic condition, it is perceived as the greatest risk to the client. The dark glasses reduce the sensitivity occurring with photophobia but do not necessarily prevent its occurrence. Taking the dose with food may decrease the rate of absorption, but may be also effective in reducing nausea and vomiting; however, this is not the greatest health promotion concern. Massaging the gums can prevent gingival hyperplasia caused by phenytoin, but is less significant than the risk of developing osteoporosis. **Cognitive Level:** Applying **Client Need:** Pharmacological and Parenteral Therapies **Integrated Process:** Nursing Process: Implementation **Content Area:** Pharmacology **Strategy:** The critical words in the question are *for some time* and *most important.* This tells you that the correct option may be one that results from long-term use and also that more than one option may be technically correct. Consider the adverse effects of the drug and choose the option that counteracts the most significant one over time. **Reference:** Wilson, B. A., Shannon, M. T., & Shields, K. M. (2012). *Pearson nurse's drug guide 2012.* Upper Saddle River, NJ: Pearson Education, pp. 1204–1208.

10 **Answer: 4** **Rationale:** Since the joints are inflamed, it will take some time to reduce the inflammation and thereby relieve the pain. The therapeutic effect of naproxen (Naprosyn) does not occur for 3–4 weeks, making 4 the correct number of weeks to identify because of the words *up to.* **Cognitive Level:** Analyzing **Client Need:** Pharmacological and Parenteral Therapies **Integrated Process:** Nursing Process: Evaluation **Content Area:** Pharmacology **Strategy:** The critical words in the stem are *up to*, meaning that the number to be provided in the answer is at the top of the possible range. Associate naproxen (Naprosyn) with a long onset, but beyond that specific drug knowledge is needed to answer the question. **Reference:** Wilson, B. A., Shannon, M. T., & Shields, K. M. (2012). *Pearson nurse's drug guide 2012.* Upper Saddle River, NJ: Pearson Education, pp. 1043–1044.

References

Abrams, A. (2009). *Clinical drug therapy: Rationales for nursing practice* (9th ed.). Philadelphia, PA: Lippincott Williams & Wilkins.

Adams, M., Holland, L., & Bostwick, P. (2011). *Pharmacology for nurses: A pathophysiologic approach* (3rd ed.). Upper Saddle River, NJ: Pearson Education.

Adams, M., & Urban, C. (2013). *Pharmacology: Connections to nursing practice* (2nd ed.). Upper Saddle River, NJ: Pearson Education.

Aschenbrenner, D., & Venable, S. (2012). *Drug therapy in nursing* (4th ed.). Philadelphia, PA: Lippincott Williams & Wilkins.

Drug facts & comparisons® (Updated monthly). St. Louis, MO: A. Wolters Kluwer.

Kee, J. (2009). *Laboratory and diagnostic tests and nursing implications* (8th ed.). Upper Saddle River, NJ: Pearson Education.

Lehne, R. (2010). *Pharmacology for nursing care* (7th ed.). St. Louis, MO: Mosby.

LeMone, P., Burke, K., & Bauldoff, G. (2011). *Medical-surgical nursing: Critical thinking in patient care* (5th ed.). Upper Saddle River, NJ: Pearson Education.

Ofirmev (acetaminophen) injection. Ofirmev (2012). Retrieved January, 2012, from www.ofirmev.com/Overview.aspx

Wilson, B. A., Shannon, M. T., & Shields, K. M. (2012). *Pearson nurse's drug guide 2012.* Upper Saddle River, NJ: Pearson Education.

ANSWERS & RATIONALES

Psychiatric Medications

11

Chapter Outline

Antipsychotics
Antidepressants

Mood Stabilizers
Sedative–Hypnotics and
   Anxiolytics

Substance Misuse

Objectives

➤ Describe the general goals of therapy when administering medications to treat psychiatric disorders.
➤ Discuss the indications for use of an antipsychotic medication.
➤ Identify the signs and symptoms and nursing management of extrapyramidal adverse effects that can occur with the administration of antipsychotic medications.
➤ List the classifications of antidepressant medications.
➤ Describe dietary restrictions associated with the use of monoamine oxidase inhibitors.
➤ Identify the indications for the use of lithium.
➤ Describe the signs and symptoms and nursing management of the adverse or toxic effects associated with the use of lithium.
➤ Discuss client teaching points related to safety and the use of sedative–hypnotics and anxiolytics.
➤ Identify the signs associated with substance misuse.
➤ Identify specific client education points related to disulfiram (Antabuse) therapy.
➤ Discuss significant client education points related to the administration of medications to treat psychiatric disorders.

NCLEX-RN® Test Prep

Use the accompanying online resource, NursingReviewsandRationales, to test yourself with hundreds of NCLEX®-style practice questions.

Review at a Glance

agranulocytosis an acute disease marked by deficit or absolute lack of granulocytic white blood cells
akathisia a subjective sense of restlessness with a need to move or pace continuously
antagonists chemicals that inhibit activity at a receptor site
anticholinergic effects effects caused by drugs that block acetylcholine receptors
dystonia rigidity in muscles that control posture, gait, or ocular movements

extrapyramidal side effects (EPSE) involuntary muscle movements resulting from effects of neuroleptic medications on extrapyramidal system; include akathisia, akinesia, dystonia, drug-induced parkinsonism, and neuroleptic malignant syndrome
metabolite results of biotransformation of a drug; most tend to be pharmacologically inactive; there are exceptions including many benzodiazepines, fluoxetine, and ethanol

neuroleptics antipsychotic medications
neuroleptic malignant syndrome (NMS) a disorder associated with sudden high fever, rigidity, tachycardia, hypertension, and decreased level of consciousness
parkinsonism masked facies, muscle rigidity, and shuffling gait; extrapyramidal side effects related to dopamine blockade

serotonin syndrome a state (agitation, sweating, confusion, fever, hyperreflexia, tachycardia, hypotension, muscle rigidity, and ataxia) that occurs when SSRIs are given concurrently with other serotonin enhancing drugs, causing an excess of serotonin in the system

synesthesia a condition in which stimulation to one sense causes a reaction in another sense, such as smelling a flavor or tasting an odor

tardive dyskinesia (TD) an extrapyramidal syndrome that includes movements such as grimacing,

buccolingual movements, and dystonia (impaired muscle tone); usually are late-onset side effects of antipsychotic agents; may be irreversible

tolerance need for an increased amount of an agent to achieve same effects

PRETEST

1 The psychiatrist prescribed chlorpromazine (Thorazine) 50 mg IM as an initial dose for a client hospitalized with psychosis. The primary focus of the nursing care should include assessment of which of the following?

1. Blood pressure and pulse
2. Decrease in psychotic symptoms
3. Ability to ambulate independently
4. Appetite and ability to eat meals

2 The home care nurse is visiting a client discharged yesterday from an inpatient unit with a prescription for a 10-day supply of olanzapine (Zyprexa) 10 mg daily. The client states a prescription refill is needed, because the prescription provided yesterday is all gone. The nurse would then assess the client for which signs? Select all that apply.

1. Headache and psychosis
2. Light-headedness and diarrhea
3. Nervousness and dizziness
4. Hypoglycemia and dehydration
5. Dizziness upon standing

3 A client reports during an initial interview that the health care provider prescribed trazodone (Desyrel) 50 mg tid. The nurse assesses for which important item in the client's health history?

1. Insomnia
2. Panic attacks
3. Mania
4. Anxiety

4 A client is discharged with a prescription for phenelzine (Nardil), a monoamine oxidase inhibitor (MAOI). Which of the following should the nurse include during client teaching? Select all that apply.

1. Written instructions on how to take daily doses of medication
2. How family members can contact appropriate health care provider
3. Written and oral information about food and drug interactions
4. That family members should administer client's medication
5. The importance of checking blood pressure and pulse daily

5 The health care provider has ordered a benzodiazepine for a 74-year-old client. The acute care nurse anticipates transcribing which medication onto the medication administration record (MAR)?

1. Diazepam (Valium)
2. Chlordiazepoxide (Librium)
3. Trazodone (Desyrel)
4. Lorazepam (Ativan)

6 Because a client is being discharged today with a prescription for lithium (Litho-Bid), the nurse collaborates with the interdisciplinary team to prevent which of the following that would most likely result in the client's readmission to an inpatient unit? Select all that apply.

1. Development of a family crisis
2. Diet regime to lose weight
3. Nonadherence to lithium (Litho-Bid) therapy
4. Development of serious illness in the family
5. Viral illness with symptoms of diarrhea and vomiting

7 A client enters the emergency department vomiting profusely and smelling of alcohol. The client states several times, "It's the medicine that's doing it; if I live through this I'll never drink again." The nurse should ask which priority assessment questions? Select all that apply.

1. "How much alcohol have you had to drink?"
2. "Are you taking antihypertensive medications?"
3. "Have you eaten today?"
4. "Are you taking disulfiram (Antabuse)?"
5. "Have you had your gallbladder removed?"

8 After several days of hospitalization on a psychiatric inpatient unit for clinical depression, the client is discharged with a prescription for imipramine (Tofranil) 75 mg by mouth daily. The nurse should include which information in client teaching? Select all that apply.

1. Change positions slowly.
2. Avoid driving until clear vision is restored.
3. Report urinary retention.
4. Cardiac dysrhythmias are uncommon.
5. Drug may decrease levels of liver enzymes.

9 After taking fluoxetine (Prozac) 20 mg by mouth every morning for 3 weeks, the client reports to the outpatient clinic today. The client reports a weight loss of 10 pounds during the last 2 weeks. Based on this assessment data, the nurse should take which action?

1. Instruct client to suspend taking dosages of this medication.
2. Instruct client to increase the daily fluid intake.
3. Consult with prescriber regarding possible need for an antiemetic.
4. Consult with prescriber regarding need to decrease the dosage.

10 Because a client is experiencing frequent, recurrent hiccups, the nurse contacts the health care provider. While the nurse waits for the prescriber to respond, the nurse would prepare for client teaching by obtaining an information sheet about which drug?

1. Risperidone (Risperdal)
2. Lorazepam (Ativan)
3. Chlorpromazine (Thorazine)
4. Thioridazine (generic)

➤ *See pages 385–388 for Answers and Rationales.*

I. ANTIPSYCHOTICS

A. Phenothiazines

1. Action and use
   a. Phenothiazines are **neuroleptics** (medications used to treat psychosis); they are also known as typical (traditional) antipsychotic agents
   b. Are divided into 3 chemical subclasses: the aliphatics, the piperidines, and the piperazines; see Table 11-1 for a complete list of neuroleptic medications
   c. Typical antipsychotics are predominantly dopamine (DA) **antagonists** (produce an effect by preventing receptor activation by endogenous regulatory molecules and drugs); thus they block postsynaptic D_2 receptors in several DA tracts in brain, although they have other synaptic effects as well; their 2 main effects are:
      1) A decrease in positive symptoms of schizophrenia (see Box 11-1 for a listing of positive and negative symptoms of schizophrenia)
      2) Production of **extrapyramidal side effects (EPSE)**: a variety of neurological disturbances resulting from dysfunction of extrapyramidal system; this may occur as a reversible side effect of certain psychotropic drugs, particularly antipsychotics; see Table 11-2 for a list of EPS manifestations and their management
   d. Psychosis is a phenomenon of brain activity; therefore effects of antipsychotic medications occur in central nervous system (CNS)
   e. Selected agents are also used as antiemetics and antihistamines; chlorpromazine is also used to treat intractable hiccups

Table 11-1 — Antipsychotic Drugs

Chemical Class & Generic (Trade) Name	Route	Uses
First Generation Agents		
Phenothiazines		
Chlorpromazine (generic)	PO, IM, R; IV rarely	Schizophrenia, schizoaffective disorders, manic phase of bipolar disorder, preoperative restlessness, antiemetic, adjunctive therapy for tetanus, intractable hiccups
Fluphenazine	PO, IM, LA	Psychotic disorders, chronic schizophrenia, behavioral complications due to mental retardation
Perphenazine (Trilafon)	PO, IM	Schizophrenia, severe nausea, and vomiting
Thioridazine (Mellaril)	PO	Schizophrenia when unacceptable response to other antipsychotics, psychotic disorders
Trifluoperazine (generic)	PO	Schizophrenia, psychotic disorders
Nonphenothiazines		
Haloperidol (Haldol)	PO, IM, LA	Tourette syndrome, chronic psychotic disorder, nonpsychotic behavioral disorder
Loxapine (Loxitane)	PO	Schizophrenia
Pimozide (Orap)	PO	Vocal and motor tics accompanying Tourette syndrome, off-label for schizophrenia
Thiothixene (Navane)	PO, IM	Psychotic disorders, schizophrenia
Second Generation (Atypical) Agents		
Aripiprazole (Abilify)	PO, IM	Schizophrenia, bipolar mania
Asenapine (Saphris)	SL	Schizophrenia, mania, or mixed episodes associated with bipolar disorder
Clozapine (Clozaril)	PO	Schizophrenia, schizoaffective disorder, reduce risk of suicidal behavior
Iloperidone (Fanapt)	PO	Acute schizophrenia
Lurasidone (Latuda)	PO	Schizophrenia
Olanzapine (Zyprexa)	PO, IM	Dementia related to Alzheimer's disease, schizophrenia, acute manic episode, agitation
Paliperidone (Invega)	PO, IM	Schizophrenia, schizoaffective disorder
Quetiapine (Seroquel)	PO	Schizophrenia, acute mania accompanying bipolar disorder
Risperidone (Risperdal)	PO, LA	Schizophrenia, mania accompanying bipolar disorder
Ziprasidone (Geodon)	PO	Schizophrenia, schizoaffective disorder, psychotic depression

PO, oral tablets, capsules; IM, intramuscular injection; R, rectal (suppository); L, oral liquid, suspension, concentrate; LA, long-acting injectable preparations.

Box 11-1

Positive and Negative Symptoms of Schizophrenia

Positive Symptoms

Hallucinations
Delusions
Disordered thinking
Combativeness
Agitation
Paranoia
Grandiosity
Illusions
Insomnia

Negative Symptoms

Social withdrawal
Emotional withdrawal
Lack of motivation
Poverty of speech
Alogia
Anergia
Anhedonia
Attention deficits
Blunted affect
Poor insight or judgment
Poor self-care

Table 11-2	Extrapyramidal Side Effects (EPSE)
Side Effects	**Nursing Interventions**
Peripheral Nervous System Effects	
Constipation	Increase fluid intake, encourage high fiber intake, provide laxatives as needed.
Dry mouth	Advise client to use sugarless hard candy or gum, sips of water frequently.
Nasal congestion	Suggest over-the-counter nasal decongestants that are safe for use with antipsychotic agents.
Blurred vision	Ask client to avoid dangerous tasks. This symptom will usually last only a short time at the beginning of treatment. Eye drops should be used for the short-term need.
Mydriasis	Advise client to report any eye pain immediately.
Photophobia	Advise client to wear sunglasses when in sunlight.
Orthostatic hypotension	Advise client to get out of chair or bed slowly, to sit before standing, and rise slowly. Observe to see if change to another antipsychotic is advisable.
Tachycardia	This is usually a reflex response to hypotension. And decreases when intervention for hypotension is effective. With clozapine, withhold dose if pulse rate is greater than 140/min.
Urinary retention	Encourage client to void when urge is present and void frequently. Catheterize for residual urine. Client should closely monitor output. Older men with benign prostatic hyperplasia are more susceptible.
Urinary hesitation	Provide privacy, encourage client to take the time to void, run water in sink or pour warm water over perineum.
Sedation	Help client to get up, get dressed, and begin the day early.
Weight gain	Advise client to maintain appropriate diet.
Agranulocytosis	There is a high incidence in clients taking clozapine. White cell counts need to be monitored weekly. If the WBC is less than 3500 cells/mm^3 prior to therapy, no treatment should begin. After treatment has begun, a WBC less than 3000 cells/mm^3 and a granulocyte count of less than 1500 cells/mm^3 indicate that treatment should be interrupted to monitor for infection. If WBC is less than 2000 cells/mm^3, and granulocyte count is less than 1000 cells/mm^3, halt therapy and do not begin treatment with drug again. If infection develops, antibiotics should be prescribed.
Central Nervous System Effects	
Akathisia	Usually develops within the first 2 months. There is an uncontrollable need to move. Occurs most often with high potency antipsychotics.
	Treatment is usually with beta blockers, benzodiazepines, and anticholinergic drugs. The antipsychotic agent should be changed to a lower potency agent.
	It is important to distinguish between akathisia and exacerbation of psychosis. If akathisia is confused with anxiety or psychotic agitation, the antipsychotic dosage would likely be increased, thereby making akathisia more intense.
Dystonias	Acute: Usually occur early in treatment, and are dangerous and severe. Oculogyric crisis or torticollis is the most common occurrence.
	Treatment includes antiparkinson drug or antihistamine immediately and offer reassurance.
	Obtain an order for IM administration when client begins treatment with antipsychotics or if in acute state of dystonia, call prescriber immediately.
	For less acute dystonias, notify prescriber when a prescription for an antiparkinson drug is warranted.
Drug-induced parkinsonism	A chronic nervous disease characterized by a fine, slowly spreading tremor, muscular weakness and rigidity, and a peculiar gait induced by some antipsychotic medications. Assess for three major symptoms: tremors, rigidity, and bradykinesia. Report to prescriber immediately. Antiparkinson drugs will be indicated.
Tardive dyskinesia (TD)	Develops in 15–20% of clients during long-term therapy. The risk is related to duration of treatment and dosage. For many clients symptoms are irreversible. Assess for signs using the Abnormal Inventory Movement Scale (AIMS). Anticholinergic agents will worsen TD, so use is contraindicated.
Neuroleptic malignant syndrome	This is a fatal side effect of antipsychotic medications. Routinely take client's temperature and encourage adequate water intake. Also routinely assess for rigidity, tremor, and similar symptoms.
Seizures	Occur in approximately 1% of clients taking antipsychotic medications.
	Clozapine causes a higher rate, up to 5% of clients taking 600–900 mg/day. For clozapine doses greater than 600 mg/day, a normal EEG should be performed. If a seizure occurs, clozapine may need to be discontinued.

Box 11-2	**High-Potency Antipsychotic Drugs**
Classification of Traditional Antipsychotics by Potency	• Fluphenazine • Haloperidol (Haldol) • Pimozide (Orap) • Thiothixene (Navane) • Trifluoperazine
	Moderate-Potency Antipsychotic Drugs • Loxapine (Loxitane) • Perphenazine (Trilafon)
	Low-Potency Antipsychotic Drugs • Chlorpromazine (Thorazine) • Thioridazine (Mellaril)

    f. Typical antipsychotics are most effective in treating "positive" symptoms of schizophrenia (behaviors and symptoms that normally seen), but are less effective in treating "negative" symptoms of schizophrenia (symptoms that develop over an extended period of time; include an absence of behaviors or features usually seen); refer again to Box 11-1 for positive and negative symptoms of schizophrenia

    g. Typical antipsychotics are not different from each other in overall clinical response at equivalent doses; thus selection of a drug is determined by extent, type, and severity of side effects produced, as well as effect of drug in a first-degree relative (see Box 11-2 for a list of antipsychotics by potency classification)

       1) A low-potency drug such as chlorpromazine can reduce risk of EPS, while a high-potency drug such as haloperidol can minimize postural hypotension, sedation, and anticholinergic effects

       2) These drugs are equally effective in treating positive symptoms of schizophrenia but are less effective in treating negative symptoms

    h. Tolerance to antipsychotic medications is very uncommon; they are also the most toxic drugs used in psychiatry

2. Common medications (refer again to Table 11-1)

    a. Chlorpromazine (Thorazine) and other antipsychotics are used primarily to treat psychotic disorders, specifically schizophrenia and other chronic mental illnesses; treatment of schizophrenia has three goals:

       1) Suppression of acute episodes

       2) Prevention of acute exacerbations

       3) Maintenance of highest possible level of functioning

    b. Selection of traditional antipsychotic drugs is based largely on side effect profile

    c. Client should not receive a drug that, because of its side effects, is likely to cause discomfort, inconvenience, or harm; for example, if a client has a history of prostatic hyperplasia or glaucoma, or is sensitive to anticholinergic drugs, a low-potency neuroleptic should not be prescribed

3. Administration considerations

    a. Typical antipsychotics effectively suppress symptoms during acute psychotic episodes, and when taken chronically, can greatly reduce incidence of relapse (a major risk in treatment of schizophrenia); but since etiology of psychotic illness is entirely unknown, the relationship of receptor blockade to therapeutic effects can only be estimated

    b. Medication effects can usually be seen in 1–2 days, but substantial improvement usually takes 2–4 weeks and full effects may not develop for several months

    c. Dosage requirements vary considerably for each client and must be adjusted as target symptoms change and side effects are monitored; initially, depending on dosage, a client receives several doses per day and total daily dose can be titrated slowly until a safe, effective dose is reached

    d. The half-life of antipsychotic drugs is greater than 24 hours, so client usually can be dosed once a day after safe, effective dose is reached

    e. Dosing for older adults requires small doses, typically 30–50% of those taken by younger clients; also poorly responsive clients may need larger doses than highly responsive clients (although very large doses are generally avoided)

    f. Positive symptoms of schizophrenia respond better than negative symptoms

    g. Antipsychotic drugs do not alter underlying pathology of schizophrenia; treatment is not curative, it offers only symptomatic relief

    h. A thorough baseline evaluation should be done, including laboratory tests and electrocardiogram (ECG), for clients beginning treatment

    i. Antipsychotic medications can also be used for clients with bipolar disorder (used to reduce acute symptoms of psychosis), and for clients who have Tourette syndrome (specifically, haloperidol can reduce severe symptoms of disease); neuroleptics suppress emesis in clients by blocking dopamine receptors in chemoreceptor trigger zone of medulla

    j. Depot antipsychotic preparations such as haloperidol and fluphenazine are long-acting injectable preparations used for long-term maintenance therapy of schizophrenia; with this form of treatment, relapse rate is usually reduced and thus is more favorable if a client needs long-term therapy; dosage should be reduced in older adults

  4. Contraindications

    a. Hypersensitivity

    b. Cross-sensitivity may exist among phenothiazines

    c. Use with caution in clients with narrow-angle glaucoma, adynamic ileus, prostatic hyperplasia, cardiovascular disease, hepatic or renal dysfunction, and seizure disorders

    d. Should not be used in clients who have CNS depression

    e. Contraindicated for comatose or severely depressed clients

    f. Also contraindicated in Parkinson disease, prolactin-dependent carcinoma of the breast, bone marrow depression, and severe hypotension or hypertension

  5. Significant drug interactions

    a. May decrease therapeutic response to levodopa

    b. May be at increased risk for **agranulocytosis**, a low white blood cell (WBC) count, when also taking antithyroid agents

    c. See Table 11-3 for additional adverse drug–drug interactions and effects

  6. Significant food interactions: use of nutmeg is contraindicated with haloperidol (Haldol); dong quai and St. John's wort increase photosensitivity; evening primrose decreases seizure threshold; kava kava increases dystonia

  7. Significant laboratory studies

    a. Before treatment is started, clients should have a complete evaluation including ECG, blood profile that includes WBC, hemoglobin, and hematocrit

    b. Ongoing monitoring is indicated to assess for decreases in WBC counts

    c. Assess liver function

  8. Side effects (refer back to Table 11-2)

    a. D_2-receptor blockade is known to be responsible for many side effects of typical antipsychotics

    b. Dopamine blockade can lead to gynecomastia, galactorrhea, amenorrhea (occasionally), and weight gain

Table 11-3 Adverse Interactions of Antipsychotics with Other Drugs

Drug	Effect of Interaction
Alcohol, antihistamines, opioids, antidepressants, sedative–hypnotics, analgesics	Additive CNS depression with other CNS depressants
Alcohol, nitrates, or antihypertensives	Additive hypotension with acute ingestion
Amoxapine, fluoxetine	↑ extrapyramidal side effects
Amphetamines	↓ antipsychotic effect
Antacids	May ↓ absorption
Anticholinergic or antiparkinson drugs	↑ anticholinergic effects; delayed onset of effects of oral doses of antipsychotics; potentially ↑ risk of hyperthermia
Barbiturates, nonbarbiturate hypnotics	Respiratory depression and ↑ sedation; ↓ antipsychotic serum levels; hypotension
Benzodiazepines	↑ sedation; respiratory depression with lorazepam and loxapine
Beta-adrenergic blocking agents (propranolol)	Effects of either or both drugs increased
Cimetidine	Chlorpromazine absorption decreased; increased sedation with chlorpromazine
Diazoxide	Can cause severe hyperglycemia
Dopaminergic antiparkinson drugs (e.g., bromocriptine)	Antagonizes the antipsychotic effect
Guanethidine	Control of hypertension is decreased
Insulin, oral hypoglycemics	Control of diabetes is weakened
L-dopa	↓ antiparkinson effect; may exacerbate psychosis
Lithium	May ↓ blood levels and effectiveness of phenothiazines
Phenobarbital	May ↑ metabolism and ↓ the effectiveness of the drug
Phenytoin	May ↑ phenytoin toxicity; ↓ antipsychotic blood serum levels
Trazodone	Additive hypotension with phenothiazines
Tricyclics	Possible ventricular dysrhythmias with thioridazine; possible ↑ blood serum levels of both; hypotension; sedation; anticholinergic effect; ↑ risk of seizures

9. Adverse effects/toxicity (refer back to Table 11-2)
   a. Most common adverse effects are sedation, orthostatic hypotension, and **anticholinergic effects** (dry mouth, blurred vision, urinary retention, photophobia, constipation, tachycardia); others include **akathisia** (uncontrollable need to move), and **parkinsonism** (set of symptoms that resembles Parkinson disease)
   b. Photosensitivity occurs; clients should take measures to protect eyes when exposed to sunlight
   c. Agranulocytosis, which is an acute deficit or absolute lack of granulocytic white blood cells (neutrophils, basophils, and eosinophils)
   d. **Neuroleptic malignant syndrome (NMS)** is characterized by catatonia, rigidity, stupor, unstable BP, hyperthermia, profuse sweating, dyspnea, and incontinence; it sometimes occurs as a toxic reaction to use of potent neuroleptic agents in therapeutic doses and may last 5–10 days after drug is discontinued; mortality rate may be as high as 20%; bromocriptine (Parlodel) and dantrolene (Dantrium) have been used to treat NMS if usual treatment for hyperthermia is ineffective; antipsychotic drug withdrawal is mandatory
   e. Low-potency drugs are more likely to cause sedation and hypotension, while high-potency drugs cause more EPS

    f. Overdoses of antipsychotic drugs are not usually fatal and treatment for attempted overdose is supportive (e.g., gastric lavage to empty stomach); it can cause severe CNS depression (somnolence to coma, hypotension, EPS); also reported are restlessness or agitation, seizures (lowered seizure threshold), hyperthermia, increased anticholinergic symptoms, and dysrhythmias

10. Nursing considerations

    !   **a.** Observe hospitalized clients take their medication so that they swallow medications and do not "cheek" them; clients may have a difficult time with "clouding" and sedating effects of antipsychotic drugs

    b. Client teaching (see following section) is a major aspect of nursing care

    c. Refer once more to Table 11-2 for more specific nursing care and teaching considerations

11. Client education

    !   **a.** Take medication as prescribed; the major relapse factor for clients with schizophrenia is discontinuing medications, which then leads to relapse and rehospitalization

    b. Take PO meds with food, milk, or a full glass of water to decrease gastric irritation

    !   **c.** Dilute most concentrates in 120 mL of distilled or acidified tap water or fruit juice just before administration

    d. Be aware of other medications that may be prescribed to treat ESP (see Box 11-3)

    e. Include family members involved in client's care and teach at a level that client or family can grasp and demonstrate knowledge acquired; provide written instructions and information about other resources, including phone contacts, if problems should arise

    f. Be aware that anticholinergic medications may decrease effectiveness of typical antipsychotics

B. Atypical antipsychotic drugs

1. Action and use

    a. The atypical antipsychotics exert both dopamine receptor subtype 2 (D_2) and serotonin receptor subtype 2 ($5HT_2$) receptor-blocking action (are DA and 5HT antagonists)

    b. Blockage of serotonin receptors is thought to liberate dopamine in cortex and may explain some reduction in negative symptoms

    !   **c.** Atypical agents cause few or no extrapyramidal symptoms, including **tardive dyskinesia (TD)** (dyskinesia is difficulty performing voluntary movement, while tardive indicates late onset—usually seen as a serious side effect of antipsychotic agents)

    !   **d.** Used to treat positive and negative symptoms of schizophrenia and other mental illnesses with psychotic features, and to treat mood symptoms, hostility, violence, suicidal behavior, and cognitive impairment seen in schizophrenia

---

Box 11-3	**Anticholinergic**
	• Benztropine (Cogentin)
Medications Used to Treat Extrapyramidal Side Effects	• Trihexyphenidyl
	Antihistamine
	• Diphenhydramine (Benadryl)
	Dopamine Agonist
	• Amantadine (Symmetrel)

  e. Provide new hope for clients with psychosis, particularly during first episode, for those who have not responded well to typical antipsychotics, or for those with dose-limiting side effects from traditional neuroleptics

2. Common medications (refer back to Table 11-1 for drug names and routes)

  a. The following are some atypical antipsychotic medications commonly used at present: clozapine (Clozaril), risperidone (Risperdal), and olanzapine (Zyprexa)

  b. Clozapine (Clozaril)

   1) Because of its serious side effect, agranulocytosis, it was released with a very rigid set of protocols including weekly blood analysis

   2) Clients are not prescribed more than a 1-week supply of medication to enforce compliance with weekly blood analysis

   3) Beneficial effects of clozapine are usually very positive for most and remarkable for others

   4) Clozapine has a greater affinity for dopamine-D_1, dopamine-D_4, and serotonin ($5HT_2$), as well as dopamine D_2 receptors

  c. Risperidone (Risperdal)

   1) Has a greater affinity for dopamine D_2 receptors and a similar antagonism of serotonin $5HT_2$

   2) Its lack of serious side effects makes it a very well-tolerated agent

   3) Has little affinity for muscarinic (i.e., cholinergic receptors), so anticholinergic side effects are minimized; neither does it appear to cause agranulocytosis, EPSEs, tardive dyskinesia, or NMS

   4) Side effects include orthostatic hypotension, insomnia, agitation, headache, anxiety, and rhinitis

  d. Olanzapine (Zyprexa)

   1) Is comparable to risperidone in efficacy of treating both positive and negative symptoms and has a comparable side effects profile

   2) Does not cause agranulocytosis; early clinical trials indicate few incidents of EPSE

  e. Newer antipsychotic medications such as paliperidone (Invega) and aripiprazole (Abilify) reduce extrapyramidal symptoms such as tardive dyskinesia, thus improving client use of medications while improving behavioral and cognitive symptoms

3. Administration considerations

  a. Clozapine is usually given 1–2 times daily and should not exceed 900 mg/day; because of the strict protocol, blood testing is done weekly; *if client does not comply, the drug will not be continued*

  b. Risperidone is usually administered PO in 1–2 daily doses; for debilitated or elderly clients or for those with renal or hepatic impairment, dosage should be reduced at onset of treatment

  c. Olanzapine is usually administered PO as well; dosage should not exceed 15 mg/day; for debilitated or nonsmoking female clients greater than 65 years, therapy should be initiated at 5 mg/day

  d. Refer back to Table 11-1 for generic and trade names, and general information about administration of antipsychotics

4. Contraindications

  a. Clozapine, risperidone, and olanzapine are all contraindicated for clients with hypersensitivity to drug; other considerations include cautious use in bone marrow depression, during severe CNS depression or coma, and during lactation

  b. Clozapine should be used cautiously with clients who have a depressed bone marrow, prostatic enlargement, narrow-angle glaucoma, malnourished state, diabetes mellitus, seizure disorder, or in clients with cardiovascular, hepatic, or renal disease; it should also be used cautiously in children less than 16 years (safety is not yet established)

     c. Risperidone should be used cautiously for older adults, debilitated clients, and those with renal or hepatic impairment, cardiovascular disease, or history of seizures, suicide attempts, or drug abuse; safety has not been established for use during pregnancy or lactation, or for use with children

     d. Olanzapine should be used cautiously with clients with liver disease or during pregnancy or lactation; safety for use with children has not yet been established

     e. For older adults or debilitated clients, or clients with known liver, renal, or cardiovascular disease, initial dosing should be lowered and ongoing monitoring should be emphasized

5. Significant drug interactions

     a. Clozapine may be decreased by concurrent use of carbamazepine (Tegretol), omeprazole (Prilosec), or rifampin (Rifadin); additive hypotension may occur with concurrent use of antihypertensives or benzodiazepines, additive CNS depression may occur with concurrent use of alcohol or other CNS depressants; atypical antipsychotics may decrease effects of levodopa or other dopamine agonists

     b. Risperidone may decrease the antiparkinson effects of levodopa or other dopamine agonists; carbamazepine increases metabolism and may decrease effectiveness of risperidone; clozapine decreases metabolism and may increase effects of risperidone; additive CNS depression may occur with other CNS depressants including alcohol, antihistamines, sedative–hypnotics, or opioids

     c. Olanzapine effects may be decreased by concurrent use of carbamazepine, omeprazole, or rifampin; additive CNS depression occurs with concurrent use of alcohol or other CNS depressants; olanzapine may also antagonize effects of levodopa or other dopamine agonists

6. Significant food interactions: none

7. Significant laboratory studies: for clients prescribed clozapine, there is a mandatory need for weekly blood tests (WBC counts) to prevent or detect agranulocytosis

8. Side effects

     a. Seizure incidence for clients taking clozapine is 3%; this is one reason that maximum dose should not exceed 900 mg/day

     b. See Table 11-4 for common side effects of atypical antipsychotics

9. Adverse effects/toxicity

     a. Some of the more serious adverse or toxic effects listed for clozapine have been discussed in previous section on side effects; other considerations include neuroleptic malignant syndrome (NMS)

     b. For clients prescribed risperidone, monitor for NMS

     c. For clients taking olanzapine, monitor for NMS and seizures

10. Nursing considerations

     a. Because of risk of fatal agranulocytosis, clozapine is reserved for clients with severe schizophrenia who have not responded to traditional antipsychotic drugs (40–60% success rate for treatment in this group)

Table 11-4 **Common Side Effects of Atypical Antipsychotics**

	Clozapine	Risperidone	Olanzapine
Extrapyramidal	None	+	+
Cardiac	+++	++	+
Sedation	++++	++	+
Anticholinergic	++++	+	++
Weight gain	+++	++	++++

Occurrence: +, least; ++++, greatest

Practice to Pass

A client taking an anti-psychotic medication asks, "What is neuro-leptic malignant syndrome?" How would the nurse describe the syndrome and its management?

b. Assist clients to adjust to changes experienced (improvement in positive and negative symptoms, ability to become more animated, and to have behavior that is more socially acceptable)

c. Usually with clients who respond well to clozapine, there is a decreased need for rehospitalization as well

d. Encourage client to void prior to administering olanzapine

11. Client education: clients will still need help with psychoeducation, social skills training, group support, and other rehabilitative interventions to improve overall level of functioning and quality of life while incorporating atypical antipsychotic drugs into life pattern

II. ANTIDEPRESSANTS

A. Tricyclics

1. Action and use
   a. Imipramine (Tofranil) was the first antidepressant drug used to treat depression (1950s) and is still used effectively today
   b. Tricyclic antidepressants (TCAs) such as imipramine block monoamine reup-take, which indicates that TCAs intensify effects of norepinephrine and serotonin; TCAs can elevate mood, increase activity and alertness, decrease a client's preoccupation with morbidity, improve appetite, and regulate sleep patterns
   c. Initial mechanism of TCAs takes about 1–3 weeks to develop while a maximum response is achieved in approximately 6–8 weeks
   d. Other uses for TCAs are to treat clients with chronic insomnia, attention-deficit/hyperactivity disorder, and panic disorder

2. Common medications (Table 11-5)
   a. Several TCAs are available that are equally effective; major differences can be found in side effects
   b. For example, doxepin has sedative effects and could be more effectively used with clients who experience insomnia
   c. Older adults and clients with glaucoma, constipation, or prostatic hyperplasia can be especially sensitive to anticholinergic effects of TCAs; therefore, a TCA such as desipramine with weak anticholinergic effects would be more appropriate with these clients

3. Administration considerations
   a. Dosing with TCAs is individualized and based on clinical response or plasma drug levels (which must be above 225 ng/ml for antidepressant effects to occur)
   b. TCAs are normally given by mouth; amitriptyline and imipramine may be given by intramuscular (IM) injection; intravenous (IV) administration is not usually used
   c. TCAs have long half-lives, so they can be taken daily in a single dose; because the half-life of individual drugs varies, client dosing is also individualized
   d. Once-a-day dosing at bedtime has several advantages, such as ease of taking as part of daily routine, promoting sleep by its sedative effect, and reducing intensity of daytime side effects

4. Contraindications
   a. Hypersensitivity to TCAs
   b. Myocardial infarction
   c. Cerebrovascular disease
   d. Clients at risk for suicide who are taking TCAs should not have access to a large quantity of the drug and should be hospitalized until risk of suicide has passed

Table 11-5	Medications Commonly Used to Treat Depression
Drug Class and Generic (Trade) Name	**Nursing Responsibilities**
Tricyclic Antidepressants (TCAs)	
Amitriptyline (Elavil) Clomipramine (Anafranil) Desipramine (Norpramin) Doxepin (Senequin) Imipramine (Tofranil) Maprotiline (Ludiomil) Nortriptyline (Pamelor) Protriptyline (Vivactil) Trimipramine (Surmontil)	• Educate the client early about potential side effects. • Inform client that side effects will diminish with time and if necessary there are management alternatives that can be implemented. • Advise client that response will take some time and continued use is essential. • Inform client that first-time treatment for major depression should continue for 6–12 months. • Warn client of a possible significant weight gain. • Monitor for improvement. If minimal or no change after 2–4 weeks it may be necessary to change drug. • Educate client and family to immediately report changes in behavior or suicidal ideation.
Selective Serotonin Reuptake Inhibitors (SSRIs)	
Citalopram (Celexa) Escitalopram (Lexapro) Fluoxetine (Prozac) Fluvoxamine (Luvox) Paroxetine (Paxil) Sertraline (Zoloft)	• Inform client to take medication as prescribed. Abrupt discontinuation of the drug is contraindicated. • Continuously monitor client for side effects or adverse effects, particularly in the area of sexual dysfunction. Client may be reluctant to discuss. • Immediately report worsening of symptoms or suicidal ideation.
Serotonin Norepinephrine Reuptake Inhibitor (SNRI)	
Desvenlafaxine (Pristiq) Duloxetine (Cymbalta) Venlafaxine (Effexor)	• Similar to SSRI, do not begin therapy within 14 days of an MAOI. • Numerous drug–drug interactions. • Educate client and family to immediately report suicidal ideation or changes in behavior. • Educate client to not abruptly discontinue the medication.
Monoamine Oxidase Inhibitors (MAOIs)	
Isocarboxazid (Marplan) Phenelzine (Nardil) Selegiline (Emsam) Tranylcypromine (Parnate)	• Educate client about the need to eat a tyramine-restricted diet. • Caution client about side effects and adverse effects of the MAOIs. • Educate client about careful use of over-the-counter or other prescription medications and be sure client understands the seriousness of the effects. • Monitor efficacy of drugs and continuously reeducate client to avoid abruptly discontinuing medication or not taking medications as prescribed.
Atypical Antidepressants	
Amoxapine Bupropion (Wellbutrin) Mirtazapine (Remeron) Nefazodone Trazodone (Desyrel) Vilazodone (Vibryd)	• Instruct client about the side effects and adverse effect of the medication, especially seizure risks at higher drug doses. • Instruct client concerning the importance of taking this and all medication as prescribed. • Instruct client to take medication as prescribed and monitor for any adverse or side effects. • Instruct client to report any signs of sexual dysfunction, especially priapism, immediately.

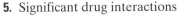

5. Significant drug interactions
  a. Combination of TCAs and a MAOI can lead to hypertensive crisis from excessive adrenergic stimulation of heart and blood vessels
  b. TCAs potentiate responses to direct-acting sympathomimetics (i.e., drugs such as epinephrine and norepinephrine); sympathetic nervous system (SNS) stimulation by these drugs can be increased because TCAs block reuptake of these drugs into adrenergic terminals, which prolongs their presence in synaptic spaces
  c. TCAs decrease responses to indirect-acting sympathomimetics (i.e., drugs such as ephedrine and amphetamine that promote release of transmitter from adrenergic nerves) because TCAs block uptake of these agents into adrenergic nerves, which prevents them from reaching their site of action within nerve terminals

    d. TCAs exert anticholinergic actions of their own; therefore, TCAs will intensify effects of other drug that have anticholinergic actions, such as antihistamines and certain over-the-counter (OTC) sleep aids; these products should be avoided while taking TCAs

    e. CNS depression caused by TCAs will add to CNS depression caused by other drugs; therefore clients taking TCAs should avoid CNS depressants, including alcohol, antihistamines, opioids, and barbiturates

    f. Increased TCA levels occur when combined with cimetidine, fluoxetine, phenothiazines, or hormonal contraceptives

6. Significant food interactions: St. John's wort is contraindicated with TCAs

7. Significant laboratory studies: assess AST, ALT levels, monitor serum drug levels to ensure they remain within therapeutic range

8. Side effects

    a. Most common undesirable effects of the TCAs are orthostatic hypotension, sedation, and anticholinergic effects

    b. Instruct client to move slowly when changing position (lying to sitting, sitting to standing, or turning) to avoid injury; monitor BP both lying and sitting if client is hospitalized

9. Adverse effects/toxicity

    a. Most serious adverse effect of TCAs is cardiac toxicity; in the absence of overdose or preexisting cardiac impairment, serious cardiotoxicity is rare

    b. To avoid adverse cardiac effects, clients over age 40 years and those with heart disease should undergo baseline ECG and then every 6 months

    c. Adverse effects of each drug are indicated in Table 11-6

10. Nursing considerations

    a. Advise clients of potential side effects and that therapeutic response will take some weeks to be established once therapy has begun; clients and families often become impatient when client is experiencing drug side effects while still having original symptoms

    b. Clients taking TCAs have highest rate of suicide after therapeutic levels achieved as compared to clients taking other types of antidepressants; family and client education about this effect should be included

    c. Refer back to Table 11-5 for nursing responsibilities with TCAs and see Table 11-6 for manifestations of common adverse effects

11. Client education

    a. Use measures to prevent orthostatic hypotension

    b. Side effects will diminish with time and symptoms will be lessened as medication regime is followed (this knowledge may enhance compliance)

    c. Utilize other available therapies as well as medications as appropriate

    d. Refer back to Tables 11-5 and 11-6 for specific teaching points

B. Monoamine oxidase inhibitors (MAOIs)

1. Action and use

    a. Because of potentially fatal food and drug interactions, this class of antidepressant is usually not a first choice to treat clients with depression unless client has atypical depression

    b. Monoamine oxidase (MAO) is an enzyme present in liver, intestinal wall, and terminals of monoamine-containing neurons; the function of MAO in neurons is to convert monoamine transmitters (norepinephrine, serotonin, and dopamine) into inactive products; in the liver and intestine, MAO serves to inactivate tyramine and other biogenic amines in food

    c. MAOIs decrease amount of monoamine oxidase in liver that breaks down amino acids tyramine and tryptophan

Table 11-6 **Most Common Adverse Effects from Antidepressant Medications**

Effect	Manifestations
1. Orthostatic hypotension	Major decrease in blood pressure with body position changes.
2. Anticholinergic	Blocks muscarinic cholinergic receptors, which produces dry mouth, blurred vision, photophobia, constipation, urinary hesitancy, and tachycardia.
3. Sedation	Sleepiness and difficulty maintaining arousal are common responses to TCAs because of blockade of histamine receptors in CNS.
4. Cardiac toxicity	TCAs can adversely affect the heart's function by decreasing vagal influence (secondary to muscarinic blockade) and acting directly on bundle of His to slow conduction.
5. Seizures	Lower seizure threshold.
6. Hypomania	Mild mania can occur.
7. Sexual dysfunction	Anorgasmia, delayed ejaculation, and decreased libido.
8. Hypertensive crisis from dietary tyramine	Although MAOIs normally produce hypotension, these drugs can cause severe hypertension if client eats tyramine-rich foods.
9. Drug interactions	Always teach clients the importance of preventing adverse drug effects and drug interactions. See individual classifications for specific nursing responsibilities.

    d. There is an antidepressant effect of MAOIs because of MAO-A in nerve terminals along with other enzymatic and chemical actions; MAOI biochemical action takes place rapidly, whereas clinical response (relief of depression) develops slowly

    e. MAOIs have been used with some success to treat bulimia and obsessive–compulsive disorders and to treat panic attacks in clients with panic disorder

2. Common medications: refer again to Tables 11-5 and 11-6 for MAOIs commonly used

3. Administration considerations: route is usually PO; see Table 11-5 for details

4. Contraindications: clients over age 60 years or those with pheochromocytoma, heart failure, liver disease, severe renal impairment, cerebrovascular defect, cardiovascular disease, or hypertension

5. Significant drug interactions

    a. Use with caution for clients taking other TCAs

    b. Taking SSRIs with MAOIs can cause **serotonin syndrome** (agitation, sweating, confusion, fever, hyperreflexia, tachycardia, hypotension, muscle rigidity, and ataxia); avoid this combination

    c. Antihypertensive drugs will potentiate hypotensive effects of MAOIs

    d. Meperidine can produce hyperthermia in clients taking MAOIs and should be avoided

    e. Instruct client to avoid all medications (prescription and nonprescription) that have not been specifically approved by health care provider

6. Significant food interactions

    a. Dietary tyramine, some other dietary constituents, and indirect-acting sympathomimetics (e.g., amphetamine, methylphenidate, ephedrine, cocaine) can precipitate a hypertensive crisis in clients taking MAOIs

    b. See Box 11-4 for lists of foods to avoid and to use cautiously while taking an MAOI

7. Significant laboratory studies: in order for antidepressant effects to occur, serum drug levels need to be maintained within a specified therapeutic range

8. Side effects

    a. Orthostatic hypotension is a common initial and sometimes persistent side effect of MAOIs

Box 11-4	**Foods to Avoid**
Foods to Avoid with Monoamine Oxidase Inhibitors	• All cheeses except cream or cottage cheese • Meats and fish: aged or cured • Fruits and vegetables: broad bean pods, tofu, soy bean extracts • Alcohol: draft beer • Other: sauerkraut, soy sauce, yeast extracts, soups (especially miso), and any nonfresh foods • Drugs: other antidepressant drugs, nasal and sinus decongestants, allergy, hay fever and asthma remedies, narcotics (especially meperidine), epinephrine, stimulants, cocaine, amphetamines **Consume with Caution** • Cheeses: mozzarella, cottage, ricotta, cream, processed • Meats and fish: chicken liver, meats, liver, herring • Fruits and vegetables: raspberries, bananas, small amounts only of avocado, spinach • Alcohol: wine • Other: monosodium glutamate, pizza, only small amounts of chocolate, caffeine, nuts, dairy products • Drugs: insulin, oral hypoglycemics, oral anticoagulants, thiazide diuretics, anticholinergic agents, muscle relaxants

   b. Edema, sexual dysfunction, and weight gain are also common and can lead to drug discontinuation

   c. Complaints of insomnia occur with all MAOIs

9. Adverse effects/toxicity: in contrast to TCAs, MAOIs cause direct CNS stimulation, which in excess can produce anxiety, agitation, hypomania, and even mania

10. Nursing considerations

   a. Provide oral and written instructions of how to avoid adverse effects of MAOIs; there are many factors to consider with client's safe use of drug because of side effects and adverse effects of MAOIs

   b. Assess client for ability to adhere to a strict dietary regime

   c. Consult with prescriber about changes in vital signs to avoid potentially fatal hypertensive crisis

   d. Instruct client not to take any prescribed or OTC medication without first consulting or notifying prescriber

11. Client education

   a. Familiarize client with symptoms of orthostatic hypotension and how to avoid injury when rising from bed or chair slowly

   b. If client is hospitalized, BP needs to be monitored regularly

   c. Educate client orally and in writing or provide a dietary consultation if appropriate for client and family in order to avoid hypertensive crisis

   d. Teach client to avoid all medications (prescribed or OTC) that have not been specifically approved by prescriber

C. Selective serotonin reuptake inhibitors (SSRIs)

1. Action and use

   a. Block reuptake of serotonin and intensify transmission at serotonergic synapses; effects can usually be seen after 1–3 weeks and are equivalent to those produced from TCAs

   b. SSRIs have same efficacy as TCAs, exhibit fewer side effects than either TCAs or MAOIs, and have a decreased time between initial dose and beginning of reduced signs and symptoms of depression

    c. All SSRIs are effective in treating obsessive–compulsive disorder (OCD), panic disorder, and bulimia nervosa

2. Common medications (refer again to Table 11-5)

3. Administration considerations

    a. SSRIs are administered orally in liquid or pulvules; older adults or those with impaired renal function should be given a low dosage with increases made cautiously

    b. Evaluate client frequently for safety and desired effects of drug

4. Contraindications

    a. Most SSRIs should not be prescribed for clients with a hypersensitivity to drug or those with severe hepatic or renal disease

    b. Caution should be used for debilitated clients or those with a history of seizure disorder or diabetes mellitus

    c. Lowered drug doses or longer dosing interval may be needed in clients with impaired hepatic function, older adults, or those receiving multiple drug therapy

5. Significant drug interactions

    a. SSRIs should not be administered with MAOIs to prevent serotonin syndrome, a hyperserotonergic state (confusion, autonomic dysfunction, muscle rigidity, ataxia) that occurs when an SSRI is given concurrently with other serotonin-enhancing drugs, causing an excess of serotonin in system

    b. If a client is on an MAOI and is changed to fluoxetine, at least 5 weeks should elapse before beginning fluoxetine; to change from fluoxetine to MAOIs, at least 2 weeks should elapse before beginning MAOI

    c. A client who is taking fluoxetine and warfarin should have warfarin level monitored closely because fluoxetine is highly bound to plasma proteins and may displace other highly bound drugs such as warfarin

    d. Fluoxetine can elevate plasma levels of TCAs and lithium and should be given cautiously when prescribed along with these other agents

6. Significant food interactions

    a. Each SSRI is individual for effect with food; fluoxetine, paroxetine, and fluvoxamine can be taken with or without food, while sertraline is slowly absorbed following oral administration; food increases extent of absorption for sertraline; yet, if there is gastric upset, drug literature recommends administration of paroxetine with food

    b. When administering a newer SSRI, consult individual drug literature

7. Significant laboratory studies

    a. Serum drug levels are not clinically useful to determine dose or monitor for toxicity

    b. Monitor CBC, differential, and bleeding time periodically throughout treatment for signs of leukopenia, anemia, or thrombocytopenia or for increased bleeding time

8. Side effects

    a. Side effect profile of SSRIs is relatively mild compared with other antidepressants; there is minimal cardiac toxicity, eliminating need for ECGs

    b. Common initial side effects of SSRIs include nausea, drowsiness, dizziness, headache, sweating, anxiety, insomnia, anorexia, and nervousness; these are generally milder and better tolerated than side effects of TCAs

9. Adverse effects/toxicity

    a. Most SSRIs are relatively safe in overdose; when taken as a single agent, SSRI overdoses are serious and can cause seizures, but complete recovery is common

    b. Sexual dysfunction, experienced by 20–40% of clients taking SSRIs, is an adverse effect that needs to be discussed with client by prescriber

10. Nursing considerations

    a. Monitor mood changes; notify prescriber if client demonstrates an increase in anxiety, nervousness, or insomnia

    b. Assess for suicidal tendencies, especially during early drug therapy

        c. Restrict amount of drug available to client to prevent overdose

        d. Monitor appetite, nutritional intake, and weight

   11. Client education

        a. Encourage client to comply with diet recommendations of health care professionals; give written and oral instructions to client and family

        b. Instruct client to notify prescriber if a rash occurs, which may indicate hypersensitivity

        c. Emphasize importance of follow-up exams to evaluate progress

        d. See also Tables 11-5 and 11-6 for points on specific SSRIs

D. Other antidepressants

   1. Action and use

        a. Trazodone (Desyrel) and bupropion (Wellbutrin) are newer antidepressant agents that have varied chemical structures and modes of action; they are not easily collapsed into a group and are thus discussed individually here

        b. Bupropion (Wellbutrin)

            1) Is similar in structure to amphetamines and can suppress appetite; it does not have cardiotoxic, anticholinergic, and antiadrenergic side effects and can therefore be used more readily with older adults; it can also be used for smoking cessation

            2) Blocks reuptake of dopamine while having only minimal reuptake effects on norepinephrine

        c. Trazodone (Desyrel)

            1) Is a second-line agent for treatment of depression; it is usually used in combination with another antidepressant and is usually prescribed to treat insomnia because of its very pronounced sedative effect

            2) Trazodone alters effects of serotonin in CNS; its antidepressant action may develop only over several weeks

        d. Venlafaxine (Effexor) and duloxetine (Cymbalta) are serotonin and norepinephrine reuptake inhibitors (SNRIs); treat depression and diabetic peripheral neuropathy

   2. Common medications: refer to Table 11-5

   3. Administration considerations

        a. Starting dose of bupropion should be no greater than 75 mg tid; because of dose-related seizure risk, never give more than 150 mg at one time; when maximum dose is required, the recommended regimen is 150 mg tid

        b. Initial dose of trazodone is usually 150 mg/day in 2 or 3 divided doses, and may be gradually increased to a maximum of 400 mg/day (outpatients) and 600 mg/day (hospitalized clients); also, a majority of drug dose may be given at bedtime to decrease daytime drowsiness and dizziness

        c. Dosages may be increased gradually for SNRIs; when taken for more than 1 week, tapering is recommended if drug needs to be discontinued

   4. Contraindications

        a. Bupropion can cause dose-related seizures

        b. Trazodone is contraindicated for clients with hypersensitivity, those recovering from myocardial infarction, or those who are using concurrent electroconvulsive therapy; it should be used cautiously in clients with cardiovascular disease or who exhibit suicidal behavior; dosage should be reduced in elderly clients or those who have severe hepatic or renal disease

        c. Recent (within 14 days) use of MAOI is a contraindication for SNRIs

   5. Significant drug interactions

        a. With bupropion there is an increased risk of adverse reactions when used with levodopa or MAOIs, and an increased risk of seizures with phenothiazines, antidepressants, theophylline, corticosteroids, OTC stimulants or anorexiants, or cessation of alcohol or benzodiazepines

    b. Trazodone may increase digoxin or phenytoin serum levels; additive CNS depression can occur with alcohol, opioids, and sedative–hypnotics; additive hypotension can occur with antihypertensive agents, acute ingestion of alcohol, or use of nitrates; concurrent use with fluoxetine increases levels and risk of toxicity from trazodone

6. Significant food interactions: do not combine with alcohol; severe reaction can occur if administered with St. John's wort

7. Significant laboratory studies

    a. Monitor hepatic and renal function closely in clients with kidney or liver impairment to prevent elevated serum and tissue bupropion concentrations

    b. For trazodone, assess CBC and renal and hepatic functioning before and periodically during treatment; slight, clinically insignificant decrease in leukocyte and neutrophil counts may occur

    c. Monitor liver function tests for SNRIs on a periodic basis or with symptoms of liver problems

8. Side effects (refer again to Tables 11-5 and 11-6)

    a. Most common side effects of bupropion are agitation and insomnia

    b. Common side effects of trazodone are sedation, orthostatic hypotension, and nausea and vomiting (N/V); in contrast to TCAs, it lacks anticholinergic actions and is not cardiotoxic; it may cause priapism (prolonged erection)

    c. SNRIs may cause sustained elevation of blood pressure; this is generally dose related

9. Adverse effects/toxicity

    a. Major adverse effect of bupropion is seizure activity; other adverse effects include headache, mania, psychoses, dry mouth, N/V, change in appetite, weight gain, weight loss, photosensitivity, hyperglycemia, hypoglycemia, and syndrome of inappropriate ADH secretion (SIADH)

    b. Overdose with trazodone is considered safer than with TCAs or MOAIs; death from overdose with trazodone alone has not been reported; adverse effects include drowsiness, confusion, dizziness, fatigue, hallucinations, headache, insomnia, nightmares, slurred speech, syncope, weakness, blurred vision, and tinnitus; also reported are hypotension, arrhythmias, chest pain, hypertension, palpitations, tachycardia, dry mouth, altered taste, constipation, diarrhea, excess salivation, flatulence, N/V, rash, hematuria, impotence, priapism, urinary frequency, anemia, leukopenia, myalgia, and tremors

10. Nursing considerations

    a. Individuals with a history of bipolar disorder taking bupropion need to be assessed for symptoms of mania

    b. Monitor BP and pulse rate before and during initial therapy with trazodone; clients with preexisting cardiac disease should have ECG monitored before and periodically during therapy to detect dysrhythmias

    c. Assess mental status and mood changes frequently; assess for suicidal tendencies, especially during early therapy; restrict amount of drug available to client

    d. Give bupropion with food to decrease GI side effects; give trazodone immediately after meals to minimize side effects (nausea, dizziness) and allow for maximum absorption

    e. Ensure that client has not taken an MAOI in last 14 days before initiating any medications in this category

11. Client education: as described in Tables 11-5 and 11-6

Practice to Pass

Describe the most common adverse effects that should be discussed with a client taking fluoxetine (Prozac).

III. MOOD STABILIZERS

A. Lithium

1. Action and use
   a. Is drug of choice for controlling manic episodes in clients with bipolar disorder and is also used for long-term prophylaxis against recurrent mania and depression
   b. Lithium is an inorganic ion that carries a single positive charge; it occurs naturally in animal tissue but has no known physiologic function; it is well-absorbed following oral administration and is distributed evenly to all tissue and body fluids
   c. Exact mechanism of action is not fully understood, but it alters many neurotransmitter functions; it may correct an ion exchange abnormality in neurons and/or may play a role in normalizing neurotransmission of norepinephrine, serotonin, dopamine, and acetylcholine
   d. Lithium is used to treat a variety of psychiatric disorders, particularly to treat effects of bipolar disorders (treatment of acute manic episodes and prophylaxis against recurrence)
2. Common medications: see Table 11-7
3. Administration considerations
   a. Precise dosing is based on serum lithium levels; 300 mg lithium carbonate contains 8–12 mEq lithium; follow prescriber instructions for dosing ranges of adults and children
   b. Lithium reduces euphoria, hyperactivity, and other symptoms of mania but does not cause sedation; mood stabilizing effects are usually seen in 5–7 days after initial doses, but full effect does not usually occur for 2–3 weeks
   c. For many clients using lithium, adjunctive therapy with a benzodiazepine can be used to provide the sedation clients need
   d. Antipsychotic medications can also be used short term to rapidly decrease symptoms of psychoses
4. Contraindications
   a. Hypersensitivity to drug, dehydration, and severe cardiovascular or renal disease; it should only be used where therapy (including blood levels) may be closely monitored; some products contain alcohol or tartrazine and should be avoided in clients with known hypersensitivity or intolerance
   b. Use cautiously in elderly or debilitated clients (decrease initial dose); also use cautiously with clients with cardiac, renal, or thyroid disease, or diabetes mellitus
5. Significant drug interactions
   a. Lithium may prolong action of neuromuscular blocking agents
   b. Neurologic toxicity may occur with haloperidol or molindone
   c. Diuretics, methyldopa, probenecid, fluoxetine, and NSAIDs may increase risk of toxicity
   d. Blood levels may be increased by angiotensin-converting enzyme (ACE) inhibitors

Table 11-7 **Commonly Used Mood-Stabilizing Drugs**

Generic (Trade) Names	Uses
Lithium carbonate (Eskalith, Lithobid)	Manic-depressive episodes, maintenance therapy for manic-depression, improvement of neutrophil counts in client receiving chemotherapy, prophylaxis of cluster headaches, hypothyroidism
Carbamazepine (Tegretol)	Seizure disorders, trigeminal neuralgia, chronic pain
Valproic acid (Depakene)	Seizure disorders, bipolar mania, prophylaxis for migraine headaches, schizophrenia, aggressive outbursts, attention deficit disorder, organic brain syndrome

  e. Lithium may decrease effects of chlorpromazine, and chlorpromazine may mask early signs of lithium toxicity

  f. Hypothyroid effects may be additive with potassium iodide or antithyroid agents

  g. Aminophylline, phenothiazines, and drugs containing large amounts of sodium increase renal elimination and may decrease effectiveness

6. Significant food interactions: large changes in sodium intake may alter renal elimination of lithium; increasing sodium intake will increase renal excretion

7. Significant laboratory studies

  a. Monitor serum lithium levels frequently because of danger of lithium toxicity, especially since therapeutic level and toxic level are very close; therapeutic range is 0.8 to 1.4 mEq/L, while toxic level is 1.5 mEq/L or greater

  b. Pre-lithium work-up

   1) Renal: urinalysis, blood urea, nitrogen (BUN), creatinine, electrolytes, 24-hour creatinine clearance

   2) Thyroid: thyroid-stimulating hormone (TSH), T_4 (thyroxine), T_3 resin uptake, T_4I (free thyroxine index)

   3) Other: fasting blood glucose, complete blood count (CBC), ECG

  c. Maintenance lithium dosing: lithium level every 3 months (for first 6 months); every 6 months reassess thyroid function and ECG; assess more often if client is symptomatic

8. Side effects

  a. Seizures, fatigue, headache, impaired memory, ataxia, confusion, dizziness, drowsiness, psychomotor retardation, restlessness, stupor

  b. Also aphasia, blurred vision, dysarthria, tinnitus, arrhythmias, ECG changes, edema, hypotension

  c. Others include abdominal pain, anorexia, bloating, diarrhea, nausea, dry mouth, and metallic taste in the mouth; also polyuria, glycosuria, nephrogenic diabetes insipidus, and renal toxicity

  d. Dermatological signs include alopecia, diminished sensation, and pruritis

  e. Also reported are hypothyroidism, goiter, hyperglycemia and hyperthyroidism, hyponatremia, leukocytosis, weight gain, muscle weakness, hyperirritability, rigidity, and tremors

9. Adverse effects/toxicity

  a. Lithium has a short half-life and high toxicity; is excreted by kidneys; sodium depletion will decrease renal excretion of lithium, which in turn will cause drug to accumulate and lead to lithium toxicity

  b. Other adverse effects with therapeutic doses include fine hand tremors, GI upset, thirst, muscle weakness; at toxic levels more adverse effects are seen, such as persistent GI upset, coarse hand tremor, confusion, hyperirritability of muscles, ECG changes, sedation, incoordination; at serum levels greater than 2.5 mEq/L, death may result

10. Nursing considerations

  a. Assess mood, ideation, and behaviors frequently; initiate suicide precautions if indicated

  b. Monitor intake and output ratios; report significant changes in totals

  c. Unless contraindicated, provide fluid intake of at least 2,000–3,000 mL/day

  d. Monitor weight at least every 3 months

  e. Assess client for signs and symptoms of lithium toxicity (vomiting, diarrhea, slurred speech, decreased coordination, drowsiness, muscle weakness, or twitching); if these occur, report before giving next dose

11. Client education

 a. Take medication exactly as directed, even if feeling well; take a missed dose as soon as remembered unless within 2 hours of next dose (6 hours if extended-release preparation used)

 b. Medication may cause dizziness or drowsiness; avoid driving, operating heavy machinery, or other activities requiring alertness until response to medication is known

 c. Low sodium levels may predispose client to toxicity; drink 2,000 to 3,000 mL fluid each day and eat a diet with consistent and moderate sodium intake to keep lithium levels stable

d. Avoid excessive amounts of coffee, tea, and cola (because of diuretic effect); avoid activities that cause excess sodium loss; notify prescriber of fever, vomiting, and diarrhea, which also cause sodium loss, and correct dehydration quickly

e. Advise client that weight gain may occur; review principles of a low-calorie diet with client

 f. Consult with prescriber before taking any OTC medications, before use of contraception, or if pregnancy is suspected

g. Review side effects and toxicity effects of medication and instruct client to report any of these to a prescriber promptly

 h. Explain to clients with cardiovascular disease or over 40 years of age the need of ECG evaluation before and periodically during therapy; report any irregular pulse, difficulty breathing, or if fainting occurs

B. Other mood stabilizing medications

1. Action and use

a. A variety of antiepileptic drugs have beneficial effects in treating bipolar disorder when lithium is ineffective, although they do not have FDA approval for this use

b. The two such medications presented here include carbamazepine (Tegretol) and valproic acid (e.g., Valproate, Depakote); they have acute antimanic and long-term mood-stabilizing effects in some clients with bipolar disorder; they are also better than lithium in treating mixed or dysphoric bipolar states and in clients who are rapid cyclers

c. When given to clients who have failed to respond to lithium, carbamazepine has had a success rate of about 60%; for treatment of acute manic episodes the mechanism by which carbamazepine stabilizes mood is unknown

d. Clinical studies indicate that valproic acid can control symptoms in acute manic episodes of mania and depression; it alters GABA-mediated neurotransmission, and this action may underlie the drug's mood-stabilizing effects

2. Common medications (refer again to Table 11-7)

3. Administration considerations

a. Carbamazepine should be started using low initial dose and then gradually increased

b. Valproic acid for treatment of acute mania is given in 2–4 divided doses initially

4. Contraindications

a. Carbamazepine is contraindicated with hypersensitivity to drug or bone marrow depression; it should be used only in pregnancy if potential benefits outweigh risks to fetus; it should be used cautiously in clients with cardiac or hepatic disease, prostatic hyperplasia, or increased intraocular pressure

b. Valproic acid is contraindicated in clients with hypersensitivity or with hepatic impairment; it should not be used with products containing tartrazine; it should be used cautiously in clients with bleeding disorders, history of liver disease, organic brain disease, bone marrow depression, renal impairment, and by children (increased risk of hepatotoxicity); safe use in pregnancy has not been established

5. Significant drug interactions

    a. Carbamazepine may decrease levels and effectiveness of corticosteroids, doxycycline, felbamate, quinidine, warfarin, oral contraceptives, barbiturates, cyclosporine, benzodiazepines, theophylline, lamotrigine, valproic acid, bupropion, and haloperidol; danazol increases blood levels; concurrent use (within 2 weeks) of MAO inhibitors may result in hyperpyrexia, hypertension, seizures, and death; verapamil, diltiazem, propoxyphene, erythromycin (should not be prescribed), clarithromycin, SSRI antidepressants, or cimetidine increases levels and may cause toxicity; may increase risk of hepatotoxicity from isoniazid; felbamate decreases carbamazepine levels but increases levels of active metabolite

    b. Carbamazepine may decrease effectiveness and increase risk of toxicity from acetaminophen, increase risk of CNS toxicity from lithium, and decrease duration of action of nondepolarizing neuromuscular blocking agents

    c. Significant drug–drug interactions for valproic acid include an increased risk of bleeding with antiplatelet agents (including aspirin, NSAIDs, tirofiban, eptifibatide, and abciximab), cefamandole, cefoperazone, cefotetan, heparin and heparin-like agents, thrombolytic agents, or warfarin; there is a decreased metabolism of barbiturates and primidone, which increases the risk for toxicity; blood levels and toxicity may be increased by carbamazepine, cimetidine, erythromycin, or felbamate; additive CNS depression with other CNS depressants, including alcohol, antihistamines, antidepressants, opioids, MAOIs, and sedative–hypnotics

    d. Large doses of salicylates (in children) increase effects of valproic acid; it may also increase or decrease effects and toxicity of phenytoin; MAOIs and other antidepressants may also lower seizure threshold and decrease effectiveness of valproates

    e. Carbamazepine, rifampin, or lamotrigine may decrease valproic acid blood levels; valproic acid may increase toxicity of carbamazepine, ethosuximide, lamotrigine, or zidovudine

6. Significant food interactions: none reported for either agent

7. Significant laboratory studies

    a. For clients receiving carbamazepine, target trough plasma levels are 6–12 mcg/mL

    b. Routine CBC, including platelet count, reticulocyte count, and serum iron should be checked weekly during first 2 months and yearly thereafter for evidence of potentially fatal blood cell abnormalities; drug should be discontinued if bone marrow depression occurs

    c. Target plasma drug level of valproic acid is 50–125 mcg/mL; clients receiving near the maximum recommended 60 mg/kg/day should be monitored for toxicity

    d. Also monitor hepatic function (LDH, AST, ALT, and bilirubin) and serum ammonia concentrations prior to and periodically during therapy with valproic acid (drug may cause hepatotoxicity); therapy should be discontinued if ammonia level becomes elevated

8. Side effects

    a. Common side effects for carbamazepine include sedation, GI disturbance, tremor, leukopenia, and hepatotoxicity

    b. Reported side effects for valproic acid include sedation, nausea, tremor, hepatotoxicity, and hair loss; nausea can be reduced by using delayed-release tablets or by applying "sprinkle" formulation to food

9. Adverse effects/toxicity

    a. Some adverse effects for carbamazepine include ataxia, drowsiness, agranulocytosis, aplastic anemia, thrombocytopenia, chills, fever, and lymphadenopathy

    b. For valproic acid some reported adverse effects include confusion, dizziness, headache, hepatotoxicity, indigestion, N/V, prolonged bleeding time, thrombocytopenia, ataxia, and paresthesia

   10. Nursing considerations
       a. Assess client frequently for seizure activity when taking carbamazepine and assess for facial pain because of possibility of trigeminal neuralgia
       b. Perform liver function tests, urinalysis, and BUN routinely and measure serum ionized calcium levels at least every 6 months or if seizure frequency increases
       c. Implement seizure precautions as indicated; administer dose with food to minimize gastric irritation; tablets may be crushed if client has difficulty swallowing—except for extended-release tablets
   11. Client education
       a. Take carbamazepine around the clock, exactly as directed; if a dose is missed, take as soon as possible but not just before next dose is due; drug should be gradually decreased to prevent seizures
       b. Report fever, sore throat, mouth ulcers, easy bruising, petechiae, unusual bleeding, abdominal pain, chills, rash, pale stools, dark urine, or jaundice to prescriber immediately
       c. Use sunscreen and protective clothing to prevent photosensitivity reactions with carbamazepine
       d. Female clients should use a nonhormonal form of contraception while taking carbamazepine
       e. Avoid activities requiring alertness; carbamazepine and valproic acid may cause dizziness or drowsiness
       f. Do not concurrently use alcohol, other CNS depressants or OTC drugs with either of these drugs without consulting prescriber first
       g. Carry information (such as a MedicAlert tag or bracelet) describing disease and medication regimen at all times
       h. Notify health care professional of drug regimen before any treatment or surgery
       i. Compliance with follow-up lab tests, eye exams, and ECGs is important
       j. Take valproic acid exactly as directed; if a dose is missed on a once-a-day schedule, take it as soon as remembered that day; if on a multiple-dose schedule, take it within 6 hours of scheduled time, then space remaining doses throughout remainder of the day; abrupt withdrawal may lead to seizures
       k. For clients taking valproic acid, notify prescriber if anorexia, severe N/V, yellow skin or eyes, fever, sore throat, malaise, weakness, facial edema, lethargy, unusual bleeding or bruising, pregnancy, or loss of seizure control occur; children less than age 2 years are especially at risk for fatal hepatotoxicity

IV. SEDATIVE–HYPNOTICS AND ANXIOLYTICS

A. Benzodiazepines
   1. Action and use
      a. Benzodiazepines (BZ) are thought to reduce anxiety because they are powerful potentiators (receptor agonists) of inhibitory neurotransmitter GABA
      b. A postsynaptic receptor site specific for BZ molecule is located next to GABA receptor; BZ molecule and GABA bind to each other at GABA receptor site, resulting in an *inhibition* of neurotransmission that results in a clinical decrease in anxiety level
      c. Most BZs are well absorbed following oral administration; because of their high lipid solubility, BZs readily cross blood–brain barrier to reach sites within CNS; most BZs undergo extensive metabolic alterations; with few exceptions, drug **metabolites** (result of drug biotransformation) are pharmacologically active so drug effects persist long after parent drug is gone from plasma (thus there may be poor correlation between plasma half-life of parent drug and duration of pharmacological effect)

Practice to Pass

The client is being discharged on lithium carbonate. What would be included in the teaching plan related to the client's medication regimen when at home?

!

    d. Major indications for use of BZs are anxiety, insomnia (sedative–hypnotic effect), and seizure disorders

    e. Other uses include alcohol withdrawal, anxiety associated with medical disease, skeletal muscle relaxation, preoperative anxiety and apprehension, substance-induced (except for amphetamines) and psychotic agitation in emergency departments or in other crisis situations; in higher doses alprazolam and clonazepam may effectively treat panic disorder and social phobia; other uses are to induce general anesthesia and to manage seizure disorders and muscle spasm

2. Common medications: see Table 11-8 for generic and trade names, dosage form, half-life, speed of onset, and approved use indications

    a. Benzodiazepines differ significantly with regard to course of action; specifically, they differ in onset of action, duration of action, and tendency to accumulate with repeated dosing

    b. Because all BZs have essentially equivalent pharmacologic actions, selection is based in large part on differences in pharmacokinetics

3. Administration considerations

    a. Benzodiazepines should be started at low doses and gradually increased as needed to achieve desired clinical response; there is a rapid onset of clinical action once an appropriate dose is achieved

Table 11-8   **Sedative–Hypnotic and Anxiolytic Medications**

Drug Class Generic and (Trade) Name	Dosage Forms	Half-Life (hr)	Speed of Onset (PO)	Approved Use Indication
Barbiturates				
Butabarbital (Butisol)	C	34–42	Short to intermediate	Hypnotic
Pentobarbital (Nembutal)	C	15–48	Long-acting	Hypnotic
Phenobarbital (Luminal)	C	80–120	Long-acting	Hypnotic
Secobarbital (Seconal)	C	15–40	Short to intermediate	Hypnotic
Benzodiazepines				
Alprazolam (Xanax)	T	12–15	Intermediate	A, AD, P
Chlordiazepoxide (Librium)	C, T, I	5–30	Intermediate	A, AW, PS
Clonazepam (Klonopin)	T	20–50	Intermediate	LGS
Clorazepate (Tranxene)	C, T, T-SR	20–80	Fast	A
Diazepam (Valium)	C-SR, T, L, I	20–80	Very fast	A, PS, SE
Lorazepam (Ativan)	T, I	10–20	Intermediate	A, PS
Oxazepam (Serax)	C, T	5–20	Intermediate to slow	A, AD, AW
Nonbarbiturate/nondiazepines				
Buspirone (Buspar)	T	2–4	Intermediate	A
Eszopiclone (Lunesta)	T	5–6	Fast	Insomnia
Zolpidem (Ambien)	T	1.5–4	Fast	Hypnotic
Benzodiazepine Antagonist				
Flumazenil (Romazicon)	I	—	Fast	R

Approved Use Indicators: A, anxiety; AD, anxiety associated with depression; AW, alcohol withdrawal; LGS, Lennox-Gastaut syndrome/seizures; P, panic disorder; PS, psychotic disorder; R, reverse moderate sedation or general anesthesia; SE, status epilepticus

Dosage Forms: C, capsule; C-SR, capsule, sustained-release; I, injection; L, oral, liquid; T, tablet; T-SR, tablet, sustained release

    b. In anxiety disorders, some anxiety reduction may be apparent almost immediately; antianxiety effect with initial dosing may not last as long as serum half-life would suggest because of drug redistributing out of the brain; with continued dosing, steady-state brain levels and sustained efficacy are achieved; for treatment of anxiety, BZs are usually dosed at bedtime or bid; only occasionally is tid dosing required

    c. For use as a hypnotic, BZs are rapidly absorbed, have a short onset of action, and a short elimination half-life, so that next-day sedation and impaired cognition are minimized (although clients may experience some sedation or "hangover effect" the next day)

    d. Treatment for insomnia should occur for as short a time as possible (not longer than 7–10 days), and should be used as an adjunct to help clients establish a regular sleep pattern along with improved sleep hygiene techniques; clients are at risk for rebound insomnia and anxiety if drugs are used for longer periods of time

  4. Contraindications

    a. BZs are contraindicated with drug sensitivity or during pregnancy or lactation because they cross blood–brain barrier and enter breast milk with ease (and develop quickly to toxic levels)

    b. BZs should not be used with clients with preexisting CNS depression, severe uncontrolled pain, or for clients with narrow-angle glaucoma

    c. BZs are readily absorbed after oral ingestion; however, intramuscular (IM) injection produces slow and inconsistent absorption for most of these drugs

    d. A convenient way of categorizing BZs is to divide them into those with short half-lives (less than 20 hours) and long half-lives (more than 20 hours) (see Table 11-8 for details); BZs with short half-life are usually preferable for use with older adult clients

    e. Because hepatic metabolism is primary mechanism for drug disposition, drugs that interfere with liver metabolism (e.g., alcohol) dangerously compound the effect of *benzodiazepines*

  5. Significant drug interactions

    a. CNS depressant actions of BZs are additive to those of other CNS depressants (e.g., alcohol, barbiturates, opioids), so although BZs are very safe when used alone, they can be extremely hazardous in combination with other depressants

      1) A combined overdose of a benzodiazepine with another CNS depressant can lead to profound respiratory depression, coma, and death

      2) Clients should be warned against use of alcohol and all other CNS depressants

    b. BZs are poorly absorbed when taken with antacids; disulfiram and cimetidine use increases plasma level of BZs that are oxidized; befazodone inhibits metabolism of alprazolam and triazolam while phenytoin increases anticonvulsant serum level; use of BZs with TCAs increases sedation, confusion, and impairs motor function; when used with MAOIs, CNS depression occurs, and succinylcholine decreases neuromuscular blockade

    c. With prolonged use of benzodiazepines, **tolerance** (increased need of drug to achieve the same effect) develops to some effects but not to others

      1) No tolerance develops to anxiolytic effects, and tolerance to hypnotic effects is generally low

      2) In contrast, significant tolerance develops to antiseizure effects

      3) Clients tolerant to barbiturates, alcohol, and other general CNS depressants show some cross-tolerance to benzodiazepines

      4) BZ can cause physical dependence, but incidence of substantial dependence is low (especially for clients taking alprazolam)

  6. Significant food interactions: none

      7. Significant laboratory studies: none unless a client is on long-term therapy with BZs; then CBC, liver, and renal function should be monitored

      8. Side effects

         a. Most common side effect is decreased mental alertness; caution clients against driving or using heavy or hazardous equipment

         b. Tolerance to most side effects quickly develops

         c. Monitor BP of inpatients routinely, withhold dose and report to prescriber a drop of 20 mmHg (systolic) while standing

         d. Other side effects include dry mouth, ataxia, dizziness, drowsiness, nausea, and withdrawal symptoms (increased anxiety, flulike symptoms, tremors)

      9. Adverse effects/toxicity: as stated earlier, use of BZs with other CNS depressants can cause fatal results; signs of overdose include somnolence, confusion, coma, diminished reflexes, and hypotension

     10. Nursing considerations

         a. Assess degree and manifestation of anxiety before client begins therapy

         b. Assess client for drowsiness, light-headedness, and dizziness periodically during treatment; these usually disappear as therapy progresses

         c. Always caution client about driving or operating hazardous machinery especially in early treatment with BZs

         d. Monitor BP, pulse, and respirations and provide supportive care as indicated

         e. Prolonged therapy may lead to psychological or physical dependence; risk is greater with larger drug doses; restrict amount of drug available to client

         f. Most BZs can be taken with food or crushed and put in food if client has difficulty swallowing

     11. Client education

         a. Take medications exactly as prescribed and do not skip or double up on missed doses; if a dose is missed, take within 1 hour or skip the dose and return to regular schedule

         b. If medication is less effective after a few weeks, check with prescriber; do not increase dose

         c. Abrupt drug withdrawal may cause sweating, vomiting, muscle cramps, tremors, and seizures

         d. Avoid use of alcohol or other CNS depressants concurrently with BZ therapy

B. Benzodiazepine antagonist

      1. Action and use

         a. Flumazenil (Romazicon) is a BZ antagonist (receptor blocker); it selectively blocks BZ receptors but does not block adrenergic or cholinergic receptors

         b. In other words, it can reverse the *sedative* effects of BZs but may not reverse BZ-induced *respiratory depression*

         c. Because it does not stimulate CNS and does not block other receptors, it can be given when BZ overdose is suspected and can also be used to reverse effects of BZs following general anesthesia

         d. A reaction occurs within 30–60 seconds after administration

      2. Common medications: flumazenil is the only drug in this class

      3. Administration considerations

         a. It does not speed up the metabolism or excretion of BZs and has a short duration of action, which poses a clinical management problem; if client responds to flumazenil, then BZs are present, but client may need vigilant, ongoing dosing and monitoring as body eliminates BZs

         b. Administration is IV: inject dose slowly over 30 seconds and repeat every minute as needed; first dose is 0.2 mg, second is 0.3 mg, and all subsequent doses are 0.5 mg; effects fade in approximately 1 hour, so additional dosing may be needed

    c. In children, 0.01 mg/kg (up to 0.2 mg); if desired level of consciousness (LOC) is not obtained after waiting an additional 45 seconds, further injections of 0.01 mg/kg can be given and repeated at 60-second intervals when necessary (up to a maximum of 4 additional times)

  4. Contraindications

    a. Hypersensitivity; clients receiving BZs for life-threatening medical problems, including status epilepticus or increased intracranial pressure; clients with serious TCA overdose

    b. Use cautiously in clients with mixed CNS depressant overdose, with history of seizures, or clients with head injury; safety has not been established for use during pregnancy, lactation, or in children less than 2 years old

  5. Significant drug interactions: none noted

  6. Significant food interactions: none noted

  7. Significant laboratory studies: none

  8. Side effects: minor side and adverse effects include dizziness, agitation, confusion, N/V, hiccups, paresthesia, rigors, and shivering

  9. Adverse effects/toxicity: principle adverse effect is precipitation of seizures, which is most likely to occur in clients taking BZs to treat epilepsy or who are physically dependent on BZs

  10. Nursing considerations

    a. Assess LOC and respiratory status before and throughout therapy

    b. Establish that client has a patent airway before administering flumazenil

    c. Observe IV site frequently for redness or irritation; give drug through a free-flowing IV infusion into a large vein to minimize pain at injection site

    d. Institute seizure precautions; seizures are more likely to occur in clients experiencing sedative–hypnotic withdrawal, who have recently received repeated doses of BZs, or who have a previous history of seizure activity; seizures may be treated with BZs, barbiturates, or phenytoin (larger than normal doses of BZs may be required)

    e. For suspected BZ overdose: if no effects are seen after giving flumazenil, consider other causes of decreased LOC (alcohol, barbiturates, opioid analgesics)

    f. Observe client for at least 2 hours after giving last dose for reappearance of sedation; hypoventilation may occur

  11. Client education

    a. Flumazenil does not consistently reverse amnesic effects of BZs; provide client and family with written instructions for postprocedure care

    b. Client may appear alert at time of discharge but sedative effects of BZs may reoccur; avoid driving or other activities requiring alertness for at least 24 hours after discharge

    c. Do not take *any* alcohol or nonprescription drugs for at least 18–24 hours after discharge

    d. Resume usual activities only when no residual effects of BZs remain

C. Barbiturates

  1. Action and use

    a. Like BZs, barbiturates bind to GABA receptor-chloride channel complex to enhance inhibitory actions of GABA and directly mimic actions of GABA; since barbiturates can directly mimic GABA, there is no ceiling to degree of CNS depression they can produce and, unlike BZs, they can readily cause death when taken in overdose

    b. Barbiturates cause relatively nonselective depression of CNS function and are prototypes of general CNS depressants; because they depress multiple aspects of CNS function, they can be used for daytime sedation, induction of sleep, suppression of seizures, and general anesthesia

!

    c. Barbiturates can cause tolerance and dependence, have a high abuse potential, and are subject to multiple drug interactions; they are powerful respiratory depressants that can readily prove fatal in overdose as well; because of these effects, they have been often been replaced by safer drugs such as the BZs

    d. Barbiturates can be grouped into three classes, based on duration of action: (1) ultrashort-acting agents, (2) short- to intermediate-acting agents, and (3) long-acting agents; duration of action is inversely related to their lipid solubility; barbiturates with highest lipid solubility have shortest duration of action; conversely, barbiturates with lowest lipid solubility have longest duration

2. Common medications (see Table 11-8)

3. Administration considerations

    a. Barbiturates are administered orally usually for daytime sedation and to treat insomnia; for general anesthesia and emergency treatment of seizures, they are usually given by IV injection; barbiturate solutions are highly alkaline and can cause pain and necrosis when injected IM, so this route is generally avoided

    b. Ability to cause generalized CNS depression underlies both therapeutic and adverse effects; as dosage is increased, responses progress from *sedation* to *sleep* to *general anesthesia*

    c. Most barbiturates can be considered nonselective CNS depressants; exceptions are phenobarbital and other barbiturates used to control seizures

    d. At hypnotic doses, barbiturates may reduce BP and heart rate; by contrast, toxic doses can cause profound hypotension and shock (from direct depressant effects on both myocardium and vascular smooth muscle)

    e. Barbiturates stimulate synthesis of hepatic microsomal enzymes (principal drug-metabolizing enzymes of liver); as a result, barbiturates can accelerate their own metabolism as well as metabolism of many other drugs

    f. Tolerance develops with repeated drug use; when taken regularly, tolerance develops to many (but not all) CNS effects; specifically, tolerance develops to sedative and hypnotic effects and to other effects that underlie barbiturate abuse

4. Contraindications: hypersensitivity, clients with overt or latent porphyria, severe hepatic/renal/respiratory dysfunction, or previous addiction to sedative–hypnotics

5. Significant drug interactions

!

    a. Drugs with CNS-depressant properties (e.g., barbiturates, benzodiazepines, alcohol, opioids, antihistamines) intensify each other's effects; if these drugs are combined, additive CNS depression can be hazardous or even fatal; warn clients emphatically not to combine barbiturates with alcohol and other CNS depressants

    b. Because barbiturates stimulate synthesis of hepatic drug-metabolizing enzymes and accelerate metabolism of other drugs, doses of *warfarin* (an anticoagulant), *oral contraceptives*, and *phenytoin* (an antiseizure agent) should be increased to account for accelerated degradation; once drug dosages are increased, they need to be gradually reregulated once barbiturate treatment ends to their previous amounts; barbiturates must be tapered and not stopped abruptly

6. Significant food interactions: none

7. Significant laboratory studies: clients on prolonged therapy (e.g., antiseizure therapy) should have hepatic and renal function and CBC evaluated periodically; also see individual agents for specific laboratory tests

8. Side effects

    a. Barbiturates have long half-lives and therefore can produce residual effects (hangover) when taken to treat insomnia; hangover can manifest as sedation, impaired judgment, and reduced motor skills; another possible effect is paradoxical excitement (especially in older adult and debilitated clients); the mechanism of this response is not known

      b. Barbiturates can intensify sensitivity to pain and may cause pain directly; their use has produced muscle pain, joint pain, and pain along nerves

  9. Adverse effects/toxicity

      a. Acute intoxication with barbiturates is a medical emergency; left untreated, overdose can be fatal; poisoning often results from attempted suicide, although it can occur by accident (usually in children or drug abusers)

      b. Acute barbiturate overdose produces a classic triad of symptoms: *respiratory depression*, *coma*, and *pinpoint pupils*, which are frequently accompanied by *hypotension* and *hypothermia*; death is likely to result from pulmonary complications and renal failure

      c. Proper management usually requires admission to an intensive care unit; barbiturate poisoning has no specific antidote, so treatment usually includes gastric lavage, induction of emesis, and use of a cathartic (to reduce absorption by accelerating drug transit through intestine); hemodialysis can remove drug that is already absorbed; forced diuresis and alkalinization of urine may facilitate drug removal via kidneys

  10. Nursing considerations

      a. With clients taking barbiturates, *always monitor respiratory status, pulse, and BP frequently*

      b. Prolonged therapy may lead to psychological or physical dependence; restrict amount of drug available to client, especially if depressed, suicidal, or with a history of addiction

      c. Always monitor client for safety, alertness, and need for help with ambulation or self-care

  11. Client education

      a. Take drug exactly as prescribed and do not discontinue without consulting prescriber

      b. May cause daytime drowsiness; avoid driving and other activities requiring alertness until response to drug is known

      c. Female clients using oral contraceptives should use an additional nonhormonal contraceptive during therapy

      d. Contact prescriber immediately if adverse or toxic signs or symptoms occur

D. Other sedative–hypnotics and anxiolytics

  1. Action and use

      a. Buspirone (BuSpar) and zolpidem (Ambien) are two sedative–hypnotics/anxiolytics that are not barbiturates or BZs

      b. Buspirone is indicated for management of anxiety; it binds to serotonin and dopamine receptors in brain and increases norepinephrine metabolism in brain; 95% of drug is bound to plasma proteins; it is extensively metabolized by liver and 20–40% is excreted in feces

      c. Buspirone differs from other anxiolytics because it reduces anxiety while producing even less sedation than BZs; its mechanism of action is unknown; major advantages are that it does not cause sedation, has no abuse potential, and does not enhance CNS depression caused by BZs, alcohol, barbiturates, and related drugs; its major disadvantage is that onset of anxiolytic effects is delayed

      d. Zolpidem is used for the short-term treatment of insomnia; it produces CNS depression by binding to GABA receptors; it has no analgesic properties, but produces sedation and induction of sleep; it is rapidly absorbed following oral administration and 92% binds to protein; is converted to inactive metabolites that are excreted by kidneys

  2. Common medications (refer again to Table 11-8)

3. Administration considerations
   a. Buspirone is well absorbed following oral dosing but undergoes extensive first-pass metabolism in liver; giving it with food delays absorption but enhances bioavailability (by reducing first-pass metabolism)
   b. Zolpidem is rapidly absorbed following oral administration and is usually given orally just before bedtime because of its rapid onset of action
4. Contraindications
   a. Buspirone and zolpidem are contraindicated for clients with a hypersensitivity to drug
   b. Buspirone is also contraindicated in severe hepatic or renal impairment and should be used cautiously in clients receiving other antianxiety agents; slowly withdraw other agents to prevent rebound phenomenon; use cautiously for clients receiving other psychoactive drugs or who are pregnant or lactating; also use cautiously with children because safety has not yet been established
   c. Zolpidem should not be used for clients with apnea; it should be used cautiously in clients with a history of previous psychiatric illness, suicide attempt, drug or alcohol abuse, impaired hepatic function or pulmonary disease, older adults, pregnant or lactating women, and children (safety has not yet been established)
5. Significant drug interactions
   a. Buspirone interacts with MAOIs, which may result in hypertension; there may be an increased risk for hepatic effects when used with trazodone; blood levels are increased with concurrent use with itraconazole or erythromycin; avoid concurrent use with alcohol
   b. For zolpidem, additive CNS depression can occur with concurrent use of other sedative–hypnotics, alcohol, phenothiazines, TCAs, opioids, or antihistamines
6. Significant food interactions: none reported with buspirone while food decreases and delays absorption of zolpidem
7. Significant laboratory studies: none since they are indicated for short-term use only
8. Side effects
   a. Buspirone is generally well tolerated; most common reactions are dizziness, nausea, headache, nervousness, light-headedness, and excitement
   b. Zolpidem has a side effect profile similar to BZs; daytime drowsiness and dizziness are most common, but only occur in about 1–2% of clients
9. Adverse effects/toxicity
   a. Buspirone is nonsedating and does not interfere with daytime activities and poses little to no risk of suicide; does not enhance depressant effects of alcohol, barbiturates, and other general CNS depressants
   b. Zolpidem is not usually associated with tolerance, dependence, or abuse because it is used for short-term treatment only, but (like other sedative–hypnotics) it can intensify effects of CNS depressants; warn clients not to combine zolpidem with alcohol or other CNS depressants
10. Nursing considerations
    a. Assess degree and manifestations of anxiety before and periodically during therapy with buspirone
    b. Buspirone does not appear to cause physical or psychological dependence or tolerance; however, clients with a history of drug abuse should be assessed for tolerance or dependence—amount of drug available to these clients should be restricted
    c. Clients changing from other antianxiety agents should receive gradually decreasing doses; buspirone will not prevent withdrawal symptoms
    d. With zolpidem, there may be a potential for physical or psychological dependence if used longer than 7–10 days; limit amount of drug available to client

!

Practice to Pass

A 72-year-old client is in the clinic today with his daughter because his wife died 1 month ago and he must move to an assisted-living apartment, being unable to live alone. The physician prescribes lorazepam (Ativan) 0.5 mg bid in the morning and at bedtime. Identify at least 3 side effects of Ativan to teach this client.

!

    e. For clients taking zolpidem, assess alertness at time of peak effect; notify prescriber if desired sedation does not occur

    f. Assess client who has pain and medicate as needed; untreated pain decreases sedative effects of zolpidem

  11. Client education

    a. As with all medications, take exactly as prescribed

    b. Buspirone and zolpidem may cause dizziness or drowsiness; avoid driving or other activities requiring alertness until response to medication is known

    c. Avoid concurrent use of buspirone and zolpidem and alcohol or other CNS depressants

    d. Do not take OTC medications without consulting prescriber

    e. With buspirone, report any chronic abnormal movements such as **dystonia** (muscle rigidity), motor restlessness, involuntary movements of facial or cervical muscles, or if pregnancy is suspected

    f. With zolpidem, go to bed immediately after taking dose because of rapid onset of action

    g. Follow-up exams are important to determine drug effectiveness

V. SUBSTANCE MISUSE

A. Alcohol

  1. Action and use

    a. Alcohol is a CNS depressant and, like barbiturates, it causes general (relatively nonselective) depression of CNS function

    b. Alcohol appears to affect CNS primarily by enhancing actions of GABA

    c. Effect of alcohol on CNS is dose dependent

      1) When dosage is low, higher brain centers (cortical areas) are primarily affected

      2) As dosage is increased, more primitive brain areas (e.g., medulla) become depressed

      3) With depression of cortical function, thought processes and learned behaviors are altered, inhibitions are released, and self-restraint is replaced by increased sociability and expansiveness; cortical depression also results in significant impairment of motor function; as CNS depression deepens, reflexes diminish greatly and consciousness becomes impaired

      4) At very high doses, alcohol produces a state of general anesthesia

    d. Tolerance to alcohol increases with alcohol use; abuse and addiction progress over time

    e. Management of withdrawal depends on degree of alcohol dependence; when dependence is mild, withdrawal can be accomplished on an outpatient basis; when dependence is great, risks of withdrawal can be fatal if medical intervention is not carried out

    f. The major objective of medically supervised withdrawal is safe and effective removal of alcohol and/or other drugs; most medical treatment includes use of BZs—chlordiazepoxide (Librium), diazepam (Valium), and lorazepam (Ativan) have been used safely; a regime of atenolol (a beta-adrenergic blocking agent) used in conjunction with BZs decreases dose of BZs necessary for safe detoxification

    g. Disulfiram is an inhibitor of enzyme *alcohol dehydrogenase*, which catalyzes a major step in breakdown of alcohol

      1) When enzyme is inhibited and client drinks alcohol, blood concentrations of toxic metabolite *acetaldehyde* increase significantly

      2) Acetaldehyde produces unpleasant symptoms of flushing, tachycardia, N/V, and hypotension

       3) In medically fragile clients, these symptoms may rarely prove life-threatening; because of associated risks, disulfiram is used only with highly selected clients in good physical health

    h. Acamprosate (Campral) interacts with CNS glutamate and GABA neurotransmitter systems to restore normal balance between excitation and inhibition of neurons

       1) Reduces alcohol cravings but without disulfiram-like reaction or alcohol aversion

       2) Used to maintain abstinence from alcohol in clients with alcoholism

2. Common medications: disulfiram (Antabuse) is the only alcohol antagonist in use; acamprosate (Campral) balances neurotransmitters to lessen alcohol craving

3. Administration considerations

    a. Disulfiram (Antabuse)

       1) Disulfiram maintenance can significantly reduce drinking; dose is typically 500 mg daily for 1–2 weeks; maintenance dosages range from 125–500 mg a day, usually taken as a single dose in the morning

       2) At least 12 hours should elapse from time of last alcohol intake and initial dose of disulfiram

       3) The relatively long half-life of disulfiram ensures that several days must elapse between stopping drug and safely drinking alcohol; this long half-life probably decreases likelihood of impulsive relapse

    b. Acamprosate (Campral)

       1) Indicated for clients with alcohol dependence but who are abstinent when treatment begins

       2) Intended to decrease alcohol cravings and significantly lowers rate of relapse

4. Contraindications: because of severity of acetaldehyde syndrome, candidates for therapy must be carefully chosen; those who lack determination to stop drinking should not be given disulfiram

5. Significant drug interactions

    a. Disulfiram causes irreversible inhibition of aldehyde dehydrogenase, the enzyme that converts acetaldehyde to acetic acid; adverse effects caused by alcohol plus disulfiram are collectively known as the *acetaldehyde syndrome*

    b. Acamprosate has no known drug interactions

6. Significant food interactions: none

7. Significant laboratory studies: obtain creatinine clearance before initiating acamprosate

8. Side effects: in absence of alcohol, disulfiram rarely causes significant effects; drowsiness and skin eruptions may occur during initial use but diminish with time

9. Adverse effects/toxicity: acetaldehyde syndrome is manifested by marked respiratory depression, cardiovascular collapse, cardiac dysrhythmias, myocardial infarction, acute congestive heart failure, convulsions, and death

10. Nursing considerations

    a. As with all medications advise client to take medication as prescribed

    b. Advise client that simultaneous use with alcohol can precipitate acetaldehyde syndrome

    c. Advise client that effects of disulfiram may persist for about 2 weeks after last dose is taken; alcohol must not be consumed until this interval is over

    d. Notify prescriber of alcohol use while taking acamprosate

11. Client education

    a. Avoid all forms of alcohol, including alcohol found in sauces and cough and cold syrups, and in after-shave lotions, colognes, and liniments

    b. Adhere to all forms of self-help groups (individual and group therapies), while using therapy to establish a recovery program

B. Opioids

1. Opioids (e.g., morphine, heroin) are major drugs of abuse and are usually Schedule II substances
2. Opioid abuse may be found in all segments of American society
3. For most abusers, initial exposure to opioids occurs either socially (illicitly) or in the context of pain management in a medical setting; only a very small percentage of those who develop an addictive pattern begin use therapeutically

 4. Opioid abuse by health care providers deserves special consideration; physicians, nurses, and pharmacists, as a group, abuse opioids to a greater extent than all other groups with similar educational backgrounds, and this is believed to be primarily the result of drug access
5. Tolerance develops with prolonged opioid use; persons tolerant to one opioid are cross-tolerant to other opioids; however, there is no cross-tolerance between opioids and general CNS depressants (e.g., barbiturates, benzodiazepines, alcohol)
6. Physical dependence is substantial with long-term use, but although opioid withdrawal syndrome can be extremely unpleasant, it is rarely dangerous
7. Opioid toxicity produces a classic triad of symptoms: respiratory depression, coma, and pinpoint pupils; withdrawal symptoms begin 6–8 hours after last dose and reach peak intensity within 48–72 hours, including craving, chills, sweating and piloerection (gooseflesh), abdominal pain and cramps, diarrhea, runny nose, and irritability
8. Naloxone (Narcan), an opioid antagonist, is the treatment of choice; it rapidly reverses all signs of opioid poisoning; dosage must be titrated carefully because excess dose can move client from a state of intoxication to one of withdrawal; because of its short half-life, naloxone must be given again every few hours until opioid has dropped to a nontoxic level
9. Nalmefene (Revex), a long-acting opioid antagonist, is an alternative to naloxone; because of its long half-life, nalmefene does not require repeated dosing; however, if dose is excessive in an opioid-dependent person, then nalmefene will put client into prolonged withdrawal
10. Methadone, an oral opioid with a long duration of action, is the agent most commonly used for easing opioid withdrawal and preventing abstinence syndrome; once stabilized on methadone, withdrawal is accomplished by administering it in gradually smaller doses; the resultant abstinence syndrome is mild, with symptoms resembling those of moderate influenza; entire process of methadone substitution and withdrawal takes about 10 days; objective of maintenance therapy is to avoid withdrawal and need to procure illicit drugs; methadone maintenance is most effective when done in conjunction with nondrug measures directed at altering patterns of drug use

C. Cocaine

1. Cocaine, extracted from coca plant, is a fine, white, odorless powder; cocaine and its offspring, crack, have caused major drug problems in the United States
2. Cocaine crosses blood–brain barrier readily, which causes an instantaneous high; when administered IV (mainlining) it is rapidly metabolized by liver, so the exhilarating "rush" does not last long; cocaine exerts both CNS and peripheral nervous system (PNS) effects because of its ability to block norepinephrine and dopamine reuptake into presynaptic neurons; it depletes these neurotransmitters
3. Cocaine can be taken orally but is poorly absorbed and has little effect by this route; it is also "snorted" (absorbed through nasal mucosa) or mixed with baking soda and ether and smoked (called *freebasing*, probably the most dangerous method of ingesting cocaine); crack is a less expensive way of using cocaine than snorting or mainlining, primarily because it is sold and marketed in smaller packages ($10 or $20 "rocks"); crack is used at every level in society, is reported to be the most addictive street drug today, and risk for overdose is extremely high; although physical dependence is less than with opioid abuse, psychological dependence is intense

4. Death from cocaine is linked to metabolic and respiratory acidosis and hyperthermia associated with prolonged seizures; tachydysrhythmias have also led to death

5. Although cocaine is highly addictive, physical withdrawal is relatively mild; psychological withdrawal is severe because drug is so pleasurable and causes an intense craving for drug; treatment is aimed at restoring depleted neurotransmitters; amino acid catecholamine precursors (such as tyrosine and phenylalanine), TCAs, and the dopamine agonist bromocriptine are 3 approaches used to increase availability of neurotransmitters

D. Cannabis (marijuana/hashish)

1. Marijuana (most widely used illegal drug in United States) is derived from Indian hemp plant *Cannabis sativa*, which has separate male and female forms; 2 most common cannabis derivatives are marijuana and hashish; major psychoactive substance in *Cannabis sativa* is delta-9-tetrahydrocannabinol (THC), which is an oily chemical with high lipid solubility

2. THC has several possible mechanisms, including activation of specific cannabinoid receptors found in various brain regions; when marijuana or hashish is smoked, about 60% of THC content is absorbed; absorption from lungs is rapid; subjective effects begin in minutes and peak in 20–30 minutes; effects from a single marijuana cigarette may persist 2–3 hours; with oral administration, absorption is only 6–20%

3. Marijuana produces 3 principal subjective effects: euphoria, sedation, and hallucinations; no other psychoactive drug produces all 3 of these; because of this singular pattern of effects, marijuana is in a class by itself

   a. Responses to low doses of THC are variable and depend on several factors including dosage size, route of administration, setting of drug use, and expectations and previous experience of user

   b. More common effects of low-dose THC include euphoria and relaxation; gaiety and a heightened sense of humor; an increased sensitivity to visual and auditory stimuli; enhanced sense of touch, taste, and smell; increased appetite and a more intense appreciation of flavor of food; distortion of time (seems to pass more slowly)

   c. Some undesirable effects of low-dose THC include impairment of short-term memory; decreased capacity to perform multiple tasks; decreased ability to drive or operate machinery; inability to distinguish time (past, present, and future); depersonalization (a sense of feeling strange about self); a decreased ability to distinguish emotions of others and reduced interpersonal interactions

   d. In higher doses, marijuana can have serious adverse psychological effects including hallucinations, delusions, and paranoia; euphoria may be replaced by intense anxiety and a dissociative state in which user feels "outside of him- or herself"

   e. In extremely high doses, marijuana can produce a state resembling toxic psychosis, which may persist for weeks; also dangerous is the use of marijuana with alcohol or other CNS depressants

4. Chronic marijuana use can produce a syndrome known as *amotivational syndrome*, characterized by apathy, dullness, poor grooming, reduced interest in achievement, and disinterest in pursuit of conventional goals

5. Other effects of marijuana include change in heart rate, orthostatic hypotension, pronounced reddening of conjunctivae, and—when used acutely—respiratory bronchodilation; when smoked chronically, effects such as bronchitis, sinusitis, and asthma can be seen; scientists believe carcinogens in marijuana smoke are more potent than tar from cigarettes

6. When used in extremely high doses, marijuana is able to produce tolerance and physical dependence; abrupt discontinuation of marijuana can lead to irritability, restlessness, nervousness, insomnia, reduced appetite, and weight loss; tremor, hyperthermia, and chills may also occur but these symptoms usually subside in 4–5 days and no symptoms of withdrawal are noted

7. Cannabinoids are sometimes used to treat N/V (more effectively than traditional antiemetics) that occur as severe side effects of cancer chemotherapy; THC has been approved for stimulating appetite in clients with AIDS

E. **Hallucinogens**

1. Use of hallucinogens, also called psychedelics or psychotomimetics, is rising again, especially among young people; these drugs alter perception; there are two basic groups of hallucinogens—natural and synthetic; see Table 11-9 for examples of hallucinogens

2. Hallucinogens can heighten awareness of reality or cause a terrifying psychosis-like reaction; users report distortions in body image, a sense of depersonalization, and/or a frightening loss of sense of reality; they have also reported seeing grotesque creatures; emotional consequences are panic, anxiety, confusion, and paranoid reactions; users have experienced frank psychotic reactions after minimal use, sometimes referred to as a "bad trip"; two most commonly used hallucinogens, LSD and PCP, are discussed here:

   a. LSD causes a phenomenon known as **synesthesia**, a blending of senses (such as smelling a color or tasting a sound); it can cause increases in BP, tachycardia, trembling, and dilated pupils; CNS effects include a sense of unreality, perceptual alteration, distortions, and impaired judgment

   b. LSD users can experience flashbacks (frightening episodes that can heighten a sense of "going crazy"); bad trips from LSD cause anxiety, paranoia, and acute panic; some clients who have experienced psychotic "breaks" from LSD have never fully recovered and a number of people have killed themselves while under influence of LSD

   c. PCP, a synthetic drug, traditionally has been used as an animal tranquilizer; the main safety risk for users is unpredictable behavior (progressing from coma to violent behavior without warning); PCP can be taken orally, IV, smoked, or snorted; it is well absorbed by all routes and effects last from 6–8 hours

   d. With PCP the user experiences a high; euphoria and peaceful feelings are the effects sought after; undesired effects of PCP can be serious; BP and heart rate are elevated; other peripheral nervous system effects include ataxia, salivation, and vomiting; a catatonic type of muscular rigidity alternating with violent outbursts may be frightening to others; psychological symptoms include hostile, bizarre behavior, a blank stare, and agitation

Table 11-9 **Categories and Examples of Drugs of Abuse**

Category	Examples
General CNS depressants	Alcohol, barbiturates (3 most widely abused are *secobarbital*, *pentobarbital*, and *amobarbital*), benzodiazepines (diazepam [Valium] is most widely abused)
Opioids	Heroin, morphine, meperidine, hydromorphone
Stimulants	Cocaine, amphetamines, nicotine
Marijuana/hashish	Can sometimes be classified with hallucinogens because of hallucination effect but is in a class by itself
Hallucinogens	LSD (lysergic acid diethylamide-25), PCP (phencyclidine), mescaline (peyote from cactus), MDA (3,4-methylenedioxyamphetamine)
Inhalants	Anesthetics (nitrous oxide, ether), nitrites (amyl nitrite, butyl nitrite, isobutyl nitrite), organic solvents (toluene, gasoline, lighter fluid, paint thinner, nail-polish remover, benzene, acetone, chloroform, and model-airplane glue)
Anabolic (androgenic) steroids	Testosterone, nandrolone decanoate (Durabolin), stanozolol (Winstrol)

    e. LSD and PCP deaths may be caused by overdose but are more likely to be linked to perceptual disorientation and unresponsiveness to environmental stimuli; hallucinogens do not produce physical dependence, so there are no withdrawal symptoms

    f. The nurse should provide a safe, calm, reassuring environment for clients detoxifying from hallucinogens

F. Inhalants

    1. Inhalants are a varied group of drugs that are inhaled; they can be divided into 3 classes: anesthetics, volatile nitrites, and organic solvents (see Table 11-9 for examples)

    2. Anesthetics produce subjective effects similar to alcohol—euphoria, exhilaration, and loss of inhibitions; the anesthetics most abused are nitrous oxide—"laughing gas"—and ether; these drugs may be popular because of ease of administration (neither requires difficult-to-obtain equipment); for nitrous oxide, ready availability also promotes use (small cylinders of drug, marketed for aerating whipping cream, can be purchased without restrictions)

    3. Nitrites (refer again to Table 11-9) are subject to abuse most often by gay men because of an ability to relax the anal sphincter, and by males in general because of a reputed ability to prolong and intensify sexual orgasm; the most pronounced effect of the nitrites is venodilation, which in turn causes a profound drop in systolic BP; the result is dizziness, light-headedness, palpitations, and possibly pulsatile headache; drug effect begins seconds after inhalation and fades rapidly; the primary toxicity is methemoglobinemia, which can be treated with methylene blue and supplemental oxygen

    4. A wide assortment of organic solvents have been inhaled to induce intoxication (see Table 11-9 for examples); these are used primarily by children and the very poor; they are administered by 3 processes

        a. "Bagging": pouring solvent into a plastic bag and inhaling vapor

        b. "Huffing": pouring solvent on a rag and inhaling vapor

        c. "Sniffing": inhaling solvent directly from its container

    5. Acute effects of organic solvents are similar to those of alcohol (euphoria, impaired judgment, slurred speech, flushing, and CNS depression); they can also cause visual hallucinations and disorientation to time and place; high doses can cause sudden death, possibly from anoxia, respiratory depression, vagal stimulation (slows heart rate), and dysrhythmias; prolonged use can cause multiple toxicities; gasoline can cause lead poisoning; chloroform is toxic to heart, liver, and kidneys; and toluene can cause severe brain damage and bone marrow depression; many solvents can cause damage to heart

    6. Management of acute toxicity is strictly supportive; objective is to stabilize vital signs because there are no antidotes for these agents

G. Anabolic (androgenic) steroids

    1. Androgens are frequently abused to enhance athletic performance; most are now regulated by Controlled Substances Act; the most widely used androgen is testosterone; there are substantial benefits for the athletes as well as many risks

    2. Steroids increase muscle mass in young males and in females of all ages and significantly increase muscle mass and strength in sexually mature males; the potential for adverse effects of androgens is significant; salt and water retention can lead to hypertension; when athletes take high doses there can be an increase in luteinizing hormone (LH) and follicle-stimulating hormone (FSH), resulting in testicular shrinkage and sterility; acne is common; reduction of HDL-cholesterol and elevation of LDL-cholesterol may accelerate development of atherosclerosis; there are potentially harmful effects to liver as well; in females, androgens can cause menstrual irregularities and virilization (growth of facial hair, deepening of the voice, decreased breast size, uterine atrophy, clitoral enlargement, and male-pattern baldness); hair loss; and irreversible voice change

3. Long-term androgen use can lead to abuse or "addiction" syndrome; characteristics include preoccupation with androgen use and difficulty in stopping use; when it is discontinued an abstinence syndrome can develop similar to that produced by withdrawal from alcohol, opioids, and cocaine

H. CNS depressants

1. Refer back to previous section on sedative–hypnotic and anxiolytic medications
2. Benzodiazepines are not likely to produce abuse in clients who do not have a history of substance dependence; they are usually abused in combination with alcohol and/ or barbiturates, which leads to CNS depression and may cause death; tolerance in those with substance dependence is rapid for sedative and euphoric effects and negligible for antianxiety effects
3. Barbiturates are frequently abused drugs among young or middle-aged users who abuse prescription drugs because they are legitimately manufactured and are available in many forms; usual route of administration is oral or IV; barbiturates have a cross-tolerance to other chemically similar drugs, including alcohol, BZs, and heroin; IV users experience a sudden warm "rush," followed by a prolonged drowsy feeling
4. Mild barbiturate intoxication is exhibited by sluggishness in coordination, emotional lability, aggressive impulses, slowness of speech, thought disorders, and faulty judgment; neurologic signs include nystagmus (involuntary eye oscillations), diplopia (double vision), strabismus (deviation of the eye), ataxic gait, positive Romberg sign (swaying of body when standing with feet close together and eyes closed), hypotonia, dysmetria (disturbance to control range of movement in muscular acts), and decreased superficial reflexes; intoxication with barbiturates is confirmed by blood tests
5. Barbiturates have potentially fatal effects; they are used frequently in accidental overdose and suicide attempts; death occurs as a result of deep coma, which progresses to respiratory arrest and cardiovascular failure; lethal doses vary widely from person to person; there is a narrow therapeutic index for sedative effects with the therapeutic dose being very close to lethal dose
6. Tolerance and withdrawal are similar to alcohol (both are CNS depressants)

I. Central nervous system stimulants

1. Amphetamines are CNS stimulants discussed here; discussion of cocaine, another CNS stimulant, can be found in a previous section
2. Amphetamines are also discussed in Chapter 10; the family of amphetamines includes dextroamphetamine, methamphetamine; when used for abuse, they are usually taken by mouth or IV; in addition, a form of dextroamphetamine known as "ice" or "crystal meth" can be smoked
3. Effects from amphetamine abuse include arousal and elevation of mood, euphoria, talkativeness, a sense of increased physical strength and mental capacity, increased self-confidence, and little or no desire for food or sleep (thus the term "uppers"); sexual orgasm is delayed, intensified, and more pleasurable
4. Some adverse effects of amphetamines can be fatal, including production of a psychotic state characterized by hallucinations and paranoid ideation; they can cause vasoconstriction and excessive stimulation of heart (sympathomimetic actions), leading to hypertension, angina pectoris, and dysrhythmias; overdose may also cause cerebral and systemic vasculitis and renal failure; vasoconstriction can be relieved by phentolamine (alpha-adrenergic blocker); cardiac stimulation can be reduced with a beta blocker (e.g., labetalol); drug elimination can be accelerated by giving ammonium chloride to acidify urine
5. Extended use of amphetamines produces a tolerance to mood elevation, appetite suppression, and cardiovascular effects; physical dependence is moderate while psychological addiction is intense; amphetamine withdrawal can produce dysphoria and a strong sense of craving; other symptoms include fatigue, prolonged sleep, excessive eating, and depression

6. A stimulant drug that is becoming less acceptable is nicotine; it is the only pharmacologically active drug in tobacco smoke other than carcinogenic tars; it exerts powerful effects on brain, spinal cord, peripheral nervous system, heart, and various other body structures; nicotine stimulates specific acetylcholine receptors in CNS including cerebral cortex, producing increases in psychomotor activity, cognitive function, sensorimotor performance, attention, and memory consolidation; as with all stimulant drugs, a period of depression follows withdrawal

7. Nicotine does not appear to induce any pronounced degree of biological tolerance; smokers seem to learn how to dose themselves so as to maintain a blood level of nicotine within a reasonably narrow range; nicotine induces both physiological and psychological dependence

8. Nicotine exerts a potent reinforcing action, especially in early phases of drug use; in the veteran smoker, the reinforcing action of repeated smoking is primarily to relieve or avoid withdrawal symptoms; in addition to CNS effects, normal doses of nicotine can increase heart rate, BP, and cardiac contractility; withdrawal from cigarettes is characterized by an abstinence syndrome, including a craving for nicotine, irritability, anxiety, anger, difficulty concentrating, restlessness, impatience, increased appetite, and insomnia; the period of withdrawal may last many months

9. See Chapter 10 for discussion of other specific CNS stimulants

Practice to Pass

The client is admitted to the unit for detoxification from alcohol. He states that his last drink was 12 hours ago. What are 4 major nursing priorities related to withdrawal from alcohol for the client?

Case Study

A 22-year-old, single male client is being discharged home today after detoxification from alcohol and cocaine. He will be taking disulfiram (Antabuse) 250 mg PO. He is scheduled to meet with the aftercare nurse tomorrow at 9:00 a.m.

1. Briefly describe the mechanism of action of disulfiram (Antabuse).
2. Describe the teaching plan the nurse will use to reinforce the adverse effects of disulfiram and alcohol use.
3. What is the purpose of taking disulfiram (Antabuse)?
4. With disulfiram (Antabuse) therapy, identify at least three other recommendations the nurse will make for inclusion in a recovery plan for the client.
5. What is the usual length of time a client will take disulfiram (Antabuse)?

For suggested responses, see page 544.

POSTTEST

POSTTEST

1. Because a client is ingesting risperidone (Risperdal) tid, the nurse instructs the unlicensed assistive personnel (UAP) to do which of the following? Select all that apply.
   1. Set the room up for bleeding precautions.
   2. Set the room up for seizure precautions.
   3. Set the room up for falls precautions.
   4. Report signs or symptoms of a psychotic break.
   5. Monitor sleeping respiratory rate.

2. When a client taking bupropion (Wellbutrin) 100 mg twice daily for 2 weeks returns to the clinic, the nurse would have which priority communication with the client?
   1. "You may now have a martini with your evening meal."
   2. "I need to listen to your heart with a stethoscope."
   3. "Has the number of your mood swings decreased?"
   4. "Are you still hearing voices?"

POSTTEST

3 Because a prescriber changed the antipsychotic drug for a client diagnosed with schizophrenia, the nurse should monitor for which intended outcome?

1. The new drug is likely to be more effective in controlling symptoms of schizophrenia.
2. The new drug is likely to become effective at a more rapid rate.
3. There should be a reduction in severity and type of side effects experienced.
4. Client should find drug easier to take and have a better taste.

4 A client taking lithium carbonate (Eskalith) is confused, agitated, has blurred vision, and is having difficulty walking. The nurse expects the lithium level drawn earlier in the day to be within which range?

1. 0.5–0.8 mEq/L
2. 1.2–1.5 mEq/L
3. 1.5–1.8 mEq/L
4. 2–3 mEq/L

5 A home health nurse is most likely to request that a prescriber consider discontinuing a phenothiazine prescribed for a client with psychosis after assessing which client data?

1. Urinary hesitation
2. White blood cell (WBC) count <3000 cells/mm^3
3. Blurred vision
4. Photophobia

6 A nurse working on an inpatient psychiatric unit would plan to monitor which of the following clients closely for neuroleptic malignant syndrome (NMS)?

1. 76-year-old female who has a typical psychotic clinical profile
2. 30-year-old male presenting with a very complex clinical profile
3. Native American who has been taking antipsychotic drugs for several months
4. Male client who has type 1 diabetes mellitus

7 Two months after beginning drug therapy with alprazolam (Xanax) 2 mg PO bid for generalized anxiety, an adult client states, "I feel much better, but I can't believe how dry my mouth gets and how dizzy and light-headed I get." Which would be the priority response by the nurse?

1. "You can use gum or candy that is sugarless to relieve some of those symptoms."
2. "The dosage of the medication will be lowered to decrease the side effects."
3. "Because the dizziness and light-headedness are side effects of the drug, avoid dangerous activities."
4. "You will need to take this medication with food from now on."

8 Because there is a higher risk of successful suicide in clients receiving selected antidepressant drugs, the nurse will plan to instruct the nursing staff to monitor clients receiving which type of antidepressant drug?

1. Selective serotonin reuptake inhibitors (SSRIs)
2. Monoamine oxidase inhibitors (MAOIs)
3. Tricyclic antidepressants (TCAs)
4. Anxiolytics

9 A 46-year-old client newly diagnosed with schizophrenia will be discharged in 5 days. The client lives in a 2-bedroom apartment with his older adult mother who is frail but self-sufficient. To promote adherence to medication therapy, the nurse would include which of the following in the care plan?

1. Teach the client and his mother how adherence to drug therapy contributes to the client's ongoing recovery process.
2. Teach the client's mother the importance of regular meals so the client can take his medication after meals.
3. Instruct the mother to be sure that the client is taking his medication daily as prescribed.
4. Teach the client that the medication regime will help him remain symptom-free indefinitely.

10 Because a client is taking a psychotropic medication, the nurse will plan to teach family members to report which of the following signs or symptoms immediately?

1. Hyperprolactinemia, gynecomastia
2. Hyperpyrexia and muscle rigidity
3. Parkinson's syndrome
4. Akathisia

➤ *See pages 385–388 for Answers and Rationales.*

ANSWERS & RATIONALES

Pretest

1 **Answer: 2** **Rationale:** Clients are admitted to the hospital because of the level of acuity of the psychosis. The primary focus of the nursing care should include reduction in the signs and symptoms of the psychosis. Monitoring for drug side effects such as tachycardia and hypotension is part of the health maintenance, but is not the focus of the nursing care. Because sedation and dizziness are common side effects of chlorpromazine, the nurse determines the safety risks to the client's health and should possibly not allow the client to ambulate alone. Appetite and food intake should improve as medication therapy takes effect and the client is better able to respond meaningfully with the environment; however, this is an indirect assessment rather than the primary focus. **Cognitive Level:** Analyzing **Client Need:** Pharmacological and Parenteral Therapies **Integrated Process:** Nursing Process: Planning **Content Area:** Pharmacology **Strategy:** Determine the relationship between the purpose of prescribing the drug and the setting. The critical words *primary focus* imply that more than one option may be of interest to the nurse and that the priority option must be selected. **Reference:** Wilson, B. A., Shannon, M. T., & Shields, K. M. (2012). *Pearson nurse's drug guide 2012.* Upper Saddle River, NJ: Pearson Education, pp. 309–312.

2 **Answer: 3, 5** **Rationale:** The nurse expects the primary possible side effects of somnolence, dizziness, insomnia, or nervousness to be compounded with excessive ingestion. Olanzapine is a newer drug approved for schizophrenia and other psychotic disorders. With ingestion of an appropriate therapeutic dose, this agent is generally well tolerated and appears devoid of serious adverse effects. Headache may occur with excessive ingestion, but psychosis is not expected to increase in intensity. Light-headedness may occur, but constipation is more likely to occur than diarrhea. Fluid retention and hyperglycemia are more likely to occur. Orthostatic hypotension is an increased risk during the initial dosing period; possible overdose would increase this risk. **Cognitive Level:** Applying **Client Need:** Pharmacological and Parenteral Therapies **Integrated Process:** Nursing Process:

Assessment **Content Area:** Pharmacology **Strategy:** Consider that the client is at risk for toxicity because of ingestion of a 10-day dose. Use knowledge of the adverse or toxic effects of this medication to make your selection. **Reference:** Wilson, B. A., Shannon, M. T., & Shields, K. M. (2012). *Pearson nurse's drug guide 2012.* Upper Saddle River, NJ: Pearson Education, pp. 1100–1102.

3 **Answer: 1** **Rationale:** Trazodone (Desyrel) is an atypical antidepressant. Because of the sedative effect it is often used more for insomnia than for depression. Alprazolam (Xanax) and diazepam (Valium) and beta-adrenergic blocking agents such as propranolol (Inderal) are used for panic attacks. Divalproex (Depakote), lithium (Litho-Bid), or lamotrigine (Lamictal) are more appropriate for mania. The same drugs used for panic attacks can be used for anxiety. **Cognitive Level:** Applying **Client Need:** Pharmacological and Parenteral Therapies **Integrated Process:** Nursing Process: Assessment **Content Area:** Pharmacology **Strategy:** First determine the possible uses for this drug. Then for this question, associate the common use of the drug with the most common side effect. **Reference:** Wilson, B. A., Shannon, M. T., & Shields, K. M. (2012). *Pearson nurse's drug guide 2012.* Upper Saddle River, NJ: Pearson Education, pp. 48–49, 448–450, 845–848, 890–893, 1284–1287, 1533–1535.

4 **Answer: 1, 2, 3, 5** **Rationale:** Monoamine oxidase inhibitors (MAOIs) such as phenelzine can interact negatively with a large number of drugs and foods, which can then place the client at great risk. For example, MAOIs taken with tricyclic antidepressants can result in seizures and hyperthermia. MAOIs taken with sympathomimetics or tyramine-containing foods such as aged cheese, avocado, and chocolate can lead to a life-threatening hypertensive crisis. Client instructions should be both written and oral. Management of most clients with mental health problems includes teaching family members when and how to notify health care providers. Depending on the degree of impairment, the family may need to assist with the drug therapy, but there is not enough information to know if this applies to this question. Thus, this option is not the priority when considering the risks inherent with use of this medication. Blood pressure and pulse should be monitored closely during initial period of administration. **Cognitive Level:** Analyzing **Client Need:** Pharmacological and Parenteral Therapies **Integrated Process:** Teaching and Learning **Content Area:** Pharmacology **Strategy:** Categorize the drug group as high drug–drug interactionist as well as high drug–food interactionist. This will help you to eliminate incorrect options easily and focus on the options that address the risks to use of this medication. **Reference:** Wilson, B. A., Shannon, M. T., & Shields, K. M. (2012). *Pearson nurse's drug guide 2012.* Upper Saddle River, NJ: Pearson Education, pp. 1192–1195.

5 **Answer: 4** **Rationale:** Because it has a shorter half-life (10–20 hours) and is not metabolized by the liver, lorazepam (Ativan) is most appropriate for use in the elderly. Because diazepam (Valium) and chlordiazepoxide (Librium) are metabolized by the liver and have longer half-lives (20–50 hours and 5–30 hours, respectively) they are contraindicated for use in older adults. Trazodone (Desyrel) is an atypical antidepressant, not a benzodiazepine. **Cognitive Level:** Analyzing **Client Need:** Pharmacological and Parenteral Therapies **Integrated Process:** Nursing Process: Planning **Content Area:** Pharmacology **Strategy:** First eliminate trazodone since it is not a benzodiazepine. Then apply knowledge of the drug profiles to the age of the client listed in the question. **Reference:** Wilson, B. A., Shannon, M. T., & Shields, K. M. (2012). *Pearson nurse's drug guide 2012.* Upper Saddle River, NJ: Pearson Education, pp. 299–301, 448–450, 898–901, 1533–1535.

6 **Answer: 3, 5** **Rationale:** Lithium (Litho-Bid) is very effective in managing bipolar disorder. Rehospitalization of a client with bipolar disorder who has the drug prescribed generally indicates the client has stopped taking the medication. Clients often do not associate "feeling better" with the drug actions, and thus think they do not need to continue the medication. Dehydration, or fluid volume deficit, can cause renal toxicity and lithium toxicity, which could require rehospitalization. A family crisis or having a seriously ill family member could impact the stability of the client's mental status; however, with appropriate counseling and drug therapy, the client should be able to cope without requiring rehospitalization. A weight loss regime would not require hospitalization. One side effect of lithium includes altered renal function that could lead to fluid retention; however, this would be more likely to cause readmission to a medical–surgical unit rather than a psychiatric unit. **Cognitive Level:** Applying **Client Need:** Pharmacological and Parenteral Therapies **Integrated Process:** Nursing Process: Planning **Content Area:** Pharmacology **Strategy:** Eliminate the options related to family crises first because they are similar. Then associate the characteristics of the health problem with the ability to comply with a drug regime. Noting the critical words *most likely*, recognize that clients with mental health problems may interpret feelings of wellness

with a cure and thus terminate drug therapy independently. **Reference:** Wilson, B. A., Shannon, M. T., & Shields, K. M. (2012). *Pearson nurse's drug guide 2012.* Upper Saddle River, NJ: Pearson Education, 890–893.

7 **Answer: 1, 2, 4** **Rationale:** Because disulfiram (Antabuse) causes the adverse reactions noted when alcohol is ingested simultaneously, the nurse should ask if the client is taking the drug. Intensity of reaction to Antabuse is generally proportional to the amount of alcohol ingested. A major life-threatening response to simultaneous ingestion of disulfiram and an alcoholic beverage includes hypotension. Ingestion of antihypertensive at the same time could compound the problem, making this a good follow-up question. Since the client is vomiting continuously, whether or not the client has eaten would not assist the nurse in managing the client's current condition. A prior history of cholecystectomy is not relevant. The client is experiencing a disulfiram reaction, not cholecystitis. **Cognitive Level:** Analyzing **Client Need:** Pharmacological and Parenteral Therapies **Integrated Process:** Nursing Process: Assessment **Content Area:** Pharmacology **Strategy:** Apply knowledge of a drug that may cause the signs and symptoms when alcohol is ingested. **Reference:** Wilson, B. A., Shannon, M. T., & Shields, K. M. (2012). *Pearson nurse's drug guide 2012.* Upper Saddle River, NJ: Pearson Education, pp. 483–485.

8 **Answer: 1, 2, 3** **Rationale:** Orthostatic hypotension, blurred vision, and urinary retention are common side effects of imipramine (Tofranil). Dysrhythmias are a common side effect rather than an uncommon one. Imipramine is more likely to increase liver enzymes rather than decrease them. **Cognitive Level:** Analyzing **Client Need:** Pharmacological and Parenteral Therapies **Integrated Process:** Teaching and Learning **Content Area:** Pharmacology **Strategy:** Specific medication knowledge is needed to answer the question. Recall that this drug is an antidepressant and consider the typical side effects to make the correct selection. **Reference:** Wilson, B. A., Shannon, M. T., & Shields, K. M. (2012). *Pearson nurse's drug guide 2012.* Upper Saddle River, NJ: Pearson Education, pp. 767–769.

9 **Answer: 3** **Rationale:** Because fluoxetine (Prozac) increases the level of serotonin, clients experience diarrhea and nausea resulting in decreased intake as well as decreased absorption of nutrients. Management of the side effects can prevent the weight loss. Abrupt discontinuance of the drug is discouraged. The client will need to increase the caloric intake but not necessarily fluid intake. The dosage should be related more to the therapeutic effect rather than the appearance of side effects. **Cognitive Level:** Applying **Client Need:** Pharmacological and Parenteral Therapies **Integrated Process:** Nursing Process: Planning **Content Area:** Pharmacology **Strategy:** Use knowledge of side effects to determine appropriate remedy. Consider that the therapeutic effect should drive decisions regarding dosage decisions to help make the correct selection. **Reference:** Wilson, B. A., Shannon, M. T., & Shields, K. M. (2012). *Pearson nurse's drug guide 2012.* Upper Saddle River, NJ: Pearson Education, pp. 1379–1381.

10 **Answer: 3** **Rationale:** Chlorpromazine (Thorazine) is not only the oldest of the antipsychotic medications, it can also be used for relief of intractable hiccups. Risperidone (Risperdal) is a benzisoxazole derivative that would not relieve hiccups. There is also no evidence that lorazepam (Ativan) or thioridazine reduces or relieves intractable hiccups. **Cognitive Level:** Applying **Client Need:** Pharmacological and Parenteral Therapies **Integrated Process:** Nursing Process: Planning **Content Area:** Pharmacology **Strategy:** Specific drug knowledge is needed to answer the question. Take time to learn this information if the question was difficult. **Reference:** Wilson, B. A., Shannon, M. T., & Shields, K. M. (2012). *Pearson nurse's drug guide 2012.* Upper Saddle River, NJ: Pearson Education, pp. 309–312, 1347–1349, 1483–1485.

Posttest

1 **Answer: 2, 5** **Rationale:** Seizures are a primary side effect of this drug so seizure precautions should be put in place. Respiratory depression and laryngospasms are side effects, so monitoring respiratory rate (while awake and asleep) would be beneficial. The client would be prone to leucopenia and risk for infection rather than decreased platelets and risk for bleeding. Falls precautions are designed for disoriented clients or for clients who have limited mobility and are not needed by the client with the information given. Reporting signs or symptoms of a psychotic break are beyond the expected competencies of UAP. **Cognitive Level:** Applying **Client Need:** Pharmacological and Parenteral Therapies **Integrated Process:** Nursing Process: Planning **Content Area:** Pharmacology **Strategy:** Note the drug in the question and determine the expected outcomes of the drug and the side or adverse effects of the drug. With the wording of the question, focus on side effects or adverse effects as being the focus of the correct option(s). **Reference:** Wilson, B. A., Shannon, M. T., & Shields, K. M. (2012). *Pearson nurse's drug guide 2012.* Upper Saddle River, NJ: Pearson Education, pp. 1347–1349.

2 **Answer: 2** **Rationale:** One of the primary side effects of bupropion (Wellbutrin) includes dysrhythmias, making assessment of the cardiac rate and rhythm most important. Ingesting alcohol with the drug may increase the development of seizures so drinking is not recommended. Bupropion is utilized for anxiety and not for depression. Antipsychotics such as clozapine (Clozaril) are prescribed for clients with hallucinations; bupropion is prescribed for anxiety. **Cognitive Level:** Applying **Client Need:** Pharmacological and Parenteral Therapies **Integrated Process:** Nursing Process: Assessment **Content Area:** Pharmacology **Strategy:** When responding to priority questions, select the option presenting the greatest risk

along with the risk with the most rapid onset. **Reference:** Wilson, B. A., Shannon, M. T., & Shields, K. M. (2012). *Pearson nurse's drug guide 2012.* Upper Saddle River, NJ: Pearson Education, pp. 200–201.

3 **Answer: 3** **Rationale:** Changing the prescription is more likely related to the type, severity, and extent of the side effects. Clinical effectiveness of most antipsychotic drugs at equivalent dosages is typically the same. The onset may be more rapid, but this is not the primary predicted outcome the nurse should monitor. Although ease of use and taste may be a factor in compliance, they would not be the primary rationale for a change in prescription. **Cognitive Level:** Applying **Client Need:** Pharmacological and Parenteral Therapies **Integrated Process:** Nursing Process: Evaluation **Content Area:** Pharmacology **Strategy:** Use principles of pharmacology related to mental health problems. Consider the common rationale for changing drugs prescribed for clients with schizophrenia. **Reference:** Kneisl, C., & Trigoboff, E. (2009). *Contemporary psychiatric-mental health nursing* (2nd ed.). Upper Saddle River, NJ: Pearson Education, pp. 208–216.

4 **Answer: 4** **Rationale:** The symptoms listed are those of lithium toxicity, and are seen when the serum level is 2–3 mEq/L. The therapeutic dose level is 1.2–1.5 mEq/L. A low dosage level of 0.5–0.8 mEq/L would not be effective in controlling manifestations of bipolar disorder but would not be an indicator of toxicity. A level 1.5–1.8 mEq/L is slightly elevated but would not produce the manifestations listed. **Cognitive Level:** Analyzing **Client Need:** Pharmacological and Parenteral Therapies **Integrated Process:** Nursing Process: Assessment **Content Area:** Pharmacology **Strategy:** Select the option that is most representative of the level in which clients are likely to experience signs or symptoms of toxicity. **Reference:** Wilson, B. A., Shannon, M. T., & Shields, K. M. (2012). *Pearson nurse's drug guide 2012.* Upper Saddle River, NJ: Pearson Education, pp. 890–893.

5 **Answer: 2** **Rationale:** Agranulocytosis is a common side effect of phenothiazines and a WBC count of 3,000 (normal 5,000–10,000) could place the client at risk for infection. Discontinuance of the drug is recommended and the client should be changed to a different drug. Since urinary hesitation is a treatable side effect, drug therapy would not need to be interrupted. Blurred vision could be managed with safety instructions and this side effect actually resolves after a short period of time. Wearing dark glasses when in sunlight will reduce the discomfort from photophobia. **Cognitive Level:** Analyzing **Client Need:** Pharmacological and Parenteral Therapies **Integrated Process:** Nursing Process: Planning **Content Area:** Pharmacology **Strategy:** Note the critical word *discontinuing* in the stem of the question. This implies a severe adverse medication effect. Look at the various options and use nursing knowledge to select the low WBC count as placing the client at greatest risk. **Reference:** Adams, M., Holland, L., & Bostwick, P. (2011).

Pharmacology for nurses: A pathophysiologic approach (3rd ed.). Upper Saddle River, NJ: Pearson Education, pp. 206–207.

6 **Answer: 2** **Rationale:** Younger male clients presenting with complex clinical profiles are more prone to neuroleptic malignant syndrome (NMS). The complexity makes it difficult to separate the syndrome from the mental health alteration. Clinical profiles are generally variable. Being female is not one of the demographic factors associated with NMS. There is no evidence that the Native American population taking antipsychotic drugs over a long period of time is more likely to develop NMS. Diabetes mellitus is associated with male schizophrenic clients who take antipsychotic drugs, but it is not necessarily associated with NMS. **Cognitive Level:** Analyzing **Client Need:** Pharmacological and Parenteral Therapies **Integrated Process:** Nursing Process: Assessment **Content Area:** Mental Health **Strategy:** The core issue of the question is what client demographics correlate most frequently with neuroleptic malignant syndrome (NMS). Use specific knowledge of risk factors for NMS and the process of elimination to make a selection. **Reference:** Kneisl, C., & Trigoboff, E. (2009). *Contemporary psychiatric-mental health nursing* (2nd ed.). Upper Saddle River, NJ: Pearson Education, p. 858.

7 **Answer: 3** **Rationale:** Without proper instructions the client may perform activities such as driving or using equipment that could lead to injury if the client was experiencing dizziness or light-headedness. Dry mouth is an uncomfortable side effect, but if unresolved would not place the client at the greatest risk. Side effects may be dose-related during early high-dose therapy, but client has been taking the drug for 2 months and "high dosage" is 8 mg/day. The medication has no known GI effects so it does not need to be taken with food. **Cognitive Level:** Analyzing **Client Need:** Pharmacological and Parenteral Therapies **Integrated Process:** Communication and Documentation **Content Area:** Pharmacology **Strategy:** Determine first that the issue of dizziness and light-headedness is more serious than dry mouth. Then compare each of the options to find the statement that provides guidance to the client to maintain safety. Another way to approach this question would be to ask, "The client would be at greatest risk if which intervention was not initiated?" **Reference:** Wilson, B. A., Shannon, M. T., Shields, K. M. (2012). *Pearson nurse's drug guide 2012.* Upper Saddle River, NJ: Pearson Education, pp. 48–49.

8 **Answer: 3** **Rationale:** Tricyclic antidepressants (TCAs) account for 70% of all deaths from intentional drug overdose. Selective serotonin reuptake inhibitor (SSRI) overdoses are serious and result in seizures, but most clients recover and these drugs are not commonly utilized for suicide. Life-threatening risks associated with monoamine oxidase inhibitors (MAOIs) include interaction with foods containing tyramine, which results in a hypertensive crisis. Anxiolytics are not a class of antidepressants; rather, they are a class of medications used to treat anxiety. **Cognitive Level:** Applying **Client Need:** Pharmacological and Parenteral Therapies **Integrated Process:** Nursing Process: Assessment **Content Area:** Pharmacology **Strategy:** Use knowledge of which drug groups clients tend to utilize most to attempt or commit suicide. **Reference:** Wilson, B. A., Shannon, M. T., & Shields, K. M. (2012). *Pearson nurse's drug guide 2012.* Upper Saddle River, NJ: Pearson Education, pp. 76–77.

9 **Answer: 1** **Rationale:** Clients with schizophrenia are at high risk for nonadherence to drug therapy. Factors contributing to nonadherence include drug side effects, nonsupportive environment, lack of understanding, and numerous other factors. Because discontinuation of medications is the primary reason for relapse and rehospitalization, it is essential for the nurse to teach both the client and his mother the importance of adhering to the medication schedule. The relationship for mental health maintenance should be a shared activity, rather than placing the burden primarily on the mother. Various factors can override drug effectiveness so this statement could provide false assurance to the client. **Cognitive Level:** Applying **Client Need:** Pharmacological and Parenteral Therapies **Integrated Process:** Teaching and Learning **Content Area:** Mental Health **Strategy:** Select the option that contributes most to maintaining the client's health. First eliminate the options that focus on the mother rather than the client. Then eliminate another option because of the unrealistic words *symptom-free indefinitely*. **Reference:** Kneisl, C., & Trigoboff, E. (2009). *Contemporary psychiatric-mental health nursing* (2nd ed.). Upper Saddle River, NJ: Pearson Education, pp. 376–377.

10 **Answer: 2** **Rationale:** Hyperpyrexia, muscle rigidity, and altered consciousness level are indicative of a life-threatening side effect called neuroleptic malignant syndrome. Immediate medical intervention is warranted. Gynecomastia is without threats but may affect the client's self-esteem. Excessive production of prolactin can result in osteoporosis over a long period of time. Parkinson's syndrome can occur because of the blockade of dopamine, but is reversible and nonurgent. Akathisia, a strong urge to pace, needs to be reported, but is nonurgent. **Cognitive Level:** Applying **Client Need:** Pharmacological and Parenteral Therapies **Integrated Process:** Nursing Process: Implementation **Content Area:** Mental Health **Strategy:** Select the option containing elements with the threat on immediate onset as well as the greatest magnitude. **Reference:** Kneisl, C., & Trigoboff, E. (2009). *Contemporary psychiatric-mental health nursing* (2nd ed.). Upper Saddle River, NJ: Pearson Education, pp. 110–139.

References

Abrams, A., Pennington, S., Lammon, C., & Goldsmith, T. (2009). *Clinical drug therapy: Rationales for nursing practice* (9th ed.). Philadelphia, PA: Lippincott Williams & Wilkins.

Adams, M., Holland, L., & Bostwick, P. (2011). *Pharmacology for nurses: A pathophysiologic approach* (3rd ed.). Upper Saddle River, NJ: Pearson Education.

Adams, M., & Urban, C. (2013). *Pharmacology: Connections to nursing practice* (2nd ed.). Upper Saddle River, NJ: Pearson Education.

American Psychiatric Association (2000). *Diagnostic and statistical manual of mental disorders, Fourth Edition, Text Revision (DSM-IV-TR).* Washington, DC: American Psychiatric Association.

Aschenbrenner, D., & Venable, S. (2009). *Drug therapy in nursing* (3rd ed.). Philadelphia, PA: Lippincott Williams & Wilkins.

Drug Facts & Comparisons® (Updated monthly). St. Louis, MO: A. Wolters Kluwer.

Karch, A. M. (2010). *Focus on nursing pharmacology* (5th ed.). Philadelphia, PA: Lippincott Williams & Wilkins.

Kee, J. (2010). *Laboratory and diagnostic tests and nursing implications* (8th ed.). Upper Saddle River, NJ: Pearson Education.

Kneisl, C., & Trigoboff, E. (2009). *Contemporary psychiatric-mental health nursing* (2nd ed). Upper Saddle River, NJ: Pearson Education.

Lehne, R. (2010). *Pharmacology for nursing care* (7th ed.). St. Louis, MO: Mosby.

LeMone, P., Burke, K., & Bauldoff, G. (2011). *Medical-surgical nursing: Critical thinking in patient care* (5th ed.). Upper Saddle River, NJ: Pearson Education.

Wilson, B. A., Shannon, M. T., & Shields, K. M. (2012). *Pearson nurse's drug guide 2012.* Upper Saddle River, NJ: Pearson Education.

Renal System Medications

Chapter Outline

NCLEX-RN® Test Prep

Use the accompanying online resource, NursingReviewsandRationales, to test yourself with hundreds of NCLEX®-style practice questions.

Objectives

➤ Describe general goals of therapy when administering renal system medications.
➤ Describe actions, side effects, and adverse effects of commonly used diuretics.
➤ Discriminate between potassium-losing and potassium-sparing diuretics.
➤ Identify significant laboratory values to monitor in the client taking a diuretic.
➤ Explore client adherence issues related to self-administration of diuretic and other urinary medications.
➤ Describe actions, side effects, and adverse effects of commonly used urinary anti-infectives, antispasmodics, and analgesics.
➤ Identify client teaching points related to medications prescribed for benign prostatic hyperplasia.
➤ Describe rationale for medications prescribed to treat acute and chronic renal failure.
➤ Identify significant client education points related to renal system medications.

Review at a Glance

anuria absence of urination and urine production (less than 400 mL/day)
benign prostatic hyperplasia (BPH) a symptom complex defined as benign adenomatous hyperplasia of peri-urethral prostate gland
bactericidal destroying or killing bacteria
baceriostasis inhibition of bacterial growth without their destruction
diuretic an agent that increases amount of urine excreted

hypertension high blood pressure
orthostatic hypotension a blood pressure fall of more than 10–15 mmHg systolic pressure or a fall of more than 10 mmHg diastole pressure and a 10–20% increase in heart rate
renin-angiotensin system a complex system in which renin, released by juxtaglomerular cells of kidney, changes angiotensinogen from liver to angiotensin I; angiotensin I is converted in lungs to angiotensin II, a powerful vasoconstrictor

that increases peripheral resistance and thereby increases blood pressure
shock severe disturbance of hemody-namics in which circulatory system fails to maintain adequate perfusion of vital organs
vasoconstriction narrowing of blood vessels in response to an internal stimulus (such as nervous system) or an external stimulus (such as cold)
vasodilation widening of blood vessels in response to an internal stimulus (such as nervous system) or an external stimulus (such as heat)

PRETEST

1 A client who is starting medication therapy with furosemide (Lasix) 20 mg PO daily asks the nurse what would be the best time of day to take the pill. What time should the nurse recommend?

1. 8:00 a.m.
2. 12 noon
3. 6:00 p.m.
4. At bedtime

2 A client with a history of renal insufficiency is experiencing a hypertensive crisis. The nurse administers which of the following prescribed diuretics?

1. Furosemide (Lasix)
2. Hydrochlorothiazide (HCTZ)
3. Chlorthalidone (Hygroton)
4. Spironolactone (Aldactone)

3 After a health care provider prescribes losartan (Cozaar), the client asks the nurse to explain the relationship(s) between the actions of the drug and the side effects. The best response by the nurse includes which of the following?

1. "Losartan inhibits calcium from crossing into the blood vessel cells, making them relax and lowering the blood pressure (BP)."
2. "Losartan directly activates chemicals in the bloodstream that will then act on blood vessel walls to dilate them."
3. "Losartan promotes the release of aldosterone, which increases urine output and lowers blood pressure (BP)."
4. "Losartan selectively blocks the binding of angiotensin II to its receptors found in many tissues."

4 A client with a chronic, dry, nonproductive cough cannot remember the name of the antihypertensive medication he has been taking. Based on the manifestation of cough, the nurse suspects that the client is most likely taking which antihypertensive drug?

1. Propranolol (Inderal)
2. Lisinopril (Prinivil)
3. Nifedipine (Procardia)
4. Bumetanide (Bumex)

5 The nurse is teaching a man recently diagnosed with hypertension about the prescribed medications. The nurse should include which statement(s) during the teaching session? Select all that apply.

1. "After you meet your weight loss goal, most medications will probably not be needed."
2. "Avoid activities that require a high level of precision until you know how you respond to medication therapy."
3. "It would be helpful to increase your fluid intake during the first few weeks of drug therapy to prevent dizziness."
4. "Your hands and feet may swell a little initially but this will go away."
5. "Report to the prescriber if you have increased difficulty experiencing an erection."

6 A 45-year-old female has been taking indapamide (generic) 2.5 mg daily. She reported to the clinic today with leg cramps and a blood pressure of 126/70. The nurse should consult with the prescriber to do which of the following?

1. Stop the indapamide.
2. Evaluate the electrolytes.
3. Switch to furosemide (Lasix).
4. Obtain order for nonsteroidal anti-inflammatory drug (NSAID).

❼ A client with hypertension and diabetes mellitus is taking hydrochlorothiazide (HCTZ). The client reports onset of an enlarged, red, painful right great toe since initiating the drug therapy. The home health nurse requests which of the following serum laboratory tests?

1. Uric acid level
2. Alanine aminotransferase (ALT)
3. Serum glucose
4. Serum sodium

❽ The health care provider prescribed oxybutynin (Ditropan) for a 65-year-old female with urinary frequency and urgency. Because of a primary side effect, the nurse teaches the client to do which of the following?

1. "Wear protective underwear."
2. "Avoid activities that may cause injury or bleeding."
3. "Carry an over-the-counter antidiarrheal agent when traveling."
4. "Rinse your mouth or use sugarless hard candy frequently."

❾ The nurse anticipates that mannitol (Osmitrol) may be prescribed for clients recently admitted to the unit with which of the following conditions? Select all that apply.

1. Pancreatitis
2. Increased intracranial pressure
3. Diarrhea
4. Increased intraocular pressure
5. Congestive heart failure

❿ Because finasteride (Proscar) was prescribed for a 45-year-old man, the nurse should include which of the following as a priority in the teaching session?

1. Use a contraceptive barrier during sexual intercourse.
2. Sexual performance level may decrease.
3. Increase daily fluid intake.
4. Take drug for one month.

➤ *See pages 422–423 for Answers and Rationales.*

I. DIURETICS

A. Loop diuretics

1. Action and use
   a. **Diuretics** (agents that increase amount of urine excreted) inhibit electrolyte reabsorption in thick ascending loop of Henle, thereby promoting excretion of sodium, water, chloride, and potassium
   b. Antihypertensive action involves renal **vasodilation** (dilation or widening of vessels), to provide a temporary increase in glomerular filtration rate (GFR) and a decrease in peripheral vascular resistance
   c. Loop diuretics are more potent than thiazide diuretics, causing rapid diuresis; this results in decreasing vascular fluid volume, cardiac output, and blood pressure (BP)
   d. Loop diuretics are considered to be "high ceiling" diuretics, which means dosage can be raised to a greater extent to cause diuresis
   e. They are used in clients with low GFR and hypertensive emergencies
   f. They are also used in clients with edema, pulmonary edema, heart failure (HF), chronic renal failure (CRF), and hepatic cirrhosis
   g. They may be used as treatment in drug overdose to increase renal elimination
2. Common medications (Table 12-1)
3. Administration considerations

   a. Take early in day to avoid nocturia
   b. Give intravenous (IV) doses slowly over 1–2 minutes; rapid injection may cause hypotension

Table 12-1 Loop Diuretics

Generic (Trade) Name	Route	Uses	Adverse Effects
Bumetanide (Bumex)	PO, IV	Hypertension, heart failure, hepatic failure, renal failure, postoperative, edema, premenstrual syndrome, disseminated cancer	Headache, dizziness, volume depletion, renal failure, dehydration, thrombocytopenia, azotemia, hypokalemia, hypochloremic alkalosis, hypocalcemia, hypomagnesemia, hyperglycemia, impaired glucose tolerance, muscle pain, rash
Ethacrynic acid (Edecrin) (rarely used)	PO, IV	Acute pulmonary edema, edema, hypertension	Fever, chills, transient deafness, malaise, confusion vertigo, volume depletion, orthostatic hypotension, hematuria, oliguria, neutropenia, azotemia, hyperuricemia, hypochloremic alkalosis, hypocalcemia, hypomagnesemia, hyperglycemia, impaired glucose tolerance, rash
Furosemide (Lasix)	PO, IV	Acute pulmonary edema, edema, heart failure, chronic renal impairment, hypertension, hypercalcemia	Fever, rash, chills, pancreatitis, vertigo, dizziness, paresthesia, restlessness, weakness, orthostatic hypotension, agranulocytosis, leukopenia, thrombocytopenia, aplastic anemia, hepatic impairment, muscle spasm, azotemia, hyperglycemia, hypocalcemia, hypomagnesemia, hypochloremic alkalosis, hypokalemia, dermatitis, photosensitivity, purpura, dilutional hyponatremia, aplastic anemia
Torsemide (Demadex)	PO, IV	Heart failure, chronic renal impairment, hepatic cirrhosis, hypertension	Dizziness, excessive thirst, gout, fatigue, insomnia, syncope, nervousness, rhinitis, chest pain, sore throat, constipation, nausea, dyspepsia, hemorrhage, hypokalemia, hypomagnesemia, hypocalcemia, hyperuricemia, hypochloremic alkalosis, cough

    c. For IV infusion, dilute in 5% dextrose in water, 0.9% sodium chloride (NaCl), or lactated Ringers; use infusion fluids within 24 hours

    d. Administer IV furosemide (Lasix) slowly, as hearing loss can occur if injected rapidly

4. Contraindications: anuria, electrolyte depletion

5. Significant drug interactions

    a. Interact with aminoglycosides causing ototoxicity

    b. Interact with digoxin (increase digoxin induced arrhythmias), indomethacin, lithium, ethacrynic acid, salicylates, and nonsteroidal anti-inflammatory drugs (NSAIDS), which may decrease efficacy of loop diuretic, tubocurarine, succinylcholine, other antihypertensives

    c. An additive effect with thiazide diuretics and thiazide-like diuretics

    d. Interact with anticoagulants (increase anticoagulant activity), propranolol (increase plasma levels of propranolol), sulfonylureas (hyperglycemia), cisplatin (ototoxicity), and probenecid

    e. Increase risk for lithium toxicity

6. Significant food interactions: taking ethacrynic acid (Edecrin) with food or milk will increase urination, licorice may lead to added loss of potassium

7. Significant laboratory studies

    a. Monitor for electrolyte imbalance especially sodium and potassium

    b. Monitor hemoglobin and hematocrit for increase due to hemoconcentration; monitor platelet count

    c. Monitor for blood dyscrasias, liver, or kidney damage

    d. Monitor blood glucose levels and lipids for possible drug interaction

    e. Monitor lithium levels, if taking lithium for elevation

Practice to Pass

The home health care nurse is visiting an older adult client who has been prescribed furosemide (Lasix). Knowing that ototoxicity is an adverse effect of loop diuretics, what symptoms should the nurse teach the client to report?

8. Side effects
   a. CNS: dizziness, headache, orthostatic hypotension, weakness
   b. GI: nausea and vomiting (N/V), abdominal pain, elevated lipids with decreased high density lipoprotein (HDL), pancreatitis, anorexia, constipation
   c. GU: excessive urination, nocturia, urinary bladder spasms
   d. Photosensitivity, sulfonamide allergy, and ototoxicity (tinnitus, hearing impairment, deafness, vertigo, and sense of fullness in ears)
   e. Skin: dermatitis, urticaria, pruritis, and muscle spasm
   f. Severe watery diarrhea is the side effect of ethacrynic acid

9. Adverse effects/toxicity
   a. Electrolyte imbalances: hyponatremia, hypochloremia, hypokalemia, hypomagnesemia, hypocalcemia, and hyperuricemia
   b. Thrombocytopenia, systemic vasculitis, interstitial nephritis, thrombophlebitis, agranulocytosis, and aplastic anemia

10. Nursing considerations
    a. Monitor vital signs for hypotension and tachycardia
    b. Monitor serum electrolytes, calcium, and uric acid levels
    c. Monitor and record body weight at regular intervals at same time of day and same scale
    d. Monitor intake and output (I & O)
    e. Assess indicators of dehydration: thirst, poor skin turgor, coated tongue
    f. Assess for inadequate tissue perfusion and weakness, decreased muscle strength, restlessness, anxiety, and agitation

11. Client education
    a. Eat foods high in potassium (such as bananas, cantaloupe) to prevent hypokalemia
    b. Restrict sodium intake; do not use salt substitutes if taking potassium supplement
    c. Avoid dehydration by avoiding alcohol and caffeine beverages and replacing fluids during exercise or hot weather
    d. Avoid exposure to intense heat as with baths, showers, and electric blankets
    e. Take small, frequent amounts of ice chips or clear liquids if vomiting
    f. Replace fluids with fruit juice or bouillon if experiencing diarrhea
    g. Diuretics increase amount and frequency of urination, so take medication in morning and afternoon to avoid nighttime urination
    h. Photosensitivity can occur while taking a loop diuretic
    i. Change position slowly to avoid dizziness and **orthostatic hypotension** (a BP fall of more than 10 to 15 mmHg systolic or more than 10 mmHg diastolic and a 10–20% increase in heart rate)
    j. Weigh self daily and report sudden weight gains or losses
    k. Report ringing in ears immediately
    l. Do not use loop diuretics while breastfeeding
    m. Eliminate licorice from diet

B. **Thiazide diuretics**
   1. Action and uses
      a. Increased urinary excretion of sodium and water by inhibiting sodium reabsorption in cortical diluting tubule of kidney
      b. Its hypotensive effect may be due to direct arteriolar vasodilation and decreased total peripheral resistance
      c. Used for edema and **hypertension** (persistent elevation of systolic BP above 140 mmHg and diastolic BP above 90 mmHg)
      d. Not effective for immediate diuresis
   2. Common medications (Table 12-2)

Table 12-2 Common Thiazide Diuretics

Generic (Trade) Name	Route	Uses	Adverse Effects
Bendroflumethiazide (Naturetin)	PO	Edema, congestive heart failure (CHF), calcium nephrolithiasis	Dizziness, vertigo, paresthesia, orthostatic hypotension, headache, blurred vision, photosensitivity, hyperglycemia, hyperuricemia, pancreatitis, gout, impotence, loss of libido
Chlorothiazide (Diuril, Microzide)	PO, IV	CHF, cirrhosis, corticosteroid and estrogen therapy, hypertension, diabetes insipidus, reduction of osteoporosis	Dizziness, vertigo, paresthesia, orthostatic hypotension, photosensitivity, rash, purpura, nausea, hyperglycemia, hyperuricemia, pancreatitis, gout, impotence, loss of libido
Chlorthalidone (Hygroton, Thalitone)	PO	CHF, cirrhosis, corticosteroid and estrogen therapy, hypertension, renal insufficiency	Dizziness, vertigo, paresthesia, fatigue, drowsiness, volume depletion, cardiac dysrhythmia, polyuria, nocturia, nausea, anorexia, diarrhea, constipation, leucopenia, agranulocytosis, pancreatitis, gouty attacks, fluid and electrolyte imbalance
Hydrochlorothiazide (Esidrix, Ezide, Hydrodiuril)	PO	CHF, cirrhosis, corticosteroid and estrogen therapy, hypertension, renal insufficiency	Dizziness, vertigo, paresthesia, orthostatic hypotension, photosensitivity, rash, purpura, nausea, hyperglycemia, hyperuricemia, pancreatitis, gout, impotence, loss of libido
Indapamide (Lozol)	PO	Edema associated with CHF, hypertension, diabetes insipidus	Dizziness, vertigo, paresthesia, weakness, headache, fatigue, volume depletion, dysrhythmia, photosensitivity, nausea, constipation, pancreatitis, polyuria, leukopenia, hypokalemia, gout, muscle cramps
Methyclothiazide (Enduron, Aquatensen)	PO	Edema associated with CHF, hypertension, diabetes insipidus	Dizziness, vertigo, paresthesia, weakness, headache, fatigue, volume depletion, dysrhythmia, photosensitivity, nausea, constipation, pancreatitis, polyuria, leukopenia, hypokalemia, gout, muscle cramps
Metolazone (Zaroxylin)	PO	Edema, CHF, hypertension, calcium nephrolithiasis	Dizziness, vertigo, paresthesia, weakness, headache, fatigue, volume depletion, dysrhythmia, photosensitivity, nausea, constipation, pancreatitis, polyuria, leukopenia, hypokalemia, gout, muscle cramps
Polythiazide (Minizide, Renese)	PO	Edema, CHF, hypertension	Dizziness, vertigo, paresthesia, weakness, headache, fatigue, volume depletion, dysrhythmia, photosensitivity, nausea, constipation, pancreatitis, polyuria, leukopenia, hypokalemia, gout, muscle cramps
Trichlormethiazide (Diureses, Metahydrin, Naqua)	PO	Edema, CHF, hypertension, calcium nephrolithiasis	Dizziness, vertigo, paresthesia, weakness, headache, fatigue, volume depletion, dysrhythmia, photosensitivity, nausea, constipation, pancreatitis, polyuria, leukopenia, hypokalemia, gout, muscle cramps

3. Administration considerations

  a. Take medication early in day to avoid nocturia
  b. Administer with food or milk to prevent GI upset
  c. Thiazide diuretics are ineffective if creatinine clearance level is less 30 mL/min
  d. Allow 2–4 weeks for maximum antihypertensive effect
  e. Metolazone is not recommended in children because safety has not been established
4. Contraindications

  a. Hypersensitivity to thiazide diuretics or sulfonamide derivatives
  b. Clients with anuria

         c. Use cautiously in client with severely impaired renal or hepatic function

         d. Contraindicated in pregnancy; women who breastfeed should not use thiazide diuretics

    5. Significant drug interactions

         a. Concomitant use with lithium will increase serum lithium levels

         b. Thiazide diuretics decrease effectiveness of hyperuricemic agents, sulfonylureas, and insulin

         c. There is an additive effect if used with loop diuretics

         d. NSAIDs cause a decreased thiazide diuretic effect

         e. Bile acid resins decrease absorption of thiazide diuretics

         f. Thiazide diuretics may increase hypersensitivity to allopurinol

    6. Significant food interactions: none reported

    7. Significant laboratory studies

         a. May alter serum electrolytes, especially lowering potassium

         b. May increase serum urate, glucose, cholesterol, triglycerides, blood urea nitrogen (BUN), and creatinine

         c. May interfere with tests for parathyroid function

         d. Decreased protein-bound iodine levels without thyroid dysfunction

    8. Side effects

         a. Dizziness, vertigo, headache, and weakness

         b. Dehydration, orthostatic hypotension, N/V, abdominal pain, diarrhea, constipation, and frequent urination

         c. Dermatitis and rash

         d. Electrolyte imbalance, impaired glucose tolerance, jaundice, muscle cramps, photosensitivity, impotence, and hyperuricemia

    9. Adverse effects/toxicity: renal failure, aplastic anemia, agranulocytosis, thrombocytopenia, and anaphylactic reaction

    10. Nursing considerations

         a. Monitor vital signs for hypotension and tachycardia

         b. Monitor serum electrolytes, calcium, and uric acid levels

         c. Monitor and record body weight at regular intervals at same time of day and same scale

         d. Monitor I & O

         e. Assess indicators of dehydration: thirst, poor skin turgor, coated tongue

         f. Assess for inadequate tissue perfusion and weakness, decreased muscle strength, restlessness, anxiety, and agitation

    11. Client education

         a. Eat foods high in potassium to prevent hypokalemia

         b. Restrict sodium intake; do not use salt substitutes if taking potassium supplement

         c. Avoid dehydration by avoiding alcohol and caffeinated beverages, and replacing fluids during exercise or hot weather

         d. Avoid exposure to intense heat as with baths, showers, and electric blankets

         e. Take small frequent amounts of ice chips or clear liquids if vomiting

         f. Replace fluids with fruit juice or bouillon if diarrhea occurs

         g. Diuretics increase amount and frequency of urination, so take doses in morning and early afternoon to avoid nighttime urination and interruption of sleep

         h. Change position slowly to avoid dizziness and orthostatic hypotension

         i. Weigh self daily and report sudden weight gains or losses

         j. If diabetic, check blood glucose periodically

Table 12-3	Common Potassium-Sparing Diuretics			
Generic (Trade) Name	**Route**	**Uses**	**Adverse Effects**
Amiloride hydrochloride (Midamor)	PO	Adjunctive therapy with thiazide and loop diuretics to treat edema and congestive heart failure (CHF), hypertension, prevention of hypokalemia	Headache, dizziness, drowsiness, fatigue, paresthesia, tremors, confusion, rash, alopecia, cough, dyspnea, hyperkalemia, decreased libido, impotence, jaundice, gastro-intestinal bleeding, muscle cramps
Spironolactone (Aldactone)	PO	Diagnosis and treatment of hyperaldosteronism; edema related to CHF, nephrotic syndrome, cirrhosis; prevention and treatment of hypokalemia; essential hypertension	Dizziness, headache, drowsiness, fatigue, rash, cramping, diarrhea, impotence, hyperkalemia, agranulocytosis, hirsutism, gynecomastia, deepened voice
Triamterene (Dyrenium)	PO	Edema related to CHF, cirrhosis, steroid-related edema, secondary hyperaldosteronism	Headache, rash, hyperkalemia, photosensitivity, nausea, vomiting, dry mouth, renal stones, interstitial nephritis

C. Potassium-sparing diuretics

1. Action and use
   a. Act directly on distal convoluted tubule to increase sodium excretion and decrease potassium secretion
   b. Used for hypertension and edema associated with HF
   c. Spironolactone is also used for detection of primary hyperaldosteronism, hirsutism, and premenstrual syndrome
2. Common medications (Table 12-3)
3. Administration considerations
   a. Take with food or milk
    b. Avoid salt substitutes
    c. Avoid excessive ingestion of foods high in potassium
   d. When administering spironolactone to children, crush tablet and mix in flavored syrup as oral suspension
4. Contraindications
   a. Serum potassium levels greater than 5.5 mEq/mL
   b. Concomitant use with other potassium-sparing diuretics
   c. Fluid and electrolyte imbalances
   d. Anuria, acute and chronic renal insufficiency, diabetic nephropathy, hypersensitivity, and impaired hepatic function
   e. Caution in client with diabetes mellitus
5. Significant drug interactions
   a. May potentiate hypotensive effects of antihypertensive medications
   b. Increased risk of hyperkalemia with other potassium-sparing diuretics
   c. May increase serum blood levels of lithium due to decreased renal clearance
   d. Reduced effect of digoxin if administered with amiloride
   e. Aspirin may slightly decrease response of spironolactone
   f. Antidiabetic drugs may need adjustment as triamterene may increase blood glucose levels
   g. Corticosteroids may increase electrolyte depletion
6. Significant food interactions: administering spironolactone with food increases its absorption

7. Significant laboratory studies
   a. Monitor electrolytes (especially potassium), creatinine, and BUN
   b. Digoxin level
   c. Triamterene may interfere with enzyme assays
8. Side effects
   a. CNS: headache, weakness, dizziness, and orthostatic hypotension
   b. GI: N/V, diarrhea, and constipation
   c. Impotence, muscle cramps, urticaria, gynecomastia, and breast soreness
   d. Dry mouth, photosensitivity, transient elevated BUN and creatinine
9. Adverse effects/toxicity
   a. Aplastic anemia and thrombocytopenia
   b. Hyperkalemia
10. Nursing considerations
    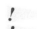
    a. Monitor vital signs and urine output
    b. Administer with meals to prevent GI upset
    c. Discontinue potassium supplements
    d. Observe closely older adult and debilitated clients for drug-induced diuresis and hyperkalemia
    e. Monitor for dehydration and electrolyte imbalance
    f. Monitor periodic serum electrolytes such as BUN and creatinine
11. Client education
    a. Take medication with food to avoid GI upset with all medications except triamterene
    b. Avoid consumption of large quantities of foods high in potassium
    c. Report any mental confusion or lethargy immediately
    d. Monitor for signs and symptoms of hyperkalemia such as nausea, diarrhea, abdominal cramps, and tachycardia followed by bradycardia
    e. Side effects usually disappear after drug is discontinued except gynecomastia may persist
    f. With spironolactone, maximal diuresis may not occur until day 3 of therapy and diuresis may continue 2–3 days after the drug is stopped
    g. Triamterene may turn urine blue
    h. Avoid salt substitutes because they contain potassium
    i. Avoid exposure to direct sunlight

D. Carbonic anhydrase inhibitors
1. Action and use
   a. Noncompetitive reversible inhibition of enzyme carbonic anhydrase, which promotes excretion of bicarbonate, sodium, potassium, and water
   b. Results in slightly acidic urine
   c. Used for treatment of edema caused by HF
   d. Used for open angle glaucoma to decrease intraocular pressure
   e. Used for treatment of epilepsy
   f. Used to treat metabolic alkalosis
2. Common medications (Table 12-4)
3. Administration considerations
   a. Increasing dose does not appear to increase diuresis
   b. Do not administer with high dose aspirin
   c. Intramuscular administration is not recommended
4. Contraindications
   a. Pregnancy
   b. Narrow angle or acute glaucoma
   c. Any situation with decreased sodium and/or potassium levels

Table 12-4 **Common Carbonic Anhydrase Inhibitors**

Generic (Trade) Name	Route	Uses	Adverse Effects
Acetazolamide (Diamox)	PO, IV	Decrease intraocular pressure in clients with open angle glaucoma, edema related to heart failure, chronic open angle glaucoma, prevention of acute mountain sickness, adjunctive therapy for seizures, paralysis, drug-induced edema	Confusion, drowsiness, paresthesias, hearing abnormalities, transient myopia, renal calculus, photosensitivity, rash, electrolyte imbalance, aplastic anemia, leukopenia, hyperchloremic acidosis, hypokalemia, hyperuricemia
Dichlorphenamide (Daranide, Oratrol)	PO	Decrease intraocular pressure in clients with open angle glaucoma	
Methazolamide (Neptazane)	PO	Decrease intraocular pressure in clients with open angle glaucoma	

     d. Marked kidney or liver dysfunction

     e. Cautionary use in client with chronic obstructive pulmonary disease (COPD) or during lactation

  5. Significant drug interactions

     a. Aspirin may cause accumulation and toxicity of acetazolamide

     b. May increase levels of cyclosporine and decreased levels of primidone

     c. Increased excretion of lithium

     d. Decreased renal clearance of amphetamines, anticholinergics, procainamide, quinidine, and tricyclic antidepressants (TCA)

  6. Significant food interactions: none reported

  7. Significant laboratory studies

     a. Obtain platelet and complete blood cell counts (CBC) prior to and periodically during therapy; may decrease hemoglobin and hematocrit

     b. Monitor serum electrolytes

     c. May cause false positive proteinuria

     d. May decrease thyroid iodine uptake

     e. May increase uric acid level

  8. Side effects

     a. Confusion, drowsiness, and paresthesias

     b. Hearing dysfunction, GI upset, polyuria, and transient myopia

     c. Electrolyte imbalance, fever, rash, renal calculus, and photosensitivity

  9. Adverse effects/toxicity

     a. Metabolic acidosis

     b. Anaphylaxis

     c. Bone marrow depression

     d. Thrombocytopenia purpura, hemolytic anemia, leukopenia, pancytopenia, and agranulocytosis

     e. Severe reactions to sulfonamides including Stevens–Johnson syndrome, toxic epidermal necrosis, fulminant hepatic necrosis, coma, and death have occurred

  10. Nursing considerations

     a. Monitor for signs and symptoms of dehydration; I & O

     b. Assess for alterations in skin integrity

     c. Assess for edema

     d. Assess vital signs and daily weight

     e. Assess cardiovascular and respiratory status

     f. Assess changes in level of consciousness and activity level

        g. Dietary assessment of high salt-containing foods

        h. Fluid restriction as ordered

   11. Client education

        a. Do not take aspirin or aspirin-containing medications

        b. Report symptoms of anorexia, lethargy, or tachypnea

        c. Use caution while driving or performing tasks that require alertness, coordination, or physical dexterity because of risk of drowsiness

        d. Monitor for signs of renal calculi

        e. Follow-up scheduled lab tests are important

        f. Weigh self daily at same time of day; report acute weight gain or loss

        g. Be aware of and avoid high-sodium foods and beverages; eat foods high in potassium instead

E. Osmotic diuretics

   1. Action and use

        a. Increase osmotic pressure of glomerular filtrate in proximal tubule and loop of Henle inhibiting reabsorption of water and electrolytes, thus promoting diuresis

        b. Used to prevent and manage acute renal failure (ARF) and oliguria

        c. Used to decrease intracranial or intraocular pressure

        d. Mannitol is used with chemotherapy to induce diuresis

   2. Common medications (Table 12-5)

   3. Administration considerations

        a. Medications are administered IV by slow infusion

        b. Urea turns to ammonia if left standing

        c. Do not infuse with blood or blood products

        d. Mannitol crystallizes at low temperatures

        e. For maximum reduction of intraocular pressure, mannitol should be given 1–1.5 hours before surgery

   4. Contraindications

        a. Severely impaired renal function, marked dehydration, breastfeeding, hepatic failure, active intracranial bleed, and anuria

        b. Severe pulmonary congestion and severe heart failure

   5. Significant drug interactions

        a. Decrease serum lithium levels

        b. Use with cardiac glycosides may cause an increased possibility of digitalis toxicity

        c. Increased effects of other diuretics

   6. Significant food interactions: none reported

   7. Significant laboratory studies: monitor BUN and electrolytes frequently

Table 12-5   **Common Osmotic Diuretics**

Generic (Trade) Name	Route	Uses	Adverse Effects
Mannitol (Osmitrol)	IV	Oliguria, acute renal impairment, edema, ascites, renal failure, hepatic failure, cardiac failure, increased intraocular pressure, increased intracranial pressure, diuresis in drug intoxication, transurethral resection of the prostate	Headaches, confusion, seizures, circulatory overload, tachycardia, chest pain, blurred vision, hypotension, hypertension, edema, thrombophlebitis, urticaria, diuresis, fluid and electrolyte imbalance, hyponatremia, pulmonary congestion, rhinitis, water intoxication
Urea (Ureaphil)	IV	Increased intracranial pressure, cerebral edema, increased intraocular pressure	Syncope, dizziness, headache, disorientation, N/V, tissue necrosis at IV site with extravasation, hyponatremia, hypokalemia, thrombophlebitis, febrile episode, hypovolemia

8. Side effects
   a. Headache, syncope, and hypotension
   b. Dry mouth, N/V, urine retention, electrolyte imbalance, and urticaria
9. Adverse effects/toxicity
   a. Seizures
   b. Thrombophlebitis
   c. Congestive heart failure
   d. Cardiovascular collapse
10. Nursing considerations
    a. Maintain adequate hydration
    b. Monitor fluid and electrolyte balance
    c. Monitor BUN
    d. Indwelling catheter should be used in comatose clients for accurate I & O
    e. Monitor I & O and vital signs hourly while on mannitol
    f. Measure daily weight
    g. Monitor renal function, fluid balance, serum, and urinary sodium and potassium levels
    h. Assess for signs of decreasing intracranial pressure if appropriate
    i. Monitor lung and heart sounds for signs of pulmonary edema
11. Client education
    a. Monitor daily weight and report sudden weight gain or loss
    b. Report immediately pain in chest or legs, shortness of breath, or apnea
    c. Change position slowly to prevent dizziness or orthostatic hypotension
    d. Drink only fluids ordered even if thirsty and/or experiencing dry mouth
    e. Have family monitor change in neuro status such as decreased level of consciousness (LOC)

Practice to Pass

Potassium supplementation has been ordered along with furosemide (Lasix) to initially treat the client with acute renal failure. The nurse teaching the client should inform her that which medications should be avoided while on Lasix?

II. POTASSIUM SUPPLEMENTS

A. Action and use
1. Potassium is the main cation in body cells
2. Acts to maintain intracellular tonicity, maintain balance with sodium across cell membranes, transmit nerve impulses, and maintain cellular metabolism
3. Help contracting cardiac and skeletal muscle, maintaining acid–base balance, and maintaining normal renal function
4. Potassium is well absorbed from GI tract and excreted largely by kidneys
5. Used to prevent and treat hypokalemia

B. Common medication names (Table 12-6)

C. Administration considerations
1. Tablet form should be taken with a full glass of water
2. Tablets are not to be crushed, chewed, or sucked; if difficulty swallowing, tablet may be broken and dissolved in water
3. Powder preparations should be mixed with 4 ounces of water or other liquid

Table 12-6 Potassium Supplements

Generic (Trade) Name	Route	Therapeutic Indications	Adverse Effects
Potassium Chloride (Kaon-Cl, K-Lor, K-Dur, Micro-K, Klotrix, K-tab)	PO, IV	Prevention and correction of potassium depletion, IV treatment of cardiac dysrhythmias associated with cardiac glycosides	Hyperkalemia, N/V, diarrhea, abdominal pain, rash, GI obstruction, ECG changes with peaked T waves, loss of P waves, ST segment depression, prolongation of QT interval

4. Potassium supplements should be taken with meals to decrease GI irritation
5. Tablets in wax matrix sometimes lodge in esophagus and cause ulceration; in cardiac clients who have esophageal compression due to enlarged left atrium, use liquid form
6. Enteric coated tablets are not recommended because of potential for GI bleeding and small bowel ulcerations
7. Parenteral potassium should be given slowly and in diluted form (often 40 mEg/L or less via peripheral vein) and infused no faster than 10 mEq/hr, even via central line

D. **Contraindications**
1. Severe renal impairment with oliguria, **anuria** (absence of urine), or azotemia
2. Untreated Addison disease
3. Acute dehydration and heat cramps
4. Hyperkalemia and form of familial periodic paralysis, as well as conditions associated with extensive tissue breakdown
5. Use cautiously with cardiac and renal disease

E. **Significant drug interactions**
1. Anticholinergics may increase risk of GI irritation and ulceration
2. Potassium-containing agents increase risk for hyperkalemia
3. Potassium is not recommended in clients with severe or complete heart block taking digoxin due to potential for arrhythmias
4. Use with potassium-sparing diuretics, angiotensin converting enzyme (ACE) inhibitors or salt substitutes containing potassium salts can cause severe hyperkalemia
5. May decrease absorption of vitamin B_{12} in GI tract

F. **Significant food interactions**
1. Foods high in potassium
2. Examples include apple juice, grapefruit, bananas, oranges, peaches, pears, raisins, broccoli, peas, tomatoes, eggplant, chicken, liver, turkey, salmon, beef, low-fat yogurt, milk, and chocolate milk

G. **Significant laboratory studies**: none reported

H. **Side effects**
1. Paresthesia of extremities, restlessness, confusion, weakness, or heaviness of legs
2. Hypotension and electrocardiogram (ECG) changes
3. Abdominal pain, N/V, and diarrhea
4. Hyperkalemia

I. **Adverse effects/toxicity**
1. Dysrhythmias or cardiac arrest
2. Respiratory paralysis

J. **Nursing considerations**
1. Monitor serum potassium, BUN, and creatinine
2. Monitor I & O
3. Monitor ECG for dysrhythmias
4. Monitor for side effects such as weakness, feeling of heaviness in legs, confusion, hypotension (signs of hyperkalemia)
5. Potassium should not be given immediately postoperatively until urine flow is established
6. Attempt to identify cause of hypokalemia
7. Assess parenteral infusion site frequently for signs of pain and inflammation

K. **Client education**
1. Foods high in potassium
2. Avoid salt substitutes while taking potassium supplements
3. Contact prescriber if swallowing problems occur
4. Monitor stools for evidence of GI bleed
5. Notify prescriber of any other prescription or over-the-counter (OTC) medications

Practice to Pass

A client has just been diagnosed with hypertension. Besides instructions regarding medication, what modifiable factors should be discussed?

6. Report diarrhea or vomiting because of increased risk for hypokalemia
7. Report immediately confusion; irregular heartbeat; numbness of feet, fingers, or lips; shortness of breath; anxiety; excessive tiredness; or weakness of legs
8. Take potassium supplement with meals to decrease GI irritation
9. Take only the prescribed amount of potassium to avoid toxicity
10. Dissolve powder, soluble tablets, or granules completely in at least 4 ounces of water or juice before drinking
11. Do not crush or chew sustained-release capsules but contents can be opened and sprinkled onto soft foods
12. Expelling a whole sustained-release tablet in stool is normal as body eliminates shell after absorbing potassium

III. ANTIHYPERTENSIVES

A. Stepped care management

1. The Seventh Report of Joint National Committee on Prevention, Detection, Evaluation, and Treatment of High Blood Pressure (JNC VII) directs practitioners to individualize each client's hypertension management to desired BP range, using BP measurements, risk factors, and target organ disease as parameters
2. Hypertension is not diagnosed on the basis of a single BP reading but is defined as a sustained elevation of systolic and/or diastolic BP
3. Consideration must be given to cost, ease of following treatment regimen, potential for drug–drug interactions, and drug side effect profile

B. Diuretics

1. JNC VII recommends thiazide diuretics as first-line therapy for hypertension
2. They reduce BP and edema by increasing urine production, enhancing water and sodium excretion
3. The most common diuretics used for hypertension are thiazide and loop diuretics (see previous discussion)
4. Other diuretics that may be used are potassium-sparing, osmotic, and carbonic anhydrase inhibitors (see previous discussion)

Practice to Pass

What routine labs need to be monitored for the hypertensive client?

C. Adrenergic inhibitors (alpha and beta blockers)

1. Action and use
   a. Alpha-adrenergic blocking agents decrease vasomotor tone to cause vasodilation and thus reduce BP
   b. Beta blockers reduce BP by preventing stimulation of beta receptors in heart by epinephrine and norepinephrine, thereby decreasing heart rate and cardiac output (CO); they also interfere with release of renin by kidneys to decrease **renin-angiotensin system** mechanism, resulting in reduced BP (see Chapter 5)
   c. Alpha blockers are used for peripheral vascular disorders, hypertension and **benign prostatic hyperplasia (BPH)** (a symptom complex defined as benign adenomatous hyperplasia of the periurethral prostate gland)
2. Common medications (Table 12-7)
3. Administration considerations
   a. Alpha blockers may cause syncope within 30 minutes to 1 hour after first dose; effect is transient and may be diminished by giving at bedtime
   b. To avoid first dose syncope, begin with a small dose
   c. Do not stop drug abruptly
4. Contraindications
   a. Alpha blockers: hypersensitivity to drug
   b. Beta blockers: hypersensitivity to drug, symptomatic bradycardia, greater than first-degree heart block, class IV heart failure, and asthma

Table 12-7 **Common Alpha-Blocker Medications**

Generic (Trade) Name	Route	Uses	Adverse Effects
Carvedilol (Coreg)	PO	Hypertension, mild to severe heart failure, left ventricular dysfunction following myocardial infarction (MI)	Dizziness, headache, fatigue, postural hypotension, depression, cerebrovascular accident (stroke), hypotension, atrioventricular heart block, bradycardia, peripheral vascular disease, thrombocytopenia, hyperkalemia, hypoglycemia
Doxazosin (Cardura)	PO	Essential hypertension	Rash, pruritis, dizziness, vertigo, headache, somnolence, drowsiness, pain, hypotension, dysrhythmia, palpitations, pharyngitis, dyspnea, arthralgia, constipation
Labetalol (Trandate/ Normodyne)	PO, IV	Hypertension, severe hypertension, hypertensive emergency	Dizziness, fatigue, headache, transient scalp tingling, orthostatic hypotension, bradycardia, ventricular dysrhythmia, N/V, diarrhea, sexual dysfunction, urinary retention, increased airway resistance
Prazosin (Minipress)	PO	Mild to moderate hypertension, BPH	Dizziness, first-dose syncope, palpitations, orthostatic hypotension, N/V, diarrhea, priapism, impotence
Terazosin (Hytrin)	PO	Hypertension, BPH	Thrombocytopenia, decreased libido, dyspnea, back pain, muscle pain, peripheral edema, atrial fibrillation, peripheral edema, nasal congestion, sinusitis, blurred vision, impotence, priapism

5. Significant drug interactions
   a. Alpha blockers
      1) Enhance hypoglycemia with insulin and oral antidiabetic agents
      2) Decrease antihypertensive effect of clonidine
      3) Prazosin and indomethacin (Indocin): decreased antihypertensive effect
      4) Prazosin and verapamil (Calan): increase serum prazosin concentration
      5) Prazosin and beta blockers: increase first dose syncope
      6) May increase digoxin level by 15%
   b. Alpha and beta blockers
      1) Additive effects with other antihypertensive medications
      2) Coreg/digoxin: increase digoxin levels
      3) Coreg or labetalol/cimetidine: increase Coreg or labetalol levels
      4) Coreg/rifampin: decrease Coreg level
6. Significant food interactions: saw palmetto (herb) produces an additive effect for BPH; butcher's broom diminishes effect of terazosin; delayed absorption of carvedilol with food
7. Significant laboratory studies
   a. Alpha blockers
      1) May cause false positive urine assays for pheochromocytoma
      2) May increase BUN, creatinine, ALT/AST, alkaline phosphatase, triglycerides, uric acid
      3) May increase or decrease glucose levels
   b. Alpha/beta blockers: may cause increased urine free and total catecholamines
8. Side effects
   a. Alpha blockers: first dose syncope, headache, drowsiness, hypotension, palpitations, impotence, nasal congestion, N/V, tachycardia
   b. Alpha/beta blockers: fatigue, orthostatic hypotension, dizziness, N/V, diarrhea, bronchospasm, muscle spasm, transient scalp tingling, hyperglycemia, upper respiratory infections, impotence, and arthralgias

9. Adverse effects/toxicity
   a. Alpha blockers: leukopenia, neutropenia, thrombocytopenia, myelosuppression, anaphylaxis, bronchospasm, and arrhythmia
   b. Alpha/beta blockers: ventricular arrhythmias, AV block, bradycardia, thrombocytopenia, and sudden death
10. Nursing considerations
    a. Monitor client for the past medical history
    b. Monitor vital signs especially BP and heart rate
    c. Monitor for manifestations of HF such as edema
    d. Monitor peripheral circulation
    e. Monitor diabetic clients for manifestations of hypoglycemia
    f. Abrupt discontinuance of medication may exacerbate angina or precipitate MI
    g. Hypotensive effects may be more pronounced in older adults
    h. Maintain safety when client is changing positions
    i. Monitor for first-dose syncope (alpha and alpha/beta blockers); give first dose at bedtime to minimize risk
11. Client education
    a. Take drug exactly as prescribed
    b. Rationale for therapy
    c. Change position slowly to prevent dizziness and falls
    d. Report any side effects to prescriber
    e. Monitor blood glucose levels and BP more frequently if taking insulin or oral antidiabetic medications
    f. Monitor weight daily and report weight gain over 5 pounds (lb) per week
    g. Avoid hazardous activities at beginning of therapy
    h. Do not stop medications without notifying prescriber
    i. Seek medical approval before taking any OTC medications
    j. Therapeutic effect may take 3–4 weeks
    k. Avoid alcohol use, excessive exercise, prolonged standing and exposure to heat due to increased risk of orthostatic hypotension

D. **Angiotensin-converting enzyme (ACE) inhibitors**
   1. Action and use
      a. Inhibit the renin-angiotensin-aldosterone mechanism by blocking conversion of angiotensin I to angiotensin II and prevent peripheral **vasoconstriction**
      b. Used to treat hypertension
      c. Are preferred drugs for kidney failure for hypertensive clients with diabetic nephropathy
      d. Are effective alone in Caucasian clients and with administration of a diuretic in African American clients
   2. Common medications (Table 12-8)
   3. Administration considerations
      a. Discontinue as soon as possible if pregnancy detected
      b. Moexipril and captopril should be taken on an empty stomach due to decreased absorption with food
   4. Contraindications
      a. Pregnancy
      b. Hypersensitivity to ACE inhibitors
      c. Avoid use with potassium supplements and potassium-sparing diuretics
   5. Significant drug interactions
      a. Potassium-sparing diuretics or potassium supplements: hyperkalemia
      b. Increased lithium concentration
      c. Increased risk of hypersensitivity with allopurinol

Practice to Pass

The client with hypertension asks if it is all right to use a salt substitute. How should the nurse respond?

Table 12-8		Common Angiotensin-Converting Enzyme Inhibitors	
Generic (Trade) Names	**Route**	**Uses**	**Adverse Effects**
Benazepril (Lotensin)	PO	Hypertension	Symptomatic hypotension, dysrhythmias, palpitations, edema, hyperkalemia, weight gain, angioedema, nonproductive cough, dyspnea, myalgia, photosensitivity, impotence, constipation, abdominal discomfort, depression, syncope, somnolence, purpura
Captopril (Capoten)	PO	Hypertension, heart failure, diabetic nephropathy, left ventricular dysfunction following MI	Renal impairment, leucopenia, agranulocytosis, pancytopenia, thrombocytopenia, hyperkalemia, angioedema of face and limbs, heart failure, dizziness, fainting, pericarditis, nephrotic syndrome, cholestatic jaundice, elevated liver enzymes, urinary frequency
Enalapril (Vasotec, Amprace, Renitec)	PO, IV	Hypertension, heart failure, asymptomatic left ventricular dysfunction	Dizziness, fatigue, headache, neutropenia, thrombocytopenia, hyperkalemia, dry persistent cough, dyspnea, angioedema, abdominal pain, constipation, decreased renal function, hypotension, vertigo, syncope
Fosinopril (Monopril)	PO	Hypertension, heart failure	Cerebrovascular accident, MI, chest pain, angina hepatitis, hyperkalemia, bronchospasm, urticaria, photosensitivity, sexual dysfunction, angioedema, dyspnea, cough, sinusitis, orthostatic hypotension
Lisinopril (Prinivil, Zestril)	PO	Hypertension, heart failure, acute MI	Hyperkalemia, muscle cramps, orthostatic hypotension, chest pain, nasal congestion, dyspnea, cough, angioedema, anaphylaxis, diminished libido
Moexipril (Univasc)	PO	Hypertension	Dizziness, fatigue, fainting, flushing, chest pain, neutropenia, hyperkalemia, myalgia, dry cough, anaphylaxis, angioedema, flulike symptoms
Quinapril (Accupril)	PO	Hypertension, heart failure	Hypertensive crisis, hyperkalemia, hemorrhage, somnolence, vertigo, light-headedness, hypotension, malaise, depression, orthostatic hypotension, angioedema, photosensitivity, back pain, exfoliative dermatitis, persistent cough, diaphoresis, vasodilation, tachycardia
Ramipril (Altace, Ramace, Tritace)	PO	Hypertension, heart failure	Seizures, dysrhythmias, myocardial infarction, hyperkalemia, angioedema, arthralgia, headache, dizziness, fatigue, light-headedness, orthostatic hypotension, insomnia, nervousness, tremors, vertigo, photosensitivity, angioedema, epistaxis, dry cough, edema, dyspepsia, gastroenteritis, diaphoresis, depression
Trandolapril (Mavik)	PO	Hypertension, heart failure, left ventricular dysfunction following acute MI	Bradycardia, dizziness, headache, fatigue, drowsiness, palpitations, edema, flushing, hypotension, palpitations, epistaxis, dry cough, throat irritation, pancreatitis, abdominal distention, neutropenia, leukopenia, hyperkalemia, angioedema, anaphylaxis, pruritis, dyspnea, upper respiratory infection

    d. May increase digoxin concentration

    e. Antacids may decrease absorption of captopril and fosinopril

    f. Indomethacin may decrease hypotensive effect

    g. Phenothiazines may increase drug effects

  6. Significant food interactions: capsicum may aggravate ACE-induced cough; black catechu will increase hypotensive effect; licorice may cause sodium retention; sodium substitutes may result in hyperkalemia; foods high in fat may impair drug absorption; administer on empty stomach

7. Significant laboratory studies
   a. Agranulocytosis and bone marrow depression
   b. May increase serum BUN and creatinine
   c. May increase liver enzymes, serum bilirubin, uric acid, and blood glucose
   d. Captopril may cause false positive urinary acetone
8. Side effects
   a. Headache, dizziness, anxiety, fatigue, insomnia, nervousness, hypotension, and palpitations
   b. Abdominal pain, N/V, constipation, persistent dry nonproductive cough, and dyspnea
   c. Rash, arthralgia, impotence, and dysgeusia (altered taste)
9. Adverse effects/toxicity
   a. Angioedema, leukopenia, agranulocytosis, pancytopenia, thrombocytopenia
   b. Cerebrovascular accident (CVA or stroke), MI, and hypertensive crisis
10. Nursing considerations
   a. Administer 1 hour before meals to increase absorption
   b. Tablets may be crushed
   c. Do not administer to pregnant or lactating women
   d. Monitor labs for increased potassium, liver enzymes, bilirubin, BUN, and creatinine, and decreased sodium levels
   e. Take BP before giving dose and monitor regularly
   f. Monitor for rashes or hives
   g. Assess for peripheral edema
   h. If the client has renal disease, monitor urine protein on a regular basis by dipstick method
   i. Diuretics should be discontinued 2–3 days before ACE inhibitor therapy
   j. Monitor white blood cells (WBC) and differential counts periodically
   k. BP is lowered within 1 hour of fosinopril with peak at 2–6 hours
11. Client education
   a. Report peripheral edema, signs of infection, facial swelling, loss of taste, or difficulty breathing
   b. Change position slowly to prevent dizziness and falls
   c. Do not skip doses or stop taking drug; it may cause serious rebound BP
   d. Seek medical approval before taking OTC medications
   e. Notify prescriber if a persistent, dry cough occurs
   f. Take antacids 2 hours before or after dose of fosinopril and captopril
   g. Avoid potassium-containing salt substitutes
   h. Monitor for bruising, petechiae, or bleeding with captopril
   i. The taste of food may be diminished during the first month of therapy
   j. Take captopril 20 minutes to 1 hour before a meal
   k. Eliminate licorice from diet
E. Angiotensin II antagonists
   1. Action and use
      a. Antagonist at angiotensin II receptor of vascular smooth muscle blocking vasoconstriction and aldosterone-secreting effects
      b. Used for hypertension
   2. Common medications (Table 12-9)
   3. Administration considerations: discontinue as soon as pregnancy is detected
   4. Contraindications
      a. Pregnancy
      b. Hypersensitivity
      c. Caution in clients with renal or hepatic disease

Table 12-9 **Common Angiotensin II Antagonist Medications**

Generic (Trade) Name	Route	Uses	Adverse Effects
Losartan (Cozaar)	PO	Hypertension, reduction of CVA risk in clients with hypertension and left ventricular hypertrophy	Dizziness, vertigo, asthenia, fatigue, headache, insomnia, angioedema, nephropathy, chest pain, diabetic vascular disease, diarrhea, anemia, hypoglycemia, weight gain, myalgia, dyspepsia, flulike symptoms, cough, bronchitis, leg pain, cellulitis, diabetic vascular disease
Valsartan (Diovan)	PO	Hypertension, heart failure	Dizziness, vertigo, fatigue, postural hypotension, syncope, pharyngitis, rhinitis, sinusitis, blurred vision, renal impairment, neutropenia, hyperkalemia, arthralgia, angioedema, upper respiratory infection, cough

5. Significant drug interactions
   a. Avoid use with potassium-sparing diuretics
   b. Diuretics may increase the risk for hypotension
   c. Losartan and phenobarbital: decreased losartan levels
   d. Losartan and cimetidine (Tagamet): increased losartan levels
   e. Indomethacin may decrease hypotensive effect
6. Significant food interactions: salt substitutes increase risk of hyperkalemia; red yeast rice may increase risk of toxicity
7. Significant laboratory studies
   a. WBC for neutropenia
   b. Electrolytes for hyperkalemia
8. Side effects
   a. Hypotension and dizziness
   b. Cough, GI upset, insomnia, nasal congestion or pharyngitis, myalgia/arthralgia, or flulike symptom
9. Adverse effects/toxicity
   a. Angioedema
   b. Hypotension
   c. Tachycardia or bradycardia
10. Nursing considerations
    a. Monitor client taking diuretics for additive hypotension
    b. Regularly assess renal function
    c. Do not administer to pregnant or lactating women
    d. Monitor potassium levels
    e. Monitor regularly BP and apical pulse
    f. Monitor WBC and differential periodically
11. Client education
    a. Do not discontinue medication abruptly
    b. Avoid salt substitutes
    c. Notify prescriber immediately if pregnancy is suspected
    d. Use nonhormonal birth control methods
    e. Report any side effects to prescriber
    f. Change positions slowly to avoid dizziness
F. **Calcium channel blockers (see Chapter 5)**
G. **Other antihypertensives**
   1. Action and use
      a. Centrally acting sympatholytics
         1) Stimulate alpha2-receptors in central nervous system (CNS) to inhibit sympathetic cardio-accelerator and vasoconstrictor centers
         2) Decrease sympathetic outflow from CNS resulting in decreased arterial BP

Table 12-10		Common Centrally and Peripherally Acting Anti-Adrenergic Medications	
Generic (Trade) Name	**Route**	**Uses**	**Adverse Effects**
Clonidine (Catapress)	PO	Essential, renal, and malignant hypertension	Anxiety, confusion, somnolence, nervousness, bradycardia, severe rebound hypertension, impotence, urinary tract infection, N/V, urinary retention, transient glucose intolerance, pruritis, dermatitis
Guanfacine hydrochloride (Tenex)	PO	Hypertension	Weakness, dizziness, sedation, headache, insomnia, tinnitus, hypokinesia, bradycardia, palpitations, substernal pain, dry mouth, constipation, impotence, testicular disorder, leg cramps, altered taste
Guanadrel sulfate (Hylorel)	PO	Hypertension, renal hypertension	

    b. Peripheral anti-adrenergics
        1) Deplete catecholamine stores in peripheral nervous system and perhaps in the CNS
        2) Decrease total peripheral resistance, heart rate, and CO
2. Common medications (Table 12-10)
3. Administration considerations

    a. Abrupt discontinuance may result in rebound hypertension
    b. Guanabenz: allow 1–2 weeks before adjusting dose
    c. Guanfacine: administer at bedtime to decrease daytime somnolence; allow 3–4 weeks before adjusting dose
    d. Methyldopa: allow 2 days for maximum response before adjusting dose
4. Contraindications
    a. Hypersensitivity for all drugs from this group
    b. Active hepatitis or cirrhosis
    c. Co-administration of methyldopa with monoamine oxidase (MAO) inhibitors
    d. History of mental depression, active peptic ulcer disease, ulcerative colitis, HF, asthma, and bronchitis (reserpine)
    e. If signs of HF occur, discontinue methyldopa
5. Significant drug interactions
    a. Clonidine/beta blockers: paradoxical hypertension
    b. Clonidine/tricyclic antidepressants: may block antihypertensive effect
    c. Methyldopa may increase effects of levodopa, lithium, haloperidol, MAO inhibitors, and sympathomimetics
    d. Methyldopa/propranolol: paradoxical hypertension
    e. Guanadrel/phenothiazines, sympathomimetics and tricyclic antidepressants: inhibit antihypertensive effect
    f. Reserpine/tricyclic antidepressants: block antihypertensive effect
    g. Additive sedation if administered with CNS depressants
6. Significant food interactions: capsicum and yohimbe may reduce antihypertensive effect
7. Significant laboratory studies
    a. Blood glucose levels
    b. A positive Coomb's test
    c. May decrease serum cholesterol and total triglycerides slightly but does not alter HDL
    d. May cause nonprogressive elevation of liver enzymes
    e. Methyldopa alters urine uric acid, serum creatinine, AST, and ALT; it may cause falsely elevated levels of urine catecholamines interfering with the diagnosis of pheochromocytoma

8. Side effects
   a. Sedation, headache, weakness, dizziness, and decreased mental acuity
   b. Involuntary choreoathetoid movements, parkinsonism, depression, nightmares
   c. Bradycardia, orthostatic hypotension, aggravation of angina, edema
   d. GI disturbance, rash, gynecomastia, galactorrhea, amenorrhea, impotence, dry mouth, weight gain
9. Adverse effects/toxicity
   a. Myocarditis, hemolytic anemia, thrombocytopenia
   b. Hepatic necrosis
   c. Severe rebound hypertension
10. Nursing considerations
    a. Administer orally; tablets may be crushed
    b. They do not need to be given with food unless GI upset occurs
    c. IV methyldopa should be given over 30–60 minutes; do not give subcutaneously or IM
    d. Transdermal systems (Clonidine) are applied to dry, hairless areas on skin of chest or upper arm
    e. Assess areas for rash
    f. Monitor labs for elevated AST, ALT, alkaline phosphatase, bilirubin, BUN, creatinine, potassium, sodium, and uric acid
    g. May prolong prothrombin times
    h. Obtain baseline BP, apical pulse, and monitor weight regularly
    i. Assess client for peripheral edema
    j. Assess for persistent drowsiness
    k. Dry mouth may contribute to development of dental caries, periodontal disease, oral candidiasis, and discomfort
    l. Do not discontinue medication abruptly
11. Client education
    a. Restrict sodium in diet if ordered and lose weight as needed; report weight gain of greater than 5 lb per week
    b. Relieve dry mouth by sipping water or chewing sugarless gum
    c. Treat nausea by eating unsalted crackers, non-cola beverages, or dry toast
    d. Change position slowly to prevent dizziness and possible falls
    e. Report mental acuity changes to prescriber
    f. Some drugs cause the urine to become darker
    g. Do not drive a car or perform hazardous activities if drug causes drowsiness
    h. Take medication as prescribed
    i. Consult prescriber before taking OTC medications
    j. Avoid alcohol or other CNS depressants medications
    k. Do not stop taking drug abruptly

IV. ANTIHYPOTENSIVES (SYMPATHOMIMETICS)

A. Action and use
1. Mimic the fight-or-flight response of the sympathetic nervous system, selectively stimulating alpha-adrenergic and beta-adrenergic receptors
2. Stimulation of alpha-adrenergic receptors results in vasoconstriction and increased systemic BP
3. Stimulation of beta-adrenergic receptors increases the force and rate of myocardial contraction
4. Used to treat **shock**

B. Common medications (Table 12-11)

Table 12-11 Common Sympathomimetic Medications

Generic (Trade) Name	Route	Uses	Adverse Effects
Norepinephrine (Levophed)	IV	Acute hypotensive state	Headache, bradycardia, hypertension, tissue sloughing with extravasation
Metaraminol (Aramine)	IV	Hypotension	Restlessness, bradycardia, tissue sloughing with extravasation
Dopamine (Intropin)	IV	Hypotension, shock	Dysrhythmias, widening QRS complex, hypotension, bradycardia, asthma attack, tissue sloughing with extravasation, anaphylaxis
Dobutamine (Dobutrex)	IV	Cardiac decompensation	Headache, increased heart rate, premature ventricular contractions, leg cramps, non-specified chest pain, N/V, anaphylaxis, sloughing with extravasation
Isoproterenol (Isuprel)	IV, IM, subQ	Bronchospasm, heart block, ventricular dysrhythmia, shock, bradycardia, mitral regurgitation	Headache, tremors, Stokes-Adams syndrome, cardiac arrest, bronchospasm, diaphoresis, tachycardia, palpitations, rapid rise and fall of BP

C. **Administration considerations**
   1. Drug must be diluted before administration
   2. Client should be attended constantly during drug administration
D. **Contraindications**
   1. Uncorrected dysrhythmias, mesenteric or peripheral vascular thrombosis
   2. Profound hypoxia, hypercapnia, hypotension due to blood volume deficit
   3. Cautionary use with those receiving MAO inhibitors or imipramine-type antidepressants
E. **Significant drug interactions**
   1. Norepinephrine interacts with general anesthesia, tricyclic antidepressants, and MAO inhibitors
   2. Beta blockers may increase potential for hypertension
   3. Diuretics decrease arterial response
   4. Atropine and tricyclic antidepressants enhance pressor effects
   5. Metaraminol/MAO inhibitors: increase vasopressor effects
F. **Significant food interactions**: rue (herb) increases inotropic potential
G. **Significant laboratory studies**
   1. Monitor serum electrolytes
   2. Monitor blood glucose levels
   3. Isoproterenol decreases sensitivity of spirometry in the diagnosis of asthma
H. **Side effects**
   1. Anxiety, weakness, dizziness, tremor, restlessness
   2. Bradycardia, tachycardia, palpitations
   3. N/V, flushing, diaphoresis, sloughing upon extravasation
   4. Azotemia, shortness of breath, and bronchospasm
I. **Adverse effects/toxicity**
   1. Severe hypertension, anaphylaxis
   2. Arrhythmias, cardiac arrest, ventricular tachycardia
   3. Stokes-Adams seizures, asthmatic episodes
J. **Nursing considerations**
   1. Reevaluate if 3–5 treatments in 6–12 hours provide minimal to no relief
   2. Carefully monitor vital signs, ECG, and I & O

3. Monitor for rebound hypertension
4. Constant infusion pump prevents sudden infusion of excessive amounts of drugs
5. Correct blood volume depletion first
6. Antidote for extravasation: 5–10 mg phentolamine mesylate (Regitine) in 10–15 mL of normal saline
7. Monitor infusion site frequently
8. Client should be attended constantly during administration
9. Protect solution from light
10. Sympathomimetics are incompatible with sodium bicarbonate

K. Client education

1. Instruct client to report adverse reactions and side effects immediately
2. Inform client that vital signs will be monitored frequently
3. Instruct client to report anginal pain while on dobutamine

V. URINARY TRACT AND BLADDER MEDICATIONS

A. Anti-infectives

1. Action and use
   a. Act as **bacteriostatic** (inhibition of the growth of bacterial without destruction) and **bactericidal** (destroying bacteria) actions
   b. Act as disinfectants within the urinary tract
   c. Used to treat urinary tract infections
2. Common medications (Table 12-12)
3. Administration considerations
   a. May take with food or milk to decrease GI upset
   b. Check renal and hepatic function before administering
   c. Oral suspension may stain teeth
   d. Complete full course of therapy

Table 12-12 Common Urinary Tract Anti-infectives

Generic (Trade) Name	Route	Uses	Adverse Effects
Methenamine (Hiprex, Mandelamine)	PO	Urinary tract infection (UTI), pyelonephritis, cystitis, residual urine, anatomical abnormalities of the urinary tract	Bladder irritation, dysuria, urgency, frequency, hematuria, nausea, headache, dyspnea, rash, elevated serum transaminase
Nalidixic acid (NegGram)	PO	UTIs caused by gram-negative bacteria, *proteus*, *klebsiella*, *enterobacter*, *Escherichia coli*	Rash, pruritis, angioedema, photosensitivity, drowsiness, weakness, headache, vertigo, dizziness, N/V, diarrhea
Nitrofurantoin (Macrodantin)	PO	UTIs caused by *Escherichia coli*, *staphylococcus aureus*, *klebsiella*, *enterobacter*, *proteus*	Stevens-Johnson syndrome, exfoliative dermatitis, urticaria, angioedema, nausea, abdominal cramps, hepatoxicity, pulmonary hypersensitivity, superinfections, brown-rust urine
Trimethoprim (Proloprim)	PO	Acute otitis media, UTIs caused by *Escherichia coli*, *proteus*, *klebsiella*, *enterobacter*, *staphylococcus*	Thrombocytopenia, leukopenia, methemoglobinemia, megaloblastic anemia, epigastric distress, N/V, diarrhea, rash, pruritus, fever
Sulfisoxazole and Phenazopyridine (Azo-Gantrisin)	PO	UTIs, acute otitis media, conjunctivitis, sexually transmitted infections	Stevens–Johnson syndrome, exfoliative dermatitis, urticaria, angioedema, nausea, abdominal cramps, hepatoxicity, pulmonary hypersensitivity, superinfections, brown-rust urine

    4. Contraindications

        a. Hypersensitivity

        b. Megaloblastic anemia and folate deficiency, renal insufficiency, and severe hepatic insufficiency

        c. Severe dehydration, anuria, oliguria, and seizure disorder

    5. Significant drug interactions

        a. Hiprex/sulfonamides: may cause formation of an insoluble precipitate in the urine

        b. Nalidixic acid/warfarin: increase the effect of warfarin

        c. Sulfonamides may increase the effects of methotrexate, phenytoin, sulfonylureas, and warfarin

        d. Trimethoprim increases the effects of phenytoin

        e. Decreased absorption of nitrofurantoin with magnesium trisilicate

    6. Significant food interactions: none reported

    7. Significant laboratory studies

        a. May increase liver enzymes and renal function tests

        b. May cause false positive urinary glucose test

        c. May cause false increase in 17 hydroxycorticosteroids, catecholamines

    8. Side effects

        a. Drowsiness, weakness, headache, dizziness

        b. Sensitivity to light, blurred vision

        c. GI distress, pruritus, rash, arthralgia

    9. Adverse effects/toxicity

        a. Seizures, increased intracranial pressure

        b. Leukopenia, thrombocytopenia, angioedema

   10. Nursing considerations

        a. Drugs work best if client is well (but not overly) hydrated

        b. Administer with meals to decrease GI distress

        c. Monitor renal and liver function, and periodic CBC levels

        d. Check urine pH before administration as some drugs work best in acidic urine

        e. Cranberry juice or vitamin C may be added to acidify the urine

        f. Monitor CNS side effects

        g. If using an oral suspension of nitrofurantoin, instruct the client to rinse mouth to avoid staining of the teeth

        h. Ingestion of large amount of fluid while taking methenamine will reduce antibacterial effects by diluting the medication and raising the urinary pH

        i. Assess client taking nitrofurantoin for pulmonary sensitivities

   11. Client education

        a. Long term therapy is common even if feeling fine

        b. Drink at least 8 glasses of water daily

        c. Take medications with meals to decrease GI distress

        d. Avoid alkalizing fluids such as milk, fruit juices, or sodium bicarbonate, and do not take with antacids

        e. Notify prescriber of any new medications

        f. Use sunscreen to avoid excessive exposure to sunlight

        g. Notify prescriber of any CNS side effects

        h. Drug may discolor the urine and this is not harmful and will disappear after the drug is discontinued

        i. Take methenamine with food

B. Antispasmodics

    1. Action and use

        a. Relax smooth muscles of the urinary tract

        b. Decrease bladder muscle spasms

Table 12-13	Common Antispasmodic Medications		
Generic (Trade) Name	**Routes**	**Uses**	**Adverse Effects**
Hyoscyamine (Cystospaz)	PO, subQ, IM, IV	Preoperatively to decrease secretions, adjunctive therapy for peptic ulcer, spastic GI disorders, cystitis, neurogenic bladder or bowel disorder, parkinsonism, biliary or renal colic, rhinitis, anticholinesterase poisoning	Palpitations, dizziness, blurred vision, dilated pupils, drowsiness, nausea, dry mouth, taste loss, constipation, urinary hesitancy, impotence, decreased sweating, anaphylaxis, fever, urticaria
Tolterodine tartrate (Detrol)	PO	Overactive bladder	Blurred vision, N/V, dyspepsia, constipation, headache, dizziness, weight gain, pain, fatigue, myopia, secondary angle closure glaucoma, increased intraocular pressure, abdominal pain
Oxybutynin chloride (Ditropan)	PO, transdermal patch	Neurogenic bladder, incontinence, urgency, frequency	Drowsiness, dizziness, blurred vision, dry mouth, nausea, urinary hesitancy, decreased sweating
Flavoxate (Urispas)	PO	Dysuria, urgency, nocturia, cystitis, prostatitis, urethritis, urethrocystitis	Nervousness, vertigo, confusion, increased ocular tension, N/V, dry mouth, tachycardia, palpitations

      c. Used to manage the disorders of the lower urinary tract associated with hyper-motility: dysuria, urgency, nocturia, suprapubic pain, frequency, and incontinence

  2. Common medications (Table 12-13)

  3. Administration considerations: administer 1 hour before antacids or antidiarrheals

  4. Contraindications

      a. Glaucoma

      b. Obstructive breathing, obstructive GI disease, severe ulcerative colitis, and myasthenia gravis

      c. Hypersensitivity to anticholinergics, paralytic ileus, unstable cardiovascular (CV) status

  5. Significant drug interactions

      a. Amantadine increases adverse anticholinergic effects

      b. Phenothiazines or haloperidol will result in decreased antipsychotic effect

      c. Antacids and antidiarrheals result in decreased absorption of hyoscyamine

      d. Additive effect with other anticholinergic drugs

  6. Significant food interactions: none reported

  7. Significant laboratory studies: none reported

  8. Side effects

      a. Headache, insomnia, drowsiness, dizziness, confusion, excitement, palpitations

      b. Blurred vision

      c. Dry mouth, GI distress, urinary hesitancy, urine retention, urticaria

  9. Adverse effects/toxicity: leukopenia

  10. Nursing considerations

      a. Monitor effect of medication

      b. Monitor for CNS manifestations

      c. Monitor I & O

  11. Client education

      a. Drowsiness and blurred vision may occur; use caution when driving or operating machinery

      b. Use hard, sugarless candy for dry mouth

    c. Avoid alcohol, which increases drowsiness

    d. Swallow pill whole and do not chew or crush

    e. Shell of medication may appear in stool

    f. Be aware of side effects and to report them to provider

C. Urinary analgesic

  1. Action and use

    a. Has a local anesthetic effect on the urinary tract mucosa

    b. Used to relieve pain with urinary tract infections or irritation

  2. Common medication: phenazopyridine (Pyridium): 100–200 mg tid

  3. Administration considerations

    a. Drug colors the urine red or orange and may stain fabrics

    b. May be used with antibiotics and should be discontinued after 2 days of antibiotic use

  4. Contraindications

    a. Hypersensitivity

    b. Renal or hepatic diseases

  5. Significant drug interactions: none reported

  6. Significant food interactions: none reported

  7. Significant laboratory studies: may alter the results of urinary dipstick

  8. Side effects

    a. Headache and vertigo

    b. Nausea and GI distress

  9. Adverse effects/toxicity

    a. Anaphylaxis

    b. Methemoglobinemia

    c. Renal and hepatic failure

  10. Nursing considerations

    a. Assess for presence of urinary tract infection (UTI)

    b. Assess urinary function and output

    c. Monitor I & O

    d. Monitor sclera for yellow tinge

    e. Ensure renal function before administering

    f. Use only as an analgesic

  11. Client education

    a. Maintain good hygiene to prevent UTI

    b. Possible side effects

    c. Drug colors the urine red-orange and may stain clothing

    d. Do not double the dose if a dose is missed

    e. Take medication with food to decrease GI distress

    f. Increase fluid intake to aid in flushing bacteria from bladder

    g. Drug may not be effective for more than 24–48 hours

    h. Notify prescriber if yellowing of the eyes develops

    i. Report symptoms that worsen or do not resolve

VI. MEDICATIONS TO TREAT BENIGN PROSTATIC HYPERPLASIA (BPH)

A. Action and use

  1. Block alpha1-receptors in prostate leading to relaxation of smooth muscles, improving urine flow, and decreasing BPH symptoms

  2. Used to increase urine flow and decrease symptoms of BPH

B. Common medications (Table 12-14)

Table 12-14 Common Medications to Treat Benign Prostatic Hyperplasia

Generic (Trade) Names	Route	Uses	Adverse Effects
Alfuzosin hydrochloride (Uroxatral)	PO	Benign prostatic hyperplasia (BPH)	Dizziness, headache, fatigue, angina, orthostatic hypotension, impotence, upper respiratory infection, bronchitis, rash, sinusitis, pharyngitis
Doxazosin (Cardura)	PO	Essential hypertension, BPH	Dizziness, vertigo, asthenia, headache, orthostatic hypotension, arrhythmias, arthralgia, myalgia, pruritis, dyspnea, tachycardia, edema, N/V, constipation
Dutasteride (Avodart)	PO	BPH	Impotence, decreased libido, ejaculation disorder, gynecomastia
Finasteride (Propecia, Proscar)	PO	BPH, male pattern baldness	Decreased libido, impotence, decreased volume of ejaculation
Prazosin hydrochloride (Minipress)	PO	Hypertension, refractory congestive heart failure, Raynaud disease, BPH	Dizziness, headache, drowsiness, palpitations, sodium and water retention, nausea, blurred vision, urinary frequency, lupus erythematosus, impotence, priapism, nasal congestion, orthostatic hypotension, tachycardia
Tamsulosin (Flomax)	PO	BPH	Dizziness, headache, insomnia, somnolence, syncope, vertigo, chest pain, orthostatic hypotension, cough, decreased libido, abnormal ejaculation, infection, tooth disorder, rhinitis, sinusitis

C. **Administration considerations**
   1. Do not handle crushed tablets if pregnant
   2. Not indicated for females or pediatric use
   3. Postural effects may occur 2–6 hours after dose
   4. If treatment is interrupted for several days, restart medication at initial dose
D. **Contraindications**
   1. Hypersensitivity
   2. Caution in clients with impaired hepatic function
E. **Significant drug interactions**
   1. May increase theophylline clearance (finasteride)
   2. Concomitant use with other antihypertensive agents or diuretics (terazosin)
   3. Do not use with alpha-adrenergic blockers (decreased blood pressure)
   4. Cimetidine may decrease alfuzosin levels
   5. Use cautiously with warfarin
   6. Doxazosin may decrease effects of clonidine
   7. Dutasteride levels increased with cimetidine, diltiazem, verapamil, ketoconazole, macrolides, and protease inhibitors
F. **Significant food interactions**: none reported
G. **Significant laboratory studies**
   1. Decrease WBC and neutrophil counts with doxazosin
   2. Decreased hematocrit, WBC, hemoglobin, total protein and albumin levels with terazosin
   3. Finasteride may decrease prostate-specific antigen (PSA), even in prostate cancer
H. **Side effects**
   1. Impotence, decreased volume of ejaculate, decreased libido, asthenia

2. Dizziness, headache, nervousness, palpitations, peripheral edema, postural hypotension, nasal congestion, myalgia
3. Diarrhea and nausea

I. Adverse effects/toxicity: hypotension, shock, and arrhythmias

J. Nursing considerations
1. Assess client for severity of symptoms
2. Provide treatment options
3. Monitor for decreased BP
4. Rule out cancer of prostate before initiating therapy
5. Monitor for concomitant medications for interactions
6. Monitor urine volume
7. Take alfuzosin with same meal each day

K. Client education
1. Change position slowly to prevent orthostatic hypotension
2. Avoid driving and hazardous tasks for first 12–24 hours or after increasing dose due to drowsiness and somnolence
3. Report side effects to prescriber
4. Take medication at same time each day
5. Women who are or may become pregnant should not handle crushed finasteride tablets due to risk of adverse effect to male fetus
6. A male client whose sexual partner is or may become pregnant should avoid exposing her to his semen or else discontinue finasteride
7. The volume of ejaculate may be decreased but does not impair fertility

VII. MEDICATIONS TO TREAT RENAL FAILURE

A. Action and use
1. Primary focus of pharmacologic management of renal failure is to restore and maintain renal perfusion and to eliminate drugs that are directly nephrotoxic
2. Diuretics to improve urinary outflow and antihypertensives have been previously discussed and are not covered in this category
3. Dopaminergic receptors cause vasodilation in the renal, mesenteric, coronary, and intracerebral vascular beds
4. Are used to increase urine flow

B. Common medications: dopamine (Intropin), 2 to 5 mcg/kg/min to increase renal perfusion; may increase to 50 mcg/kg/min IV to raise blood pressure

C. Administration considerations
1. Administered IV using an infusion device to control the rate of flow
2. Administered into a large vein to prevent possibility of extravasation
3. Hypovolemia should be corrected before initiation of dopamine therapy
4. Decrease dose as soon as hemodynamic condition is stabilized
5. Do not mix with other medications
6. Discard solutions after 24 hours

D. Contraindications
1. Uncorrected tachydysrhythmias, pheochromocytoma, or ventricular fibrillation
2. Caution in use with occlusive vascular disease, cold injuries, diabetic endarteritis, and arterial embolism

E. Significant drug interactions
1. MAO inhibitors may prolong and intensify the effect of dopamine
2. Beta blockers antagonize cardiac effects
3. General anesthetics may cause ventricular arrhythmias and hypertension
4. Diuretics may result in increased diuretic effects

F. **Significant food interactions**: none reported

G. **Significant laboratory studies**: increased catecholamines and increased serum glucose levels

H. **Side effects**

1. Headache, tachycardia, angina, palpitations, hypotension, bradycardia, vasoconstriction, widening of QRS complex

2. N/V, piloerection, azotemia

I. **Adverse effects/toxicity**: anaphylaxis, asthmatic episodes, severe hypertension

J. **Nursing considerations**

1. Carefully monitor I & O

2. Assess infusion site frequently for extravasation; use 5–10 mg phentolamine mesylate (Regitine) in 10–15 mL of normal saline as an antidote

3. Monitor vital signs, cardiac output, and ECG frequently

4. Monitor for side effects

K. **Client education**: report side effects and monitor vital signs and I & O

VIII. HEMATOPOIETIC GROWTH FACTOR

A. **Action and use**

1. Used to stimulate red blood cell (RBC) production

2. Reverses anemia associated with chronic renal failure (CRF)

B. **Common medication**: epoetin alfa (Epogen, Procrit), subQ/IV 300–500 units/kg/dose 3 times/wk

C. **Administration considerations**

1. Initial effects can be seen within 1 to 2 weeks

2. Hematocrit (Hct) reaches normal levels (30 to 33%) in 2–3 months

3. Do not shake solution

4. IV administration: Epoetin alfa may be given undiluted by direct IV as a bolus dose

D. **Contraindications**

1. Uncontrolled hypertension

2. Known hypersensitivity to mammalian cell-derived products and albumin

E. **Significant drug interactions**: none reported

F. **Significant food interactions**: none reported

G. **Significant laboratory studies**

1. CBC with differential and platelet count

2. Monitor BUN, creatinine, phosphorus, and potassium

3. Monitor partial thromboplastin time (APPT)

4. Evaluate transferrin and serum ferritin prior to initiation of therapy

H. **Side effects**

1. Hypertension

2. Headache, seizure

3. Iron deficiency, sweating

I. **Adverse effects/toxicity**

1. Thrombocytosis, clotting of AV fistula

2. Bone pain, arthralgias

J. **Nursing considerations**

1. Blood pressure may rise during early therapy as Hct increases; notify prescriber of a rapid rise in Hct greater than 4 points in 2 weeks

2. Do not give with any other drug solution

3. Use only one dose per vial, and do not reenter vial

4. Inspect solution for particulate matter prior to use

5. Monitor for hypertensive encephalopathy in clients with CRF during period of increasing Hct

*   6. Client may require additional heparin during dialysis to prevent clotting of vascular access

K. Client education

*   1. Self-monitor vital signs, especially BP
*   2. Headache is a common adverse effect; it should be reported if it is severe
*   3. Avoid driving or other hazardous activity because of possible seizure activity, especially during first 90 days of therapy
*   4. It is important to keep all follow-up appointments

IX. MEDICATIONS TO PREVENT ORGAN REJECTION

A. Cyclosporine (Neoral)

1. Is an immunosuppressant
2. Acts on T lymphocytes to suppress production of interleukin-2
3. Used to prevent rejection of allogeneic kidney transplant
4. Oral administration is preferred
5. Blood levels should be monitored frequently
6. Administer prednisone concurrently
7. Client should be instructed to monitor for signs of infection
8. Grapefruit juice can raise cyclosporine levels, thus increasing the risk of toxicity
9. Client should be instructed to mix the concentrated medication solution with milk, chocolate milk, or orange juice just before administration
10. Side effects: N/V, hypertension, tremor, hirsutism, depression, and anaphylactic shock
11. Dose: oral route, 14–18 mg/kg beginning 4–12 hours before transplantation and continued for 1–2 weeks after surgery

B. Azathioprine (Imuran)

1. Is a cytotoxic medication
2. Suppresses cell-mediated and humoral immunity
3. Used with cyclosporine to help suppress transplant rejection
4. Can cause neutropenia
5. Side effects: N/V, bone marrow depression, agranulocytosis, and secondary infection
6. Dose: PO, 3–5 mg/kg/day initially, may reduce to 1–3 mg/kg/day

C. Muromonab-CD3 (Orthoclone OKT3)

1. Is an antibody
2. Used to prevent acute allograft rejection of kidney transplants
3. Side effects: N/V, chest pain, and dyspnea
4. Dose: IV, 5 mg/day administered in less than 1 minute for 10–14 days

Case Study

A 51-year-old male has a 164/120 blood pressure reading when taken at a health fair. The nurse refers him to his physician and he gives her permission to call his physician. The physician orders lisinopril (Prinivil, Zestril) 10 mg PO daily.

1. What should the client be taught about the administration of lisinopril?
2. What type of diet should the client adhere to?

3. What are the adverse effects of lisinopril?
4. What is the action of lisinopril?

For suggested responses, see pages 544–545.

POSTTEST

1 A nurse administering tamsulosin (Flomax) to a client would expect to note which therapeutic outcomes of drug therapy? Select all that apply.

1. Hypotension
2. Syncope
3. Decreased urethral obstruction
4. Increased urine flow
5. Decreased urinary frequency

2 After phenazopyridine (Pyridium) is prescribed for a client, the nurse teaches the client which of the following items of information?

1. Continue taking drug until infection is resolved.
2. Long-term use of drug requires no follow-up.
3. With appropriate hydration, it is safe to perform breastfeeding.
4. Report sign of yellow-tinged skin or sclera.

3 A client's blood pressure (BP) has continued to drop despite administration of IV fluids. The client asks why an infusion of IV dopamine (Intropin) is being started. What response(s) by the nurse would be most appropriate? Select all that apply.

1. "This medication helps to increase the heart rate."
2. "Dopamine increases the ability of the heart muscle to contract."
3. "It increases smaller blood vessel constriction, which moves more blood into larger vessels."
4. "This drug increases blood flow to the kidneys, which helps to increase your blood pressure."
5. "This medication relaxes the arteries near the heart."

4 A 63-year-old client who has lost 30 lbs, who exercises regularly, and who has changed dietary habits becomes upset when the nurse states that antihypertensive and diuretic drug therapy needs to be continued. What is the most appropriate response by the nurse?

1. "Age-related structural changes in the body are associated with hypertension, not just living habits."
2. "You need to continue taking the drugs just as a precautionary measure."
3. "Would you like the health care provider to write a prescription to help you with your nerves?"
4. "Do you recall our first teaching session when I explained this to you?"

5 A client who recently began antihypertensive drug therapy states she needs to go to the pharmacy to buy an over-the-counter (OTC) product to treat a common cold. The home health nurse should provide which most helpful instruction first?

1. "Buy a generic brand of medicine because it is more cost effective and they act in similar ways."
2. "Do not purchase a product that contains aspirin."
3. "Read the label carefully and avoid products with pseudoephedrine."
4. "Many of the common products are contraindicated if you are taking medication for high blood pressure."

6 A client taking spironolactone (Aldactone) for hypertension reports to the ambulatory clinic with bilateral edema in the lower legs. After receiving the laboratory test results, the nurse instructs the licensed practical/vocational nurse (LPN/LVN) to withhold the additional dose that was just ordered because of which value?

1. Blood glucose 160 mg/dL
2. Sodium 142 mEq/L
3. Blood urea nitrogen 18 mg/dL
4. Serum potassium 6.0 mEq/L

7 Because a client is scheduled to receive a 10 mg/kg dose of cyclosporine over a period of 6 hours, the nurse instructs the licensed practical/vocational nurse (LPN/LVN) to perform which priority activity?

1. Call central processing department for an infusion pump.
2. Measure client's blood pressure.
3. Administer antiemetic prior to initiation of medication.
4. Ensure that epinephrine 1:1000 is readily available on unit or at bedside.

8 While screening an elementary school's faculty for hypertension, the nurse detects high blood pressure in a 32-year-old female client. What question is most appropriate for the nurse to ask the client at this time?

1. "Are you currently taking an oral contraceptive?"
2. "Is there a lot of psychological stress in your life right now?"
3. "Do you realize that you will probably need medication therapy?"
4. "Have you had your total cholesterol level checked?"

9 The nurse is providing information to a client who has started drug therapy with sulfisoxazole (Gantrisin). Which instruction would be the highest priority of the nurse to provide?

1. "Check the urine pH to prevent crystals from forming in the urine."
2. "Report sudden onset of fever, pruritis, and malaise."
3. "Restrict your oral fluid intake to an amount between 500 and 1,000 mL/day."
4. "Keep your urine at an alkaline level."

10 Because a health care provider prescribed hydralazine (Apresoline) for a client with hypertension, the nurse should include in a teaching plan information about which unique side effect?

1. Declining blood pressure
2. Decreased white blood cell (WBC) count
3. Increased cardiac workload
4. Orthostatic hypotension

➤ *See pages 424–425 for Answers and Rationales.*

POSTTEST

ANSWERS & RATIONALES

Pretest

1 **Answer: 1** **Rationale:** If the nurse is to advise the client appropriately, knowledge of pharmacokinetics is necessary. For example, onset: 20–60 mins; peak: 60–70 mins; duration: 2 hrs; elimination: 50% every 24 hrs. Since clients may not respond as expected, the client should ingest the drug as early as possible to prevent nocturia resulting in disruption of the client's sleep. Therefore, 8:00 a.m. is the best answer. While 12 noon is a more appropriate time than 6:00 p.m. or bedtime, it is not the best time. Since 50% will remain in the body, a cumulative effect could disrupt the client's sleep–rest pattern. An onset of 20–60 mins would result in a direct interruption of the sleep–rest pattern. **Cognitive Level:** Applying **Client Need:** Pharmacological and Parenteral Therapies **Integrated Process:** Teaching and Learning **Content Area:** Pharmacology **Strategy:** Associate the drug actions and pharmacokinetics with the client's lifestyle. Knowing the drug is a diuretic will help to avoid times that would result in nocturia. **Reference:** Wilson, B. A., Shannon, M., & Shields, K. (2011). *Pearson nurse's drug guide 2011.* Upper Saddle River, NJ: Pearson Education, pp. 689–690.

2 **Answer: 1** **Rationale:** Furosemide, a loop diuretic, is the drug of choice for clients with renal insufficiency because it results in renal and peripheral vasodilation, increased renal blood flow, a temporary increase in glomerular filtration rate (GFR) and decreased peripheral vascular resistance. Hydrochlorothiazide may be utilized in the client with CRF, but does not increase renal blood flow. Chlorthalidone's actions are similar to hydrochlorothiazide. Because of the risk of hyperkalemia, spironolactone is contraindicated in clients with reduced renal function. **Cognitive Level:** Analyzing **Client Need:** Pharmacological and Parenteral Therapies **Integrated Process:** Nursing Process: Implementation **Content Area:** Pharmacology **Strategy:** Associate furosemide (Lasix) with immediate or rapid reduction in the central circulation volume. Recall also that it is a high-ceiling drug, which means that the dosage can be increased to aid in achieving sufficient results. These two concepts should help you to choose correctly. **Reference:** Wilson, B. A., Shannon, M., & Shields, K. (2011). *Pearson nurse's drug guide 2011.* Upper Saddle River, NJ: Pearson Education, pp. 683–684.

3 **Answer: 4** **Rationale:** Losartan (Cozaar) is an angiotensin II antagonist that prevents the binding of angiotensin II (a potent vasoconstrictor) to its receptors. This reduces blood pressure. Inhibition of calcium influx is more representative of calcium channel blockers, such as nifedipine (Procardia), which cause the arteries to relax. Losartan is not a direct vasodilator; rather, it works by inhibiting angiotensin II. Losartan does not promote release of aldosterone; aldosterone leads to sodium and water retention, which in turn would raise blood pressure (BP). **Cognitive Level:** Applying **Client Need:** Pharmacological and Parenteral Therapies **Integrated Process:** Teaching and Learning **Content Area:** Pharmacology **Strategy:** Apply knowledge of the process of blood pressure maintenance with the drug's actions. Recall that drugs that end in *sartan* are angiotensin II inhibitors to make it easier to make the correct selection. **Reference:** Wilson, B. A., Shannon, M., & Shields, K. (2011). *Pearson nurse's drug guide 2011.* Upper Saddle River, NJ: Pearson Education, p. 917.

4 **Answer: 2** **Rationale:** A dry, persistent, tickling, and nonproductive cough is a common side effect of angiotensin-converting enzyme (ACE) inhibitors such as lisinopril (Prinivil). This drug side effect subsides after the drug is discontinued. Dizziness is a common side effect associated with many antihypertensive medications, including beta blockers such as propranolol (Inderal). They can also cause a reduction in pulse rate. Cough and wheezing can occur with calcium channel blockers such as nifedipine (Procardia) but they are not as common as dizziness and lightheadedness. Dehydration is more common with diuretics such as bumetanide (Bumex). **Cognitive Level:** Analyzing **Client Need:** Pharmacological and Parenteral Therapies **Integrated Process:** Nursing Process: Assessment **Content Area:** Pharmacology **Strategy:** Note the critical words *most likely* in the stem of the question. This tells you that more than one option might be partially correct but that just one option is clearly the better answer. Select the drug category (ACE inhibitors) that is known to have a cough of unknown origin as a side effect. **Reference:** Wilson, B. A., Shannon, M., & Shields, K. (2011). *Pearson nurse's drug guide 2011.* Upper Saddle River, NJ: Pearson Education, pp. 683–684.

5 **Answers: 2, 4, 5** **Rationale:** Initially, reduction of blood pressure (BP) using medications can result in drowsiness related to hypotension. Clients should avoid activities that could place them in danger. Antihypertensive medication that redistributes central circulating volume to the periphery often results in peripheral edema. Many antihypertensive medications cause erectile dysfunction. Weight loss will contribute to reduction of hypertension, but hypertension is a chronic disease that will not resolve with weight loss alone. Increased fluid intake may be needed if the client is ingesting diuretics and becomes dehydrated. Dehydration will not place the client at immediate risk. **Cognitive Level:** Applying **Client Need:** Pharmacological and Parenteral Therapies **Integrated Process:** Teaching and Learning **Content Area:** Pharmacology **Strategy:** Apply knowledge of the physiological changes associated with drug management of hypertension.

The wording of the question tells you that the correct options are also correct statements. Evaluate each option in terms of whether it is a true or false statement and select the true ones as the answers to the question. **Reference:** Adams, M. P., & Koch, R. W. (2010). *Pharmacology: Connections to nursing practice.* Upper Saddle River, NJ: Pearson Education, pp. 546–577.

6 **Answer: 2** **Rationale:** Indapamide is a thiazide diuretic that may cause hypokalemia. Because the function of potassium involves the action potential of smooth muscles such as arteries, hypokalemia can result in irregular muscle contractions. Hence, muscle weakness and leg cramps can occur. Since the cause of the signs and symptoms is manageable and the problems do not significantly impact the client's health, terminating the drug is not necessary. Furosemide (Lasix) is a loop diuretic that can also result in hypokalemia. Since the leg cramps are the result of hypokalemia, a nonsteroidal anti-inflammatory drug (NSAID) is not the appropriate treatment for the symptom. **Cognitive Level:** Analyzing **Client Need:** Pharmacological and Parenteral Therapies **Integrated Process:** Nursing Process: Implementation **Content Area:** Pharmacology **Strategy:** First determine that indapamide is a diuretic. Then correlate the category of the drug with potential side effects that could result in leg cramps. **Reference:** Wilson, B. A., Shannon, M., & Shields, K. (2011). *Pearson nurse's drug guide 2011.* Upper Saddle River, NJ: Pearson Education, pp. 790–791.

7 **Answer: 1** **Rationale:** Hyperuricemia is a side effect of thiazide diuretics and this could lead to symptoms resembling gout (such as an enlarged, painful great toe). An increase in liver enzymes such as alanine aminotransferase (ALT) is not associated with thiazide diuretics. Clients may experience hyperglycemia but this is more likely related to the comorbidity of diabetes mellitus than to a drug side effect, and pain from diabetic neuropathy (if present) is not likely to occur in the toe. The drug is more likely to cause hypokalemia than a change in sodium level. **Cognitive Level:** Applying **Client Need:** Pharmacological and Parenteral Therapies **Integrated Process:** Nursing Process: Planning **Content Area:** Pharmacology **Strategy:** The core issue of the question is knowledge that symptoms of gout can occur with thiazide diuretics because of an increase in uric acid level. Eliminate the option referring to the liver first, based on location of symptoms and the option related to blood glucose for the same reason. Choose correctly between the remaining 2 by recalling that potassium is the electrolyte of concern, or by associating the client's symptoms with an elevated uric acid level. **Reference:** Wilson, B. A., Shannon, M., & Shields, K. (2011). *Pearson nurse's drug guide 2011.* Upper Saddle River, NJ: Pearson Education, pp. 749–751.

8 **Answer: 4** **Rationale:** Oxybutynin (Ditropan) is an antispasmodic used for urinary incontinence and bladder spasms. It causes anticholinergic side effects such as dry mouth, constipation, urinary hesitancy, and decreased gastroenteritis motility. For this reason the client needs to use measures to counteract dry mouth. Wearing protection is an appropriate action for urinary incontinence, but retention and hesitancy is associated with this drug. The drug has no effect on the clotting process so there is no unusual risk of injury. The anticholinergic actions are more likely to cause constipation than diarrhea. **Cognitive Level:** Applying **Client Need:** Pharmacological and Parenteral Therapies **Integrated Process:** Teaching and Learning **Content Area:** Pharmacology **Strategy:** First recall that oxybutynin (Ditropan) is an antispasmodic that causes anticholinergic effects. Then evaluate each option to find the recommendation that matches the side effects of this drug. **Reference:** Wilson, B. A., Shannon, M., & Shields, K. (2011). *Pearson nurse's drug guide 2011.* Upper Saddle River, NJ: Pearson Education, pp. 1147–1149.

9 **Answer: 2** **Rationale:** Mannitol (Osmitrol) may be prescribed for clients with increased intracranial pressure or increased intraocular pressure by causing diuresis. It would not be prescribed for clients with pancreatitis, diarrhea, and congestive heart failure. Clients with pancreatitis would not experience a benefit from a drug that promotes diuresis, and mannitol is known to precipitate pulmonary edema and heart failure because of its osmotic action. **Cognitive Level:** Applying **Client Need:** Pharmacological and Parenteral Therapies **Integrated Process:** Nursing Process: Implementation **Content Area:** Pharmacology **Strategy:** Consider first that mannitol (Osmitrol) is an osmotic diuretic. Then systematically review each option to determine which health problems would benefit from a state of diuresis. **Reference:** Lehne, R. A. (2010). *Pharmacology for nursing care* (7th ed.). St. Louis, MO: Saunders, p. 451.

10 **Answer: 1** **Rationale:** Finasteride (Proscar) is an androgen inhibitor that may be used to treat enlarged prostate. It reduces the serum levels of testosterone, resulting in decreased prostate gland size and indirectly improving the flow of urine during voiding. Because of the risk of abnormalities to the fetus, pregnant women or women of childbearing age should not be exposed to semen fluid of a male taking finasteride. The decreased serum level of testosterone may result in decreased libido, but is not as relevant as the risk to the developing fetus. Because of urinary stasis that accompanies enlarged prostate, the client should increase fluid intake to prevent infection. Once again, however, this is not as relevant as the health of a developing fetus. It may take 6–12 months to reach full therapeutic effectiveness so 3 weeks is too short a time frame. **Cognitive Level:** Analyzing **Client Need:** Pharmacological and Parenteral Therapies **Integrated Process:** Teaching and Learning **Content Area:** Pharmacology **Strategy:** Recall first that finasteride (Proscar) is an androgen inhibitor, and then associate fetal deformities with the drug. **Reference:** Wilson, B. A., Shannon, M., & Shields, K. (2011). *Pearson nurse's drug guide 2011.* Upper Saddle River, NJ: Pearson Education, pp. 144–145.

ANSWERS & RATIONALES

Posttest

1 **Answers: 3, 4, 5** **Rationale:** Therapeutic outcomes of tamsulosin (Flomax) would include decreased urethral obstruction, increased urine flow, and decreased urinary frequency. Hypotension and syncope are adverse effects of tamsulosin. **Cognitive Level:** Analyzing **Client Need:** Pharmacological and Parenteral Therapies **Integrated Process:** Nursing Process: Evaluation **Content Area:** Pharmacology **Strategy:** The critical words in the question are *therapeutic outcomes*. With this in mind, select the options that are intended effects of the drug. **Reference:** Lehne, R. A. (2010). *Pharmacology for nursing care* (7th ed.). St. Louis, MO: Saunders, p. 782.

2 **Answer: 4** **Rationale:** Phenazopyridine (Pyridium) is a urinary tract analgesic that may be ordered alone or may be combined with an antibiotic appropriate for urinary tract infections. Yellow-tinged skin is a sign of drug accumulation related to renal impairment. This sign should be reported to the prescriber if noted. Although it may be manufactured in combination with an antibiotic, it could also be discontinued after pain with urination is relieved, often after 1–2 days of antibiotic therapy. Any drug that is used long term would require follow-up, but this drug is used on a short-term basis. The safety of the drug during breastfeeding is unsubstantiated. **Cognitive Level:** Applying **Client Need:** Pharmacological and Parenteral Therapies **Integrated Process:** Teaching and Learning **Content Area:** Pharmacology **Strategy:** Associate the characteristics of the drug with the significant risks to the client. Frequently, medication questions seek to determine knowledge of adverse effects and the action needed if they occur. **Reference:** Wilson, B. A., Shannon, M., & Shields, K. (2011). *Pearson nurse's drug guide 2011*. Upper Saddle River, NJ: Pearson Education, pp. 1211–1212.

3 **Answers: 2, 3, 4** **Rationale:** Dopamine (Intropin) increases blood pressure by increased cardiac contractility, which increases cardiac output leading to increased blood pressure (BP). Increased vasoconstriction of small blood vessels results in increased movement of blood from the periphery to the central circulating volume, resulting in increased BP. Increased blood flow to the kidneys enhances the renin-angiotensin system resulting in increased vasoconstriction, leading to increased blood pressure. Without appropriate filling and emptying as well as appropriate contractility, the blood pressure would not increase significantly. Dopamine does not relax blood vessels near the heart. **Cognitive Level:** Analyzing **Client Need:** Pharmacological and Parenteral Therapies **Integrated Process:** Teaching and Learning **Content Area:** Pharmacology **Strategy:** Associate the dynamics of blood pressure maintenance with the drug's actions. **Reference:** Wilson, B. A., Shannon, M., & Shields, K. (2011). *Pearson nurse's drug guide 2011*. Upper Saddle River, NJ: Pearson Education, pp. 493–495.

4 **Answer: 1** **Rationale:** Atherosclerosis associated with aging and excessive fat intake is associated with hypertension. Continuing the antihypertensive drug therapy is not prophylactic but rather meets the client's current needs. There is not enough information to know whether the client needs an antianxiety medication, and it could be considered demeaning for the nurse to suggest this because the client is upset about the need for antihypertensive therapy. The nurse needs to address the client's current concern rather than referring back to an earlier teaching session. **Cognitive Level:** Applying **Client Need:** Pharmacological and Parenteral Therapies **Integrated Process:** Communication and Documentation **Content Area:** Pharmacology **Strategy:** Correlate the etiologies and client demographics with appropriate management of hypertension. **Reference:** Adams, M. P., & Koch, R. W. (2010). *Pharmacology: Connections to nursing practice*. Upper Saddle River, NJ: Pearson Education, pp. 567–569.

5 **Answer: 3** **Rationale:** Some clients will experience an increased blood pressure with over-the-counter (OTC) cold preparations containing pseudoephedrine as this ingredient causes vasoconstriction. Therefore, clients should avoid taking these products if on antihypertensive drug therapy. Generic brands contain the same medications but generally cost less, but cost should be considered only after the proper medication is identified. Avoiding aspirin would be appropriate if allergies exist or if overlapping characteristics exist, but this information is not in the question. While it is true that many products cannot be used, the statement is vague and cannot be applied by the client without further information. **Cognitive Level:** Applying **Client Need:** Pharmacological and Parenteral Therapies **Integrated Process:** Teaching and Learning **Content Area:** Pharmacology **Strategy:** Correlate the actions of the components of most over-the-counter (OTC) cold remedies with hypertension. **Reference:** Adams, M. P., & Koch, R. W. (2010). *Pharmacology: Connections to nursing practice*. Upper Saddle River, NJ: Pearson Education, pp. 567–569.

6 **Answer: 4** **Rationale:** Spironolactone (Aldactone) is a potassium-sparing diuretic. Potassium levels greater than 5.1–5.5 mEq/L (normal 3.5–5.1 mEq/L) are contraindicated with spironolactone because of the high risk for experiencing signs of hyperkalemia. The glucose level is above normal but unrelated to the characteristics of the drug. The sodium level and the BUN are within normal limits (135–145 mEq/L and 8–22 mg/dL, respectively). **Cognitive Level:** Analyzing **Client Need:** Management of Care **Integrated Process:** Nursing Process: Implementation **Content Area:** Pharmacology **Strategy:** To answer this question correctly, recall normal laboratory values and eliminate 2 options because they are normal values. Then consider that diuretics are likely to affect electrolyte levels to choose correctly. **Reference:** Wilson, B. A., Shannon, M., & Shields, K. (2011). *Pearson nurse's drug guide 2011*. Upper Saddle River, NJ: Pearson Education, p. 1653.

7 **Answer: 4** **Rationale:** Although anaphylaxis is considered rare, the enormity of the risk warrants proper preparation. The nurse should ensure that epinephrine is readily available while the drug is infusing. The client should be monitored closely during the first 30 minutes, especially for a hypersensitivity reaction. Infusion pump guards against rapid infusion that could result in rapid nephrotoxicity, but this activity could be performed by unlicensed personnel so it is not the highest priority for the LPN/LVN to do. Since hypertension is a common side effect, a baseline pressure is needed, but this does not supersede the risk for allergy as a priority. Vomiting is a common side effect, but this does not have the highest priority either. **Cognitive Level:** Analyzing **Client Need:** Management of Care **Integrated Process:** Nursing Process: Planning **Content Area:** Pharmacology **Strategy:** Note the critical word *priority* in the question. This tells you that more than one or all options may be technically correct but that one is better than the others. Use knowledge of the characteristics of the drug, the safety precautions needed during administration, and the role of the LPN to make a selection. **Reference:** Wilson, B. A., Shannon, M., & Shields, K. (2011). *Pearson nurse's drug guide 2011.* Upper Saddle River, NJ: Pearson Education, pp. 381–382.

8 **Answer: 1** **Rationale:** Oral contraceptives are the most common cause of secondary hypertension in females of reproductive age. Although the actual cause of hypertension is unknown, psychological stress may be associated with it, but this is not currently considered a primary cause. It is too early to tell if the client will need medication therapy or whether lifestyle changes alone will be effective treatment. Hyperlipidemia tends to contribute to hypertension across populations but again this is not the priority question of concern. **Cognitive Level:** Analyzing **Client Need:** Pharmacological and Parenteral Therapies **Integrated Process:** Nursing Process: Assessment **Content Area:** Pharmacology **Strategy:** Note the critical words *most appropriate* in the stem of the question. This tells you that more than one answer may be technically correct but that one is better than the others. Refer to

the gender and age of the client to help make a selection. **Reference:** Adams, M. P., & Koch, R. W. (2010). *Pharmacology: Connections to nursing practice.* Upper Saddle River, NJ: Pearson Education, p. 567.

9 **Answer: 2** **Rationale:** Early signs of hypersensitivity require immediate intervention, so the client should report sudden onset of fever, pruritis, or malaise. Checking the urine pH decreases the potential for stone formation, a very painful but not life-threatening problem. Fluid intake should produce 1,500 mL/day, and the client needs to take in at least 2 liters of fluid per day. The medication is more soluble in alkaline urine, but attending to a hypersensitive reaction takes priority. **Cognitive Level:** Analyzing **Client Need:** Pharmacological and Parenteral Therapies **Integrated Process:** Teaching and Learning **Content Area:** Pharmacology **Strategy:** Note the syllable *sulf* in the drug and associate this with a sulfa drug, which has high allergenic potential. Correlate this with the signs and symptoms in the correct option and the immediacy of need. **Reference:** Wilson, B. A., Shannon, M., & Shields, K. (2011). *Pearson nurse's drug guide 2011.* Upper Saddle River, NJ: Pearson Education, p. 1453.

10 **Answer: 2** **Rationale:** A major side effect that is relatively unique to hydralazine (Apresoline) as an antihypertensive agent is agranulocytosis. A declining blood pressure is an expected effect of drug therapy. If the drug is effective, it should decrease cardiac workload because of reduced afterload. Orthostatic hypotension can occur but is not unique to this medication—it is common for most antihypertensive drugs. **Cognitive Level:** Analyzing **Client Need:** Pharmacological and Parenteral Therapies **Integrated Process:** Nursing Process: Planning **Content Area:** Pharmacology **Strategy:** The critical word in the question is *unique.* Eliminate one option first because it is a false statement. Choose correctly from the remaining options by eliminating the intended effect of the drug and the common (nonunique) side effect in another option. **Reference:** Wilson, B. A., Shannon, M., & Shields, K. (2011). *Pearson nurse's drug guide 2011.* Upper Saddle River, NJ: Pearson Education, pp. 731–732.

References

Abrams, A. (2009). *Clinical drug therapy: Rationales for nursing practice* (9th ed.). Philadelphia, PA: Lippincott Williams & Wilkins.

Adams, M., Holland, L., & Bostwick, P. (2011). *Pharmacology for nurses: A pathophysiologic approach* (3rd ed.). Upper Saddle River, NJ: Pearson Education.

Adams, M., & Urban, C. (2013). *Pharmacology: Connections to nursing practice* (2nd ed.). Upper Saddle River, NJ: Pearson Education.

Aschenbrenner, D., & Venable, S. (2012). *Drug therapy in nursing* (4th ed.). Philadelphia, PA: Lippincott Williams & Wilkins.

Drug Facts & Comparisons® (Updated monthly). St. Louis, MO: A. Wolters Kluwer.

Karch, A. M. (2010). *Focus on nursing pharmacology* (5th ed.). Philadelphia, PA: Lippincott Williams & Wilkins.

Kee, J. (2009). *Laboratory and diagnostic tests and nursing implications* (8th ed.). Upper Saddle River, NJ: Pearson Education.

Lehne, R. (2010). *Pharmacology for nursing care* (7th ed.). St. Louis, MO: Mosby, Inc.

LeMone, P., Burke, K. M., & Bauldoff, G. (2011). *Medical-surgical nursing: Critical thinking in patient care* (5th ed.). Upper Saddle River, NJ: Pearson Education.

Wilson, B. A., Shannon, M. T., & Shields, K. M. (2012). *Pearson nurse's drug guide 2012.* Upper Saddle River, NJ: Pearson Education.

ANSWERS & RATIONALES

13 Reproductive System Medications

Chapter Outline

Estrogens
Progestins
Androgens
Anabolic Steroids

Medications for Erectile
    Dysfunction
Contraceptives
Fertility Medications

Medications for Labor and
    Delivery
Emergency Contraceptives

 NCLEX-RN® Test Prep

Use the accompanying online resource,
NursingReviewsandRationales, to test
yourself with hundreds of NCLEX®-style
practice questions.

Objectives

➤ Describe general goals of therapy when administering medications
  associated with the reproductive system.
➤ Discuss side effects and adverse effects of estrogens, progestins,
  and androgens.
➤ Describe nursing considerations related to medications used to
  treat erectile dysfunction.
➤ Discuss effects of oxytocin (Pitocin) on the uterus.
➤ Identify indications, contraindications, side effects, and adverse
  reactions of ergonovine (Ergotrate) and methylergonovine
  (Methergine).
➤ Identify action and use for ritodrine (Yutopar).
➤ Identify indications, contraindications, side effects, and adverse
  reactions of magnesium sulfate.
➤ Describe specific nursing considerations when administering
  magnesium sulfate.
➤ List significant client education points related to reproductive
  system medications.

Review at a Glance

anabolic steroid an androgen with
anabolic properties, rarely prescribed but
often abused by athletes to increase
muscle mass
androgen a medication that
induces or increases male
hormone-like effects

cryptorchidism a congenital condition characterized by failure of testis to
descend into scrotum
hepatotoxic toxic to liver
Homan's sign calf pain on dorsiflex-
ion of foot often caused by deep vein
thrombosis

hypogonadism underdevelopment
of gonads
priapism painful penile erection that
does not spontaneously subside

PRETEST

1 The health care provider at an outpatient clinic is considering prescribing sildenafil (Viagra) for a 61-year-old client. The nurse would make it a priority to discuss which item in the client's health history with the prescriber?

1. Coronary artery disease (CAD) with nitroglycerin use
2. Renal impairment with elevated creatinine level
3. Blurred vision of unknown etiology
4. Gout managed with allopurinol (Zyloprim)

2 The pregnant client is being prepared for initiation of labor with oxytocin (Pitocin). The nurse concludes that the client has adequate understanding when the client verbalizes the medication will have which action? Select all that apply.

1. Cause an increase in blood pressure to provide adequate oxygen for the baby
2. Cause the uterus to contract harder and more often
3. Start contractions that will be almost continuous until the baby is born
4. Be given through the IV in small continuous amounts that can be adjusted as needed
5. Cause the client to be in real labor

3 The client with preterm labor is receiving magnesium sulfate (generic) intravenously. Because of an early side effect, the nurse should perform which of the following assessments?

1. Deep tendon reflexes
2. Decreased respiratory rate
3. Nervousness and tremors
4. Nausea and diarrhea

4 To better help a client understand the action of clomiphene (Clomid), the nurse should include which of the following in the care plan of a female client who will begin taking the drug?

1. Teach normal process of conception.
2. Explain uterine involution process.
3. Teach the client to keep a record of daily temperatures.
4. Explain function of female hormones.

5 The client taking an estrogen–progestin (Ortho Tri-Cyclen) combination oral contraceptive calls the clinic reporting that she has forgotten her pills for the last 2 days. What medication directions should the nurse provide?

1. "Take 2 pills today and 2 pills tomorrow, then 1 pill daily for the rest of the pill pack."
2. "Take 2 pills today, and then 1 each day until the pill pack is finished."
3. "Notify health care provider of the missed dosage."
4. "Stop taking the pills and use condoms until the next menses, then restart a new pill pack."

6 The perinatal nurse is assigned to several clients. The nurse anticipates that which client is most likely to be a candidate for drug therapy with terbutaline (Brethine)?

1. Client at 27 weeks' gestation who has regular uterine contractions
2. Client at 41 weeks' gestation with irregular uterine contractions
3. Postpartum hemorrhage following delivery
4. Client at 38 weeks' gestation with hypertension and seizures

7 Because a hypertensive client is experiencing post-partal hemorrhage, the nurse anticipates that the health care provider will most likely prescribe which drug to treat the hemorrhage?

1. Ergonovine (Ergotrate)
2. Methylergonovine (Methergine)
3. Oxytocin (Pitocin)
4. Carboprost tromethamine (Hemabate)

8 The nurse is reviewing the health history of a client who is to begin therapy with a combined oral contraceptive drug. Which findings in the client's history should the nurse address with the client? Select all that apply.

1. Use of St. John's wort for depression
2. Smoking cessation over 10 years ago
3. Frequent migraine headaches
4. Follows a vegan diet
5. Cholecystectomy 3 months ago

9 After testosterone cypionate (Andronate) is prescribed for a 16-year-old male client diagnosed with hypogonadism, the client asks, "Why do I need these hormones anyway?" The nurse should provide which description of the relationship between hypogonadism and Andronate?

1. "Testosterone is necessary to prevent your muscles from atrophying."
2. "This medication is a form of testosterone. Your doctor can best explain it to you."
3. "Testosterone prevents your body from becoming feminine looking."
4. "This medication will increase your testosterone to a normal level."

10 The nurse determines a client with endometriosis understands the purpose of the newly prescribed danazol (Cyclamen) when the client makes which statement?

1. "It suppresses pituitary output of the follicle-stimulating hormone (FSH)."
2. "I'll need to take this medication for the rest of my life."
3. "I have to administer injections weekly."
4. "This medication will relieve hot flashes."

➤ *See pages 449–450 for Answers and Rationales.*

I. ESTROGENS

A. Action and use

1. Hormone replacement therapy (HRT) after spontaneous or surgically induced menopause
2. Relieves symptoms of menopause such as hot flashes, night sweats, sleep disturbances, and vaginal dryness; protects against coronary heart disease and osteoporosis
3. Used to treat female **hypogonadism**, a condition characterized by underdevelopment of the gonads
4. Adjunctive therapy for osteoporosis (oral or transdermal forms only)
5. Used in men to decrease the progression of prostate carcinoma

B. Common medications (Table 13-1)

C. Administration considerations

1. Report symptoms of menopause to provider for dosage adjustment
2. Dose should be given with food to reduce nausea
3. Intravenous (IV) estrogen is given slowly by direct IV injection at a rate of 5 mg/min
4. Rapid IV injection may cause skin flushing
5. Estradiol transdermal should be applied to clean, dry area on the trunk of the body (including buttocks and abdomen)
6. Replace patch according to schedule
7. Cream form of the medication should be applied deeply into vagina, to assist in retention
8. Intravaginal ring (Estring) should be placed near cervix and checked for placement periodically

D. Contraindications

1. Current undiagnosed vaginal bleeding
2. History of breast cancer
3. Cautious use in smokers
4. Cautious use in women with history of deep vein thrombosis (DVT) or thrombophlebitis
5. Use cautiously with severe renal or hepatic disease

Table 13-1   **Common Estrogens**

Generic (Trade) Names	Route	Uses	Adverse Effects
Estradiol (Alora, Climara, Divigel, Elestrin, others)	PO, IM, transdermal patch, intravaginal	Vasomotor symptoms, hypoestrogenism from hypogonadism, castration, primary ovarian failure, atrophic vaginitis, kraurosis vulvae, palliative therapy for advanced inoperable breast or prostate cancer, osteoporosis prevention	Thromboembolism, increased risk of endometrial cancer, hepatic adenoma, increased risk of breast cancer, breast changes, gynecomastia, abnormal PAP smear, increased appetite, weight gain, jaundice, gallbladder disease, nausea, vomiting, diarrhea, bloating, cervical erosion, altered cervical secretions, uterine fibromas, increased risk of endometrial cancer, myopia, breakthrough bleeding, testicular atrophy, impotence, hypercalcemia, urticaria, melasma, hair loss, dermatitis
Conjugated estrogens, synthetic (Cenestin, Premarin)	PO	Hormonal imbalance with bleeding, vaginal atrophy, castration, primary ovarian failure, palliative therapy for inoperable prostate cancer, palliative therapy for breast cancer, osteoporosis prevention	
Estropipate (Ogen)	PO, intravaginal	Vulvar and vaginal atrophy, ovarian failure, castration, hypogonadism, osteoporosis prevention	Depression, seizures, headache, migraine headache, dizziness, pulmonary embolism, myocardial infarction, thromboembolism, cerebrovascular accident, edema, nausea, vomiting, abdominal cramps, bleeding, endometrial cancer, breast cancer, erythema multiforme, breast engorgement, porphyria, breast enlargement, hirsutism
Esterified estrogens (Estratab, Menest)	PO	Inoperable prostate cancer, metastatic breast cancer, hypogonadism, castration, ovarian failure, vasomotor menopausal symptoms, atrophic vaginitis, urethritis, osteoporosis prevention	Headache, dizziness, seizure, depression, edema, thromboembolism, hypertension, thrombophlebitis, pulmonary embolism, cerebrovascular accident, breast and endometrial cancer, amenorrhea, abnormal menstrual flow, hirsutism, hepatic adenoma, gallbladder disease, gynecomastia, weight changes, breast changes, breakthrough bleeding, pancreatitis, myopia, astigmatism, testicular atrophy, uterine fibromas

E. **Significant drug interactions**
   1. May create need to increase doses of warfarin, oral hypoglycemic agents, or insulin
   2. Increased risk of hepatotoxicity when estrogens are taken with drugs that are hepatotoxic
   3. May increase risk of toxicity with cyclosporine
   4. Barbiturates, St. John's wort, and rifampin may decrease effectiveness of estrogens
   5. Increased effects possible with ginseng
   6. Red clover and black cohosh my interfere with estrogen therapy (they have weak estrogenic effects)
F. **Significant food interactions:** none reported
G. **Significant laboratory studies**
   1. May increase levels of high density lipoproteins (HDL), phospholipids, and triglycerides in blood
   2. May decrease low density lipoprotein (LDL) and total cholesterol levels
   3. May increase bone density
H. **Side effects**
   1. Increased skin pigmentation when exposed to sunlight; chloasma
   2. Weight gain and fluid retention
   3. Nausea (oral forms)

     4. Change in libido and increased breast tenderness

     5. Headaches, moodiness, and hypertension

     6. Amenorrhea, breakthrough bleeding

!   **I. Adverse effects/toxicity**

     1. May increase risk of breast cancer

     2. Endometrial cancer risk increases if uterus is intact and there is no concurrent progestin use

J. Nursing considerations

!   **1.** Assess blood pressure (BP) prior to and periodically during use

     2. Monthly self–breast exams and annual mammograms are recommended

     3. In clients with breast cancer and bone metastasis, severe hypercalcemia (greater than 15 mg/dL) may be caused by estradiol therapy

     4. Nausea frequently occurs in the morning, but disappears after 1 or 2 weeks of treatment; administer dose with meals or at bedtime to decrease nausea

     5. Monitor for thromboembolic events

     6. Monitor blood sugar in diabetic clients

!   **K. Client education**

     1. Correct dosage and route of administration, including how often to change transdermal patches

     2. Take medication with food if nausea occurs, usually at beginning of therapy

     3. Cigarette smoking increases risk of thrombus formation

     4. Report signs of fluid retention (edema, weight gain)

     5. When taken cyclically, vaginal bleeding will likely occur during the week each month when the estrogen is withheld

     6. Remain lying down for 30 minutes after administration of vaginal creams

     7. Place cream deep into vagina, avoid douching, and wash applicator with warm, soapy water after use

     8. Use panty liners or mini-pads, but avoid use of tampons with vaginal creams

     9. Instruct client to report positive **Homan's sign**, which is calf pain on dorsiflexion of the foot, possibly caused by formation of clots in the vein; also assess for limited leg movement

     10. Caution client that risk of blood clot formation is high with use of morning-after pill; teach signs of thrombophlebitis such as tenderness, swelling, redness in extremity, and pain; assess for sudden severe chest pain that could indicate pulmonary embolism

     11. Instruct client to take medications exactly as prescribed

     12. Encourage smoking cessation (smoking increases risk of cardiovascular events)

II. PROGESTINS

A. Action and use

     1. Cause the endometrium to change from proliferative to secretory in the latter half of the menstrual cycle in preparation for implantation of an embryo

     2. Decrease mid-cycle bleeding in peri- and postmenopausal women or in women with dysfunctional uterine bleeding

     3. Used to treat postmenopausal syndrome

     4. Used to treat amenorrhea, breast cancer, and renal cancer

B. Common medications (Tables 13-2 and 13-3)

C. Administration considerations

     1. Must be discontinued immediately if pregnancy is suspected

     2. Intramuscular (IM) injection should be given deeply; injection site may be irritated

!   **3.** Oral capsules contain peanut oil; they should not be given to clients with allergy to peanuts

---

Practice to Pass

The client has been started on estradiol (Estrace), and asks how to use this medication. How do you respond?

Table 13-2 Common Progestins

Generic (Trade) Name	Route	Therapeutic Indications	Adverse Effects
Medroxyprogesterone (Provera)	PO, IM, subQ	Abnormal uterine bleeding caused by hormonal imbalance, endometrial or renal cancer, contraception, paraphilia	Dizziness, migraine headache, depression, nervousness, pulmonary embolism, jaundice, tremors, gallbladder disease, thrombophlebitis, hypertension, edema, breakthrough bleeding, intolerance to contact lenses, hyperglycemia, weight gain, rash, pain, decreased libido, breast tenderness, breast enlargement, hypersensitivity reaction, uterine fibromas, nausea, vomiting
Norethindrone acetate (Aygestin, Errin, Jolivette, Nora-BE, Nor-QD)	PO	Amenorrhea, abnormal uterine bleeding, endometriosis, pregnancy prevention	
Megestrol acetate (Megace)	PO	Breast, renal cell, and endometrial cancer, severe weight loss, anorexia, and cachexia in clients with HIV/AIDS and cancer	Vaginal bleeding, breast tenderness, headache, increased appetite, weight gain, abdominal pain, nausea, vomiting
Progesterone (Prometrium, others)	IM	Primary and secondary amenorrhea, functional uterine bleeding, contraception, premenstrual syndrome, prevention of premature labor	Loss of vision, migraine headaches, depression, dizziness, insomnia, rash, acne pruritis, breakthrough bleeding, amenorrhea, cervical erosion, thromboembolism, thrombotic disease, decreased glucose tolerance, hepatic adenoma, edema, breast enlargement or tenderness, increase in sodium and chloride excretion, photosensitivity, jaundice, bradycardia, somnolence, syncope, spontaneous abortion, pelvic infection

Table 13-3 Common Estrogen-Progestin Hormone Replacement Medications

Generic (Trade) Name	Route	Therapeutic Indications	Adverse Effects
Conjugated estrogens with medroxyprogesterone (Prempro)	PO	Relief of menopausal symptoms, osteoporosis prevention	Breakthrough bleeding, breast tenderness, weight gain, hypertension, nausea, vomiting, dysmenorrhea, vaginal candidiasis, thromboembolic disease
Ethinyl estradiol and norethindrone acetate (Activella)	PO	Relief of menopausal symptoms, osteoporosis prevention with women who have an intact uterus	Breakthrough bleeding, breast tenderness, weight gain, hypertension, nausea, vomiting, dysmenorrhea, vaginal candidiasis, thromboembolic disease
Estradiol with norgestimate (Prefest)	PO		
Ethinyl estradiol with norethindrone (Activella)	Transdermal patch	Relief of menopausal symptoms	

D. **Contraindications**
1. Pregnancy
2. Cautious use with current or past history of depression
E. **Significant drug interactions:** decreased effectiveness when taken concomitantly with anti-epileptic medications; decreased medroxyprogesterone levels with aminoglutethimide, barbiturates, primidone, rifampin, rifabutin, and topiramate
F. **Significant food interactions:** increased caffeine levels if caffeine is ingested; use with St. John's wort may cause bleeding between menses and reduced efficacy

G. Significant laboratory studies
1. Increased LDL
2. Decreased HDL
3. Abnormal liver function tests
4. May affect coagulation, thyroid, and endocrine function

H. Side effects
1. Depression
2. Male-pattern baldness
3. Increased or decreased libido
4. Insomnia and somnolence
5. Fluid retention, edema, weight gain
6. Nausea, vomiting
7. Amenorrhea, changes in menstrual flow

I. Adverse effects/toxicity
1. Change in menstrual flow, amenorrhea, and breast changes
2. Edema
3. Cholestatic jaundice

J. Nursing considerations
1. Prior to administration in clients with current or history of depression, make certain a plan is in place to deal with worsening or recurrent depressive symptoms
2. A thorough physical examination should be done with special attention to pelvic organs, breasts, and hepatic function
3. A Pap test should be done prior to initiation of therapy and every 6–12 months while client is taking the medication
4. Monitor vital signs, including blood pressure (BP)
5. Monitor intake and output (I & O)

K. Client education
1. How to use medication and the timing of use
2. Possible side effects and symptoms to report, such as sudden severe headache, vomiting, dizziness, fainting, pain in calves, acute chest pain, and dyspnea
3. Postmenopausal women might resume cyclical vaginal bleeding
4. Perform routine breast self-examinations
5. Monitor BP and I & O
6. Avoid exposure to ultraviolet (UV) light
7. Diabetic clients should monitor glucose levels closely
8. Client should take medication with food if GI upset occurs
9. Smoking increases risk of cerebrovascular and cardiovascular adverse effects

III. ANDROGENS

Practice to Pass

A 16-year-old male client with hypogonadism is starting testosterone enanthate (Andropository) therapy. You are developing a plan of care for this client. What information should be included in the plan regarding the effects of this medication?

A. Action and use
1. **Androgens** are steroids that stimulate the action of endogenous hormones
2. Used primarily to treat male androgen (testosterone) deficiency in men with delayed puberty, hypogonadism, oligospermia, **cryptorchidism** (a congenital condition characterized by failure of the testis to descend into the scrotum), or orchiectomy
3. Used for hormone replacement therapy in women who experience decreased energy and libido
4. Used to suppress tumor growth in androgen-sensitive breast cancer
5. Danazol (Danocrine) is used to treat endometriosis and fibrocystic breast disease in women

B. Common medications (Table 13-4)

Table 13-4 Common Androgens

Generic (Trade) Name	Route	Uses	Adverse Effects
Danazol (Danocrine, Cyclomen)	PO	Endometriosis, fibrocystic breast disease, hereditary angioedema, precocious puberty, gynecomastia, hemolytic anemia, thrombocytopenia	Pseudotumor cerebri, hirsutism, dizziness, headache, sleep disorder, menstrual disturbances, hepatic damage (rare), thrombophlebitis, thromboembolism, fluid retention, weight gain, hypoestrogenic effects
Fluoxymesterone (Halotestin)	PO	Hypogonadism, inoperable breast cancer in women	Aggressiveness, hirsutism, insomnia, irritability
Methyltestosterone (Android, Testred)	PO, buccal	Cryptorchidism	
Testosterone (Androderm, others)	Gel, transdermal, buccal, pellets	Hypogonadism, hypogonadotropic hypogonadism, delayed puberty, inoperable breast cancer, metastatic mammary cancer	Dizziness, sleep disorders, fatigue, headache, rash, dermatitis, acne, hirsutism, deepening of voice, weight gain, clitoral hypertrophy, testicular atrophy, nausea, hepatocellular carcinoma, fluid retention, polycythemia, leucopenia, hypercalcemia, chills, premature closure of epiphyses
Testosterone cypionate (Depo-Testosterone)	IM, subQ implant, transdermal		
Testosterone enanthate (Delatestryl)	IM, subQ implant, transdermal patch		

C. Administration considerations
1. Medically indicated androgen use will often result in virilization and side effects must be monitored closely
2. Buccal tablets should not be chewed or swallowed
3. Testoderm should be applied to scrotal skin; dry shave the area
4. Androderm should be applied to nonscrotal skin; apply to clean dry area of back, abdomen, upper arms, or thighs
5. Use very cautiously in children because of the bone maturation effects
6. Can reduce blood glucose levels, thus reducing insulin requirements in the diabetic client
7. IM preparations may crystallize at low temperatures; therefore the vial may need warming and shaking to re-dissolve the crystals

D. Contraindications
1. Pregnancy and lactation
2. Heart failure (HF), renal and liver failure
3. Enlarged prostate

E. Significant drug interactions
1. Increased action of warfarin, can cause bleeding
2. Increased action of oral hypoglycemic agents, insulin, and glucocorticoids
3. Additive **hepatotoxicity** (toxic to liver) when administered with other hepatotoxic medications
4. Increase the effect of imipramine (increased paranoid symptoms)

F. Significant food interactions: none reported

G. Significant laboratory studies
1. Complete blood count (CBC): hemoglobin (Hgb) and hematocrit (Hct) will increase in women
2. Decrease in HDL and increase in LDL levels

Practice to Pass

A client has admitted to using illegally obtained anabolic steroids IM with his athletic teammates for the past 2 years. How would you explain to the client the laboratory studies that the physician will likely order, and why they are needed?

H. Side effects

1. In both genders are dose-related, including lowered voice, edema, acne, change in libido, increased facial hair growth, and increase in aggressive tendencies
2. In male: gynecomastia, oligospermia, impotence, decreased ejaculatory volume, and urinary urgency
3. In female: menstrual irregularities, enlarged clitoris, breast size decrease, male pattern baldness, deepening of voice, and increase in oiliness of skin

I. Adverse effects/toxicity

1. Androgens will increase male sex characteristics in pre-pubertal boys; x-ray examination of the epiphyseal growth plate must be done every 6 months in pre-pubescent boys
2. **Priapism** (painful penile erection) may also occur
3. Polycythemia may develop

J. Nursing considerations

1. Assess client for edema, weight gain, and any changes in skin
2. Assess lung and heart sounds
3. Assess client for signs of liver dysfunction
4. Evaluate client for signs of depression
5. Assess client for the presence of secondary sexual characteristics

K. Client education

1. Apply transdermal patches to shaved skin
2. Monitor weight twice weekly and report increase
3. Notify prescriber if fluid retention develops
4. Be aware of signs of virilization as side effects
5. Women who are sexually active should use a nonhormonal (barrier) contraceptive while on therapy
6. Take medication with meals or a snack

IV. ANABOLIC STEROIDS

A. **Action and use:** developed to replace androgens

B. **Common medications (Table 13-5)**

C. **Administration considerations**
1. **Anabolic steroids** are androgens with anabolic properties and are rarely prescribed, but are commonly abused by athletes in an attempt to enhance performance
2. Medically indicated androgen use will often result in virilization, and side effects must be monitored
3. High doses of androgens are occasionally used to treat breast cancer

D. **Contraindications**
1. During pregnancy and lactation
2. Contraindicated with HF, renal and liver failure, and enlarged prostate

E. **Significant drug interactions**
1. Increased action of warfarin, oral hypoglycemic agents, insulin, and glucocorticoids
2. Additive hepatotoxicity when administered with other hepatotoxic medications

F. **Significant food interactions:** none reported

G. **Significant laboratory studies**
1. May cause increase in serum aspartate aminotransferase (AST)
2. May increase bilirubin level
3. May suppress clotting factors II, V, VII, and X
4. Hgb and Hct will increase in female
5. HDL cholesterol level will decrease and LDL cholesterol level will increase

H. **Side effects**
1. In both genders: lowered voice, edema, acne, change in libido, increased facial hair growth, and increase in aggressive tendencies

Table 13-5 Common Anabolic Steroids

Generic (Trade) Name	Route	Uses	Adverse Effects
Oxandrolone (Oxandrin)	PO	Adjuvant therapy to enhance weight gain, offset protein catabolism when administering corticosteroids, short stature associated with Turner syndrome, HIV-associated muscle weakness, alcoholic hepatitis	Insomnia, confusion, phallic enlargement, hirsutism, inhibition of testicular function, clitoral enlargement, epididymitis, liver failure, intra-abdominal hemorrhage, increased blood lipid levels, sodium and water retention, acne, premature closure of epiphyses, abdominal fullness, loss of appetite, burning of tongue, increased risk of benign prostatic hyperplasia (BPH)
Oxymetholone (Anadrol-50)	PO	Anemia related to deficiency in red blood cell production, acquired or congenital aplastic anemia, myelofibrosis and hypoplastic anemia due to myelotoxic drugs	

    2. In male: gynecomastia, oligospermia, impotence, and decreased ejaculatory volume
    3. In female: menstrual irregularities, enlarged clitoris, decreased breast size, male pattern baldness; voice changes and hair growth patterns are not reversible after discontinuation of use

I. Adverse effects/toxicity
    1. Hepatotoxicity, especially when used with other hepatotoxic effects
    2. Abusers of anabolic steroids often share needles, increasing the incidence of hepatitis B and C and HIV transmission

J. Nursing considerations
    1. Assess client athletes from junior high through adulthood (especially football players, bodybuilders, weightlifters, sprinters, and endurance sport participants) for anabolic steroid abuse
    2. Assess client for edema, weight gain, and skin changes
    3. Assess lung and heart sounds
    4. Assess clients for signs of liver dysfunction
    5. Evaluate clients for signs of depression
    6. Assess client for the presence of secondary sexual characteristics

K. Client education
    1. Risks of using anabolic steroids if obtained and used illegally
    2. Risks of sharing needles if illegal use
    3. Risks of contamination when using non–U.S.-manufactured or veterinary quality substances
    4. Notify health care provider if using these medications
    5. Anabolic steroids raise cholesterol level and lower male sperm counts
    6. Females may experience menstrual irregularities

V. MEDICATIONS FOR ERECTILE DYSFUNCTION

A. Actions and use
    1. Enhance normal erectile response to sexual stimuli through inhibition of phosphodiesterase type 5 (PDE5)
    2. Increase corpus cavernosus arterial inflow and decrease venous outflow, resulting in erection
    3. Used for erectile dysfunction

B. Common medications (Table 13-6)

C. Administration considerations
    1. Sildenafil (Viagra) should not be used more than once per day
    2. Alprostadil (Caverject) should not be used more than once per 24 hours and up to 3 times per week

Table 13-6 **Common Medications for Erectile Dysfunction**

Generic (Trade) Name	Route	Adverse Effects
Sildenafil citrate (Viagra)	PO	Sudden cardiac arrest, ventricular dysrhythmias, hemorrhagic stroke, transient ischemic attack, flushing, hypotension, temporary vision loss, ocular redness, increased intraocular pressure (IOP), retinal bleeding, diarrhea, dyspepsia, respiratory infection, flulike syndrome
Tadalafil (Cialis)	PO	Headache, flushing, nasal congestion, dyspepsia, back pain, limb pain, myalgia
Vardenafil hydrochloride (Levitra)	PO	Headache, dizziness, flushing, rhinitis, sinusitis, dyspepsia, nausea, back pain, flulike symptoms
Alprostadil (Caverject Muse)	IV, transurethral pellets	Cardiac arrest, seizures, penile pain, rash, fibrosis, erection, priapism, apnea, respiratory distress

3. Alprostadil: reconstitute using 1 mL of diluent of bacteriostatic or sterile water
4. Alprostadil (Muse) should not be used more than twice in 24 hours

D. Contraindications
1. Clients with cardiovascular diseases, MI, cerebrovascular accident (CVA), or dysrhythmias within 6 months
2. CHF and unstable angina
3. With use of nitroglycerine or other nitrates
4. Hypertension (BP greater than 170/110) or hypotension (BP less than 90/50)

E. Significant drug interactions
1. Life-threatening hypotension can occur with concurrent use of nitroglycerine or nitroprusside
2. Increased adverse effects with antidepressants
3. Alprostadil increases risk of bleeding if used concurrently with warfarin
4. Do not take alpha blockers within 4 hours of anti-impotency medications
5. Erythromycin, itraconazole, ketoconazole will increase vardenafil levels
6. Nitrates enhance hypotensive effects and should not be used concurrently
7. Levodopa and papaverine may interfere with levodopa in clients with Parkinson's disease

F. Significant food interactions: grapefruit juice may increase levels but delay absorption, high-fat meals reduce peak drug levels, hawthorne (herb) increases vasodilator effects

G. Significant laboratory studies: none reported

H. Side effects
1. Ecchymosis and painless fibrotic nodules in the corpus cavernosus may occur with injections
2. With transurethral administration: a dull penile pain, prolonged erection (4 to 6 hours)
3. Sildenafil: headache, blurred vision, flushing, dyspepsia, and nasal congestion

I. Adverse effects/toxicity
1. Priapism may occur and must be treated as a medical emergency
2. Upper respiratory infection and urinary tract infection (UTI)
3. Urethral bleeding
4. Increased motor activity

J. Nursing considerations
1. Obtain a thorough medical history of clients experiencing erectile dysfunction, especially history of cardiovascular disease
2. Obtain accurate history of onset of the problem to assess for possible psychological cause since not all cases of sexual dysfunction are truly erectile dysfunction
3. Sildenafil (Viagra) is the most prescribed medication in the United States, and has been presented as a panacea for all sexual problems in the population
4. Sildenafil is usually taken 1 hour prior to sexual activity

Practice to Pass

The client has been experiencing erectile dysfunction. He asks if sildenafil (Viagra) is the only medication that can be used to treat his condition. How do you answer?

K. Client education

1. How to inject papaverine into corpus cavernosum using a ³/₈-inch, 27- or 28-gauge needle 1-mL syringe
2. Instruct client to insert transurethral pellets with a plastic introducer about 1½ inches into the urethra
3. Maximum use of the medication in a 24-hour time block and in each week
4. Take sildenafil 1 hour prior to sexual activity
5. Report chest pain or palpitations immediately if taking sildenafil
6. Eating a high-fat meal before taking sildenafil may delay onset of drug action
7. Do not take these medications with other drugs containing nitrates
8. Eliminate grapefruit from diet because of interaction with medications for erectile dysfunction

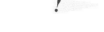

VI. CONTRACEPTIVES

A. Action and use

1. Decrease the incidence of ovulation to prevent conception
2. Thin the endometrial lining of the uterus, decreasing the incidence of implantation if fertilization takes place
3. Decrease fallopian tube ciliary peristalsis, which decreases the likelihood of an ovum meeting a sperm
4. Thicken cervical mucus, preventing sperm from penetrating into the uterine cavity
5. Used as a means of birth control
6. NuvaRing is the only vaginal contraceptive containing estrogen and progesterone; it is a 5-cm diameter ring inserted for 3 weeks, followed by a ring-free week allowing for withdrawal bleeding
7. Two IUDs, or intrauterine devices, are available
   a. ParaGard is a non-hormonal Copper T device which creates an ionic charge in the uterus, making it deadly to sperm; it can be left in place up to 10 years
   b. Mirena is a levonorgestrel releasing system which thickens cervical mucus, making it impenetrable to sperm; it can be left in place for 5 years

B. Common medications (Table 13-7)

C. Administration considerations

1. If an adolescent has not yet attained maximum growth, estrogen may cause the epiphyseal plates to close

Table 13-7 Common Contraceptives

Type	Estrogen	Progestin	Brand Name
Combination orals	Ethinyl estradiol, mestranol	Norethindrone, ethynodiol acetate, levonorgestrel, desogestrel, norgestrel, norgestimate	Triphasil, Tri-Cyclen, Tri-Norinyl, Desogen, Demulen, Ovrette, Mircette, LoEstrin, Ovcon, Nordette, Lybrel, Seasonale, Nordette, Yasmin, Yaz
Progestin-only orals	N/A	Norethindrone	Micronor, Nor-QD
Combination injectable	Estradiol cypionate	Medroxyprogesterone acetate	Lunelle
Progestin-only injectable	N/A	Medroxyprogesterone acetate	Depo-Provera
Progestin-only intradermal	N/A	Levonorgestrel	Norplant
Progestin only intrauterine device	N/A	Levonorgestrel releasing system	Mirena, Norgestrel
Spermicidal agents: creams, foams, jellies, sponge, and suppositories	N/A	Non-oxynol-9	Today sponge

2. Estrogen may decrease milk supply

3. Smokers older than 35 years of age are recommended to either quit smoking or use another method of birth control due to increased risk of deep vein thrombosis (DVT)

4. Dosing schedule is usually based on a 28-day menstrual cycle

5. Infertility and amenorrhea may persist as long as 18 months after repeated injections of Depo-Provera

6. The FDA added a black box warning in 2004 for Depo-Provera, warning that users may lose significant bone mineral density, which may be greater with increasing duration of use

7. The levonorgestrel-releasing intrauterine system devices (commonly referred to as IUDs) may be left in place up to 5 years

8. Spermicides are available in creams, foams, jellies, suppositories, and sponges; Non-oxynol-9 has a 1-hour duration of action; reapply if coitus extends beyond this time; the sponge releases the drug slowly and provides up to 24 hours protection

D. Contraindications

1. Estrogen-containing and progestin-only methods are contraindicated in females with a history of CVA, DVT, and with known or suspected breast, ovarian, or endometrial cancer

2. In 2010 the CDC advised postpartum women avoid use of combined hormonal contraceptives during the first 21 days after delivery due to a high risk for venous thromboembolism (VTE); women with a risk for VTE should wait until more than 42 days postpartum

E. Significant drug interactions

1. Progestin efficacy decreases in presence of anti-epileptic medications

2. Most antibiotics such as ampicillin, isoniazid, nitrofurantoin, rifampin, penicillin V, sulfonamides, and tetracyclines will decrease effectiveness of contraceptives

3. Increased effects of benzodiazepines, beta blockers, caffeine, corticosteroids, and theophylline occur

F. Significant food interactions: none reported

G. Significant laboratory studies

1. Progestin other than desogestrel increases total cholesterol and LDL

2. Desogestrel decreases total cholesterol and increases HDL

3. Thyroid stimulating hormone (TSH) will become slightly elevated while on combination oral contraceptive therapy (OCT)

H. Side effects

1. Estrogen-containing methods: cyclical weight gain, increased skin pigmentation, breast enlargement and tenderness, and irritability

2. Progestin-containing methods: decreased libido, depression, acne, and male pattern hair loss

3. The symptoms of possible complications of combination OCT form the acronym ACHES: **A**bdominal pain (liver tumor formation), **C**hest pain, **H**eadache, and **E**ye problems (embolus), and **S**evere leg pain (thrombophlebitis)

4. Loss of bone mineral density with Depo-Provera

5. Vaginal dryness, vaginitis, and toxic shock syndrome with contraceptive sponge

I. Adverse effects/toxicity

1. Spotting, change in menstrual flow, amenorrhea

2. Nausea, vomiting, abdominal cramps, bloating

3. Headaches, depression, edema

J. Nursing considerations

1. No single hormonal contraceptive method works best for all females

2. Finding the right combination and dosage of hormones may occur by trial-and-error

3. Encourage smokers to quit because of increased risk of DVT, especially after age 35

4. Monitor for signs and symptoms of thrombophlebitis (calf pain, possible redness and warmth and possible edema in affected leg)

5. Administer IM Depo-Provera deep into a large muscle

K. Client education

1. Take OCT exactly as directed

2. Methods of using different OCTs

    a. Combination orals: take one pill daily at the same time each day; the last 5–7 days of the pills are inert; withdrawal bleeding may occur during the last 5–7 days

    b. Progestin-only orals: take one pill each day at exactly the same time; each pill is a medicated pill; there is no week off hormones; bleeding will be irregular or may not occur

    c. Medroxyprogesterone acetate (Depo-Provera): bleeding will be irregular until the second or third dose is given; after the third dose, most females develop amenorrhea

3. Do not miss doses

4. Follow schedule below for missed dose

    a. If 1 dose is missed, take 2 tablets the next day

    b. If 2 doses are missed, take 2 tablets as soon as remembered with the next pill or take 2 tablets daily for the next 2 days; use a back-up method such as condom for the rest of the pill pack

    c. If 3 doses are missed, begin a new compact of tablets starting on day 1 of the cycle after the last pill was taken; use a back-up contraceptive method

5. Report prolonged vaginal bleeding or amenorrhea

6. Wait at least 3 months before becoming pregnant after stopping OCT

7. Conduct breast self-examination monthly

8. Instruct clients on Depo-Provera to increase intake of calcium-containing foods

9. Spermicides have low levels of effectiveness when used alone; use with barrier method such as condom or diaphragm

10. When using a contraceptive sponge, moisten with water to activate spermicide; insert high into vaginal to cover cervix; leave in place for 6 hours after intercourse; may provide protection for up to 24 hours, but remove by 30 hours after insertion to avoid toxic shock syndrome

Practice to Pass

The client is considering beginning combination oral contraceptive pills. What questions do you need to ask as part of her medical history?

VII. FERTILITY MEDICATIONS

A. Action and use

1. Used when an infertility workup determines that the cause of an inability to conceive after 12 months of unprotected intercourse is due to lack of ovulation

2. Will stimulate ovulation or follicular maturation

B. Common medications (Table 13-8)

C. Administration considerations

1. Ovulation induction agents are expensive and can cost over $1,000 per cycle

2. Multifetal pregnancy will occur in 12–20% of cases, mostly twins

3. Clients should start with smaller doses, and then increasing dosages will be used if the cycle does not achieve ovulation

D. Contraindications

1. Inability to keep track of the dosing schedule

2. Lack of access to emergency medical care

3. Primary ovarian failure

4. Hepatic dysfunction

E. Significant drug interactions:

1. Butyrophenones, phenothiazines, and methyldopa may increase prolactin levels, which may interfere with fertility

F. Significant food interactions: none reported

Table 13-8 | Common Medications for Female Infertility

Generic (Trade) Name	Route
Bromocriptine (Parlodel)	PO
Clomiphene (Clomid, Milophene, Serophene)	PO
Danazol (Danocrine)	PO
FSH- and LH-Enhancing Drugs	
Chorionic gonadotropin HCG (Ovidrel, others)	IM
Follitropin alfa (Gonal-F), follitropin beta (Follistim)	subQ
Menotropins (Menopur, Repronex)	subQ
Urofollitropin (Bravelle)	subQ
GnRH Antagonists	
Cetrorelix acetate (Cetrotide)	subQ
Ganirelix (generic)	subQ
GnRH Analogs/Agonists	
Goserelin (Zoladex)	subQ implant (endometriosis and advanced carcinoma)
Leuprolide (Lupron, others)	subQ infertility; IM endometriosis
Nafarelin (Synarel)	Intranasal

G. **Significant laboratory studies:** none reported
H. **Side effects**
   1. Ovarian hyperstimulation syndrome is more common in female with polycystic ovaries
   2. Nausea and vomiting, constipation, bloating, abdominal pain
   3. Transient blurring, diplopia, photophobia
   4. Vasomotor flushes, breast discomfort
   5. Headache, fatigue, dizziness, vertigo
   6. Tachycardia, phlebitis
   7. Blurred vision, diplopia, photophobia
I. **Adverse effects/toxicity**
   1. Ovarian enlargement resulting in lower abdominal or pelvic pressure or pain
   2. Tenderness or infection of injection site
   3. Heavy menses, exacerbation of endometriosis
   4. Mental depression
   5. Insomnia
J. **Nursing considerations**
   1. Make certain that the client understands the potential for multi-fetal pregnancy
   2. Full diagnostic measures are important if abnormal bleeding occurs
   3. Client should have an ophthalmic examination at regular intervals if clomiphene is prescribed more than 1 year
   4. Client with pelvic pain should be assessed carefully
K. **Client education**
   1. Techniques for medication administration
   2. Take medication at same time every day
   3. Be aware of side effects and the importance of reporting them
   4. If there is a response, ovulation usually occurs 4 to 10 days after last day of treatment
   5. The incidence of multiple births is increased as high as 6 times normal
   6. Be aware of treatment regimen including probable office visits for ultrasound examination of the ovaries

7. Client should have intercourse at least every other day beginning on the fifth day after the last dose of clomiphene (Clomid), or the day prior to chorionic gonadotropin administration and 3 days following
8. If a medication dose is missed:
   a. Take medication as soon as possible
   b. If not remembered until time for next dose, double the dose, then resume regular dosing schedule
   c. If more than 1 dose is missed, notify the prescriber

VIII. MEDICATIONS FOR LABOR AND DELIVERY

A. Oxytocics

1. Action and use
   a. Initiate or improve uterine contraction at term
   b. Facilitate involution in the treatment or prevention of postpartum hemorrhage
   c. Used to stimulate letdown reflex in nursing mothers and relieve pain from breast engorgement
2. Common medications (Table 13-9)
3. Administration considerations
   a. Only oxytocin (Pitocin) is Food and Drug Administration (FDA) approved for use during labor
   b. Methylergonovine (Methergine) is used only for postpartum control of excessive bleeding and hemorrhage
   c. Oxytocin should never be administered by more than one route at a time
   d. Diluted IV oxytocin solution should be administered continuously
   e. Pitocin IV preparation: for inducing labor, 10 units (1 mL) of Pitocin in 1 liter of D_5W or normal saline (NS) to give 10 milliunits/mL; for postpartum bleeding, 10 to 40 units in 1 liter of D_5W or NS provides 10 to 40 milliunits/mL
   f. The nurse should have a clear understanding of when medication is to be administered in relation to delivery
4. Contraindications
   a. Methylergonovine is contraindicated with hypertension and should be avoided, if possible, in clients planning to breastfeed, as they inhibit lactation
   b. Contraindicated in unfavorable fetal position or presentations that are undeliverable
   c. Fetal distress in which delivery is not imminent
   d. Prematurity, placenta previa
   e. Previous surgery of uterus or cervix including cesarean section
5. Significant drug interactions: oxytocin and vasoconstrictors may cause severe hypertension

Table 13-9 **Common Oxytocic Medications**

Generic (Trade) Name	Route	Therapeutic Indications	Adverse Effects
Oxytocin (Pitocin)	IV	Induce or stimulate labor, reduce postpartum bleeding, incomplete abortion, oxytocin challenge test to assess fetal distress in high-risk pregnancy	Subarachnoid bleed, seizures, coma, water intoxication, hypertension, arrhythmias, tetanic uterine contractions, abruption placentae, impaired uterine blood flow, increased uterine motility, anaphylaxis, anoxia, asphyxia, bradycardia
Methylergonovine (Methergine)	IM, IV, PO	Management of delivery of the placenta, postpartum atony and hemorrhage, uterine stimulation in the second stage of labor	Dizziness, headache, tinnitus, diaphoresis, transient hypertension, palpitations, chest pain, dyspnea, nausea, vomiting

6. Significant herbal/food interactions: Ephedra use with oxytocin may cause hypertension
7. Significant laboratory studies: oxytocin intrapartum increases unconjugated fetal bilirubin
8. Side effects
    a. Methylergonovine (Methergine): significant increase in systolic and diastolic BP, chest pain
    b. In fetus: bradycardia or other dysrhythmias, hypoxia, intracranial hemorrhage, trauma from too rapid propulsion through pelvis
    c. In mother: nausea and vomiting, postpartum hemorrhage, pelvic hematoma
    d. All oxytocics will cause uterine cramping when administered postpartum
9. Adverse effects/toxicity
    a. Uterine tetany leading to fetal demise
    b. Uterine rupture has been documented with overdose
    c. Newborns exposed to oxytocin in utero have higher incidence of hyperbilirubinemia
10. Nursing considerations
    a. Antepartum and intrapartum: monitor uterine contraction pattern, fetal heart rate (FHR), and BP
    b. Postpartum: monitor lochia and BP
    c. Massage the injection site after deep injection of oxytocin into deltoid muscle to assist quick absorption
    d. Obtain baseline tracing of uterine contraction and FHR prior to medication
    e. Increase IV dosage of oxytocin only after assessing contraction, FHR, maternal BP and heart rate
    f. Do not increase rate of oxytocin once the desired contraction pattern is achieved (contraction frequency of 2–3 minutes lasting 60 seconds)
    g. Oxytocin should be discontinued if contraction frequency is less than 2 minutes or duration is more than 90 seconds
    h. Breastfeeding should be delayed by at least 24 hours after oxytocin is discontinued
    i. Oxytocin has antidiuretic action; monitor client for water intoxication
11. Client education
    a. Indication for administration
    b. Route of administration and possible side effects
    c. Report sudden headache

B. **Ergot alkaloids**
1. Action and use
    a. Used to control postpartum hemorrhage
    b. Cause clonic contractions
2. Common medication: ergonovine (Ergotrate), 0.2 mg IV over 60 seconds only in emergency, more commonly given IM
3. Administration considerations: causes rebound uterine relaxation
4. Contraindications
    a. Contraindicated in hypersensitivity to ergot medication
    b. Cautious use with hypertension, unstable angina, recent myocardial infarction
5. Significant drug interactions: none reported
6. Significant food interactions: none reported
7. Significant laboratory studies: none reported
8. Side effects
    a. Significant increase in systolic and diastolic BP
    b. Uterine cramping
    c. Decreased milk production
9. Adverse effects/toxicity
    a. Hypertension

!　　　　　　**b.** Ergotism or overdose: nausea, vomiting, weakness, muscle pain, insensitivity to cold, paresthesia of extremities

!　　　**10.** Nursing considerations: closely monitor lochia and blood pressure after administration

11. Client education

    a. Indication for administration

    b. Route of administration and possible side effects, such as cramping

    c. Report increased blood loss, increased temperature, or foul-smelling lochia

    d. Perform pad count to monitor bleeding

    e. Do not smoke because of increased/additive vasoconstriction with ergonovine use

C. Prostaglandins

1. Action and use

    a. To terminate pregnancy from 12th week through second trimester

!　　 **b.** Dinoprostone (Prepidil, Cervidil) has FDA approval only for cervical ripening prior to labor induction

    c. Carboprost tromethamine (Hemabate) has FDA approval only for control of postpartum bleeding

2. Common medications (Table 13-10)

3. Administration considerations

!　　 **a.** Client should remain in supine position for 10 minutes after administration of dinoprostone

    b. Before dinoprostone, client should receive anti-emetic and antidiarrheal medications

4. Contraindications

    a. Use with caution in hypertension and with history of asthma

    b. Use of dinoprostone during labor has been documented to cause uterine rupture and fetal demise

    c. Acute pelvic inflammatory disease

    d. History of pelvic surgery

5. Significant drug interactions: none reported

6. Significant food interactions: none reported

7. Significant laboratory studies: none reported

8. Side effects

    a. Diarrhea, nausea, vomiting, possible increase in BP

    b. Uterine cramping

Table 13-10　**Common Prostaglandins Used During Pregnancy**

Generic (Trade) Name	Route	Therapeutic Indications	Adverse Effects
Carboprost tromethamine (Hemabate)	IM	Pregnancy termination 13–20 weeks, evacuation of uterus for missed abortion or fetal death during second trimester, postpartum hemorrhage	Flushing, hypotension, nausea, cough, dyspnea, perforated uterus, vaginal and uterine pain, endometriosis, incomplete abortion
Dinoprostone (prostaglandin E2 or PGE2) (Cervidil, others)	Vaginal suppository, gel, or insert	Termination of pregnancy, cervical ripening	Headache, dizziness, syncope, hypotension, vomiting, diarrhea, nausea, perforated uterus, uterine rupture, uterine and vaginal pain, coughing, dyspnea, endometriosis, incomplete abortion
Misoprostol (Cytotec)	PO	Prevention of non-steroidal anti-inflammatory induced gastric ulcers, abortifacient	Nausea, diarrhea, abdominal pain, flatulence, dyspepsia, miscarriage, cramping, spotting, dysmenorrhea, hypermenorrhea, headache

       c. Tension headache

       d. Flushing, cardiac dysrhythmias

   9. Adverse effects/toxicity

       a. Hypertension

       b. Uterine tetany may develop with pre-labor or intrapartum administration

       c. Uterine rupture

  10. Nursing considerations

       a. Prenatal: follow manufacturer's instructions for placement of medication; client must remain recumbent for up to 20–30 minutes after administration, and have fetal monitoring during this time

       b. Postpartum: monitor lochia and BP, be prepared for client to develop diarrhea

       c. Ensure adequate hydration when administering dinoprostone

       d. When administering carboprost, arrange pretreatment for nausea and vomiting prior to drug administration

  11. Client education

       a. Prenatal: report long or continuous contractions, as uterine tetany may develop; count fetal movement as an indicator of fetal well-being; monitor uterine tone and client temperature

       b. Postpartum: route of administration and possible side effects

D. Uterine relaxants

   1. Action and use

       a. Inhibit contractions and therefore arrest labor for at least 48 hours so that corticosteroids (betamethasone) can be given to facilitate fetal lung maturity

       b. Used for cessation of contractions to allow intrauterine fetal resuscitation when uterine hyperstimulation is present

       c. Used to delay delivery in preterm labor

   2. Common medications (Table 13-11)

   3. Administration considerations

       a. Medication is started at lowest possible dose and increased as indicated until contractions cease

       b. Be certain about recommended dose

       c. If GI symptoms occur, advise client to take the medications with food

       d. Dilute IV terbutaline by adding each 5 mg to 1,000 mL D_5W or NS to yield a concentration of 5 mcg/mL

       e. Infuse the medication via microdrip and infusion pump

   4. Contraindications

       a. Known fetal anomaly incompatible with life

       b. Beta-adrenergics contraindicated in presence of pulmonary edema

Table 13-11   **Common Uterine Relaxant Medications**

Generic (Trade) Name	Category	Route	Notes
Terbutaline sulfate (generic)	Beta-adrenergic	subQ, IV, PO	Not FDA-approved for preterm labor but most commonly used medication
Nifedipine (Procardia)	Calcium-channel blocker	PO	Not FDA-approved for preterm labor but commonly used; may cause oligohydramnios
Indomethacin (Indocin)	NSAID	Rectal, PO	Not FDA-approved for preterm labor but used as third line; increased risk of fetal complications
Magnesium sulfate	mineral	IV infusion	Monitor reflexes and respiratory and cardiovascular status

    c. Cautious use if cervix is dilated greater than 5 cm or if gestational age is less than 20 or greater than 36 weeks

    d. Severe hypertension and coronary artery disease (CAD)

5. Significant drug interaction:

    a. Increased incidence of pulmonary edema when used concurrently with corticosteroids (betamethasone) for fetal lung maturity acceleration

    b. Additive cardiovascular effects when given with sympathomimetic drugs

    c. Antagonistic effects when given with beta blockers

6. Significant food interactions: caffeine will increase side effects of beta-adrenergics

7. Significant laboratory studies: beta-adrenergics will cause hyperglycemia, worse with concomitant corticosteroid use

8. Side effects

    a. Beta-adrenergics: maternal and fetal tachycardia, palpitations, tremors, jitteriness, and anxiety, hypertension

    b. May cause or exacerbate constipation

    c. Nausea and vomiting, anorexia

    d. Hyperglycemia, hypokalemia

9. Adverse effects/toxicity

    a. Beta-adrenergics: pulmonary edema

    b. Nifedipine (Procardia) and indomethacin (Indocin) can cause oligohydramnios

    c. Indomethacin (Indocin) can cause premature closure of the ductus arteriosus leading to fetal death

10. Nursing considerations

    a. Beta-adrenergics: if client continues on to deliver after receiving uterine relaxant medications, be prepared with oxytocic for treatment of postpartum hemorrhage

    b. Monitor vital signs and I & O

    c. Nifedipine (Procardia): avoid grapefruit juice during administration (interferes with effect)

    d. Use indomethacin for a short period of time (2–3 days)

    e. If mother uses terbutaline during pregnancy, monitor the neonate for hypoglycemia

11. Client education

    a. Possible side effects and coping strategies

    b. Purpose and use of oral medications and importance of taking them on time

    c. Nifedipine (Procardia): encourage client change position slowly due to possible orthostatic hypotension

    d. How to self-monitor pulse

    e. Consult prescriber prior to taking over-the-counter (OTC) medications

E. Magnesium sulfate

1. Action and use

    a. When given parenterally, it acts as central nervous system (CNS) depressant and also depresses smooth, skeletal, and cardiac muscle function

    b. Used to arrest preterm labor and to prevent or to treat seizures with preeclampsia and eclampsia

2. Administration considerations

    a. It is used in conjunction with beta adrenergics, which increases risk of pulmonary edema

    b. A 4-gram loading dose is often utilized, which must be given over 20–30 minutes via infusion pump

    3. Contraindications

        a. Preterm labor

        b. Fetal anomaly incompatible with life

        c. Pulmonary edema or CHF

        d. Anuria, renal failure

        e. Organic CNS disease

    4. Significant drug interactions: none reported

    5. Significant food interactions: none reported

    6. Significant laboratory studies: none reported

     7. Side effects

        a. Flushed warm feeling, drowsiness

        b. Decreased deep tendon reflexes

        c. Decreased hand grasp strength

        d. Fluid and electrolyte imbalance, hyponatremia

        e. Nausea and vomiting

    8. Adverse effects/toxicity

         a. Lack of deep tendon reflexes and/or hand grasp

        b. Respiratory depression leading to respiratory arrest

    9. Nursing considerations

         a. Check patellar reflex prior to dose

        b. Monitor hand grasps, deep tendon reflexes, respiratory rate, and serum levels

        c. IV infusion flow rate is generally adjusted to maintain urine flow of at least 30 to 50 mL/h, monitor I & O carefully

        d. Monitor IV site closely to avoid extravasation

        e. Monitor vital signs

        f. Take accurate daily weight

  10. Client education

        a. Side effects of medication

        b. Report signs of preeclampsia including headache, epigastric pain, and visual disturbance

        c. Report any signs of confusion

IX. EMERGENCY CONTRACEPTION

    A. Plan B

        1. It is the only currently available emergency contraception designed to be taken as soon as possible after unprotected intercourse; it is less effective if taken more than 72 hours after coitus

        2. It contains 750 mcg of levonorgestrel; 1 pill taken initially, followed by a second pill 12 hours later; it prevents ovulation if taken correctly

        3. It is available OT for women 17 years and older; a prescription must be obtained for those younger than 17 years

        4. It is dispensed by the pharmacist; pharmacies may not have this drug in stock due to insufficient demand or pharmacists may refuse to dispense it based on moral grounds

    B. Considerations

        1. Side effects include nausea, vomiting, dizziness, abdominal pain, fatigue, and irregular menses

        2. It is not to be used in place of a primary form of birth control

Case Study

The pregnant client with preeclampsia has been scheduled to have labor induced after cervical ripening. The client is planning to breastfeed her infant.

1. What medications can be used for cervical ripening, and how are they administered?

2. How will the labor be induced physiologically?

3. The client delivered 5 minutes ago and is now experiencing a postpartum hemorrhage. What medication(s) would you anticipate the physician ordering for administration at this time?

4. The client has seized. What medication should you prepare to administer?

5. A few days postpartum, the client asks what hormonal methods of contraception she can use. How do you answer her question?

For suggested responses, see page 545.

POSTTEST

1 A client beginning oral contraceptive therapy with desogestrel and ethinyl estradiol (Desogen) asks the nurse why 2 different drugs are needed in the pill. Which explanation by the nurse is best?

1. "Desogestrel is a weak estrogen and progestin combination that requires additional estrogen to work."
2. "Together the hormones prevent the ovum from maturing and the sperm from penetrating through the cervical mucus."
3. "Estrogens alone would prevent pregnancy, but progestins are added so that spotting doesn't occur."
4. "Taking each hormone separately would prevent most pregnancies, but the combination taken together in one pill is more effective."

2 Several clients in an outpatient clinic have requested prescriptions for sildenafil (Viagra). The nurse anticipates having to inform which client that the request has been denied by the prescriber?

1. Client diagnosed with type 2 diabetes mellitus
2. Client taking medication therapy for angina pectoris
3. Client with benign prostate hypertrophy (BPH) who is being managed medically
4. Client who has chronic sinusitis with flare-ups in the spring

3 The nurse determines the client has understood teaching when she makes which statement about clomiphene (Clomid)?

1. "This medication will help make me ovulate."
2. "I'll take this medicine orally for one month."
3. "The medication prepares the wall of the uterus for fertilization."
4. "My husband is going to ask if he can ingest the medication as well."

4 The nurse concludes that which client is most likely to have testosterone transdermal (Androderm) prescribed for his condition?

1. A 45-year-old with status-post bilateral vasectomy
2. A 17-year-old with status-post right cryptorchidism repair
3. A 23-year-old with status-post varicocele repair
4. A 32-year-old with status-post bilateral orchidectomy

5 Because the client is being prepared for labor induction with oxytocin (Pitocin), the nurse instructs the licensed practical/vocational nurse (LPN/LVN) to report which of the following? Select all that apply.

1. Sudden rise in blood pressure
2. Changes in discomfort level immediately after drug is initiated
3. Gain of more than 5 lbs during the last month
4. Sensation of nausea without vomiting
5. Changes in level of consciousness

6 The nurse determines teaching on the levonorgestrel–releasing intrauterine delivery system (Mirena) has been effective when the client makes which statement?

1. "These devices are 100% effective."
2. "I can keep this device in place for up to 5 years."
3. "I will need to use a barrier method of birth control in addition to this device."
4. "I will have the device removed every 2 years and replaced."

7 After a female client taking an estrogen–progestin combination (Demulen) reports by phone a sudden onset of blurred vision, the nurse at the outpatient clinic should ask what most appropriate question?

1. "Is there someone there with you?"
2. "When was last time you had your eyeglasses prescription changed?"
3. "When is your next appointment with your gynecologist?"
4. "Do you have problems with migraine headaches?"

8 The client who has a history of asthma and who is in preterm labor received 2.5 mg of terbutaline sulfate (Brethine) subcutaneously. After the client expresses concern about the health care provider's competency, the nurse would make which most appropriate reply?

1. "The health care provider wanted to make sure you didn't have asthma problems and early labor."
2. "I'm sure the health care provider has a very good reason for ordering Brethine."
3. "What do you normally take to control your asthmatic attacks?"
4. "Brethine causes the respiratory tract to relax as well as the uterine wall."

9 The nurse should consult with the health care provider after noting that testosterone enanthate (Delatestryl) has been prescribed for which of the following clients?

1. A 16-year-old with moderate acne
2. A 32-year-old client with an increased prostatic antigen level (PSA)
3. A 66-year-old with melanoma
4. A 65-year-old male with high-density lipoprotein (Apo-I) level of 88 mg/dL

10 After dinoprostone (Prepidil) is administered to a client, a nurse plans to monitor for which of the following?

1. Fetal heart tones on a client that had difficulty conceiving
2. Initiation of contractions for a client desiring a therapeutic abortion
3. Initiation of lactation for a client interested in breastfeeding
4. Early signs and symptoms of pregnancy

➤ *See pages 451–452 for Answers and Rationales.*

ANSWERS & RATIONALES

Pretest

1 **Answer: 1** **Rationale:** Nitroglycerin is commonly used to manage signs and symptoms of coronary artery disease (CAD). A client with CAD who takes sildenafil (Viagra) is at risk for sudden cardiac death because of additive hypotension. Although the drug is contraindicated in clients with severe renal impairment, outcomes of using this drug would not place the client at immediate risk. Blurred vision is a side effect of the drug and could place the client at risk when performing certain activities but is not as life-threatening as a cardiac arrest. Although gout is a side effect of the drug, it does not compare to the risk of cardiac arrest. There is no known negative interaction between allopurinol (Zyloprim) and sildenafil. **Cognitive Level:** Analyzing **Client Need:** Pharmacological and Parenteral Therapies **Integrated Process:** Communication and Documentation **Content Area:** Pharmacology **Strategy:** The critical word in the question is *priority*. This tells you that more than one option may be partially or completely correct but that one is more important than the others. Correlate the drug action that both drugs have in common (vasodilation) to select the correct option. **Reference:** Wilson, B. A., Shannon, M., & Shields, K. (2012). *Pearson nurse's drug guide 2012.* Upper Saddle River, NJ: Pearson Education, pp. 1381–1383.

2 **Answer: 2, 4, 5** **Rationale:** Synthetic oxytocin (Pitocin) enhances endogenous oxytocin. It is administered as a dilute solution of 10 or 20 units in 1 liter IV fluid via infusion pump, with a goal of increasing the frequency, duration, and amplitude of contractions. It also increases the intensity and regularity of uterine contractions. The drug is initiated at a minimal rate to start labor and is administered with increased increments until labor is well established. Hypertension is a side effect of the drug and not a reason to administer it. Contractions that are almost continuous would result in hypoxia, which would damage the fetus and possibly cause uterine rupture. **Cognitive Level:** Analyzing **Client Need:** Pharmacological and Parenteral Therapies **Integrated Process:** Teaching and Learning **Content Area:** Pharmacology **Strategy:** Note the wording of the question indicates that more than one option is likely to be correct. Note the words *further teaching* to identify that the correct options are statements that are factually incorrect. Select the options most indicative of danger to the fetus. **Reference:** Wilson, B. A., Shannon, M., & Shields, K. (2012). *Pearson nurse's drug guide 2012.* Upper Saddle River, NJ: Pearson Education, pp. 1333–1335.

3 **Answer: 1** **Rationale:** Because IV magnesium sulfate acts as a central nervous system (CNS) depressant, it is prescribed to reduce risk of or to treat seizure activity in an eclamptic or preeclamptic client. The side effects are drowsiness, flushing, heaviness in the limbs, and decreased deep tendon reflexes. Decreased respiratory rate related to depressed neuromuscular function is a sign of magnesium toxicity. The nurse monitors the client to *prevent* toxicity. **Cognitive Level:** Applying **Client Need:** Pharmacological and Parenteral Therapies **Integrated Process:** Nursing Process: Assessment **Content Area:** Pharmacology **Strategy:** The critical words in the question are *early side effects.* This tells you the correct answer is an option that represents a mild change rather than an extreme one. Next associate the function of magnesium with the neurological side effects to choose correctly. **Reference:** Wilson, B. A., Shannon, M., & Shields, K. (2012). *Pearson nurse's drug guide 2012.* Upper Saddle River, NJ: Pearson Education, pp. 915–917.

4 **Answer: 1** **Rationale:** Clomiphene (Clomid) stimulates the production of lutein hormone (LH) and follicle-stimulating hormone (FSH), and therefore increases ovulation in women with anovulatory infertility. Clomiphene is used to treat absence of pregnancy rather than returning the uterus to its normal status. Information about female hormones is appropriate for the client experiencing infertility problems, but does not address the drug specifically. **Cognitive Level:** Applying **Client Need:** Pharmacological and Parenteral Therapies **Integrated Process:** Nursing Process: Planning **Content Area:** Pharmacology **Strategy:** Answer the critical thinking question: What normal reproductive function does clomiphene (Clomid) enhance? **Reference:** Wilson, B. A., Shannon, M., & Shields, K. (2012). *Pearson nurse's drug guide 2012.* Upper Saddle River, NJ: Pearson Education, pp. 349–350.

5 **Answer: 1** **Rationale:** When 2 pills are missed, the client should "catch up" by taking 2 pills per day for 2 days and then 1 pill daily until finishing the pill pack. This will keep her cycle controlled and minimize the chance of midcycle bleeding. The half-life of the drug is 3–27 hours. Since the client could ovulate when missing 2 or more pills, a backup method such as condoms should be utilized for the rest of the cycle. To prevent midcycle bleeding, the client should take two tablets for 2 days instead of 1 day. **Cognitive Level:** Applying **Client Need:** Pharmacological and Parenteral Therapies **Integrated Process:** Nursing Process: Implementation **Content Area:** Pharmacology **Strategy:** The core issue of the question is how many doses of an oral contraceptive can safely be missed. To determine the correct option, consider the relationship between the half-life of the drug and maintenance of the therapeutic level. **Reference:** Wilson, B. A.,

Shannon, M., & Shields, K. (2012). *Pearson nurse's drug guide 2012.* Upper Saddle River, NJ: Pearson Education, pp. 583–586.

6 **Answer: 1** **Rationale:** Terbutaline (Brethine) is a beta-adrenergic medication utilized for tocolysis in the treatment of preterm labor. It stimulates beta$_2$-receptors in uterine smooth muscle, reducing intensity and frequency of uterine contractions and lengthening the gestation period. If a drug is needed to regulate contractions, it is more likely to be oxytocin (Pitocin). Since terbutaline is used to interrupt preterm labor, it could decrease or eliminate the contractions. Oxytocin rather than terbutaline is used for postpartal hemorrhage. An antiepileptic drug such as magnesium sulfate should be administered to a client with signs and symptoms of eclampsia. **Cognitive Level:** Applying **Client Need:** Pharmacological and Parenteral Therapies **Integrated Process:** Nursing Process: Planning **Content Area:** Pharmacology **Strategy:** Specific drug knowledge is needed to answer the question. Correlate the drug's action with the client's need. **Reference:** Wilson, B. A., Shannon, M., & Shields, K. (2012). *Pearson nurse's drug guide 2012.* Upper Saddle River, NJ: Pearson Education, pp. 1462–1464.

7 **Answer: 3** **Rationale:** Oxytocin (Pitocin) is used to control postpartum hemorrhage and promotion of postpartum uterine involution. It causes the least increase in blood pressure of *all* of these oxytocic medications, and considering the history of the client, this drug would be used first in this case. Methylergonovine (Methergine) may result in a severe hypertensive crisis. Ergonovine (Ergotrate) may raise or lower the blood pressure (BP). If the client is receiving antihypertensives, it could place client at risk for hypotension (consider that this client is already at risk for shock because of postpartal hemorrhage). **Cognitive Level:** Analyzing **Client Need:** Pharmacological and Parenteral Therapies **Integrated Process:** Nursing Process: Planning **Content Area:** Pharmacology **Strategy:** The critical words *most likely* indicate that more than one option may be partially correct but that one is a better choice than the others. The core issue in this question is which drug will stop the bleeding while raising the blood pressure the least. Thus, you need to consider which drug will be effective while minimizing the risk to the client. **Reference:** Wilson, B. A., Shannon, M., & Shields, K. (2012). *Pearson nurse's drug guide 2012.* Upper Saddle River, NJ: Pearson Education, pp. 1333–1335.

8 **Answer: 1, 3** **Rationale:** St. John's wort and many oral antibiotics can decrease the estrogenic effects of oral contraceptives and therefore decrease the efficacy of the pills. Side effects of oral contraceptives include headaches, nausea, cramping, bloating, changes in menstrual flow, and amenorrhea. Oral contraceptives also increase the risk for thromboembolic events, especially in clients with a history of same or who smoke. The use of oral contraceptives is associated

with cholelithiasis and gall bladder disease, but since the client has had her gall bladder removed, this is not a concern. Following a vegan diet would not interfere with the actin of combined oral contraceptives, but the client taking Depo-Provera should increase intake of dairy and calcium-containing foods. **Cognitive Level:** Analyzing **Client Need:** Pharmacological and Parenteral Therapies **Integrated Process:** Nursing Process: Implementation **Content Area:** Pharmacology **Strategy:** Recall specific information about oral contraceptives and their side effects. Correlate the client's risk factors for an increase in these side effects to choose the correct options. **Reference:** Wilson, B. A., Shannon, M., & Shields, K. (2012). *Pearson nurse's drug guide 2012.* Upper Saddle River, NJ: Pearson Education, pp. 583–586.

9 **Answer: 4** **Rationale:** Testosterone is responsible for development of male sex organs and the secondary sex characteristics, and facilitates growth of bone and muscle. In cases of hypogonadism, too little testosterone is naturally produced. Supplementation may be required to achieve normal hormone levels. Testosterone contributes to muscle development but this is not its only action. **Cognitive Level:** Analyzing **Client Need:** Pharmacological and Parenteral Therapies **Integrated Process:** Teaching and Learning **Content Area:** Pharmacology **Strategy:** Associate the functions of testosterone with the client's need. Use the process of elimination to omit inappropriate responses, and then choose the option that is most complete. **Reference:** Wilson, B. A., Shannon, M., & Shields, K. (2012). *Pearson nurse's drug guide 2012.* Upper Saddle River, NJ: Pearson Education, pp. 1466–1469.

10 **Answer: 1** **Rationale:** Danazol (Cyclamen) is an androgen used in the treatment of endometriosis. It suppresses pituitary output of follicle-stimulating hormone (FSH) and lutein hormone (LH), which interrupts the progress and pain of endometriosis. The usual period of administration is 3–6 months extending up to 9 months, if needed. Because of potential liver damage, the client would not take it on a lifelong basis. Danazol is only given orally. One of the side effects of danazol is hot flashes. **Cognitive Level:** Applying **Client Need:** Pharmacological and Parenteral Therapies **Integrated Process:** Teaching and Learning **Content Area:** Pharmacology **Strategy:** The critical words in the question are *endometriosis* and *purpose*, which tells you that the correct option is the one that explains the reason for the use of the drug in a client with endometriosis. Eliminate 2 options first because they are not purposes of the medication. Of the remaining 2 options, choose the correct option because hot flashes are not associated with endometriosis. **Reference:** Wilson, B. A., Shannon, M., & Shields, K. (2012). *Pearson nurse's drug guide 2012.* Upper Saddle River, NJ: Pearson Education, pp. 401–403.

ANSWERS & RATIONALES

Posttest

1 **Answer: 2** **Rationale:** Combining the hormones offers 2 processes that interrupt conception. Progestins thicken cervical mucous to prevent sperm penetration, follicular maturation, and ovulation. Estrogen prevents the luteinizing hormone (LH) surge that stimulates ova maturation. Additional estrogen is not needed. Progestins are added to reduce sperm penetration, not to prevent spotting. Combining the 2 ingredients in 1 pill is more economical rather than effective, but the statement is too vague to have the greatest use to the client. **Cognitive Level:** Analyzing **Client Need:** Pharmacological and Parenteral Therapies **Integrated Process:** Teaching and Learning **Content Area:** Pharmacology **Strategy:** Correlate the drug actions with the therapeutic purposes. Eliminate the false statements first and then choose the most specific option from those remaining. **Reference:** Wilson, B. A., Shannon, M., & Shields, K. (2012). *Pearson nurse's drug guide 2012.* Upper Saddle River, NJ: Pearson Education, pp. 583–586.

2 **Answer: 2** **Rationale:** Nitrates are the most common drugs used in management of angina. Current evidence indicates clients taking nitrates should not ingest sildenafil (Viagra) at the same time because a sudden drop in blood pressure could occur that could lead to sudden death. No endocrine alterations such as diabetes mellitus are associated with the drug, and a diagnosis of diabetes would not be a contraindication for use of sildenafil. Finasteride (Proscar) used to treat benign prostate hypertrophy (BPH) may cause impotence and may decrease the effectiveness of sildenafil, but it is not as significant as the risk of cardiac arrest. Sildenafil may worsen chronic sinusitis, but is not as significant as cardiac arrest. **Cognitive Level:** Analyzing **Client Need:** Pharmacological and Parenteral Therapies **Integrated Process:** Nursing Process: Assessment **Content Area:** Pharmacology **Strategy:** The core issue of the question is identification of a client at particular risk if taking sildenafil (Viagra). Recall that this drug has vasodilating effects and use the process of elimination to select the client in whom vasodilation could pose added risk. **Reference:** Wilson, B. A., Shannon, M., & Shields, K. (2012). *Pearson nurse's drug guide 2012.* Upper Saddle River, NJ: Pearson Education, pp. 1381–1383.

3 **Answer: 1** **Rationale:** Clomiphene (Clomid) induces ovulation through stimulation of luteinizing hormone (LH) and follicle-stimulating hormone (FSH). It is taken orally in 50 mg dosage for 5 days each month, beginning on day 5 of the menstrual cycle. Clomiphen does not prepare the uterine wall for fertilization. Use of this drug by male clients has occurred but lacks scientific evidence, so therefore this is not the best response. **Cognitive Level:** Applying **Client Need:** Pharmacological and Parenteral Therapies **Integrated Process:** Nursing Process: Evaluation **Content Area:** Pharmacology **Strategy:** Correlate the drug category with the client's statement. The drug is categorized as an ovulation stimulant. **Reference:** Wilson, B. A., Shannon, M., & Shields, K. (2012). *Pearson nurse's drug guide 2012.* Upper Saddle River, NJ: Pearson Education, pp. 347–348.

4 **Answer: 4** **Rationale:** Orchidectomy is removal of the testicle, which would require hormone replacement. Vasectomy is severing of the vas deferens to prevent the passage of sperm during ejaculation. Cryptorchidism repair is correction of an undescended testicle and would not require hormone replacement. Varicocele repair involves repair of a blood vessel and would require no hormone replacement. **Cognitive Level:** Applying **Client Need:** Pharmacological and Parenteral Therapies **Integrated Process:** Nursing Process: Planning **Content Area:** Pharmacology **Strategy:** Associate the syllable *andro* for *androgen* with the testicles. Recall that it is a male reproductive hormone to help make the correct selection. **Reference:** Wilson, B. A., Shannon, M., & Shields, K. (2012). *Pearson nurse's drug guide 2012.* Upper Saddle River, NJ: Pearson Education, pp. 1466–1468.

5 **Answer: 1, 5** **Rationale:** One common side effect of oxytocin (Pitocin) is hypertensive episodes, so blood pressure should be closely monitored. Subarachnoid hemorrhage is a side effect of the drug and level of consciousness should be monitored. Nausea may occur, as well as an increase in discomfort once the therapy is initiated, but these do not signal the nurse of a serious threat. Weight gain may reflect fluid retention in the later months of pregnancy. **Cognitive Level:** Applying **Client Need:** Pharmacological and Parenteral Therapies **Integrated Process:** Nursing Process: Planning **Content Area:** Pharmacology **Strategy:** Align side effects with management of the client's needs. **Reference:** Wilson, B. A., Shannon, M., & Shields, K. (2012). *Pearson nurse's drug guide 2012.* Upper Saddle River, NJ: Pearson Education, pp. 1133–1135.

6 **Answer: 2** **Rationale:** Mirena is a levonorgestrel–releasing intrauterine system used for contraception. It releases 20 mcg/day of levonorgestrel over a period of 5 years, at which time it needs to be removed. **Cognitive Level:** Analyzing **Client Need:** Pharmacological and Parenteral Therapies **Integrated Process:** Nursing Process: Planning **Content Area:** Pharmacology **Strategy:** Recall knowledge of intrauterine devices and their duration of action. **Reference:** Adams, M., & Koch, R. (2010). *Pharmacology: Connections to nursing practice.* Upper Saddle River, NJ: Pearson Education, p. 1212.

7 **Answer: 1** **Rationale:** Sudden onset of blurred vision may indicate blood clot formation and subsequent pressure on the optic nerves. Hypercoagulation is a common side effect of estrogen derivatives. The client could become suddenly unable to communicate or seek assistance. Sudden onset of blurred vision is not commonly associated with the development of a refractory problem. The client is in need of immediate health care unrelated to gynecologic assessment. Clients with migraine headaches often have blurred vision before an attack; however, since the nurse is aware of the risks associated with an estrogen–progestin combination (Demulen), the high-risk possibilities should be pursued first. **Cognitive Level:** Applying **Client Need:** Pharmacological and Parenteral Therapies **Integrated Process:** Nursing Process: Implementation **Content Area:** Pharmacology **Strategy:** Correlate the client's reported symptom with the drug characteristics and side effects. Select the option that provides the greatest degree of safety. **Reference:** Wilson, B. A., Shannon, M., & Shields, K. (2012). *Pearson nurse's drug guide 2012.* Upper Saddle River, NJ: Pearson Education, pp. 583–586.

8 **Answer: 4** **Rationale:** Terbutaline sulfate (Brethine) is categorized as a selective beta$_2$-adrenergic stimulant that results in smooth muscle relaxant of the respiratory tract as well as the uterine muscles. Therefore, it is used to treat both bronchospasms as well as premature labor. Asking the client what is used normally to control asthmatic attacks does not address the client's concern and it also provides no actual information. The primary issue is for the nurse to communicate the appropriate information regarding the use of Brethine to treat preterm labor. **Cognitive Level:** Analyzing **Client Need:** Pharmacological and Parenteral Therapies **Integrated Process:** Communication and Documentation **Content Area:** Pharmacology **Strategy:** Correlate the differences between common use of the drug and the common physiological processes existing between respiratory function and uterine contraction. **Reference:** Wilson, B. A., Shannon, M., & Shields, K. (2012). *Pearson nurse's drug guide 2012.* Upper Saddle River, NJ: Pearson Education, pp. 1462–1464.

9 **Answer: 2** **Rationale:** Testosterone is contraindicated in a client suspected of having prostate cancer. Although further assessment is warranted, an increased prostatic antigen level (PSA) may indicate prostate cancer exists. Acne is believed to be stimulated by androgenic hormones and the testosterone could contribute to this, but this is not as much a concern as the client with an elevated PSA level. Etiological factors associated with melanoma include genetic predisposition, sun exposure, and the presence of moles. Ingestion of testosterone can result in hyper-cholesterolemia, but this lipoprotein level is within normal limits. **Cognitive Level:** Applying **Client Need:** Pharmacological and Parenteral Therapies **Integrated Process:** Nursing Process: Planning **Content Area:** Pharmacology **Strategy:** Compare and contrast the client characteristics with the characteristics of the drug. Specific drug knowledge is needed to make the correlation. **Reference:** Wilson, B. A., Shannon, M., & Shields, K. (2012). *Pearson nurse's drug guide 2012.* Upper Saddle River, NJ: Pearson Education, pp. 1466–1468.

10 **Answer: 2** **Rationale:** Dinoprostone (Prepidil) is a form of prostaglandin E2 and is used for cervical ripening. It is commonly used as an abortifacient. The client who had difficulty conceiving would be most interested in carrying the fetus to full term so the drug would not be given to this client. Since it is an abortifacient, breastfeeding does not correlate with the drug's actions. **Cognitive Level:** Applying **Client Need:** Pharmacological and Parenteral Therapies **Integrated Process:** Nursing Process: Assessment **Content Area:** Pharmacology **Strategy:** Associate the characteristics of the drug with the needs of the client and use the process of elimination to make a selection. **Reference:** Wilson, B. A., Shannon, M., & Shields, K. (2012). *Pearson nurse's drug guide 2012.* Upper Saddle River, NJ: Pearson Education, pp. 475–476.

References

Abrams, A. (2009). *Clinical drug therapy: Rationales for nursing practice* (9th ed.). Philadelphia, PA: Lippincott Williams & Wilkins.

Adams, M., Holland, L., & Bostwick, P. (2011). *Pharmacology for nurses: A pathophysiologic approach* (3rd ed.). Upper Saddle River, NJ: Pearson Education.

Adams, M. P., & Urban, C. Q. (2013). *Pharmacology: Connections to nursing practice* (2nd ed.). Upper Saddle River, NJ: Pearson Education.

Aschenbrenner, D., & Venable, S. (2012). *Drug therapy in nursing* (4th ed.). Philadelphia, PA: Lippincott Williams & Wilkins.

Drug Facts & Comparisons® (Updated monthly). St. Louis, MO: A. Wolters Kluwer.

Karch, A. M. (2010). *Focus on nursing pharmacology* (5th ed.). Philadelphia, PA: Lippincott Williams & Wilkins.

Kee, J. (2009). *Laboratory and diagnostic tests and nursing implications* (8th ed.). Upper Saddle River, NJ: Prentice Hall.

Lehne, R. (2010). *Pharmacology for nursing care* (7th ed.). St. Louis, MO: Mosby, Inc.

LeMone, P., Burke, K., M. & Bauldoff, G. (2011). *Medical-surgical nursing: Critical thinking in patient care* (5th ed.). Upper Saddle River, NJ: Pearson Education.

Lilley, L. L., Collins, S. R., et al. (2011). *Pharmacology and the nursing practice* (6th ed.). St. Louis, MO: Mosby, Inc.

Centers for Disease Control and Prevention (CDC). Update to CDC's *U.S. medical eligibility criteria for contraceptive use, 2010*: Revised recommendations for the use of contraceptive methods during the postpartum period. *MMWR. Morbidity and Mortality Weekly Report.* (2011). 60 (26), 878–883.

ANSWERS & RATIONALES

Respiratory System Medications

14

Chapter Outline

Bronchodilators
Inhaled Corticosteroids
Inhaled Nonsteroidals

Leukotriene Modifiers
Antihistamines

Medications to Control
    Bronchial Secretions
Oxygen

Objectives

➤ Describe general goals of therapy when administering respiratory system medications.
➤ Discuss action, contraindications, side effects, and adverse/toxic effects of bronchodilators.
➤ Identify client teaching points related to the administration of inhaled respiratory medications.
➤ Identify nursing considerations related to the administration of intravenous bronchodilators.
➤ Discuss nursing considerations when administering antihistamines, decongestants, expectorants, antitussives, and mucolytics.
➤ Identify signs and symptoms of oxygen toxicity.
➤ Describe nursing considerations related to the administration of oxygen.
➤ Identify client education points related to safety and home care use of oxygen.
➤ List significant client education points related to respiratory system medications.

NCLEX-RN® Test Prep

Use the accompanying online resource, NursingReviewsandRationales, to test yourself with hundreds of NCLEX®-style practice questions.

Review at a Glance

acute asthma attack bronchospasm with shortness of breath, wheezing, and cough

adrenergic agonist medication that exerts same effects as sympathetic nervous system

anticholinergic effect caused by blockade of acetylcholine receptors that inhibits transmission of parasympathetic nervous system impulses

antihistamine a medication used to treat allergic symptoms that competes with histamine for receptor sites to block action

of histamine; result is to inhibit smooth muscle contraction, decrease capillary permeability, decrease salivation and tear formation, and inhibit vascular permeability and edema formation

antitussive a medication that aids in quieting a nonproductive, ineffective cough

atelectasis incomplete lung expansion or collapse of alveoli

catecholamine an agent released from adrenal medulla in response to sympathetic nervous system stimulation

decongestant medication that relieves nasal stuffiness by shrinking swollen nasal mucous membranes

expectorant a medication used to aid clients with sputum production during cough

histamine substance released from mast cells and basophils in response to stimuli, such as in allergic reactions or cellular injury; effects of histamine include bronchoconstriction

hypoxemia deficiency of oxygen in arterial blood

PRETEST

hypoxia a state in which insufficient oxygen is available to meet needs of body cells and tissues

inhaler device used for administration of a medication by inhalation

interleukin plasma protein that increases during inflammatory process

lacrimal a term referring to glands or ducts involved with secretion of tears

leukotrienes substances released when client is exposed to an allergen and experiences an allergic response; they cause inflammation, bronchoconstriction, and mucus production

mast cell type of cell involved in hypersensitivity reactions; many are found in skin, nasal region, and lungs;

they contain histamine, kinins, chemotactic factors, leukotrienes, prostaglandins, and thromboxanes; irritants or allergens cause breakdown of mast cells, causing release of bronchoconstrictive and inflammatory substances, resulting in airway edema, bronchospasm, and excess mucus production

mucolytic a medication administered by inhalation to liquefy respiratory secretions

nebulizer a device used for inhalation medications that produces a fine spray or mist

neutrophils white blood cells that increase in concentration in response to inflammation or infection

noncatecholamine not from sympathetic nervous system

opioid narcotic agent that acts on central nervous system to reduce pain perception

rhinitis inflammation of nasal mucous membrane

status asthmaticus severe asthma that cannot be controlled with typical medications; symptoms persist in spite of treatment efforts

sympathomimetic medication that mimics effect of sympathetic nervous system

xanthines medications that lead to bronchodilation by inhibiting the enzyme phosphodiesterase (PDE) and thereby increasing cyclic adenosine monophosphate

PRETEST

1 After the nurse administers albuterol (Proventil) to a 24-year-old client with symptoms of an acute asthma attack, which of the following outcomes is best?

1. Relief of wheezing
2. Respiratory rate decreased from 34 to 22
3. Dyspnea rating scale decreased from 9 to 6
4. Oxygen saturation of 82%

2 The nurse should question an order for epinephrine (Primatene) for the treatment of acute bronchitis when the client has which of the following health problems?

1. Asthma
2. Coronary artery disease
3. Hypotension
4. Bradycardia

3 A client receiving theophylline (Theo-Dur) asks the nurse why a specific item was removed from the food tray. Which of the following is the best response?

1. "Peas contain a chemical that can reduce the effects of the drug."
2. "Brown beans are high in protein and can increase the effects of the drug."
3. "Milk is high in calcium and increases the cardiac rate."
4. "Coffee contains caffeine, which can increase the drug level more quickly."

4 After assessing a client with chronic obstructive pulmonary disease (COPD) who is being treated with beclomethasone dipropionate (Beclovent) via oral inhaler, which clinical manifestations would the nurse conclude are side effects of this medication? Select all that apply.

1. Excess salivation
2. Delayed healing
3. Oral fungal infection
4. Fluid retention with weight gain
5. Decreased respiratory rate

5 Because a client on the inpatient unit is having an acute asthma attack, the nurse is most likely to administer which of the following medications with an appropriate order?

1. Aminophylline (Truphylline)
2. Albuterol (Proventil)
3. Cromolyn disodium (Intal)
4. Cromolyn (generic)

6 The nurse is evaluating the effectiveness of client teaching about home medication administration. Which statement by the client indicates that more teaching is needed related to zafirlukast (Accolate)?

1. "I will take the drug a few weeks before I expect to notice an improvement in my symptoms."
2. "I will use this medication when I have the symptoms of an acute asthma attack."
3. "I will increase my fluid intake while I am taking this medication."
4. "I will plan to take my medicine one hour before meals."

7 Which statement would the nurse include when teaching a client about loratadine (Claritin)?

1. "This medication may make you feel nervous."
2. "It will take this medication a few hours before it becomes effective."
3. "This medication will help in an acute asthma attack."
4. "Be sure to take this medication on an empty stomach."

8 Under which circumstance should the nurse suspend IV administration of phenylephrine (Neo-Synephrine) and consult with the health care provider?

1. After 3 days of continuous use
2. If client develops hypertension or tachycardia
3. If client develops a dry, irritated oral cavity
4. If client develops rebound congestion

9 Because of a potential side effect of guaifenesin (Robitussin), the nurse at the outpatient clinic instructs the client to perform which of the following?

1. Consider using over-the-counter (OTC) antiemetic.
2. Report increased production of respiratory secretions.
3. Follow medication with a sip of water.
4. Take aspirin 625 mg for temperature elevation.

10 A client with acute bronchitis is apprehensive because the flaps on the nonrebreather oxygen mask close during exhalation. The nurse should make which of the following adjustments?

1. None, because the mask is functioning properly.
2. Change client to a nasal cannula.
3. Replace nonrebreather mask with a new one.
4. Call the respiratory therapist.

➤ *See pages 481–483 for Answers and Rationales.*

I. BRONCHODILATORS

A. Beta adrenergics

1. Action and use
   a. Act as sympathetic nervous system (SNS) **adrenergic agonists**; raise intracellular levels of cAMP (cyclic adenosine monophosphate), which dilates constricted bronchi and bronchioles by relaxing smooth muscle
   b. Medications that lead to bronchodilation stimulate beta$_2$-adrenergic receptors in smooth muscle of bronchi and bronchioles
   c. Medications can have alpha, beta$_1$, or beta$_2$ activity; beta$_1$-adrenergic receptors increase heart rate and force of myocardial contraction
   d. Used during an **acute asthma attack**, which is characterized as bronchospasm with shortness of breath and wheezing, for quick airway dilation; used also for emphysema, acute and chronic bronchitis, and relief of bronchospasm; alpha-adrenergic stimulators can act as a decongestant due to constriction of blood vessels in nasal cavity
   e. Beta adrenergic agents can be classified as **catecholamines** released from adrenal medulla in response to stimulation of SNS or **noncatecholamines**, which are not released by SNS; all beta adrenergic agents stimulate beta$_2$ receptors; catecholamines affect both alpha and beta receptors and cause cardiovascular effects

2. Common medications (Table 14-1)

a. Selective beta$_2$ agonists are preferred drugs for bronchial smooth muscle dilation as they produce fewer cardiac side effects

b. Albuterol (Proventil, Ventolin, Proventil Repetabs, Volmax): predominately a beta$_2$ stimulator; given PO or by inhalation; it is not as likely to cause cardiac side effects and is used for prevention and treatment of bronchoconstriction

c. Ipratroprium bromide (Atrovent): has **anticholinergic** effect or sympathetic nervous system effect; given by inhalation

d. Levalbuterol (Xopenex): short-acting beta$_2$ agonist used for prevention and treatment of bronchoconstriction; it is given by nebulizer and is not as likely to cause cardiac side effects

e. Ephedrine: alpha and beta stimulant and therefore causes nasal decongestion; given PO, IM, IV, or subQ

f. Epinephrine (Adrenalin, Primatene, Bronkaid, Bronitin, Medihaler-Epi): alpha and beta stimulant; given subQ, IM, or by inhalation; epinephrine has beta1-adrenergic action causing increased heart rate and increased force of myocardial contraction

g. Ethylnorepinephrine (Bronkephrine): alpha and beta stimulant, given IM or subQ

h. Isoetharine (Arm-a-Med Isoetharine): beta$_1$ and beta$_2$ stimulant; given by inhalation

i. Isoproterenol (Isuprel, Medihaler-Iso); beta$_1$ and beta$_2$ stimulant; given IV, sublingual, or by inhalation; used for short-acting bronchodilation effect but also has cardiac stimulant effects

Table 14-1	**Common Beta-Adrenergic Agents**		
Generic (Trade) Name	**Route**	**Therapeutic Indications**	**Adverse Effects**
Albuterol sulfate (Proventil, Ventolin, VoSpire)	Inhalation Nebulizer PO	Relief of bronchospasm, asthma, exercise-induced bronchospasm	Nervousness, restlessness, tremors, pain, bronchospasm, chest pain, angina, palpitations, hypertension, hypokalemia, hyperglycemia
Arformoterol (Brovana)	Nebulizer	COPD including chronic bronchitis and emphysema	
Formoterol (Foradil, Perforomist)	Inhalation Nebulizer	Asthma prophylaxis, relief of bronchospasm	
Indacaterol (Arcapta Neohaler)	Inhalation	COPD including chronic bronchitis and emphysema	
Levalbuterol (Xopenex)	Nebulizer Inhalation	Bronchospasm in reversible obstructive pulmonary disease	Increased cough, dyspepsia, hyperglycemia, anxiety, dizziness, headache
Metaproterenol (generic)	Inhalation	Bronchial asthma, emphysema	Nervousness, anxiety, tremors, headache, insomnia, arrhythmias, angina, hypertension, bronchospasm, changes in blood pressure
Salmeterol (Serevent)	Inhalation	Bronchospasm, asthma	
Pirbuterol acetate (Maxair)	Inhalation	Bronchospasm, asthma	
Terbutaline (Brethine)	PO	Bronchospasm, bronchial asthma	Angina, tremors, arrhythmias, nervousness, tachycardia, nausea, vomiting, hyperglycemia
Ipratropium (Alti-Ipratropium, Apo-Ipravent, Atrovent, Novo-Ipramide) (anti-cholinergic)	Inhalation or Nebulizer	Bronchospasm related to chronic obstructive pulmonary disease, chronic bronchitis, emphysema	Blurred vision, acute eye pain, bitter taste, dry oropharyngeal membranes, hoarseness, cough, nasal dryness, urinary retention, headache

    j. Metaproterenol (Alupent, Metaprel): beta$_2$ stimulant; given PO or by inhalation; causes cardiac and CNS stimulation in higher doses

    k. Pirbuterol (Maxair): beta$_2$ stimulant; given by inhalation; short-acting beta$_2$ agonist used for prevention and treatment of bronchoconstriction; not as likely to cause cardiac side effects

    l. Salmeterol (Serevent): beta$_2$ stimulant; given by inhalation; used very commonly because of 12-hour duration of action; used for prophylaxis of acute bronchoconstriction

    m. Terbutaline (Brethine): beta$_2$-adrenergic agonist; long-acting bronchodilator; administered PO, subQ, or by inhalation

    n. Ipratroprium bromide/albuterol sulfate (Combivent): combination product

3. Administration considerations

    a. May see adverse effects with albuterol, bitolterol, levalbuterol, and pirbuterol if used too frequently because they lose beta$_2$ specific actions at larger doses (so beta$_1$ receptors are stimulated and the result can be elevated heart rate, nausea, anxiety, palpitations, and tremors)

    b. Epinephrine, ephedrine, and ethylnorepinephrine can be used as a nasal decongestant due to alpha stimulation

    c. Use with caution in young children and monitor for tremors, restlessness, hallucinations, dizziness, palpitations, tachycardia, and gastrointestinal (GI) difficulties

    d. Epinephrine is given subcutaneously for bronchoconstriction; effects are usually seen in 5 minutes and may last up to 4 hours

    e. Salmeterol is not used in an acute asthma attack because of slow onset of action (20 minutes); not to be dosed more often than every 12 hours due to 12-hour duration of action

4. Contraindications

    a. Albuterol is contraindicated in clients with hypersensitivity to drug as well as those with tachyarrhythmias and severe coronary artery disease

    b. Contraindicated with hypersensitivity to **sympathomimetics**, which mimic effect of SNS

    c. Sympathomimetics are used with caution in clients with cardiovascular disease because of potential for increasing myocardial oxygen demand

    d. Use caution in clients with hypertension, diabetes mellitus, seizures, and hypothyroidism

    e. Avoid use with monoamine oxidase (MAO) inhibitors and sympathomimetics

    f. Children under 12 should not use inhalations of albuterol, bitolterol, metaproterenol, and terbutaline

    g. Avoid use of extended-release albuterol in children under age 12 years

    h. Catecholamines should not be used in clients with tachydysrhythmias

5. Significant drug interactions

    a. Concurrent use of MAO inhibitors may lead to hypertensive crisis

    b. Use with other sympathomimetics may cause additive adrenergic effects

    c. The action of beta agonists is antagonized by beta-adrenergic blocking agents and therefore therapeutic effects may be minimized

    d. Potassium-losing diuretics may increase risk of hypokalemia

    e. Cardiac glycoside toxicity may occur with concurrent use of cardiac glycosides and beta-adrenergic agents, especially in presence of hypokalemia

    f. These drugs can potentiate therapeutic and adverse effects of other bronchodilators

    g. Use with digoxin may lead to decreased digoxin levels

    h. Effects of sympathomimetics can be intensified by thyroid hormone, decongestants, and some antihistamines

6. Significant food interactions: none reported

7. Significant laboratory studies
    a. Sympathomimetics can stimulate liver production of glucose
    b. Sympathomimetics can exacerbate symptoms of hyperthyroidism
8. Side effects
    a. When beta$_1$ receptors are stimulated, client may experience nervousness, tremors, increased heart rate, and increased blood pressure
    b. With alpha- and beta-adrenergic stimulation, client may experience insomnia, restlessness, anorexia, tremors, cardiac stimulation, and vascular headache
    c. With nonselective beta agonists, client may experience cardiac stimulation, tremors, anginal pain, and vascular headache
    d. With beta$_2$-adrenergic agents, client may experience hypotension, vascular headache, and tremors
    e. Muscle tremors are most frequent side effect of terbutaline
    f. Additional side effects may include hypokalemia, hyperglycemia, nausea, vomiting, chest pain, and arrhythmias
    g. Paradoxic bronchospasm and urinary retention may also occur
9. Adverse effects/toxicity
    a. CV: tachyarrhythmias, chest pain
    b. CNS: restlessness, agitation, nervousness, and insomnia
10. Nursing considerations
    a. Monitor elderly clients carefully
    b. Monitor vital signs, especially heart rate and blood pressure when administering beta agonists (because of cardiovascular effects)
    c. Ensure proper use of metered dose inhaler (MDI) for maximum benefit
    d. Use appropriate diluent when giving medications
    e. If ordered, ensure that chest physiotherapy and postural drainage are done after client has received dose of expectorant, bronchodilator, mucolytic, or anti-inflammatory drug and that client is having intended response of expectorating mucus
    f. Ask client about current medications (including OTC and herbal products) and about any history of drug allergies
    g. At times, use of multiple drugs is effective and dosages of each can be reduced
    h. Note amount, color, and character of sputum
    i. Monitor baseline pulmonary function tests periodically throughout drug therapy to determine effectiveness of therapy
    j. Administer oral medications with meals to decrease GI irritation
    k. Solutions may remain diluted for 24–48 hours
    l. Monitor blood glucose levels in diabetic clients
    m. Avoid intramuscular (IM) injections
11. Client education
    a. Monitor blood glucose level closely in diabetic clients because some medications, especially epinephrine, may elevate blood glucose levels; an adjustment in maintenance doses of antidiabetic agents may be indicated
    b. Contact prescriber prior to taking OTC drugs to ensure there is no potential interaction
    c. Report chest pain, palpitations, seizures, headaches, hallucinations, or blurred vision to prescriber
    d. Do not take more than prescribed dose because of risk of hypertension, tachycardia, dysrhythmias, and angina
    e. Record prn use of these drugs, noting date, time, symptoms, and whether or not symptoms subsided
    f. Use inhaled preparations properly; have client give a return demonstration; see Box 14-1 and Figure 14-1

The correct steps in administering medication with a metered-dose inhaler (MDI) are as follows:

- Insert the medication firmly into the inhaler.
- Remove the cap and hold the inhaler upright.
- Shake the inhaler for 3–5 seconds to ensure even mixing of medication in propellant.
- Tilt the head back slightly and hold the inhaler upright.
- Position the inhaler 1–2 inches away from the open mouth or attach it to a spacer or holding chamber. If a medicine chamber is used, seal the lips around the mouthpiece.
- Press on the inhaler while beginning to breathe in slowly through mouth.
- Breathe in slowly and deeply for 3–5 seconds.
- Hold the breath for 8–10 seconds as able to allow the medication to move down into airways.
- Wait 1–3 minutes as per product directions before the next inhalation if another inhalation is ordered.
- Rinse the mouth with water and blow the nose.
- Use mild soap and water to clean the mouthpiece. Allow to air dry.
- Store the inhaler at room temperature.

Figure 14-1

Proper Use of a Metered Dose Inhaler

 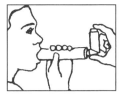 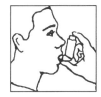

A. Open mouth with inhaler 1 to 2 inches away.

B. Use spacer/holding chamber (which is recommended especially for young children and for people using corticosteroids).

C. In the mouth. Do not use for cortico-steroids.

D. NOTE: Inhaled dry powder capsules require a different inhalation technique. To use a dry powder inhaler, it is important to close the mouth tightly around the mouthpiece of the inhaler and to inhale rapidly.

    g. Using a spacer enables more medication to reach site of drug action in lungs, and less is deposited in mouth and throat

    h. Care of nebulizer and/or inhaler

        1) Wash and dry inhaler and nebulizer tubing and apparatus daily

        2) White vinegar can be used to rinse nebulizer tubing

        3) Read and follow manufacturer's instructions about use, storage, and cleaning of equipment

    i. Wait 1–3 minutes (some references suggest 3–5 minutes) between inhalations of aerosol medications

    j. Avoid eye contact with inhaler spray

    k. Anticipated response to a nebulizer or inhalation treatment is absence of wheezing and dyspnea

    l. Take medication exactly as ordered; do not double dosage or increase frequency of doses

    m. Avoid contact with an allergen that tends to cause bronchoconstriction; avoid contact with smoke and other irritants, such as aerosol hair spray, perfumes, and cleaning products

    n. Increase fluid intake if not contraindicated by other diseases

o. Recognize symptoms of respiratory difficulty (such as activity intolerance and waking at night with asthma symptoms) so that intervention can begin as soon as possible

p. Avoid caffeine as this may increase nervousness and insomnia of broncho dilating drugs

q. An inhaled bronchodilator is the treatment of choice in an acute asthma attack

r. Do not break, chew, or crush extended-release tablets

s. Nervousness and tremors may be experienced when a medication is newly administered but frequently decrease over time

B. Xanthines

1. Action and use

a. **Xanthines** inhibit enzyme phosphodiesterase (PDE), which breaks down cAMP (cyclic adenosine monophosphate), and thereby increases amounts of cAMP, leading to bronchial dilation due to smooth muscle relaxation

b. Increase catecholamine levels, inhibiting calcium ion movement into smooth muscle, inhibiting prostaglandin synthesis, and inhibiting release of bronchoconstrictive substances from leukocytes and **mast cells** (which contain histamine, prostaglandins, and thromboxanes)

c. Cause bronchodilation and thereby increase ability of cilia to clear mucus from airways

d. Used to treat bronchoconstriction associated with COPD (diseases such as chronic bronchitis, asthma, and emphysema) and other chronic respiratory disorders

e. Have a slow onset of action and therefore are utilized to prevent asthma attacks rather than treat them; can be used during an asthma attack if it is mild to moderate

f. Can be used as an additional treatment in pulmonary edema by decreasing vascular permeability and paroxysmal nocturnal dyspnea (PND)

g. Are useful for symptom control of clients with asthma and reversible bronchospasm (may occur in clients with chronic bronchitis and emphysema)

h. Used to treat **status asthmaticus**, which is characterized by severe asthma that cannot be controlled with typical medications (use IV theophylline if client has not responded to faster-acting beta agonist)

2. Common medications (see Table 14-2)

3. Administration considerations

a. Administer cautiously to older adults because of potential for increased sensitivity

b. Administer xanthines cautiously to children over 6 months of age

c. Monitor carefully blood levels and therapeutic response to medication to avoid potential toxicity

d. Xanthines exhibit a direct stimulating effect on CNS, which may be enhanced in children

Practice to Pass

A client is admitted to the emergency department with inspiratory and expiratory wheezes, dusky color, and pulse oximetry of 88%. What is the appropriate action of the nurse in the emergency department?

Table 14-2 **Common Xanthines**

Generic (Trade) Names	Route	Uses	Adverse Effects
Aminophylline (Truphylline)	PO, IV	Bronchial asthma, Cheyne-Stokes respirations	Nausea, vomiting, diarrhea, dizziness, restlessness, depression, unresponsiveness, proteinuria, increased AST, tachycardia, hyperglycemia, hypotension
Dyphylline (Lufyllin)	PO	Acute bronchospasm with asthma and COPD	
Theophylline (Theophylline, others)	PO, IV	Bronchial asthma	

e. Therapeutic range of theophylline is 10 to 20 mcg/mL

f. Use correct diluent and proper time of administration when giving parenterally

g. Use cautiously in clients with cardiovascular disorders

h. Theophylline is metabolized in liver; some excretion occurs via kidneys

i. Theophylline dosages should be based on lean body weight because it does not enter adipose tissue

j. Theophylline can enter breast milk and cross placenta

k. Children metabolize drug faster than adults

l. Theophylline metabolism is slowed by hepatic failure

m. Aminophylline is administered at a rate no faster than 25 mg/min because of potential for cardiovascular collapse

n. Dosages are often started low and titrated up as needed for relief of symptoms

o. Adults who smoke cigarettes and children metabolize these medications more quickly and therefore may need higher doses for therapeutic effects

p. Theophylline levels may be increased in liver disease, congestive heart failure (CHF), and acute viral infections because of impaired metabolism

4. Contraindications

a. Avoid use when there is known hypersensitivity to xanthines

b. Avoid use in clients with tachydysrhythmias

c. Contraindicated in clients with a history of peptic ulcer disease and GI disorders including acute gastritis because of increased gastric acid secretion

d. Use cautiously in clients with cardiovascular disorders

e. Theophylline can cause seizures and is therefore not given to clients with seizure disorders unless bronchospasm is unresponsive to other treatments

f. Theophylline is contraindicated in clients with hyperthyroidism because it can exacerbate the disease

5. Significant drug interactions

a. Levels of xanthines increase if taken with allopurinol, cimetidine, erythromycin, flu vaccine, and oral contraceptives

b. Sympathomimetics can intensify cardiac and CNS stimulation

c. Metabolism of theophylline is increased with smoking

d. Phenytoin, rifampin, barbiturates, carbamazepine, phenytoin, and phenobarbital increase metabolism of theophylline

6. Significant food interactions: limit drinks and foods containing caffeine because of increased drug levels

7. Significant laboratory studies

a. Adverse effects are more severe with drug levels of 20 to 25 mcg/mL

b. Adverse cardiac effects are more frequently seen with drug levels above 30 mcg/mL

c. Seizures may be seen with drug levels above 40 mcg/mL

8. Side effects

a. Nausea, vomiting, anorexia, and gastroesophageal reflux during sleep

b. Sinus tachycardia, extrasystoles, palpitations, and ventricular dysrhythmias

c. Hyperglycemia and transient increased urination

9. Adverse effects/toxicity

a. CNS: tremors, dizziness, hallucinations, restlessness, agitation, headache, and insomnia

b. GI: nausea and vomiting

c. CV: palpitations, tachydysrhythmias, chest pain, and tachycardia

10. Nursing considerations

a. Assess for toxicity; note symptoms of restlessness, insomnia, irritability, tremors, nausea, and vomiting

Practice to Pass

A client comes to the clinic with results of lab work that was drawn earlier that day. The theophylline level is 25 mcg/mL. The client has diabetes and his BUN is 52 mg/dL and creatinine level is 2.1 mg/dL. What actions should the nurse take?

b. Restlessness is a symptom of a toxic reaction; however, it could signal hypoxia, and nurse should assess client for this

c. Monitor for adverse effects (tremors, restlessness, hallucinations, and dizziness) in all clients, especially in children

d. Monitor for cardiovascular side effects of palpitations and tachycardia

e. Carefully monitor clients with a history of cardiac disorder

f. Do not crush or allow client to chew sustained-release forms

g. Refrigerate suppository forms

h. Utilize appropriate diluent when administering medications

i. Ask client about current medications (including OTC and herbal products) and history of any allergies

j. Children may exhibit hyperactive behavior with administration of theophylline because of CNS stimulation

11. Client education

a. Do not chew or crush sustained-release forms (irritating to gastric mucosa)

b. Mechanism of drug action, usage, and side effects

c. Do not omit or double-up on doses; take exactly as prescribed

d. Suppository forms should be refrigerated

e. Notify prescriber if suppositories cause rectal burning, itching, or irritation

f. Notify prescriber if palpitations, nausea, vomiting, weakness, dizziness, chest pain, or convulsions occur

g. Monitor blood levels

h. Avoid use of caffeine as this could lead to an additive effect with xanthines

i. Avoid contact with allergen that tends to cause allergic response if possible; avoid contact with smoke and other respiratory irritants such as aerosol hair spray, perfumes, and cleaning products

j. Increase fluid intake if no contraindication with other disease process

k. Take medications even when there are no symptoms of asthma

l. Inform prescriber prior to taking OTC medication

m. Take medications with food if GI symptoms develop

II. INHALED CORTICOSTEROIDS

A. Action and use

1. Exact mechanism of action is unknown; however, it is thought that inhaled cortico-steroids stabilize membranes of cells that release bronchoconstricting substances such as **histamine** and thereby decrease release of these substances

2. Cell membranes of **neutrophils** (white blood cells that increase in concentration in response to inflammation) are stabilized and therefore inflammation-causing substances are not released; the result is decreased inflammation and bronchodilation

3. Reducing inflammation decreases mucosal edema and mucous secretions and thereby decreases bronchoconstriction

4. Inhaled corticosteroids may have a role in increasing responsiveness of bronchial smooth muscle to beta-agonist drugs

5. These agents appear to be involved in inhibiting movement of fluid and protein into tissues as well as inhibiting production of prostaglandins, **leukotrienes** (substances released after exposure to an allergen), and **interleukins** (plasma proteins that increase during inflammatory process)

6. These agents also promote mobilization of mucus by increasing mucociliary action

7. Used in chronic asthma to decrease inflammation and therefore decrease airway obstruction and are used prophylactically, not during acute attack

8. Aid in treatment of bronchospastic disorders when bronchodilators are not completely effective; are not used to treat acute bronchospasm
9. Used to treat chronic bronchitis, COPD, and cystic fibrosis

B. **Common medications (Table 14-3)**
C. **Administration considerations**

!   1. Proper technique is essential when administering medications by inhalation route
2. Chemical structures of inhaled corticosteroids have been slightly altered so there is not as much systemic absorption and therefore less likelihood of systemic side effects
3. Beclomethasone has greater anti-inflammatory action and causes fewer side effects than dexamethasone
!   4. If client is also taking a systemic corticosteroid, dose may need to be decreased with addition of inhaled corticosteroids
5. Beclomethasone, flunisolide, and fluticasone are available as nasal solutions for treatment of allergic rhinitis
6. Monitor for impaired bone growth in children receiving inhaled corticosteroids

D. **Contraindications**
!   1. Clients with known allergy
2. Clients with psychosis, fungal infection, acquired immunodeficiency syndrome (AIDS), tuberculosis, and idiopathic thrombocytopenia
!   3. Children under age of 2 years
4. Use cautiously in clients with diabetes, glaucoma, osteoporosis, ulcers, renal disease, CHF, myasthenia gravis, seizure disorders, inflammatory bowel disease, hypertension, thromboembolic disorders, or esophagitis
5. Use with caution in clients with infections due to potential for suppressed immune system

E. **Significant drug interactions**
1. There are relatively few drug interactions because these inhalers work locally rather than systemically
!   2. May need to adjust dose of antidiabetic agents secondary to potential for elevation of blood glucose levels when corticosteroids are administered orally
3. Rifampin, barbiturates, and phenytoin cause a decreased corticosteroid effect

F. **Significant food interaction**: none reported

Table 14-3   **Inhaled Corticosteroid Medications**

Generic (Trade) Name	Route	Uses	Adverse Effects
Beclomethasone (Qvar)	Inhalation Intranasal	Bronchial asthma, allergic rhinitis	Dry mouth, sore throat, cough, hoarse voice, candidiasis of mouth or throat, hypersensitivity, Cushing syndrome with overdose (hypercorticism)
Budesonide (Pulmicort)	Dry powder inhaler	Asthma, allergic rhinitis	
Ciclesonide (Alvesco)	Inhalation Intranasal	Allergic rhinitis	
Flunisolide (AeroBid)	Intranasal	Allergic rhinitis	
Fluticasone (Flovent)	Inhalation Intranasal	Asthma	
Mometasone (Asmanex)	Dry powder inhaler	Asthma	
Triamcinolone acetonide (Azmacort)	Inhalation Intranasal	Pulmonary emphysema, pulmonary fibrosis, bronchial asthma, allergic rhinitis	

G. Significant laboratory studies
1. There may be a decreased response to skin test antigens
2. Skin testing should be postponed if possible until after corticosteroid therapy

H. Side effects
1. Pharyngeal irritation and sore throat
2. Coughing
3. Dry mouth
4. Oral fungal infections
5. Sinusitis

I. Adverse effects/toxicity
1. Adrenocortical insufficiency, fluid and electrolyte disturbances, nervous system effects, and endocrine effects if absorbed systemically
2. Increased susceptibility to infection, dermatologic effects, and osteoporosis
3. Diarrhea, nausea, vomiting, and stomach upset
4. Headache, fever, dizziness, angioedema, rash, urticaria, and paradoxical bronchospasm
5. **Rhinitis** or inflammation of mucous membranes of nose, menstrual disturbances, and palpitations

J. Nursing considerations
1. Ask client about current medications (including OTC and herbal products) and history of any allergies
2. Monitor respiratory status and lung sounds for effectiveness of therapy
3. Teach client to report early signs of respiratory difficulty (such as activity intolerance and awakening with asthma symptoms)
4. Monitor for hyperglycemia
5. Monitor growth in children
6. Assess for adrenal insufficiency when changing from systemic corticosteroid to inhalation route
7. Chronic use of inhaled corticosteroids can predispose client to osteoporosis
8. Rinse mouth after use of medication because oropharyngeal candidiasis and/or hoarseness can occur
9. Assess sputum color and viscosity for signs of infection

K. Client education
1. Use medications as prescribed; do not overuse
2. Use metered dose **inhaler** or **nebulizer** as instructed and keep equipment clean and in working order per manufacturer's guidelines
3. Inhale bronchodilator drug before corticosteroid when both are ordered; wait prescribed interval between puffs and rinse mouth after use of inhalation device
4. Pediatric clients may need a physician's order to keep this inhaler with them at school
5. Do not abruptly stop taking this medication; taper dose slowly over a 2-week period under direction of a prescriber
6. Wear a MedicAlert bracelet or necklace identifying steroid use
7. Be aware of symptoms of steroid use, including moon face, acne, increased fat pads, increased edema; notify prescriber if these symptoms arise
8. Report signs of decreased amounts of steroid levels including nausea, dyspnea, joint pain, weakness, and fatigue
9. Report weight gain of more that 5 pounds in a week
10. Avoid smoking and contact with allergens that trigger allergic response if possible
11. Learn to recognize respiratory difficulty early so treatment can begin promptly
12. Take drug at approximately same time each day for maximal effectiveness
13. Use inhaled corticosteroids as maintenance drugs; they are ineffective in acute bronchospasm or asthma attack

Practice to Pass

A client is newly diagnosed with chronic obstructive pulmonary disease (COPD). The medications that are to be taken at home include albuterol (Proventil) and beclomethasone dipropionate (Beclovent). What client teaching is needed related to these medications?

III. INHALED NONSTEROIDALS

A. Action and use

1. These agents stabilize mast cells so bronchoconstrictive and inflammatory substances are not released when stimulated with an allergen; therefore, inflammation is limited

2. Used to prevent and treat inflammation of airways; decreasing inflammation decreases mucosal edema and mucous secretions and thereby decreases bronchoconstriction

3. Used for prophylaxis of acute asthma attacks

4. Used also for prevention and treatment of allergic rhinitis

B. Common medications (Table 14-4)

1. Cromolyn (Intal): oral spray or nebulizer solution for oral inhalation; Nasalcrom is the nasal spray form of cromolyn

2. Nedocromil: is no longer available by inhalation; different formulation available as ophthalmic drops

C. Administration considerations

1. Reduction in dose of bronchodilators and corticosteroids may be indicated with use of these drugs

2. Use with caution in clients with impaired hepatic or renal function

3. Administer by inhalation

4. Nasal solution is used for prevention and treatment of allergic rhinitis

5. It may take 3 weeks of daily dosing to see therapeutic effects

D. Contraindications

1. Not to be used in acute bronchospasm or status asthmaticus

2. It is contraindicated in clients with hypersensitivity

3. Use with caution in clients with impaired renal or hepatic function; lower dosages may be required

E. Significant drug interactions: none reported

F. Significant food interactions: none reported

G. Significant laboratory studies: none reported

H. Side effects (see Table 14-4)

I. Adverse effects/toxicity (see Table 14-4)

J. Nursing considerations

1. Ask client about current medications (including OTC and herbal products) and history of any allergies

2. Coronary artery disease (CAD) and/or dysrhythmias may be aggravated by any propellants in aerosols; therefore, use with caution in clients with cardiac dysrhythmias

3. Pulmonary function testing may be ordered prior to administering these medications

4. Perform respiratory assessment to monitor effectiveness of therapy

5. If dose is ordered intranasally, assess for rhinitis (stuffiness, rhinorrhea, or runny nose)

Table 14-4	**Inhaled Nonsteroidal Medications: Mast Cell Stabilizers**		
Generic (Trade) Name	**Route**	**Therapeutic Indications**	**Adverse Effects**
Cromolyn disodium (Intal, Nasalcrom)	Inhalation Intranasal	Bronchial asthma, bronchospasm, allergic rhinitis	Headache, nasal irritation and stinging, sneezing, irritation to the throat and trachea, cough, unpleasant taste, erythema, parotitis, bronchospasm, epistaxis, flushing
Nedocromil sodium (Alocril)	Ophthalmic	Allergic conjunctivitis	Dizziness, headache, nausea, vomiting, cough, pharyngitis, rhinitis, fatigue, dyspepsia

6. Doses of other asthma medications may be reduced after 2–4 weeks of therapy with inhaled nonsteroidal drugs
7. Client may require pretreatment with bronchodilator while using these inhalers
8. Do not use cloudy solution

K. Client education
1. Take medications exactly as prescribed
2. Be familiar with drug action, usage, and side effects
3. Proper use of inhaler ensures maximal effectiveness of medication; use spacer as appropriate
4. Record frequency and severity of asthma attacks
5. It may take 2–4 weeks to see results of medication
6. Rinse mouth after taking medication to avoid dry mouth
7. Do not take during an acute attack as symptoms may be aggravated
8. Bronchodilator should be taken optimally 20–30 minutes prior to taking cromolyn; see individual product literature; always wait a minimum of 3–5 minutes between inhalations
9. Cromolyn can be administered 15–60 minutes prior to contact with known allergens to reduce reaction to allergens
10. With intranasal drug use, clear nasal passages prior to use

IV. LEUKOTRIENE MODIFIERS

A. Action and use
1. Leukotrienes are substances that are released when a client is suffering from an allergic response to an allergen
2. Leukotrienes cause inflammation, bronchoconstriction, and mucus production that leads to coughing, sneezing, and shortness of breath
3. Leukotriene modifiers work by blocking action of leukotrienes by preventing them from attaching to receptors in circulating cells and cells in lungs
4. Bronchoconstriction is prevented by inhibition of smooth muscle contraction of bronchial airways
5. These medications are a newer class of asthma medications and provide relief of inflammatory symptoms of asthma; they are referred to as anti-inflammatory drugs
6. Leukotriene modifiers are used for prophylaxis and chronic treatment of asthma in adults and children over age of 12; they are not used in managing an acute asthma attack

B. Common medications (Table 14-5)
1. Zileuton (Zyflo): inhibits enzyme 5-lipoxygenase and therefore blocks production of leukotrienes; is given orally
2. Zafirlukast (Accolate): blocks specific leukotrienes called cysteinyl leukotrienes that are thought to be mediators of asthma; inflammation in lung is prevented; classified as a leukotriene receptor antagonist
3. Montelukast (Singulair): inhibits leukotriene receptors and is classified as a leukotriene receptor antagonist; is given orally

C. Administration considerations
1. They are used in adults and children 12 and over
2. It may take a week before therapeutic effects are seen
3. They have localized effects in lungs
4. They are used alone or in combination with corticosteroids
5. Zafirlukast cannot be taken during lactation as it is excreted in breast milk
6. Montelukast and zafirlukast are taken orally, metabolized in liver, and excreted in feces

Table 14-5 Leukotriene Modifiers

Generic (Trade) Names	Route	Therapeutic Indications	Adverse Effects
Montelukast sodium (Singulair)	PO	Asthma, allergic rhinitis	All: headache, sore throat, nausea, diarrhea, elevated AST (hepatotoxicity), and for roflumilast—weight loss and psychiatric problems including risk of suicide
Roflumilast (Daliresp)	PO	Asthma	
Zafirlukast (Accolate)	PO	Asthma, urticaria	
Zileuton (Zyflo)	PO	Asthma	

7. Zileuton is metabolized by liver and excreted in urine
8. Monitor hepatic aminotransferase enzymes when administering zileuton; discontinue medication if levels elevate to 5 times the norm or if liver dysfunction develops

D. **Contraindications**
　1. Zileuton is contraindicated in clients with liver disease and with elevations of transaminase (3 times the norm)
　2. All are contraindicated in clients with hypersensitivity

E. **Significant drug interactions**
　1. Theophylline, warfarin, and propranolol levels increase when administered with zileuton
　2. Warfarin, tolbutamide, phenytoin, and carbamazepine levels increase when administered with zafirlukast
　3. Decreased levels of zafirlukast are seen with concurrent administration of erythromycin
　4. Increased levels of zafirlukast are seen with concurrent administration of aspirin
　5. Calcium channel blockers have increased effect with zafirlukast
　6. Phenobarbital and phenytoin may decrease available montelukast due to initiation of hepatic metabolism

F. **Significant food interaction**: food decreases absorption of zafirlukast and zileuton

G. **Significant laboratory studies**
　1. Monitor serum theophylline levels if used concurrently due to decreased theophylline clearance when taking zileuton
　2. Monitor prothrombin time (PT) or international normalized ratio (INR) when client on zafirlukast or zileuton and warfarin as PT/INR may be elevated

H. **Side effects**
　1. Headaches may occur with all drugs
　2. Zileuton may also cause dyspepsia, nausea, and insomnia
　3. Zafirlukast may cause nausea and diarrhea
　4. Zileuton and zafirlukast cause dizziness, which could increase risk of falls or other injury

I. **Adverse effects/toxicity**
　1. Limited information is available for zileuton because the drug is relatively new
　2. Hepatotoxicity (zileuton)

J. **Nursing considerations**

　1. Be sure drug is prescribed for chronic, not acute, treatment of asthma
　2. Ask client about current medications (including OTC and herbal products) and history of any allergies
　3. Caution client that it takes about a week to see improvement in symptoms

4. Assess respiratory status to evaluate effectiveness of therapy
5. Monitor liver function tests for elevated AST and ALT levels
6. Singulair should be administered in evening

K. Client education

1. Drugs may take a week before therapeutic effects are seen
2. Mechanism of action, usage, and potential side effects of prescribed drug
3. Take medications exactly as prescribed
4. Avoid contact with specific allergen if possible
5. Drugs help prevent some of symptoms of asthma; they are not intended to be used for acute attacks
6. Liver function studies may be needed
7. Increase fluid intake if not contraindicated because of other disease processes
8. Take zafirlukast 1 hour before or 2 hours after meals
9. Montelukast and zileuton may be taken with or without food
10. Use caution when driving or operating machinery with zafirlukast and zileuton because these drugs can cause dizziness

V. ANTIHISTAMINES

A. Action and use

1. The action of these drugs is to block or inhibit action of histamine
   a. They work best early in the response as they do not displace histamine from receptors
   b. **Antihistamines** compete with histamine for receptor sites so that action of histamine can be blocked; thus, they do not prevent histamine release or reduce amount released
2. Antihistamines reduce effects of histamine (vasodilation, contraction of smooth muscles, increased GI and respiratory secretions, increased capillary permeability, increased heart rate and CNS transmission); therefore, antihistamines inhibit smooth muscle contraction (respiratory system, blood vessels, and GI tract), decrease capillary permeability, decrease salivation and tear formation, and inhibit vascular permeability and edema formation
3. Antihistamines cause bronchial smooth muscle relaxation
4. They reduce bronchial, salivary, gastric, nasal, and **lacrimal** (tear) secretions
5. Antihistamines reduce itching (urticaria)
6. Antihistamines are used to treat allergies, allergic rhinitis (hay fever), allergic conjunctivitis, allergic contact dermatitis, vertigo, motion sickness, insomnia, allergic reactions, cough, and sneezing and runny nose due to common cold
7. Used in treatment of anaphylactic shock
8. Can be used as prevention or treatment for allergic reactions to medications

B. Common medications (Table 14-6)

1. Nonsedating antihistamines (Table 14-6) include azelastine (Astelin), cetirizine (Zyrtec), desloratadine (Clarinex), fexofenadine (Allegra), and loratadine (Claritin)
   a. Cetirizine is a metabolite of hydroxyzine but causes less drowsiness
   b. These second-generation antihistamines cause less sedation than first-generation antihistamines
   c. They are selective for peripheral H1 receptors and do not cross blood–brain barrier
   d. Second-generation medications have a rapid onset of action after oral administration

Table 14-6 **Second-Generation or Nonsedating Antihistamines**

Generic (Trade) Names	Route	Uses	Adverse Effects
Azelastine (Astelin)	Intranasal	Rhinitis	All: dry mouth, nausea, dizziness, headache, hypersensitivity, hypotension, paradoxical excitation Drowsiness (cetirizine) Bitter taste in mouth (olopatadine)
Cetirizine (Zyrtec)	PO		
Desloratadine (Clarinex)	PO		
Fexofenadine (Allegra)	PO		
Levocetirizine (Xyzal)	PO		
Loratadine (Claritin)	PO		
Olopatadine (Patanase)	PO		

2. Traditional antihistamines (Table 14-7) have sedative effects because they work peripherally as well as centrally; first generation H1 receptor antagonists bind to central and peripheral H1 receptors and can cause CNS depression (drowsiness or sedation) or stimulation (anxiety or agitation)
   a. CNS stimulation is more likely to occur in high doses and especially in children
   b. These drugs also have anticholinergic effects such as dry mouth, urinary retention, constipation, and blurred vision
C. **Administration considerations**
   1. Antihistamines treat symptoms but not the cause of the problem
   2. Antihistamines may cause drowsiness
   3. Antihistamines should not be used for treatment of an acute asthma attack or lower respiratory disorder
   4. Most antihistamines are tolerated better when taken with meals
   5. Brompheniramine (Dimetane), chlorpheniramine, and diphenhydramine are all available over the counter
   6. Hydroxyzine is effective with pruritis
   7. Most antihistamines are metabolized by liver
   8. Azelastine is topically applied to nasal mucosa and action peaks in 2–3 hours; it does not tend to cause drowsiness but does leave an unpleasant taste in mouth
   9. Hydroxyzine causes profound drowsiness; diphenhydramine has a high incidence of drowsiness and anticholinergic effects
   10. Antihistamines may be used as a premedication prior to administration of blood products to decrease likelihood of allergic reactions

Table 14-7 **Selected First-Generation Antihistamines**

Generic (Trade) Name	Route	Uses	Adverse Effects
Chlorpheniramine (Chlor-Trimeton)	PO	Rhinitis	Drowsiness, sedation, dizziness, disturbed coordination, epigastric distress, thickening of bronchial excretions, tinnitus, labyrinthitis, palpitations, hypotension, hemolytic anemia
Diphenhydramine (Benadryl)	PO		
Hydroxyzine (Vistaril)	PO		
Meclizine (Antivert)	PO	Vertigo	Drowsiness, confusion, euphoria, nervousness, hypotension, urinary frequency, respiratory depression, death

11. Oral antihistamines act in 15–60 minutes and last 4–6 hours; sustained-release medications last 8–12 hours
12. A rapid acting agent should be used with an acute allergic reaction
13. Longer-acting agents give more consistent relief with chronic allergic conditions

D. **Contraindications**
1. Hypersensitivity
2. Astemizole should be used with caution in clients with liver dysfunction because of potential for elevation in blood levels and potential cardiac malfunction
3. Loratadine is contraindicated in acute asthma treatment and in conditions affecting lower respiratory tract
4. Diphenhydramine should not be given to nursing mothers or clients with conditions of lower respiratory tract
5. Antihistamines should be used cautiously if clients have a history of increased intraocular pressure, cardiac or renal disease, hypertension, bronchial asthma, stenosing peptic ulcer disease, prostatic hyperplasia, convulsive disorders, or during pregnancy
6. Promethazine should not be used in children with hepatic disease, Reye syndrome, history of sleep apnea, or family history of sudden infant death syndrome (SIDS)
7. Diphenhydramine is not recommended for use with infants or for children with chickenpox or flulike infections

E. **Significant drug interactions**
1. Astemizole should not be used concurrently with erythromycin, ketoconazole, or itraconazole as this can lead to cardiac arrest and ventricular dysrhythmias
2. Anticholinergic effects are more pronounced if taken with tricyclic antidepressants, antipsychotic agents and some antiparkinson agents
3. Ethyl alcohol, anti-anxiety agents, tricyclic antidepressants, antipsychotic agents, opioid analgesics, sedative hypnotics, and MAO inhibitors increase effects of first-generation sedating antihistamines
4. Loratadine blood levels are increased when taken with azithromycin, clarithromycin, erythromycin, fluconazole, itraconazole, ketoconazole, miconazole, and cimetidine
5. Azelastine levels will be increased when administered with cimetidine

F. **Significant food interactions**
1. Licorice and loratadine should not be taken together because of potential prolongation of QT interval
2. Coffee and tea may reduce drowsiness caused by these medications
3. Alcohol or other CNS depressants will reduce alertness if taking sedating antihistamine

G. **Significant laboratory studies**: antihistamines can mask positive skin test results

H. **Side effects**
1. Drowsiness is the main side effect; however, children can experience paradoxical excitement with antihistamines
2. Anticholinergic side effects include dry mouth and nose, changes in vision, difficulty urinating, and constipation
3. CNS: sedation from drowsiness to deep sleep, dizziness, syncope, muscular weakness, unsteady gait, paradoxical excitement (especially in older adults), restlessness, insomnia, and nervousness
4. GI: anorexia, nausea, vomiting, diarrhea, constipation, and jaundice
5. Urinary retention, impotence, vertigo, visual disturbances, blurred vision, tinnitus, hypotension, syncope, and headache

I. **Adverse effects/toxicity**
1. Seizures can result from CNS effects
2. Dysrhythmias, palpitations, and cardiac arrest

3. Agranulocytosis, hemolytic anemia, leukopenia, thrombocytopenia, and pancytopenia
4. Overdose in children can cause hallucinations, convulsions, and death

J. Nursing considerations

1. Assess client's current medications (including OTC and herbal products) and history of any allergies
2. Assist client to determine factors that precipitate allergic reactions and to identify symptoms caused by allergens
3. Assess client for drowsiness and dizziness especially during first few days of therapy
4. Encourage increased fluid intake of 2,000–3,000 mL/day unless contraindicated by another condition
5. Give antihistamines prior to contact with allergen if possible
6. Administer sedating antihistamines at bedtime to help with side effect of drowsiness
7. Administer IM antihistamines deeply into large muscles
8. IV injection should be over a few minutes
9. May cause false negative results on allergy skin tests; client should discontinue use 72 hours prior to testing
10. Cetirizine, loratadine, and fexofenadine may be used in children over age 6

K. Client education

1. Take medications exactly as prescribed and contact prescriber before taking any OTC or herbal products
2. Be aware of potential side effects of specific drug
3. Avoid contact with allergen responsible for reaction if possible; if unable, take medication prior to exposure
4. Do not crush or chew sustained-release tablets
5. Do not take more than one medication at a time
6. Do not operate heavy machinery or participate in other hazardous activities while taking a sedating antihistamine
7. Do not use alcohol or other CNS depressants while taking this type of medication
8. Contact physician if excessive sedation, confusion, dizziness, fainting, rapid heart rate, or hypotension occur
9. Rinse mouth and use hard sugarless candy to relieve dry mouth
10. Antihistamines may dry and thicken respiratory tract secretions and make them difficult to expectorate; increase fluid intake to 2 liters daily to decrease their viscosity
11. Take nonsedating antihistamines with meals to decrease stomach upset
12. Take loratadine on an empty stomach to increase absorption
13. Avoid prolonged exposure to sunlight and use sunscreen to reduce risk of sunburn
14. Take sedating medication at bedtime to reduce drowsiness, which should become less significant after repeated doses
15. Do not take antihistamines for 72 hours prior to allergen skin testing to reduce likelihood of false negative results

Practice to Pass

A 22-year-old college student comes to the university clinic because of problems with allergies. He is started on fexofenadine (Allegra). What teaching should the nurse in the clinic initiate?

VI. MEDICATIONS TO CONTROL BRONCHIAL SECRETIONS

A. Nasal decongestants

1. Action and use
   a. **Decongestants** relieve nasal stuffiness by shrinking swollen nasal mucous membranes
   b. Adrenergic agents (sympathomimetics) do this by vasoconstriction, decreasing blood flow to nasal mucosa and thereby reducing swelling
   c. Nasal steroids act as anti-inflammatory agents by suppressing inflammatory response

     d. Used to relieve nasal congestion and nasal discharge caused by acute or chronic rhinitis (common cold), sinusitis, hay fever, and other allergies

     e. May be used to decrease local blood flow prior to nasal surgery

     f. May be used to aid visualization of nasal mucosa during diagnostic exams because of effect of decreasing blood flow

2. Common medications (Table 14-8)

3. Administration considerations

     a. Nasal decongestants can be applied topically (with sprays or drops) or can be administered orally

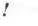   **b.** Sustained use of topical decongestants (longer than 3 days or in excessive amounts) can cause rebound congestion; therefore, oral agents should be used if needed for longer than 3 days

     c. Topical decongestants are potent decongestants with prompt onset of action

     d. Topical decongestants are preferred if client has cardiovascular disease because of decreased likelihood of cardiovascular side effects

4. Contraindications

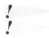   **a.** Avoid use when client has known hypersensitivity

     b. Adrenergic agents are contraindicated in clients with hypertension and CAD

     c. Clients with nasal mucosal infection should not take nasal steroids

     d. Decongestants should not be taken during pregnancy or lactation

     e. Contraindicated in clients taking tricyclic antidepressants or MAO inhibitors

     f. Use cautiously in clients with cardiac dysrhythmias, hyperthyroidism, diabetes mellitus, glaucoma, prostatic hyperplasia, and insomnia

5. Significant drug interactions

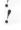   **a.** Possible increased toxicity with sympathomimetics

      b. Possible increased sympathetic effect when given concurrently with MAOIs (i.e., severe hypertensive crisis)

     c. Beta blockers decrease effects of decongestants

     d. Concurrent use with digitalis agents can cause dysrhythmias

     e. Decongestants decrease effectiveness of antihypertensive agents

     f. Increased effect of nasal decongestants is seen with use of cocaine, digoxin, general anesthetics, antihistamines, epinephrine, ergot alkaloids, methylphenidate, MAOIs, thyroid preparations, and xanthines

6. Significant food interactions: none reported

7. Significant laboratory studies: none significant

Table 14-8   **Nasal Decongestants**

Generic (Trade) Name	Route	Uses	Adverse Effects
Naphazoline (Privine)	Intranasal	Nasal congestion	Oral: dry mouth, headache, insomnia, CNS stimulation, tremors, dysrhythmias, tachycardia, hypertension, difficulty voiding Nasal: temporary nasal irritation, dryness, burning, sneezing, headache, rebound congestion
Oxymetazoline (Afrin)			
Phenylephrine (Afrin, others)			
Tetrahydrozoline (Tyzine)			
Xylometazoline (Otrivin)			
Pseudoephedrine (Sudafed)	PO		

8. Side effects
    a. Local nasal mucosal irritation and dryness
    b. Rarely nervousness, insomnia, palpitations, and tremors
    c. Rebound congestion is common
9. Adverse effects/toxicity
    a. If a topical decongestant is absorbed, it can cause cardiovascular disturbances such as hypertension and tachycardia
    b. CNS disturbances can occur if topical decongestant is absorbed and these include headache, nervousness, dizziness, confusion, delirium, and insomnia
    c. Muscle tremors, nausea, vomiting, appetite loss, and urinary retention
10. Nursing considerations
    a. Ask client about current medications (including OTC and herbal products) and history of any allergies
    b. Assess client for other medical history to determine potential for possible side effects; older adults with significant cardiac disease should avoid nasal decongestants because they are at high risk for hypertension, dysrhythmias, nervousness, and insomnia
    c. Assess client for history of open-angle glaucoma
    d. For administration of nose drops, have client lie down or sit with neck hyperextended to instill medication
    e. Wash medication dropper after each use to prevent contamination
    f. Client should sit and squeeze nasal spray container once and avoid touching nares with spray dispenser; tip of dispenser should be rinsed after each use
    g. Observe client for decrease in nasal congestion
    h. Observe for tachycardia, hypertension, and cardiac dysrhythmias; also observe for rebound nasal congestion, (after 3 days) chronic rhinitis, and ulceration of nasal mucosa
    i. Question prescriber about need to change from nasal decongestant to oral drug if needed for longer than 3 days (rebound congestion)
11. Client education
    a. Take medications exactly as prescribed
    b. Recognize potential side effects, especially palpitations, insomnia, restlessness, and nervousness; report these to prescriber if they occur
    c. Do not use alcohol or other CNS depressants while taking this medication
    d. Do not operate heavy machinery while taking this medication
    e. Avoid use of caffeine while taking this medication as it can cause nervousness, tremors, and insomnia
    f. Avoid smoking because it increases secretions and decreases ciliary action
    g. Avoid exposure to crowds to minimize spread of disease
    h. Increase fluid intake to 2,000 to 3,000 mL per day unless contraindicated by another medical condition
    i. Nasal congestion in infants can decrease ability to suck effectively; application of a nasal solution prior to feeding can increase infant's ability to feed
    j. Avoid eating or drinking for 30 minutes after topical (nasal) medication administration
    k. Practice good hand hygiene
    l. Rinse droppers and spray bottles after each use to avoid contamination
B. **Expectorants**
    1. Action and use
        a. **Expectorants** increase fluid flow in respiratory tract and reduce viscosity of secretions to aid in removal of secretions by cough reflex and ciliary action

    b. They are used for relief of nonproductive cough associated with common cold, bronchitis, laryngitis, and influenza; they also thin secretions

    c. Guaifenesin (glyceryl guaiacolate) (Robitussin, Guiatuss, Humibid, and others): most common oral expectorant

2. Common medications (Table 14-9)

3. Administration considerations

    a. Use with caution in elderly or debilitated clients

    b. Use with caution in clients with asthma and respiratory insufficiency

    c. Not used as commonly as in past because of questionable effectiveness

4. Contraindications: iodide expectorants are contraindicated in clients with thyroid problems because of potential for altered thyroid function

5. Significant drug interactions: iodinated products may produce hypothyroid effects when given with lithium

6. Significant food interactions: none significant

7. Significant laboratory studies: guaifenesin may interfere with results of color tests for 5-hydroxyindoleacetic acid and vanillylmandelic acid

8. Side effects

    a. Nausea, vomiting, and gastric irritation

    b. Rash

9. Adverse effects/toxicity

    a. CNS: dizziness and headache

    b. GI: nausea and vomiting

    c. Skin: rash

10. Nursing considerations

    a. Ask client about current medications (including OTC and herbal products) and history of any allergies

    b. Increase fluid intake to 2–3 liters per day, if not contraindicated by another condition, to assist in liquefying secretions

    c. Assess respiratory status to evaluate medication effectiveness

11. Client education

    a. Take medications exactly as prescribed and be aware of potential side effects

    b. Use effective coughing techniques to mobilize secretions

    c. Do not drive or operate heavy machinery while taking this medication because of risk for dizziness

    d. Do not use alcohol or other CNS depressants while taking this medication

    e. Report a fever or a cough lasting longer than a week to health care provider

    f. Increase fluid intake if not contraindicated by other disease processes

    g. Avoid smoking as this increases secretions and decreases ciliary action

    h. Avoid drinking fluids for 30 minutes after taking this medication

C. Antitussives

1. Action and use

    a. **Opioid** (narcotic) and nonopioid **antitussives** suppress cough reflex by directly affecting cough center; nonopioid antitussives do this without CNS suppression of opioid antitussives

Table 14-9   Expectorants

Generic (Trade) Name	Route	Uses	Adverse Effects
Guaifenesin (Organidin, Robitussin)	PO	Dry, nonproductive cough related to mucus in the respiratory tract	Headache, dizziness, rash, nausea, vomiting, gastrointestinal discomfort
Terpin hydrate elixir	PO	Dry, nonproductive cough related to mucus in the respiratory tract	Headache, dizziness, rash, nausea, vomiting, gastrointestinal discomfort

      b. Peripherally acting agents (glycerin, ammonium chloride) have local anesthetic effects to decrease irritation of pharyngeal mucosa; they are available in gargles, lozenges, and syrups; lozenges increase saliva flow and therefore suppress cough

      c. They are used to stop a nonproductive cough or a dry, hacking, and nonproductive cough that interferes with rest and sleep

2. Common medications (Table 14-10)

3. Administration considerations

      a. Swallow benzonatate capsules whole

      b. There is a potential for addiction and CNS and respiratory depression with opioid antitussives

      c. Most antitussives are given in a liquid form or as oral tablets

      d. Antitussives in syrup form may soothe irritated mucosa in pharynx

      e. Dextromethorphan is preferred over codeine as it provides desired effect without use of opioids; it is available in many OTC products and does not require a prescription

4. Contraindications

      a. Dextromethorphan is contraindicated if client has asthma, emphysema, or consistent headaches

      b. Hypersensitivity

      c. Codeine preparations are contraindicated in clients with respiratory depression, increased intracranial pressure, severe liver or renal disease, hypothyroidism, adrenal insufficiency, or seizure disorders

      d. Cautious use of nonopioid agents is recommended for clients with seizure disorders, hypotension, glaucoma, and prostatic hyperplasia

5. Significant drug interactions

      a. Opioid antitussives may potentiate action of sedating drugs such as anesthetic agents, tranquilizers, hypnotics, alcohol, MAOIs, and tricyclic antidepressants

      b. Dextromethorphan should not be given with MAOIs

      c. Avoid use of dextromethorphan with selegiline because of risk of confusion, coma, and hyperpyrexia

      d. Medications that increase antitussive effects of codeine include CNS depressants such as alcohol, anti-anxiety agents, barbiturates, and sedative hypnotics

6. Significant food interactions: use of parsley and dextromethorphan can produce serotonin syndrome

7. Significant laboratory studies: none significant

Table 14-10 **Antitussives**

Generic (Trade) Name	Route	Uses	Adverse Effects
Nonopioid			
Benzonatate (Tessalon, Tessalon Perles)	PO	Nonproductive cough	Sedation, headache, dizziness, hallucinations, burning of the eyes, constipation, nausea, GI upset, numbness of the chest, pruritis
Dextromethorphan hydrobromide (Robitussin, Novahistine DM)	PO	Nonproductive cough	Respiratory depression
Opioid			
Guaifenesin and codeine (Robitussin AC)	PO	Cough	Hypotension, bradycardia, respiratory depression

8. Side effects
   a. Dizziness, headache, drowsiness or sedation, nausea, vomiting, constipation, pruritus, nasal congestion, dry mouth, blurred vision, and sweating
   b. Dependence and respiratory depression with codeine
   c. Dry mouth, palpitations, thickened respiratory mucus, anorexia, urinary retention or frequency, diarrhea, photosensitivity, and dysuria with nonopioids
   d. Nasal congestion and burning of eyes with benzonatate

9. Adverse effects/toxicity
   a. Opioid agents: hypotension, bradycardia, and respiratory depression
   b. CNS: dizziness, headache, and sedation
   c. GI: nausea, constipation, and GI upset

10. Nursing considerations
    a. Ask client about current medications (including OTC and herbal products) and history of any allergies
    b. Assess for inability to cough effectively from excessive cough suppression
    c. Monitor for listed side effects; assess for respiratory depression and possible drug dependence with opioid antitussive
    d. Cough may be a useful diagnostic tool and protective measure for client; therefore, antitussives should be used only cautiously for irritating, nonproductive, and ineffective cough
    e. Use cautiously in older adults

11. Client education
    a. Take medication exactly as prescribed
    b. Be aware of potential side effects
    c. Do not operate heavy machinery or other activities requiring alertness while using these types of medications
    d. Avoid alcohol and other CNS depressants while taking these medications
    e. Notify physician if client has a cough that lasts longer than a week, a persistent headache, fever, or rash
    f. Do not drink liquids for 30–35 minutes after taking a chewable tablet or a lozenge
    g. Avoid smoking because it increases secretions and decreases ciliary action
    h. For excessive respiratory secretions, teach client coughing, deep breathing, and benefits of ambulation
    i. Liquefy secretions with increased oral intake up to 2,000–3,000 mL/day unless contraindicated

D. **Mucolytics**

1. Action and use
   a. **Mucolytics** are administered by inhalation to liquefy (thin) mucus in the respiratory tract
   b. They are used with sinusitis and the common cold
   c. Aid in removal of viscous secretions
   d. An oral form of acetylcysteine (Mucomyst) can be used to treat acetaminophen overdose

2. Common medications (Table 14-11)

3. Administration considerations
   a. Not used as commonly anymore because of questionable effectiveness
   b. These drugs are nebulized using a face mask or a mouth piece; can be instilled into a tracheostomy
   c. Acetylcysteine is effective one minute after inhalation; maximal effect is in 5–10 minutes
   d. Acetylcysteine is effective immediately after direct instillation

Practice to Pass

An 80-year-old client is admitted to the hospital. She is lethargic with a respiratory rate of 8 breaths per minute and cyanosis around the lips. When questioning the daughter, she tells the nurse that her mother has had a nonproductive cough for about 2 weeks and has been taking Dimetane-DC. What are the appropriate nursing actions?

Table 14-11	Mucolytic Medications		
Generic (Trade) Name	**Route**	**Uses**	**Adverse Effects**
Acetylcysteine (Mucomyst)	Nebulizer (inhalation)	Abnormal, viscid, or viscous mucous secretions related to acute and chronic bronchopulmonary disease	Nausea, stomatitis, bronchospasm, rhinorrhea, urticaria
Dornase alfa (Pulmozyme)	Nebulizer (inhalation)	Management of respiratory symptoms related to cystic fibrosis	Pharyngitis, increased cough, dyspnea, rhinitis, wheezes, conjunctivitis

4. Contraindications
    a. Use with caution for asthmatic clients
   b. Proteolytic enzymes are contraindicated in asthmatic clients due to allergy potential
   c. Contraindicated in client with hypersensitivity to these agents
5. Significant drug interactions
   a. Activated charcoal limits effectiveness of acetylcysteine
   b. Mucomyst is incompatible with tetracyclines, erythromycin, lactobionate, amphotericin B, and ampicillin sodium
6. Significant food interactions: none significant
7. Significant laboratory studies: none significant
8. Side effects
   a. Oral irritation and sore throat
   b. Cough
   c. Nausea and vomiting
   d. Headaches
9. Adverse effects/toxicity: bronchospasm
10. Nursing considerations
     a. Ask client about current medications (including OTC and herbal products) and history of any allergies
    b. Administer medications as prescribed
     c. May cause bronchospasm and are therefore usually given with bronchodilators
    d. Suction client if cough is ineffective
    e. Rinse mouth after therapy to decrease oropharyngeal irritation
    f. Discard unused medication after 4 days
11. Client education
    a. Take medication exactly as prescribed
    b. Be aware of potential side effects
    c. Increase fluid intake to thin secretions unless contraindicated by other disease processes
    d. Avoid smoking as this increases secretions and decreases ciliary action

VII. OXYGEN

A. Indications
1. **Hypoxia**, deficiency of oxygen (O_2) in cells and tissues, and **hypoxemia**, deficiency of O_2 in arterial blood, are indications for use of supplemental oxygen
2. Some conditions in which O_2 therapy is indicated include conditions associated with decreased arterial PO_2 levels (pulmonary edema), decreased cardiac output (myocardial infarction), decreased blood oxygen-carrying capacity (anemia), and increased O_2 demand (sepsis, sustained fever)

B. Types of delivery systems

1. Nasal cannula (nasal prongs): most common form of O_2 delivery
   a. Two prongs go into nostrils and tubing attaches to oxygen source and flowmeter
   b. Client can eat and talk with a nasal cannula
   c. Oxygen can be administered at a rate ranging from 1 L/min to 6 L/min
   d. Dryness of mucous membranes can occur
2. Nasal catheter: inserted into throat through a nostril and should be changed to other nostril every 8 hours; not used frequently because of client discomfort; gastric distention sometimes occurs
3. Oxymizer: a nasal cannula with a reservoir that can deliver higher concentrations of O_2 than a regular cannula without use of a mask; delivers approximately twice the amount of O_2 of a regular cannula
4. Face mask: a mask that fits over client's mouth and nose
   a. Simple face mask: flow rate is 5–10 L/min with O_2 delivery capabilities of 40–60%
   b. Partial rebreather mask: consists of a face mask with a reservoir bag; some of the air client exhales goes into reservoir bag and is mixed with 100% O_2 for next inhalation; this system permits conservation of O_2 and can deliver 70–90% O_2 at rates of 6–15 L/min
   c. Nonrebreather mask: delivers highest concentration of O_2 by mask; no exhaled air goes into reservoir bag; reservoir bag contains O_2, which client breathes in with inspiration; exhaled air goes out through side vents and can deliver 60–100% O_2 at flow rates of 6–15 L/min
   d. Venturi mask: percentage of O_2 to be administered is adjusted by a dial at end of mask; amount of air pulled into system varies with needed amount of O_2; gives precise oxygen concentrations

C. Oxygen toxicity

1. Lung tissue can be damaged from prolonged exposure to high O_2 concentrations; exact amount of O_2 and length of time required to cause O_2 toxicity varies with different clients depending on degree of underlying lung disease; some sources say that lung damage can occur with O_2 delivery of greater than 50% for longer than 24–48 hours
2. **Atelectasis** or alveolar collapse can result with O_2 administration at rates of 60% for more than 36 hours or 90% for more than 6 hours
3. Acute respiratory distress syndrome (ARDS) can result from breathing 80 to 100% oxygen for longer than 24 hours
4. Symptoms of O_2 toxicity begin as a nonproductive cough, substernal chest pain, gastrointestinal upset, and dyspnea; as it worsens, client develops decreased vital capacity, decreased lung compliance, and hypoxemia; atelectasis, pulmonary edema, and pulmonary hemorrhage can result if problem is not reversed
5. Oxygen should be weaned as soon as possible and according to client's SaO_2 level

D. Administration and nursing considerations

1. Oxygen therapy can be anxiety-provoking; provide sufficient explanation and allow client to express anxieties
2. Flow rate is measured in liters per minute; it is a measure of amount of O_2 delivered but is not completely accurate, because there is loss of O_2 content with leaking and mixing with room air
3. Oxygen analyzers are available to measure amount of O_2 client inhales, and this is recommended every 4 hours to provide precise measurement of percentage of O_2 client is receiving

4. Clients with COPD should not receive O_2 at high percentages because higher levels of O_2 in bloodstream can cause hypoventilation; a COPD client's drive to breathe is from low levels of O_2 tension; a client with COPD can usually tolerate a rate of up to 2 L/min by nasal cannula

5. Check O_2 delivery system frequently to ensure proper functioning

6. Oxygen should be humidified when client is receiving O_2 at a rate higher than 2 L/min

7. A face mask should fit client's face to avoid unnecessary leakage of O_2; if mask is too snug, skin irritation can occur

8. Masks can be replaced with a nasal cannula during mealtime with a physician's order

9. The reservoir bag on a partial rebreather should deflate slightly with inspiration

10. Provide reassurance if client becomes claustrophobic

11. Flaps on sides of nonrebreather mask should be open during expiration and closed during inhalation

12. Monitor SaO_2 with pulse oximeter during oxygen administration; with physician order, O_2 may be titrated to achieve desired SaO_2 level

13. Assess for signs and symptoms of hypoxia and respiratory distress; also assess for changes in vital signs and color changes

14. Monitor arterial blood gases (ABGs) per physician order

15. Normal arterial O_2 levels decrease with age

16. Provide oral care for client comfort because of potential for drying of mucous membranes

17. Identify clients at high risk for development of O_2 toxicity

E. **Client education**

1. Prepare client for noise that occurs with flow of O_2

2. Avoid open flames with O_2 administration due to flammable nature of O_2

3. Ensure there are not frayed electrical cords near O_2 so there is no chance of a spark causing combustion

4. Smoking is prohibited when O_2 therapy is being utilized

5. Inform client that O_2 delivery can cause dryness of mouth and nasal mucosa

6. Remove O_2 when client uses an electric razor

7. Continue O_2 therapy at home as prescribed by physician

8. Keep O_2 tank in holder and away from direct sunlight to reduce effects of heat

9. Instruct client signs of hypoxia and to report them to physician

Case Study

R. C. is a 14-year-old girl with newly diagnosed asthma. She will be using albuterol (Ventolin) and beclomethasone (Beclovent) inhalers. You are the nurse working in the doctor's office where R. C. comes for her check-ups.

1. What teaching does R. C. need about albuterol?

2. What teaching does R. C. need about beclomethasone?

3. What developmental issues related to a newly diagnosed illness should you anticipate, and how will you respond?

4. What are the anticipated effects and the side effects of the medications?

5. What assessment will you do when R. C. comes for office visits to assess how she is dealing with her disease and its treatment?

For suggested responses, see page 545–546.

POSTTEST

1 Because the symptoms have worsened, the mother of a 6-year-old child with asthma informs the nurse that the child is using metaproterenol (Alupent) more frequently. The nurse is most likely to caution the parent about which of the following adverse effects?

1. Nervousness and tachycardia
2. Lethargy and bradycardia
3. Decreased blood pressure and dizziness
4. Increased blood pressure and fatigue

2 What statements best indicate to the nurse that the client understood instructions about self-administration of salmeterol (Serevent)? Select all that apply.

1. "I will use this medication every 6 hours."
2. "If my symptoms are not better within 20 minutes, I should notify my health care provider."
3. "Although it will remain regular, this medicine may increase my heart rate."
4. "This drug is supposed to prevent an asthma attack, but is not good for treating one."
5. "I will take a dose of this medicine when I notice I am wheezing."

3 A client takes oxtriphylline (Choledyl) for chronic obstructive pulmonary disease (COPD). Which explanation by the nurse accurately represents the drug's characteristics?

1. "The medicine increases your heart rate to increase the release of oxygen."
2. "The drug relaxes the lung tissue so that oxygen will pass across it easier."
3. "The medicine is used to dilate your airways and make it easier for you to breathe."
4. "The medicine thins the secretions in your lungs and makes it easier for you to cough."

4 A health care provider prescribed theophylline (Theo-Dur) 0.4 mg/kg every 6 hours for a client. Which of the following would lead the nurse to consult with the prescriber?

1. Concurrent history of Cushing disease
2. History of narcolepsy
3. Concurrent diagnosis of hyperthyroidism
4. Current state of hypothermia

5 Because a client with chronic obstructive pulmonary disease (COPD) had been taking triamcinolone acetamide (Azmacort) 8 mg PO qid (4 times daily) at home and is currently receiving dexamethasone (Decadron) 4 mg IV q4h in the hospital, the nurse should anticipate which of the following in relation to these 2 medications?

1. Increase in the dose of triamcinolone
2. Scheduling the drugs so they peak at different times
3. Increase in symptoms with administration of the 2 drugs
4. Smaller dose of triamcinolone and/or dexamethasone

6 The nurse withholds the currently scheduled drug dose after noting that a client with which health problem is receiving fluticasone aerosol (Flovent)?

1. AIDS
2. Asthma
3. Chronic obstructive pulmonary disease
4. Systemic lupus erythematosus

7 A homebound client who has a history of asthma and was recently started on cromolyn sodium (Intal) has a 3-week-old newborn at home. The case manager would give which priority instruction to the home health aide?

1. "Teach the client to pace activities of daily living (ADLs)."
2. "Encourage the client to wear a mask when mowing the lawn."
3. "Recommend that the client avoid individuals with upper respiratory infections."
4. "Report if breastfeeding is observed during your visit."

8 Which of the following goals is *most likely* to be included by the nurse in the care plan for a client who is taking zileuton (Zyflo)?

1. Client will manage lethargy commonly associated with drug.
2. Client will manage constipation commonly associated with the drug.
3. Client will manage headaches commonly associated with the drug.
4. Client will demonstrate ability to manage the signs and symptoms of asthma.

---

9 After administering promethazine (Phenergan) 12.5 mg intravenously to an 80-year-old client for nausea, the nurse instructs the nursing unlicensed assistive personnel (UAP) to perform which of the following?

1. Provide client with nonskid slippers for ambulation.
2. Teach client how to use emergency cord in the bathroom.
3. Place a chair next to client's bed to reduce potential falls.
4. Instruct client to remain in bed with top half rails up.

---

10 The nurse selects which of the following as the most appropriate nursing diagnosis for a client who is receiving oxymetazoline (Afrin)?

1. Impaired Gas Exchange
2. Chronic Pain
3. Impaired Tissue Integrity
4. Disturbed Sleep Pattern

➤ *See pages 483–484 for Answers and Rationales.*

ANSWERS & RATIONALES

Pretest

1 **Answer: 1** **Rationale:** The symptoms of an acute asthma attack are related to constriction of the airway, which leads to dyspnea, wheezing, increased respiratory rate, and declining oxygen saturation. Albuterol (Proventil) is a beta-adrenergic agent or sympathomimetic that relaxes the smooth muscles of the bronchial tree, resulting in bronchodilation and relief of wheezing. The respiratory rate should return to normal (12–20 per minute in an adult), making a respiratory rate of 34 to 22 slightly above the normal range. An intensity rating scale can be used for dyspnea, just as it is used for pain, and so a reduction from 9 to 6 is inadequate. The normal oxygen saturation level is 95 to 100%, making an oxygen saturation of 82% suboptimal. **Cognitive Level:** Analyzing **Client Need:** Pharmacological and Parenteral Therapies **Integrated Process:** Nursing Process: Evaluation **Content Area:** Pharmacology **Strategy:** Correlate the primary outcome of the disease process with the drug action. Because of the critical word *best* in the question, choose the option that has data that has fully returned to within normal limits. **Reference:** LeMone, P., Burke, K., & Bauldoff, G. (2011). *Medical-surgical nursing: Critical thinking in patient care* (5th ed.). Upper Saddle River, NJ: Pearson Education, pp. 1232–1238.

2 **Answer: 2** **Rationale:** Because adrenergic agents such as epinephrine (Primatene) increase oxygen consumption as well as increase the workload on the myocardium, they are contraindicated in clients with cardiovascular disease. Because epinephrine causes arterial constriction, which results in decreased inflammation, it is often utilized during acute asthmatic attacks and would not be contraindicated in a client with asthma. Because of the sympathomimetic action, it may increase the blood pressure, which might then aid a client who has hypotension and increase the heart rate, which would be helpful to a client with bradycardia. **Cognitive Level:** Applying **Client Need:** Pharmacological and Parenteral Therapies **Integrated Process:** Nursing Process: Planning **Content Area:** Pharmacology **Strategy:** The critical words are *question an order*, indicating that the correct answer represents a contraindication or hazard with the use of epinephrine (Primatene). Correlate the drug category (sympathomimetic) with the various options and use the process of elimination to choose the one that could have an adverse effect because of impaired coronary circulation. **Reference:** Wilson, B. A., Shannon, M., & Shields, K. (2010). *Pearson nurse's drug guide 2010.* Upper Saddle River, NJ: Pearson Education, p. 561.

3 **Answer: 4** **Rationale:** The actions of theophylline (Theo-Dur) are similar to the sympathetic response, which results in increased heart rate. Food items, such as coffee or tea, contain stimulants such as caffeine that can have an additive effect with theophylline. Peas, beans, and milk do not contain a chemical that could result in heightened adverse effects of the drug (as with the correct option) or result in inadequate drug action.

Cognitive Level: Applying **Client Need:** Pharmacological and Parenteral Therapies **Integrated Process:** Teaching and Learning **Content Area:** Pharmacology **Strategy:** Questions that include a drug and one or more foods are highly likely to be looking for either an additive drug effect or a diminished drug effect when the drug and food are taken together. With this in mind, consider the elements that the foods and the drug have in common and the potentially combined outcomes. **Reference:** Wilson, B. A., Shannon, M., & Shields, K. (2010). *Pearson nurse's drug guide 2010*. Upper Saddle River, NJ: Pearson Education, p. 1500.

4 **Answer: 2, 3** **Rationale:** Delayed healing is related to the decreased inflammatory response. Because corticosteroids such as beclomethasone dipropionate (Beclovent) reduce the immune response, a potential side effect of an inhaled corticosteroid is an oral fungal infection. Because inhaled corticosteroids generally do not cause fluid retention and weight gain, these are not common side effects. Inhaled corticosteroids can cause dry mouth. Asthma is believed to be an abnormal inflammatory response to an irritant. Because the drug decreases inflammation, a decreased respiratory rate is expected. **Cognitive Level:** Applying **Client Need:** Pharmacological and Parenteral Therapies **Integrated Process:** Teaching and Learning **Content Area:** Pharmacology **Strategy:** Associate glucocorticoids with the outcomes of a reduced immune response and fluid retention. **Reference:** Wilson, B. A., Shannon, M., & Shields, K. (2010). *Pearson nurse's drug guide 2010*. Upper Saddle River, NJ: Pearson Education, p. 158.

5 **Answer: 2** **Rationale:** Albuterol (Proventil) is an adrenergic bronchodilator that generally results in immediate relief of an acute asthmatic attack. The onset of aminophylline (Truphylline) is 15–20 minutes and could be utilized for an acute attack if bitolterol was not available. Cromolyn is a mast cell stabilizer and is a prophylactic agent that inhibits the release of bronchoconstricting histamines. The onset is several days to 1 week after the first dose and would not be indicated for use in a client with a need for immediate bronchodilation. **Cognitive Level:** Applying **Client Need:** Pharmacological and Parenteral Therapies **Integrated Process:** Nursing Process: Planning **Content Area:** Pharmacology **Strategy:** Select the option that identifies the drug with the most rapid onset. Eliminate 2 options first as not immediate acting and select 1 option from the remaining 2 choices because of the suffix *olol*, which indicates a beta-adrenergic effect. Specific nursing knowledge of the various drugs and the time of onset is needed to answer the question. **Reference:** Wilson, B. A., Shannon, M., & Shields, K. (2010). *Pearson nurse's drug guide 2010*. Upper Saddle River, NJ: Pearson Education, p. 29.

6 **Answer: 2** **Rationale:** Zafirlukast (Accolate) is a leukotriene modifier. This class of medications is indicated for the prophylaxis and chronic treatment of asthma.

Because leukotriene modifiers are not used during an acute attack, this response indicates that the client needs more teaching. "I will take the drug a few weeks before I expect to notice an improvement in my symptoms" is a correct response because the onset of action occurs at 1 week. Fluid intake should increase to liquefy secretions and assist the client with expectoration. To promote absorption, this medication should be taken 1 hour before meals or 2 hours after meals. **Cognitive Level:** Applying **Client Need:** Pharmacological and Parenteral Therapies **Integrated Process:** Nursing Process: Evaluation **Content Area:** Pharmacology **Strategy:** The wording of the question tells you that the correct option is an incorrect statement. Select the option that is most opposite the characteristics of the drug. **Reference:** Wilson, B. A., Shannon, M., & Shields, K. (2010). *Pearson nurse's drug guide 2010*. Upper Saddle River, NJ: Pearson Education, p. 1619.

7 **Answer: 4** **Rationale:** Loratadine (Claritin) should be taken on an empty stomach to increase absorption. Although it does not cause drowsiness at the level as earlier antihistamines, it is more likely to cause drowsiness than nervousness. The onset of action is approximately one hour. It acts to reduce the inflammatory response by competing for histamine 1 (H_1) receptor sites within the mucous membranes, which would not reduce bronchoconstriction occurring with asthma. **Cognitive Level:** Applying **Client Need:** Pharmacological and Parenteral Therapies **Integrated Process:** Teaching and Learning **Content Area:** Pharmacology **Strategy:** Specific drug knowledge is needed to answer the question. Use the process of elimination to identify the option closest to appropriate administration of this drug. **Reference:** Wilson, B. A., Shannon, M., & Shields, K. (2010). *Pearson nurse's drug guide 2010*. Upper Saddle River, NJ: Pearson Education, p. 921.

8 **Answer: 2** **Rationale:** Because phenylephrine (Neo-Synephrine) is a sympathomimetic, it has the potential to produce cardiovascular side effects such as sustained hypertension and tachycardia. If this occurs, the drug should be discontinued and the health care provider notified. Because of the risk of thinning of nasal mucous membranes due to prolonged vasoconstriction (which could result in increased risk of nosebleed), oral agents should be used for long-term therapy. Often, decongestants cause a dry mouth, but the client should use hard, sugarless candy rather than discontinuing the medication. Rebound congestion is more likely to occur with nasal spray decongestants. **Cognitive Level:** Applying **Client Need:** Pharmacological and Parenteral Therapies **Integrated Process:** Nursing Process: Planning **Content Area:** Pharmacology **Strategy:** Answer the critical thinking question, "What potential outcomes of phenylephrine (Neo-Synephrine) are likely to place the client at the *greatest* risk?" **Reference:** Wilson, B. A., Shannon, M., & Shields, K. (2010). *Pearson nurse's drug guide 2010*. Upper Saddle River, NJ: Pearson Education, p. 1232.

9 **Answer: 1** **Rationale:** Guaifenesin (Robitussin) is an expectorant with potential side effects such as nausea, vomiting, gastric irritation, rash, dizziness, and headache. Since the drug is an expectorant, the purpose is to reduce the viscosity of respiratory secretion to increase mobilization of the secretions. The client should take the medication with a full glass of water unless contraindicated. Because the drug can potentially inhibit platelet function, aspirin may increase the risk of bleeding. **Cognitive Level:** Applying **Client Need:** Pharmacological and Parenteral Therapies **Integrated Process:** Teaching and Learning **Content Area:** Pharmacology **Strategy:** Recall that guaifenesin (Robitussin) is an expectorant and the side effects of this drug frequently affect the GI tract. Next correlate the common side effects with the most appropriate remedy. **Reference:** Wilson, B. A., Shannon, M., & Shields, K. (2010). *Pearson nurse's drug guide 2010.* Upper Saddle River, NJ: Pearson Education, pp. 734–735.

10 **Answer: 1** **Rationale:** A nonrebreather mask has a 1-way valve between the mask and the reservoir along with 2 flaps over the exhalation ports. This design allows the client to draw oxygen from the reservoir bag during inhalation and the flaps to close to prevent room air from entering during exhalation. Changing the equipment should not be done without a new order. A nasal cannula is utilized for clients with chronic lung disease. The nonrebreather mask is used to treat clients with unstable breathing patterns that may be in need of intubation. The mask is functioning properly so there is no need to replace it or call the respiratory therapist. **Cognitive Level:** Applying **Client Need:** Pharmacological and Parenteral Therapies **Integrated Process:** Nursing Process: Implementation **Content Area:** Pharmacology **Strategy:** Apply knowledge of the purposes of the flaps on a nonrebreather mask with the appropriate nursing intervention. **Reference:** Smith, S. F., Duell, D. J., & Marin, B. C. (2011). *Clinical nursing skills: Basic to advanced skills* (8th ed.). Upper Saddle River, NJ: Pearson, p. 1264.

Posttest

1 **Answer: 1** **Rationale:** Potential side effects of this medication are stimulation of the central nervous system (CNS) and cardiovascular (CV) system. Excessive administration may result in excessive side effects. It is not likely, but lethargy and bradycardia may occur with increased doses, especially in a 6-year-old child. Decreased blood pressure and fatigue are not consistent with either CNS or CV stimulation. **Cognitive Level:** Applying **Client Need:** Pharmacological and Parenteral Therapies **Integrated Process:** Teaching and Learning **Content Area:** Pharmacology **Strategy:** Recall that sometimes the adverse effects of medications are too much of the action that was originally expected. Since this drug is a sympathetic nervous system stimulant, align excess sympathetic nervous system stimulation with an increased frequency in use. **Reference:** Wilson, B. A.,

Shannon, M., & Shields, K. (2010). *Pearson nurse's drug guide 2010.* Upper Saddle River, NJ: Pearson Education, pp. 975–976.

2 **Answer: 2, 4** **Rationale:** The drug should begin to take effect within 20 minutes. Use of salmeterol (Serevent) is prophylactic. It is dosed every 12 hours because of the 12-hour duration. Although salmeterol is predominately a beta₂ stimulant, occasionally it may cause tachycardia. It is not used for treatment of acute attack. **Cognitive Level:** Applying **Client Need:** Pharmacological and Parenteral Therapies **Integrated Process:** Nursing Process: Evaluation **Content Area:** Pharmacology **Strategy:** Recall first that this medication is a sympathetic nervous system stimulant. Beyond that, specific drug knowledge is needed to answer the question. Since multiple choices can be made in this question, consider that there is more than one correct option but that not all of them will apply. **Reference:** Wilson, B. A., Shannon, M., & Shields, K. (2010). *Pearson nurse's drug guide 2010.* Upper Saddle River, NJ: Pearson Education, pp. 1387–1388.

3 **Answer: 3** **Rationale:** Oxtriphylline (Choledyl) is a xanthine bronchodilator, and the mechanism of action is to increase the amount of cyclic adenosine monophosphate (cAMP), which leads to bronchial dilation related to the relaxation of smooth muscle. Xanthines can increase heart rate and force of myocardial contraction, but that is not the rationale for the administration of the medication. The drug does not increase permeability of lung tissue. Thinning of secretions is more commonly associated with expectorants. **Cognitive Level:** Analyzing **Client Need:** Pharmacological and Parenteral Therapies **Integrated Process:** Teaching and Learning **Content Area:** Pharmacology **Strategy:** Recall the primary outcome of chronic obstructive pulmonary disease (COPD) and the appropriate drug action needed to reduce the effects of the disease. **Reference:** Wilson, B. A., Shannon, M., & Shields, K. (2010). *Pearson nurse's drug guide 2010.* Upper Saddle River, NJ: Pearson Education, pp. 1155–1166.

4 **Answer: 3** **Rationale:** Because tachycardia is a common side effect of theophylline (Theo-Dur), it is *contraindicated* in clients with hyperthyroidism. Cushing disease has no overlapping signs or symptoms with the characteristics of the drug. Theophylline may stimulate the client with narcolepsy, thereby reducing the problem rather than aggravating it. Metabolic processes are likely to be below normal with hypothermia. The drug is not likely to have an adverse effect. **Cognitive Level:** Analyzing **Client Need:** Pharmacological and Parenteral Therapies **Integrated Process:** Nursing Process: Planning **Content Area:** Pharmacology **Strategy:** Correlate the drug category with possible side effects along with diseases that result in the same signs or symptoms. **Reference:** Wilson, B. A., Shannon, M., & Shields, K. (2010). *Pearson nurse's drug guide 2010.* Upper Saddle River, NJ: Pearson Education, pp. 1498–1500.

5 **Answer: 4** **Rationale:** Both of these medications are corticosteroids. Because of the increased risks of adverse effects such as hyperglycemia, hypertension, infection, hypervolemia, and many others, a *decrease* in the dose of one or both drugs may be needed. Because the actions and side effects could be compounded (placing the client at significant risk), the drug doses should not be increased. Since the suppressive effects by dexamethasone is 36–54 hrs with triamcinolone ranging from 18–36 hrs, the effects of the drugs are likely to overlap. The nurse needs to intervene rather than assess for additional symptoms. **Cognitive Level:** Applying **Client Need:** Pharmacological and Parenteral Therapies **Integrated Process:** Nursing Process: Planning **Content Area:** Pharmacology **Strategy:** Note first that both of the drugs in the question are corticosteroids. Recall the actions, side effects, and contraindications to compare and contrast the drugs and then reason that one or both drugs need to have a reduction in dose to avoid adverse effects. **Reference:** Wilson, B. A., Shannon, M., & Shields, K. (2010). *Pearson nurse's drug guide 2010.* Upper Saddle River, NJ: Pearson Education, pp. 1560–1562.

6 **Answer: 1** **Rationale:** Corticosteroids such as fluticasone aerosol (Flovent) suppress the immune system. The administration of these drugs is *contraindicated* in a client who has a suppressed immune system as in AIDS. Fluticasone is commonly used in the treatment of asthma. It may be utilized in the treatment of chronic obstructive pulmonary disease (COPD). Corticosteroids are sometimes utilized in the treatment of joint pain and stiffness associated with systemic lupus erythematosus (SLE). **Cognitive Level:** Applying **Client Need:** Pharmacological and Parenteral Therapies **Integrated Process:** Nursing Process: Planning **Content Area:** Pharmacology **Strategy:** The wording of the question tells you that the correct answer is a condition with which a corticosteroid is contraindicated. Recall that this drug class suppresses immune function and then look for an option that represents an issue with immune function. **Reference:** Wilson, B. A., Shannon, M., & Shields, K. (2010). *Pearson nurse's drug guide 2010.* Upper Saddle River, NJ: Pearson Education, p. 1647.

7 **Answer: 4** **Rationale:** This drug should be used with caution in lactating women. A health care provider should be consulted prior to the client breastfeeding while on this drug. Because of the risk to the newborn, this is the most relevant point. The client does also need to pace activities to prevent excessive oxygen demand. Reducing exposure to elements likely to cause an asthma attack is appropriate. An infectious process may increase the risk of an asthma attack. Of all the options, however, the most important instruction relates to the risks inherent in breastfeeding. **Cognitive Level:** Analyzing **Client Need:** Pharmacological and Parenteral Therapies **Integrated Process:** Communication and Documentation **Content Area:** Pharmacology **Strategy:** Note the critical terms *newborn* and *priority.* These tell you that the presence of an infant has relevance to the question and that

more than one option is likely to be a correct statement. Consider the adverse effects of the drug to choose correctly. **Reference:** Wilson, B. A., Shannon, M., & Shields, K. (2010). *Pearson nurse's drug guide 2010.* Upper Saddle River, NJ: Pearson Education, p. 388.

8 **Answer: 3** **Rationale:** Headache is one of the *most common* side effects associated with the drug. The client is more likely to be restless and nervous than to be lethargic and to have dyspepsia rather than constipation. The goal is to reduce or alleviate the signs and symptoms, rather than to help the client learn to live with them. **Cognitive Level:** Applying **Client Need:** Pharmacological and Parenteral Therapies **Integrated Process:** Nursing Process: Planning **Content Area:** Pharmacology **Strategy:** Recall that the drug causes vasodilation, which may result in conditions similar to migraine episodes. Use this information and the process of elimination to make a selection. **Reference:** Wilson, B. A., Shannon, M., & Shields, K. (2010). *Pearson nurse's drug guide 2010.* Upper Saddle River, NJ: Pearson Education, p. 1626.

9 **Answer: 4** **Rationale:** Promethazine (Phenergan) is a traditional antihistamine that causes drowsiness because it works centrally as well as peripherally. The client should be kept in bed with half side rails up until the effects of the drug wear off (2–8 hours) to promote client safety. The effects may be heightened by the client's age. Using nonskid slippers does not provide the greatest safety measure. The client will be impaired by the medication and less capable of understanding or remembering instructions and should not be left alone in the bathroom. The client should not get out of bed for at least 2–8 hours; this may be longer because of client's age. **Cognitive Level:** Applying **Client Need:** Pharmacological and Parenteral Therapies **Integrated Process:** Nursing Process: Planning **Content Area:** Pharmacology **Strategy:** Recall first that this drug is a traditional antihistamine that can cause drowsiness as a side effect. Note next the client's age to reason that this risk may be heightened further. Then choose the option that represents nursing care to avoid adverse drug effects. **Reference:** Wilson, B. A., Shannon, M., & Shields, K. (2010). *Pearson nurse's drug guide 2010.* Upper Saddle River, NJ: Pearson Education, pp. 1300–1302.

10 **Answer: 4** **Rationale:** Oxymetazoline (Afrin) is a nasal decongestant. Insomnia is a side effect of the drug. After administration, many clients experience pain and burning in the nasal passages, but not chronic pain. The nasal congestion is not significant enough to interfere with gas exchange. The nasal passages may be irritated because of the inflammatory response, but this is not related to the presence of the drug. **Cognitive Level:** Analyzing **Client Need:** Pharmacological and Parenteral Therapies **Integrated Process:** Nursing Process: Diagnosis **Content Area:** Pharmacology **Strategy:** Recall the specific side effects of the drug to arrive at the correct nursing diagnostic label. **Reference:** Wilson, B. A., Shannon, M., & Shields, K. (2010). *Pearson nurse's drug guide 2010.* Upper Saddle River, NJ: Pearson Education, pp. 1159–1160.

References

Abrams, A. (2008). *Clinical drug therapy: Rationales for nursing practice* (9th ed.). Philadelphia, PA: Lippincott Williams & Wilkins.

Adams, M., Holland, L., & Bostwick, P. (2011). *Pharmacology for nurses: A pathophysiologic approach* (3rd ed.). Upper Saddle River, NJ: Pearson Education.

Aschenbrenner, D., & Venable, S. (2009). *Drug therapy in nursing* (3rd ed.). Philadelphia, PA: Lippincott Williams & Wilkins.

Drug Facts & Comparisons® (Updated monthly). St. Louis, MO: A. Wolters Kluwer.

Karch, A. M. (2009). *Focus on nursing pharmacology* (5th ed.). Philadelphia, PA: Lippincott Williams & Wilkins.

Kee, J. (2009). *Laboratory and diagnostic tests and nursing implications* (8th ed.). Upper Saddle River, NJ: Pearson Education.

Kee, J., Hayes, E., & McCuiston, L. (2011). *Pharmacology: A nursing process approach* (5th ed.). St. Louis, MO: Elsevier Science.

Lehne, R. (2010). *Pharmacology for nursing care* (7th ed.). St. Louis, MO: Mosby.

LeMone, P., Burke, K., & Bauldoff, G. (2011). *Medical-surgical nursing: Critical thinking in patient care* (5th ed.). Upper Saddle River, NJ: Pearson Education.

Wilson, B. A., Shannon, M. T., & Shields, K. M. (2012). *Pearson nurse's drug guide 2012*. Upper Saddle River, NJ: Pearson Education.

15 Visual and Auditory Medications

Chapter Outline

Medications to Treat Glaucoma

Mydriatics and Cycloplegics

Anti-Inflammatory and Anti-Infective Medications for the Eye

Anesthetic Medications for the Eye

Auditory Medications

NCLEX-RN® Test Prep

Use the accompanying online resource, NursingReviewsandRationales, to test yourself with hundreds of NCLEX®-style practice questions.

Objectives

➤ Describe general goals of therapy when administering visual or auditory medications.

➤ Describe actions and uses of mydriatic, miotic, and cycloplegic medications.

➤ Explain the mechanism of action of medications used to treat glaucoma.

➤ Describe drug-induced ototoxicity.

➤ Identify medications that cause ototoxicity.

➤ Identify correct procedures for administering visual and auditory medications.

➤ List significant client education points related to administering visual or auditory medications.

Review at a Glance

aqueous humor fluid formed by ciliary body; contained in anterior and posterior chambers of eye; bathes and feeds posterior surface of cornea, lens, and iris

cerumen substance secreted by glands at outer third of ear canal; if accumulated, may cause obstruction of ear canal; also called "earwax"

cornea protective anterior covering of eye; normally is transparent and allows light to enter

cycloplegia paralysis of ciliary muscle

external ear outer ear (pinna) and external auditory canal

intraocular pressure pressure within the eye

keratitis inflammation of cornea; usually caused by trauma, microorganisms, or immune-mediated responses

miosis constriction of pupils caused by contraction of sphincter muscle alone or in combination with relaxation of dilator muscle

mydriasis dilation of pupils caused by contraction of dilator muscle and relaxation of sphincter muscle

narrow-angle glaucoma an acute form of glaucoma characterized by increased intraocular pressure caused by impaired rate of outflow of aqueous humor; also called angle-closure or closed-angle glaucoma

open-angle glaucoma a chronic form of glaucoma that leads to a change in appearance of optic disk and results in visual loss as cup of disk becomes enlarged; increased intraocular pressure may or may not be associated with this

disorder; open-angle glaucoma is most common type

photophobia intolerance to light

systemic absorption entry of drug into body and circulating fluids

tonometry a measurement of tension, such as intraocular tension or pressure; used to detect glaucoma

tympanic membrane thin partition of transparent tissue between external auditory canal and middle ear

uveitis an intraocular inflammatory disorder; may involve iris, ciliary body, choroids, retina, or cornea

vertigo sensation of moving around in space or spinning; also called "dizziness"

PRETEST

1 Which is the priority of the nurse in assessing a client prior to administering the first dose of an ophthalmic medication?

1. Client's understanding of purpose of medication
2. Client's level of consciousness (LOC)
3. Client's history of medication allergies
4. Client's understanding of drug action

2 A nurse concludes that a client can safely self-administer ophthalmic medications after the client demonstrates which of the following techniques? Select all that apply.

1. Pulls lower lid down and instills medication directly onto cornea
2. Pulls lower lid down and instills medication into conjunctival sac
3. Pulls lower lid up and instills medication directly onto the eye
4. Applies gentle pressure to inner canthus for 30 seconds after medication administration
5. Cleanses exudates from eye before instillation of medication

3 The external ear canal of a client with an ear infection is obstructed due to swelling. The nurse should instruct the client to use which of the following techniques for otic medication administration? Select all that apply.

1. Insert gauze ear wick and apply medication to wick.
2. Wait until swelling subsides before instilling medication.
3. Request change in the route of medication.
4. Insert dropper past the edematous canal.
5. Avoid using pressure to insert tip of the fluid container.

4 A client with open-angle glaucoma is being treated with acetazolamide (Diamox) 250 mg tablets by mouth twice daily. Which statements made by the client to the nurse indicate a need for further teaching? Select all that apply.

1. "I can take the medication with milk."
2. "I should take the medication in the morning."
3. "I should have a yearly complete blood count."
4. "I can crush the tablet and mix it in juice."
5. "I should avoid foods containing high potassium such as bananas."

5 A client has a new prescription for the carbonic anhydrase inhibitor dorzolamide (Trusopt) for the treatment of glaucoma. The client asks the nurse how the medication will affect the disease. The nurse's best response includes which information?

1. Medication decreases production of aqueous humor.
2. Medication causes pupil constriction.
3. Medication increases the production of aqueous humor.
4. Medication increases the outflow of aqueous humor.

6 A client with a history of asthma is describing symptoms that began after starting drug therapy with pilocarpine (Isopto Carpine) to treat glaucoma. The nurse concludes that which symptom indicates a side effect associated with systemic absorption of this drug?

1. Dry mouth
2. Increased blood pressure
3. Wheezing
4. Constipation

7 The nurse concludes that a 68-year-old client understands proper otic medication administration after observing the client perform which of the following techniques? Select all that apply.

1. Client pulls pinna down and back before administering medication.
2. Client pulls pinna up and back before administering medication.
3. Client places dropper into the ear canal before administering medication.
4. Client tilts head toward the affected side before administering medication.
5. Client gently massages the anterior ear area after medication administration.

8 The nurse concludes that a client newly diagnosed with glaucoma knows the purpose for the prescribed beta-adrenergic blocker timolol (Timoptic) when the client makes which statement?

1. "This eyedrop will reduce the intraocular pressure."
2. "I can stop using the eyedrop once my intraocular pressure is normal."
3. "The medicine will help to increase my intraocular pressure."
4. "This eyedrop is the only treatment available for glaucoma."

9 Before administering preoperative medications to a client with a history of glaucoma, the nurse would question which medication order?

1. Atropine (generic)
2. Diphenhydramine (Benadryl)
3. Hydroxyzine (Vistaril)
4. Retelase recombinant (Retavase)

10 The nurse would question an order for brinzolamide (Azopt), a carbonic anhydrase inhibitor, for a client who has which disorder listed in the health history portion of the medical record?

1. Hypertension
2. Chronic renal failure
3. Liver disease
4. Osteoporosis

➤ See pages 505–507 for Answers and Rationales.

I. MEDICATIONS TO TREAT GLAUCOMA

A. Prostaglandin analog

1. Action and use
   a. Increases aqueous humor outflow
   b. Used in management of open-angle glaucoma and ocular hypertension
2. Common medications (Table 15-1)
3. Administration considerations
   a. Administer 5 minutes apart from other antiglaucoma ophthalmic medications
   b. If pilocarpine (Isopto Carpine) is included in drug regimen, it should be administered 1 hour after administration of prostaglandin agonist
   c. May be used in conjunction with other agents to lower intraocular pressure
4. Contraindications: hypersensitivity to latanoprost or benzalkonium

Table 15-1	Prostaglandin Agents for Glaucoma	
Generic (Trade) Name	**Therapeutic Indications**	**Adverse Effects**
Bimatoprost (Lumigan)	Glaucoma	Stinging sensation in eye, sensation of foreign body in eye, darkened iris, longer and thicker lashes, flu or respiratory infection, muscle or joint pain

  5. Significant drug interactions: none reported
  6. Significant food interactions: none reported
  7. Significant laboratory studies: none reported
  8. Side effects
     a. Blurred vision, photophobia, burning, stinging, and itching
     b. Longer, thicker, darker eyelashes
  9. Adverse effects/toxicity
     a. Conjunctival hyperemia
     b. Increasing iris pigmentation
 10. Nursing considerations
     a. Assess for hypersensitivity to latanoprost or benzalkonium chloride
     b. Assess for burning, itching, and stinging after initial administration of medication
 11. Client education
     a. Drug may cause an increase in iris pigmentation
     b. Do not exceed once-a-day dose
     c. Remove contact lenses before use and for 15 minutes after instillation of medication
     d. Report symptoms of burning, itching, and stinging after administration to prescriber
     e. Proper self-administration of ophthalmic medications

B. Beta blockers (beta-adrenergic antagonists)
  1. Action and use
     a. Decrease production of **aqueous humor** (fluid formed by ciliary body in eye)
     b. Reduce **intraocular pressure** (pressure within eyeball) in **open-angle glaucoma** (a change in appearance of optic disk resulting in visual loss)
     c. Exact mechanism of action is unknown
  2. Common medications (Table 15-2)
  3. Administration considerations
     a. Available in ophthalmic solution and ophthalmic suspension
     b. Drugs cross placenta, enter breast milk
     c. Use nasolacrimal occlusion to minimize **systemic absorption** (entry of drug into body and circulating fluids)
     d. Administer with caution to clients receiving cardiovascular agents such as anti-hypertensives and antidysrhythmics
     e. May mask symptoms of hyperthyroidism
     f. Drug may be $beta_1$ selective (cardiac), $beta_2$ selective (pulmonary), or both $beta_1$ and $beta_2$ selective
     g. Because it is $beta_1$ selective, betaxolol (Betoptic) is usually the drug of choice for clients with pulmonary disease

Table 15-2   **Beta-Adrenergic Blocking Agents for Ophthalmic Use**

Generic (Trade) Name	Therapeutic Indications	Adverse Effects
Betaxolol (Betoptic)	Ocular hypertension, open-angle glaucoma	Bradycardia, congestive heart failure Dysrhythmias, sinoatrial or atrioventricular nodal block Tachycardia Dry eyes, conjunctivitis Dizziness or vertigo Pulmonary edema Cerebrovascular accident (CVA or stroke) Constipation, nausea, or vomiting Gastric pain Impotence or decreased libido

4. Contraindications
   a. Hypersensitivity
    b. Sinus bradycardia or second- or third-degree heart block
   c. Cardiogenic shock or congestive heart failure (CHF)
   d. Do not administer with other beta blockers (additive effect)
   e. Use cautiously in clients with renal failure, diabetes, asthma, and chronic obstructive pulmonary disease (COPD)
5. Significant drug interactions
   a. Beta-blocking agents may be absorbed systemically, although risk is minimal; review client's current medications to avoid drug–drug interactions; most drug interactions occur as result of systemic absorption
   b. Systemic absorption of ophthalmic beta blockers increases effects of insulin, verapamil, prazosin, clonidine, and nonsteroidal anti-inflammatory drugs (NSAIDs)
   c. Adverse cardiovascular effects may occur when beta-adrenergic blockers are used in combination with other cardiovascular agents such as antihypertensives and antidysrhythmics
    d. Use of these agents with ophthalmic epinephrine may decrease effectiveness
6. Significant food interactions: none reported
7. Significant laboratory studies: if systemic absorption occurs, glucose or insulin tolerance tests may be affected
8. Side effects
   a. Primarily local reactions: eye irritation, burning, stinging
   b. Rare occurrences of allergic reaction, eye inflammation, **photophobia** (intolerance to light), burning, stinging, pruritis, blurred vision, and rashes
9. Adverse effects/toxicity
   a. Systemic adverse reactions or toxicity affecting cardiovascular system include bradycardia or tachycardia, CHF, dysrhythmias, hypotension, and edema of lower extremities
   b. Systemic adverse reactions or toxicity affecting respiratory system include wheezing, cough, exacerbation of asthma, and bronchospasm
   c. Systemic adverse reactions or toxicity affecting central nervous system (CNS) include weakness, ataxia, confusion, and depression
   d. Systemic adverse reactions or toxicity affecting gastrointestinal (GI) symptom include nausea and vomiting
10. Nursing considerations
    a. Obtain baseline vital signs and neurologic status
    b. Obtain baseline vision and intraocular pressure data
    c. Assess for cardiovascular disease, renal failure, diabetes mellitus, lactation, or thyrotoxicosis
    d. Assess for signs and symptoms of hypersensitivity such as burning, itching, redness, and swelling occurring after drug administration
    e. Refer to Box 15-1 for procedure for administering ophthalmic medications
11. Client education
    a. Beta-blocking agents may mask symptoms of hypoglycemia in clients with diabetes mellitus
    b. Inform health care provider if surgery is being considered; gradual withdrawal of beta-blocking agent 48 hours before surgery may be required (withdrawal is controversial)
    c. Have routine eye examinations and measurement of intraocular pressure (IOP)
    d. Do not stop medication unless instructed to do so by prescriber
    e. Report symptoms of breathing difficulty, swelling of extremities, slow heart rate
    f. Avoid driving if weakness or dizziness occur as drug side effects

Box 15-1	
Administration of Ophthalmic Medications	**Instillation of Eye Drops**

Instillation of Eye Drops
- Wash hands and apply gloves
- Cleanse exudates from eye(s) if necessary
- Tilt client's head toward the side of the affected eye
- Gently pull lower eyelid down, have client look up (this forms a "sac")
- Instill drops in the sac formed by lower lid, *not* onto the eye
- Unless specifically indicated otherwise, apply gentle pressure for 30 seconds to 1 minute over the inner canthus next to the nose. This prevents absorption through the tear duct and drainage of the medication
- Unless specifically indicated otherwise, the client should close the eye(s) gently. Avoid squeezing the eye(s) tightly, as this forces the medication out

Instillation of Eye Ointment
- Follow the same procedure for instillation of eye drops, except that the ointment is expressed directly into the conjunctival sac from the inner canthus to the outer canthus
- Unless specifically indicated otherwise, the client should close the eye(s) and gently massage the eye(s) to distribute the medication

Note: To avoid contamination and risk of infection, do not touch the dropper or tube to the eye, eyelashes, or any other surface. Remove contact lenses before instilling ophthalmic medications.

     g. Wear dark glasses and avoid bright light if photophobia is present
     h. Proper procedure for instillation of ophthalmic medications
C. Adrenergic medications (alpha-adrenergic agonists), also known as sympathomimetics
    1. Action and use
      a. Decrease production of aqueous humor
      b. Decrease intraocular pressure
      c. Exact mechanism of action is unknown
      d. Used in management of open-angle glaucoma, often in combination with other drugs
      e. Used in management of glaucoma secondary to **uveitis** (intraocular inflammatory disorder)
      f. Used to produce **mydriasis** (pupil dilation) for ocular examination
      g. Used to produce local hemostasis during eye surgery to control bleeding
    2. Common medications (Table 15-3)

Table 15-3 Adrenergic Agonist Agents for Ophthalmic Use

Generic (Trade) Name	Uses	Adverse Effects
Apraclonidine (Iopidine)	Increased IOP related to chronic open-angle glaucoma	Blurred vision, unsteady gait, chest pain, dizziness, depression, arrhythmias, numbness of extremities, edema of the eyelids, facial edema, redness of eyelids, eye tearing
Brimonidine tartrate (Alphagan)		Eye irritation, eye edema, blurred vision, photosensitivity, arrhythmias, wheezing, dyspnea, chest pain
Dipivefrin (Propine)		
Epinephrine borate (Epinal)	Conjunctivitis, bleeding control during surgery; produces mydriasis	Transient stinging on initial instillation of eye, conjunctival hyperemia, headache, brow ache, blurred vision, photophobia, deposits on the cornea
Hydroxyamphetamine/ Tropicamide (Paremyd)	Eye dilation before eye examination	Blurred vision, chest pain, confusion, dizziness, faintness, irregular heartbeat, dyspnea, sweating, weakness, fatigue
Tetrahydrozoline hydrochloride (Visine, Murine plus)	Redness of eyes, minor irritations	Ocular irritation, photophobia, blurred vision

3. Administration considerations

 a. Administer with caution to clients with cardiovascular disease, hypertension, asthma, diabetes mellitus, hyperthyroidism, and parkinsonism

 b. Onset of action for epinephrine is 1 hour; peak effect occurs in 4–8 hours; if epinephrine hydrochloride (Epifrin, Glaucon) is used in conjunction with miotics, instill miotic first

 c. Onset of action for dipivefrin (Propine) is 30 minutes; peak effect in 1 hour

 d. Assess for sensitivity to sulfites

 e. Avoid concurrent use with MAOIs

 f. Drugs cross placenta, enter breast milk

 g. Do not administer ophthalmic solution that contains precipitates or has turned brown

4. Contraindications

 a. Not for treatment of **narrow-angle glaucoma** or abraded **cornea** (protective anterior covering of the eye) because pupil dilation will further restrict ocular fluid outflow, precipitating an acute attack of glaucoma

 b. Hypersensitivity to epinephrine

 c. Epinephrine is contraindicated with use of contact lenses

5. Significant drug interactions

 a. Significant drug interactions are related to systemic absorption of adrenergic agonists

 b. Systemic absorption may result in adverse cardiovascular reactions and adverse CNS reactions, especially in clients with cardiovascular disease

 c. Systemic absorption of adrenergic agonists interferes with actions of beta-blocking agents and some antihypertensive agents

6. Significant food interactions: none reported

7. Significant laboratory studies: none reported

8. Side effects

 a. Local reactions include eye pain and stinging on initial instillation

 b. CNS side effects include headache, blurred vision, brow ache, photophobia, and difficulty with night vision

 c. Rebound **miosis** (constriction of pupils) may occur with phenylephrine

 d. Older adults with cardiac disease may experience blood pressure (BP) elevations with phenylephrine

9. Adverse effects/toxicity: systemic adverse effects are unusual, but may occur especially in clients with cardiovascular disease; symptoms include confusion, tachycardia, hypertension, diaphoresis, and tremors

10. Nursing considerations

 a. Obtain history of allergies or hypersensitivity to specific agents

 b. Be alert for vasovagal episode with bradycardia, pallor, nausea, and pain

 c. Obtain baseline vital signs

 d. Obtain baseline vision and intraocular pressure data

 e. Assess cardiac, respiratory, and renal function routinely

11. Client education

 a. Drugs may discolor contact lenses

 b. Do not blink for at least 30 seconds after instilling medication

 c. Report a decrease in visual acuity, floating spots, sensitivity to light, eye redness, or headache to health care provider

 d. Proper self-administration of ophthalmic medications

D. Cholinergic agents (miotics, cholinesterase inhibitors)

1. Action and use

 a. Increase outflow of aqueous humor, decrease resistance to aqueous flow

 b. Produce miosis

Table 15-4	Cholinergic Agents for Ophthalmic Use	
Trade (Generic) Name	**Uses**	**Adverse Effects**
Carbachol (Carboptic)	Glaucoma, miosis during surgery	Ataxia, confusion, seizures, coma, respiratory failure, hypotension, death
Echothiophate iodide (Phosphaline iodide)	Open-angle glaucoma, accommodative esotropia	Conjunctival thickening, chest pain, arrhythmia, ocular irritation
Pilocarpine hydrochloride (Adsorbocarpine, Isopto, Carpine)	Acute or chronic glaucoma	Burning of eye, tearing, ciliary spasm, hypertension, nausea, vomiting, pulmonary edema, salivation, sweating, bronchial spasm, respiratory failure

    c. Used in treatment of open-angle and angle-closure glaucoma

    d. Used to facilitate miosis before ophthalmic examination or after ophthalmic surgery

    e. Generally used for clients who fail to respond to first-line agents (such as prostaglandin analogs or beta blockers)

2. Common medications (Table 15-4)

3. Administration considerations

    a. Drug crosses placenta, enters breast milk

    b. Do not administer ophthalmic solution that contains precipitates or has turned brown

    c. Pilocarpine can be stored at room temperature

4. Contraindications

    a. Acute iritis

    b. Conditions in which pupillary constriction is not desirable

5. Significant drug interactions: concurrent use with beta-adrenergic blocking agents may increase risk of cardiovascular reactions

6. Significant food interactions: none reported

7. Significant laboratory studies: none reported

8. Side effects

    a. Visual blurring, myopia, irritation, brow pain, and headache

    b. Systemic reactions include abdominal pain, bronchoconstriction, diarrhea, hypotension, nausea, vomiting, diuresis, diaphoresis, exacerbation of asthma

9. Adverse effects/toxicity

    a. Toxic effects produce ataxia, confusion, seizures, coma, respiratory failure, hypotension, and death

    b. Prolonged use of cholinergics may lead to retinal detachments, obstruction of tear drainage, and cataracts

    c. Acute toxicity is reversible by intravenous (IV) administration of atropine (anticholinergic agent) as an antidote

10. Nursing considerations

    a. Obtain baseline vital signs and neurologic status

    b. Obtain baseline vision and intraocular pressure data

    c. Assess for cardiovascular disease, renal failure, diabetes, lactation, or thyrotoxicosis

    d. Assess for signs and symptoms of hypersensitivity such as burning, itching, redness, and swelling occurring after medication administration

11. Client education

    a. Difficulty adjusting quickly to changes in illumination may occur as a result of miosis

    b. Proper self-administration of ophthalmic medications

Table 15-5 Carbonic Anhydrase Inhibitors

Generic (Trade) Name	Route	Uses	Adverse Effects
Acetazolamide (Diamox)	PO	Increased IOP related to open-angle glaucoma	Drowsiness, Stevens–Johnson syndrome, transient myopia, N/V, hyperchloremic acidosis, hypokalemia, aplastic anemia, renal calculi, bone marrow depression
Brinzolamide (Azopt)	Ophthalmic		Headache, dry eyes, altered taste
Dorzolamide hydrochloride (Trusopt)	Ophthalmic		Altered taste, fatigue, dizziness, ocular burning, keratitis, conjunctivitis, photophobia, bronchospasm, dyspnea, angioedema
Methazolamide (Neptazane)	PO		Photophobia, photosensitivity, urticaria, anorexia, vomiting, constipation, bone marrow depression, hepatic insufficiency

E. Carbonic anhydrase inhibitors
   1. Action and use
      a. Converted to epinephrine, lowering intraocular pressure by decreasing aqueous production
      b. Oral carbonic anhydrase inhibitors are used to treat open-angle, secondary, and angle-closure glaucoma
      c. Ophthalmic carbonic anhydrase inhibitors are used to treat open-angle glaucoma and ocular hypertension
      d. Commonly used preoperatively in intraocular surgery
   2. Common medications (Table 15-5)
   3. Administration considerations
      a. Oral acetazolamide (Diamox) is administered for maintenance
      b. IV route is used preoperatively or to rapidly reduce increased intraocular pressure
      c. Observe for signs of hypokalemia and hyperglycemia
      d. To minimize nocturia, schedule doses early in day
      e. Administer with caution to clients with adrenocortical insufficiency
   4. Contraindications
      a. Hypersensitivity to antibacterial sulfonamides
      b. Chronic noncongestive angle-closure glaucoma
      c. Hyponatremia, hypokalemia, or other electrolyte imbalances
      d. Hepatic or renal dysfunction
   5. Significant drug interactions
      a. Interference with renal excretion of quinidine, salicylates, lithium
      b. Carbonic anhydrase inhibitors decrease excretion of amphetamines, mecamylamine (Inversine), and quinidine, which could result in prolonged duration of drug actions
   6. Significant food interactions: none reported
   7. Significant laboratory studies
      a. False-positive results in tests for urinary protein
      b. Monitor sodium, potassium, bicarbonate levels for imbalances
      c. May increase uric acid level
      d. May decrease thyroid iodine uptake, WBC count
   8. Side effects
      a. Oral agents: anorexia, diarrhea, diuresis, nausea, vomiting, lethargy, weakness, weight loss, metallic bitter taste, and paresthesia of fingers, hands, and toes
      b. Topical agents: topical allergic reaction, photosensitivity, superficial **keratitis** (inflammation of the cornea)

Practice to Pass

A client with open-angle glaucoma is having the medication regimen changed to acetazolamide (Diamox). What important teaching and information do you provide to the client?

9. Adverse effects/toxicity
   a. Stevens–Johnson syndrome with acetazolamide (Diamox)
   b. Bone marrow depression with acetazolamide
   c. Acidosis
   d. Blood dyscrasias
   e. Hypokalemia
10. Nursing considerations
    a. Potential exacerbation of renal stones; monitor renal function
    b. Monitor for fluid volume depletion related to diuresis
    c. Monitor intake and output (I & O), skin turgor, mucous membranes, and weight
    d. Monitor urinalysis, complete blood cell count (CBC), electrolytes
11. Client education
    a. Unless contraindicated, eat a diet high in potassium and low in sodium
    b. Unless contraindicated, increase fluid intake to at least 2 liters per day to decrease risk of renal stones
    c. Report changes in urine color, rashes, fever
    d. Proper self-administration of ophthalmic medications
    e. Monitor weight for weight loss and report to prescriber
    f. Report symptoms of bone marrow toxicity such as weakness, unusual bleeding, numbness, or tingling of extremities

F. **Immunomodulators**
   1. Action and use
      a. Used to increase tear production if the cause of dry eye is inflammation
      b. Immunosuppressant
   2. Common medication: cyclosporine (Restasis)
   3. Administration considerations: with concurrent use of ophthalmic NSAIDS, tear production is *not* increased
   4. Contraindications: administer cautiously in clients with decreased immune function
   5. Significant drug interactions: none noted
   6. Significant food interactions: none noted
   7. Significant laboratory studies: renal studies in case of systemic absorption
   8. Side effects: immunosuppression and nephrotoxicity (if systemically absorbed)
   9. Adverse effects/toxicity: irritation, blurred vision
   10. Nursing considerations: gently mix the emulsion prior to use
   11. Client teaching: adverse effects/toxicity

II. MYDRIATICS AND CYCLOPLEGICS

A. **Anticholinergics**
   1. Action and use
      a. Produce mydriasis
      b. Produce **cycloplegia** (paralysis of ciliary muscle)
      c. Used in treatment of ocular pain secondary to inflammatory disorders such as uveitis and keratitis
      d. Used to relax ciliary muscle to improve measurement of refractive errors
      e. Used preoperatively and postoperatively for intraocular surgery
   2. Common medications (Table 15-6)
   3. Administration considerations
      a. Use with caution in clients with primary glaucoma
      b. Use with caution in clients with predisposition to angle-closure glaucoma
      c. Apply ointment several hours before vision examination
      d. Compress lacrimal duct during administration and for 2–3 minutes after administration

Practice to Pass

A client receiving pilocarpine (Isopto Carpine) ophthalmic solution for glaucoma is prescribed latanoprost (Xalatan) for concurrent therapy with the pilocarpine. What teaching and information do you provide to this client?

Table 15-6	Mydriatic and Cycloplegic Agents for Ophthalmic Use	
Generic (Trade) Name	**Uses**	**Adverse Effects**
Atropine sulfate	Mydriasis, inflammation of iris and uveal tract	Transient stinging, dry mouth, vomiting, nausea, bradycardia, palpitations, tachycardia, increased IOP, photophobia, urinary hesitancy, heat prostration, decreased sweating
Cyclopentolate (Cyclogyl)	Mydriasis, cycloplegia	Allergic reaction, conjunctivitis
Homatropine (Isopto Homatropine) Scopalamine hydrobromide	Mydriasis, inflammation of iris and uveal tract	Transient stinging, dry mouth, vomiting, nausea, bradycardia, palpitations, tachycardia, increased IOP, photophobia, urinary hesitancy, heat prostration, decreased sweating
Tropicamide (Mydriacyl)	Mydriasis, cycloplegia	Allergic reaction, conjunctivitis
Hydroxyamphetamine/ Tropicamide (Paremyd)	Mydriasis	Blurred vision, headache, dizziness, enlarged pupils, tachycardia, nervousness, stomach pain, vomiting, photosensitivity, nausea, flatulence, dyspepsia

4. Contraindications
    a. Severe systemic reactions to atropine
    b. Hypersensitivity to anticholinergic drugs
5. Significant drug interactions: results from systemic absorption; decreases effectiveness of phenothiazines and haloperidol
6. Significant food interactions: none reported
7. Significant laboratory studies: none reported
8. Side effects
    a. Local: blurred vision, photophobia, allergic lid reactions
    b. Systemic: confusion, delirium, drowsiness, dry mouth, flushing, and tachycardia
9. Adverse effects/toxicity
    a. Hallucinations, tachycardia, slurred speech, psychiatric and behavioral problems, fever, respiratory depression, coma
    b. Acute glaucoma can be precipitated by pupillary dilation; if not recognized and treated, acute glaucoma can result in blindness
    c. Dry mouth and tachycardia may be symptoms of scopolamine toxicity
10. Nursing considerations
    a. Obtain baseline intraocular pressure and vision status data
    b. Combination drugs produce greater mydriasis
    c. Systemic side effects are more pronounced in infants and children with blond hair and blue eyes
    d. Monitor for tachycardia, confusion, slurred speech, dry mouth, dry skin, weakness, drowsiness
11. Client education
    a. Mydriasis may last from 3 days (scopolamine) to 12 days (atropine)
    b. Blurred vision may occur
    c. Wear dark sunglasses and avoid bright light for photophobia
    d. Intraocular pressure and vision should be monitored over course of therapy
    e. Withhold medication if experiencing tachycardia or dry mouth (symptoms of toxicity) and report these symptoms to prescriber
    f. Use sugarless hard candy to combat dry mouth
    g. Proper self-administration of ophthalmic medications
 B. **Adrenergics:** refer to Section I-B Medications to Treat Glaucoma

III. ANTI-INFLAMMATORY AND ANTI-INFECTIVE MEDICATIONS FOR THE EYE

A. Nonsteroidal anti-inflammatory drugs (NSAIDs)

1. Action and use
   - a. In general, used for pain and inflammation following surgery
   - b. Flurbiprofen (Ocufen) and suprofen (Profenal) are used to inhibit intraoperative miosis
   - c. Diclofenac (Voltaren) is used to treat postoperative inflammation after cataract extractions
   - d. Ketorolac (Acular) is used to treat conjunctivitis and seasonal allergic ophthalmic pruritis
2. Common medications (Table 15-7)
3. Administration considerations
   - a. Systemic effect may be produced if absorbed
   - b. NSAIDs have potential to cause increased bleeding; therefore, clients with increased bleeding tendencies should be monitored closely
4. Contraindications
   - a. Sensitivity to aspirin or phenylacetic acid derivatives
   - b. Sensitivity to systemic NSAIDs
5. Significant drug interactions: none reported
6. Significant food interactions: St. John's wort (herb) and ciprofloxacin lead to increased photosensitivity
7. Significant laboratory studies: potential to cause increased bleeding; monitor CBC and coagulation studies
8. Side effects: local—transient burning or stinging on application, itching, allergic reaction, pain, and redness
9. Adverse effects/toxicity: bleeding
10. Nursing considerations: assess for hypersensitivity symptoms such as burning, itching, redness, and swelling occurring administration of dose
11. Client education
    - a. NSAIDs may potentiate bleeding in clients with known bleeding tendencies
    - b. Proper self-administration of ophthalmic medications

B. Antibacterial, antifungal, and antiviral agents

1. Action and use
   - a. Antibacterial agents are used to treat bacterial infections such as conjunctivitis, blepharitis, keratitis, uveitis, and hordeolum (sty)
   - b. Antifungal agents are used to treat fungal blepharitis, conjunctivitis, and keratitis
   - c. Antiviral agents are used to treat herpes simplex virus keratitis and herpes simplex virus keratoconjunctivitis
2. Common medications (Table 15-8)

Table 15-7 Nonsteroidal Anti-Inflammatory Agents for Ophthalmic Use

Generic (Trade) Name	Uses	Adverse Effects
Diclofenac sodium (Voltaren)	Postoperative inflammation after cataract surgery	Headache, dizziness, dyspepsia, ophthalmic effects, renal impairment, anaphylactic shock, constipation
Flurbiprofen (Ocufen)	Constriction of pupil prior to surgery	Eye irritation
Ketorolac tromethamine (Acular)	Relief of ocular itching, postoperative inflammation after cataract surgery	Eye irritation
Suprofen (Profenal)	Inhibit intraoperative miosis	Eye irritation

Table 15-8 Antibacterial, Antifungal, and Antiviral Agents for Ophthalmic Use

Generic (Trade) Name	Uses	Adverse Effects
Bacitracin (AK Tracin)	Eye infection caused by staphylococcus	Blurring of vision
Chloramphenicol (Chloroptic)	Eye infection for susceptible organisms when less dangerous anti-infectives are ineffective	Bone marrow hypoplasia, irritation, burning, itching, angioneurotic edema, superinfection, aplastic anemia
Ciprofloxacin (Cipro HC Otic, Cioxan)	Eye infection for susceptible organisms when less dangerous anti-infectives are ineffective, otitis externa	Dry eye, eye pain, keratopathy
Erythromycin (Ilotycin)	Superficial ocular infections, ophthalmia neonatorum caused by Gonorrhoeae or trachomatis	Edema, urticaria, dermatitis, angioneurotic edema, irritation, burning, itching at application site
Gentamicin sulfate (Garamycin, others)	Superficial ocular infections	Transient irritation, burning, stinging, itching, angioneurotic edema, urticaria, maculopapular dermatitis, photosensitivity, superinfection
Ofloxacin (Floxin Otic, Ocuflox)	Bacterial conjunctivitis, otitis externa from *E. coli, P. aeruginosa, S. aureus*	Visual disturbances
Polymyxin B (Polymyxin B Sterile Ophthalmic)	Bacterial infection caused by *Proteus aeruginosa*	Eye irritation, blurred vision, itching, stinging, burning
Sulfisoxazole (Gantrisin)	Conjunctivitis, corneal ulcer, superficial ocular infection	Stevens–Johnson syndrome, nausea, vomiting, abdominal pain, headache, hematuria, crystalluria, agranulocytosis, photosensitivity, alopecia
Tobramycin sulfate (Tobrex ophthalmic)	Superficial ocular infection	Pain, irritation, superinfection, ocular toxicity, hypersensitivity, erythema, punctuate keratitis
Trifluridine (Viroptic)	Keratoconjunctivitis, epithelial keratitis	Burning, stinging, palpebral edema, epithelial keratopathy, keratitis sicca, hyperemia, increased IOP
Vidarabine (Vira-A)	Varicella zoster virus, cytomegalovirus, vaccinia, and HBV	Increased IOP glaucoma, cataracts

3. Administration considerations
  a. If indicated, obtain culture specimen from eye(s) before administering first dose of medication
  b. Remove exudates from eyes before administering dose
4. Contraindications: hypersensitivity
5. Significant drug interactions
  a. Paraaminobenzoic acid (PABA) reduces the action of sulfonamides (sulfacetamide sodium)
  b. Ophthalmic anesthetics should not be administered within 30 minutes of sulfonamides (sulfacetamide sodium)
  c. Sulfonamides are incompatible with thimerosol and silver preparations
6. Significant food interactions: none reported
7. Significant laboratory studies: monitor CBC and coagulation studies in clients with potential for bleeding
8. Side effects
  a. Local: dermatitis, itching, stinging, swelling
  b. Systemic: chloramphenicol (Chloroptic) may cause blood dyscrasias
9. Adverse effects/toxicity
  a. Stevens–Johnson syndrome, systemic lupus erythematosus (SLE) with sulfacetamide sodium
  b. Blood dyscrasias with chloramphenicol

Practice to Pass

A client with an eye infection has crusty drainage in and around the eye. Before administering the prescribed ophthalmic solution, what nursing measures do you implement?

Table 15-9 **Common Corticosteroid Agents for Ophthalmic Use**

Generic (Trade) Name	Uses	Adverse Effects
Dexamethasone (Maxidex)	Conjunctivitis	Cataracts, glaucoma
Prednisone	Ophthalmic disorders	Cushing syndrome, hyperglycemia, muscle weakness, nausea, vomiting, dyspepsia, increased appetite, delayed wound healing, superinfection, cataracts, glaucoma, thrombus formation

   10. Nursing considerations
       a. Monitor infected eye(s) for pain, drainage, redness, and swelling
       b. Monitor for unusual bleeding or bruising with chloramphenicol
       c. Idoxuridine (Stoxil, Herplex) and trifluridine (Viroptic) should be stored in cool place or refrigerated
   11. Client education
       a. Inform prescriber of photosensitivity, redness, or swelling
       b. Inform prescriber of increased drainage, pain, or if no improvement is seen within a few days
       c. Proper self-administration of ophthalmic medications
C. **Corticosteroids**
   1. Action and use: management of allergic and inflammatory ophthalmic disorders of conjunctiva, cornea, and anterior segment of eye
   2. Common medications (Table 15-9)
   3. Administration considerations
       a. Corticosteroids should be used for short-term treatment only
       b. Use with caution in clients with cataracts and chronic open-angle glaucoma
   4. Contraindications: hypersensitivity and corneal abrasion
   5. Significant drug interactions: corticosteroids may mask hypersensitivity reactions to other drugs
   6. Significant food interactions: none reported
   7. Significant laboratory studies: none reported
   8. Side effects: local—stinging after application
   9. Adverse effects/toxicity: visual disturbances, headache, and eye pain
   10. Nursing considerations
       a. Corticosteroids may mask symptoms of infection and hypersensitivity reactions
       b. Corticosteroids may increase susceptibility to infection
   11. Client education
       a. Avoid use of contact lenses during and for the prescribed time after use of corticosteroid therapy
       b. Do not discontinue medication without instructions from prescriber
       c. Have eye(s) examined periodically for progress
       d. Proper self-administration of ophthalmic medications

IV. ANESTHETIC MEDICATIONS FOR THE EYE
A. **Action and use**
   1. Prevent initiation and transmission of nerve impulses
   2. Used to prevent pain during procedures such as **tonometry** (measurement of intra-ocular tension, used to detect glaucoma), subconjunctival injections, removal of foreign bodies, and removal of sutures
B. **Common medications**
   1. Proparacaine hydrochloride (Alcaine, Ophthaine): 1–2 drops of 0.5% solution (single dose) to affected eye(s)
   2. Tetracaine hydrochloride (Pontocaine): 1–2 drops of 0.5–1% solution (single dose) to affected eye(s)

C. Administration considerations
　1. Rapid onset within 20 seconds, and duration is 15–20 minutes
　2. Tetracaine hydrochloride can cause systemic toxicity
D. Contraindications: hypersensitivity
E. Significant drug interactions: may interact with ophthalmic cholinesterase inhibitors, increasing risk of toxicity
F. Significant food interactions: none reported
G. Significant laboratory studies: none reported
H. Side effects: proparacaine (Ophthaine, Ophthetic) causes allergic contact dermatitis, cycloplegia, conjunctival congestion, delayed corneal healing
I. Adverse effects/toxicity
　1. CNS excitation symptoms: blurred vision, dizziness, nervousness, restlessness, trembling
　2. CNS depression (follows CNS excitation): dyspnea, drowsiness, dysrhythmias
J. Nursing considerations
　1. To protect cornea, apply eye patch until blink reflex has returned
　2. Assess for hypersensitivity symptoms such as burning, itching, stinging
K. Client education: do not touch or rub the eye until anesthesia has worn off

V. AUDITORY MEDICATIONS

A. Antibiotics for the ear
　1. Action and use
　　a. Used to manage infections of **external ear** (external auditory canal surface)
　　b. Chloramphenicol (Chloromycetin Otic) is used to treat infections caused by such organisms as *Enterobacter aerogenes*, *Escherichia coli*, *Haemophilus influenzae*, *Pseudomonas aeruginosa*, and others
　2. Common medications
　　a. Chloramphenicol (Chloromycetin Otic): 2–3 drops instilled in ear canal every 6–8 hours
　　b. Gentamicin sulfate otic solution (Garamycin): 3–4 drops instilled in ear canal 3 times daily
　　c. Note: otic preparation of gentamicin sulfate has not been approved by Food and Drug Administration (FDA); prescribers in United States use the *ophthalmic* preparation for otic infections
　3. Administration considerations
　　a. Unless contraindicated, warm ear drops by running medication bottle under warm water, immersing bottle in a cup of warm water, or by holding bottle in the hand or pocket for 30 minutes prior to administration
　　b. Assess client's baseline hearing status
　　c. Assess client for ear drainage, earache, erythema, pain, and **vertigo** (dizziness)

　　d. Assess that ear canal is clear and not impacted with **cerumen** (earwax) before medication administration
　　e. Assess for intact **tympanic membrane** (thin membrane between external auditory canal and middle ear)
　4. Contraindications
　　a. Hypersensitivity
　　b. Perforation of tympanic membrane

　5. Significant drug interactions: none reported
　6. Significant food interactions: none reported
　7. Significant laboratory studies: assess for blood dyscrasias with chloramphenicol

8. Side effects
   a. Local: burning, rash, redness, swelling, blurred vision
   b. Systemic: hypersensitivity reaction
9. Adverse effects/toxicity
   a. Hypersensitivity reaction
   b. Rare occurrence of systemic hematologic toxicity
10. Nursing considerations
    a. Assess for signs of hypersensitivity such as burning, rash, redness, and swelling after administration of dose
    b. Discontinue use if hypersensitivity reaction occurs
    c. Monitor auditory canal for drainage and pain
    d. Monitor for hearing disturbances
11. Client education
    a. Inform health care provider of increased pain, drainage, or no improvement in symptoms within a few days of treatment
    b. Refer to Box 15-2 for instillation of otic medications

B. Corticosteroids
1. Action and use
   a. Used for antibacterial, antifungal, and anti-inflammatory effects
   b. Used for antipruritic and antiallergic effects
2. Common medications (Refer to Table 15-10)
3. Administration considerations
   a. Assess client's hearing status
   b. Assess client for ear drainage, earache, erythema, pain, and vertigo

   c. Assess that ear canal is clear and not impacted with cerumen before medication administration
   d. Assess for intact tympanic membrane
   e. May be given in combination with antibiotics to treat infections of external ear canal or mastoid cavity
4. Contraindications
   a. Hypersensitivity to sulfites
   b. Perforation of tympanic membrane
5. Significant drug interactions: none reported
6. Significant food interactions: none reported
7. Significant laboratory studies: none reported
8. Side effects: corticosteroids may mask infection or exacerbate an existing infection

Table 15-10	Corticosteroid Agents for Otic Use	
Generic (Trade) Name	**Uses**	**Adverse Effects**
Betamethasone (Betnesol) Hydrocortisone (Cortamed) Dexamethasone (Decadron) Hydrocortisone with acetic acid Hydrocortisone with alcohol Hydrocortisone with acetic acid and benzethonium	Bacterial, antifungal, anti-inflammatory conditions of ear	Cushing syndrome Hyperglycemia Muscle weakness Nausea and vomiting Dyspepsia Increased appetite Delayed wound healing Superinfection Cataracts Glaucoma Thrombus formation

Box 15-2	**For instillation of eardrops in older children and adults:**
Administration of Otic Medications	• Assess the ear canal for cerumen or edema • Tilt client's head toward the unaffected side • Gently pull the pinna of the ear up and back • Instill the eardrops—*do not* insert dropper into the ear canal • Gently massage the area anterior to the ear to facilitate entry of the drops into the ear canal
	For instillation of eardrops in children 3 years and younger:
	• Assess the ear canal for cerumen or edema • Tilt client's head toward the unaffected side • Gently pull the pinna of the ear slightly down and back • Instill the eardrops—*do not* insert dropper into the ear canal • Gently massage the area anterior to the ear to facilitate entry of the drops into the ear canal

9. Adverse effects/toxicity: corticosteroids may mask infection or exacerbate an existing infection
10. Nursing considerations: assess for hypersensitivity after administration of dose
11. Client education
    a. Have hearing monitored for duration of treatment
    b. Inform health care provider of new onset of ear drainage, heat, fever, odor, or pain
    c. Inform health care provider if no improvement is seen within a few days of treatment
    d. Refer to Box 15-2 for administration of otic medications

C. **Other medications (over-the-counter medications)**
    1. Action and use
       a. Acetic acid (alcohol, glycerin, or propylene glycol) is used after swimming or bathing to restore normal acid pH to the ear canal
       b. Glycerin, mineral oil, and olive oil are used as emollients to relieve itching and burning in ear
       c. Propylene glycol enhances antibacterial effects and acidity of acetic acid
       d. Carbamide peroxide is an antibacterial agent used to help remove accumulated cerumen
    2. Common medications (refer to Table 15-11)
    3. Administration considerations: generally considered safe and effective
    4. Contraindications: hypersensitivity; otherwise generally considered safe

Table 15-11 **Common Over-the-Counter (OTC) Agents for Otic Use**

Drug Name	Usual Adult Dosage
Hydrocortisone, propylene glycol, alcohol, benzyl benzoate (Earsol-HC Drops)	Instill 3–4 drops 2–3 times daily, or saturate a cotton wick and insert into ear canal. Moisten wick every 4–6 hours with 3–5 drops of solution. Remove wick after 24 hours and use prescribed amount of drops 3–4 times daily.
Boric acid and isopropyl alcohol (Aurocaine 2)	Follow package directions.
Carbamide peroxide (Auro Ear Drops)	
Carbamide peroxide and glycerin (Dent's Ear Wax Drops, others)	
Isopropyl alcohol (Aurocaine 2)	
Isopropyl alcohol in glycerin (Swim-Ear Drops)	

Practice to Pass

A client returns to the clinic complaining that the medication prescribed for an ear infection "runs right back out of my ear." What assessment and instructions do you provide for this client?

!

5. Significant drug interactions: none reported
6. Significant food interactions: none reported
7. Significant laboratory studies: none reported
8. Side effects: generally considered safe without side effects
9. Adverse effects/toxicity: generally considered safe without side effects
10. Nursing considerations: assess for hypersensitivity
11. Client education
    a. Seek evaluation by health care provider if symptoms do not improve within several days
    b. Inform health care provider if adverse reactions occur or if symptoms worsen
    c. Refer to Box 15-2 for administration of otic medications

D. Medications that cause ototoxicity
1. Analgesics: aspirin and other salicylates, NSAIDs
2. Antibiotics: aminoglycosides, clarithromycin, erythromycin, vancomycin
3. Antineoplastic agents: cisplatin, mechlorethamine
4. Loop diuretics: bumetanide (Bumex), ethacrynic acid (Edecrin), furosemide (Lasix)

Case Study

A client with newly diagnosed open angle glaucoma is prescribed betaxolol (Betoptic). The client also has a history of pulmonary disease.

1. How does the nurse explain glaucoma and the purpose of the medication to this client?

2. The client expresses concern about the new medication and the possible interference with the treatment and course of the preexisting pulmonary disease. What information should be provided to the client?

3. What information does the client need regarding the side effects and signs and symptoms of hypersensitivity to betaxolol (Betoptic)?

4. What instructions does the nurse provide specifically related to the potential side effect of photophobia?

5. What instructions does the client need regarding proper administration of ophthalmic medications?

For suggested responses, see page 546.

POSTTEST

POSTTEST

1 A client has NPH insulin (Humulin N) and carteolol (Ocupress) listed on the medication administration record. The nurse considers that which outcome has the most immediate significance and should be given first priority?

1. Blood pressure is within normal limits (WNL).
2. Serum glucose is within normal limits (WNL).
3. Headache is controlled with nonsteroidal anti-inflammatory drugs (NSAIDs).
4. Diarrhea is controlled with loperamide (Imodium).

2 The nurse concludes that a client understands instructions about how to self-administer a prescribed otic solution when the client makes which statement?

1. "I place the bottle of medication under cool running water before using."
2. "I place the bottle of medication under warm running water before using."
3. "I warm the bottle of medication in the microwave before using."
4. "I warm the bottle of medication in my hand for 5 minutes before using."

POSTTEST

POSTTEST

3 After a nurse provides instructions about betaxolol (Betoptic) to a client with a history of chronic obstructive pulmonary disease (COPD), the client asks, "How can eyedrops affect my lungs?" The nurse's best response includes which of the following information?

1. Medication does not have any effects on the pulmonary system.
2. Client is only at risk if prescribed ophthalmic medication is cardioselective.
3. Client is at risk if Betoptic is given at the same time as the oral medications taken for pulmonary disease.
4. If ophthalmic medication is systemically absorbed, it can have the same systemic effects as other beta-blocking agents.

4 A client telephones the outpatient clinic and reports severe ear pain that ceased suddenly when copious drainage came from the ear. The client wants to instill remnants of a 2-month-old otic antibiotic prescription left over from a previous ear infection. Which is the best response by the nurse?

1. "See a health care provider. Do not treat the ear."
2. "If the medication has been stored properly, it should be okay to instill."
3. "Begin treatment and seek help if no improvement is seen within 2 days."
4. "The shelf life of otic medications is 3 months; therefore, the medication would be safe to use."

5 The nurse's evaluation reveals that a client is demonstrating appropriate technique for instilling ophthalmic medication when the client does which of the following?

1. Cleanses crust from eye by applying petroleum jelly and wiping with a washcloth
2. Cleanses crust from eye by wiping from the inner canthus outward with a cotton ball
3. Cleanses crust with mild soapy water using 434 gauze
4. Cleanses crust with a cotton-tipped swab

6 Because a prescription of gentamicin sulfate (Garamycin) for an ear infection reads "for ophthalmic use," the client refuses to instill the medication. After verifying the prescription with the client's chart, what is the most appropriate conclusion by the nurse?

1. An error is likely in the dispensing of the medication since the clinician is treating an otic infection.
2. It is an accepted and safe practice in the United States for clinicians to prescribe ophthalmic gentamicin for otic use.
3. An error was likely committed by the clinician in prescribing the medication.
4. The client requires further teaching on proper medication administration.

7 Because a client with glaucoma is scheduled for removal of a cataract from the left eye, the nurse anticipates an order from the surgeon to administer which of the following drugs?

1. Atropine sulfate (generic)
2. Glycopyrrolate (Robinul)
3. Acetazolamide (Diamox)
4. Pralidoxime (Protopam)

8 A client is receiving an ophthalmic anesthetic agent prior to removal of sutures. The nurse would consider including which of the following items as a priority of nursing care?

1. Measures to protect the airway
2. Measures to reduce hypersensitivity
3. Measures to control body temperature
4. Measures to protect the eye

9 A client with narrow angle glaucoma informs the nurse at an outpatient clinic that a colonoscopy is scheduled later in the week. After hearing the client make which of the following statements, the nurse concludes that the client needs no additional instruction?

1. "I will tell the surgeon and the nursing staff of my glaucoma and the medication I am taking."
2. "I will stop taking my medication 2 days before the colonoscopy."
3. "I will omit part of the preparation for the procedure to prevent the loss of fluid."
4. "Since the procedure involves my intestines, I won't worry about the problem I have with my eyes."

10 An unlicensed assistive personnel (UAP) tells the nurse that a client who underwent detached retina repair today (using a gas preparation) rang the call bell to report sudden severe pain accompanied by nausea. The nurse considers that which of the following actions would be contraindicated at this time?

1. Administer prescribed analgesia and antiemetic.
2. Perform an assessment of the eye.
3. Position head with the affected eye up.
4. Position client on the abdomen.

➤ *See pages 507–508 for Answers and Rationales.*

ANSWERS & RATIONALES

Pretest

1 **Answer: 3** **Rationale**: Assessment of allergies and reactions to medications is essential when administering a new medication. Hypersensitivity responses can occur with ophthalmic medications, and severe adverse reactions may occur with hypersensitivity to the medication because it may be systemically absorbed. Knowledge of the purpose of a drug is not unique to ophthalmic drugs. Assessment of level of consciousness (LOC) would not override the risks of a topical allergic reaction or the risks of systemic responses to the medications. Teaching about the drug's action is very important but should follow assessment. **Cognitive Level**: Analyzing **Client Need**: Pharmacological and Parenteral Therapies **Integrated Process**: Nursing Process: Assessment **Content Area**: Pharmacology **Strategy**: The critical words in the question are *first dose*. Use principles of safety in medication administration to consider that a risk for allergy is present whenever a client receives a new medication. Correlate this risk with the likely reaction to choose the option that indicates the critical assessment. **Reference**: Adams, M., Holland, L., & Bostwick, P. (2011). *Pharmacology for nurses: A pathophysiologic approach* (3rd ed.). Upper Saddle River, NJ: Pearson Education, p. 769.

2 **Answer: 2, 5** **Rationale**: Because placing medications in the conjunctival sac ensures retention of the medication as well as exposure to a highly vascular area, the correct technique for administration of ophthalmic medications includes pulling the lower eyelid down and instilling medication into the conjunctival sac. Cleaning exudates from eye before instillation of medication promotes the absorption of medication. Applying gentle pressure to inner canthus for 30 seconds to 1 minute after medication administration prevents absorption through the tear duct and subsequent drainage of medications. Placing medications directly on the cornea can be extremely painful and can cause tissue injury. The dose should be deposited so that the maximum amount of medication is retained with the lowest risk of systemic absorption and the least risk of discomfort. **Cognitive Level**: Applying

Client Need: Pharmacological and Parenteral Therapies **Integrated Process**: Nursing Process: Evaluation **Content Area**: Pharmacology **Strategy**: Select the option most likely to result in retaining the medication within the eye for the longest period of time and that also promotes absorption of medication. **Reference**: Adams, M., Holland, L., & Bostwick, P. (2011). *Pharmacology for nurses: A pathophysiologic approach* (3rd ed.). Upper Saddle River, NJ: Pearson Education, pp. 25–26.

3 **Answer: 1, 5** **Rationale**: When an external ear canal is obstructed by edematous tissue, a gauze wick is inserted past the edematous segment. The medication is then applied to the outside wick, allowing the medication to be absorbed along the path of the wick. Forcing the tip of the container or forcing the stream of liquid could result in damage to the ear canal or ear drum. The occluded canal is related to the infection and probably will not subside without intervention. Topical medications are prescribed because it provides direct contact with the microorganism. Since an alternative to expensive systemic medications exists, it is the best method. Insertion of an object into a canal without visualization is an unsafe technique. Since an infected ear is usually very painful, forcing an object into the canal would be painful. **Cognitive Level**: Applying **Client Need**: Pharmacological and Parenteral Therapies **Integrated Process**: Nursing Process: Implementation **Content Area**: Pharmacology **Strategy**: Evaluate each option considering its effect on tissue that is edematous and most likely uncomfortable. Select the options that are most likely to achieve the goal while protecting the safety of the client. **Reference**: Adams, M., Holland, L., & Bostwick, P. (2011). *Pharmacology for nurses: A pathophysiologic approach* (3rd ed.). Upper Saddle River, NJ: Pearson Education, pp. 25–26.

4 **Answer: 3, 5** **Rationale**: One primary side effect of acetazolamide (Diamox) is reduced function of the bone marrow, which may result in decreased platelets, RBCs, and WBCs. Since the signs and symptoms of adverse bone marrow effects can be vague, the client should have regular blood counts performed several times during the year. A high potassium diet should be encouraged (unless there is a specific contraindication), as Diamox can cause hypokalemia. To minimize gastrointestinal distress, the client may take the medication with milk. Acetazolamide is taken in the morning to avoid nocturnal diuresis. It reduces intraocular pressure, which is related to increased formation of aqueous humor formation. The client may crush the tablet and mix it with juice. **Cognitive Level:** Applying **Client Need:** Pharmacological and Parenteral Therapies **Integrated Process:** Teaching and Learning **Content Area:** Pharmacology **Strategy:** Specific knowledge of adverse effects of acetazolamide (Diamox) is needed to answer the question. Associate the drug with the side effect of hematological alterations and hypokalemia to help make the correct selection. **Reference:** Wilson, B. A., Shannon, M. T., & Shields, K. M. (2012). *Pearson nurse's drug guide 2012.* Upper Saddle River, NJ: Pearson Education, pp. 11–14.

5 **Answer: 1 Rationale:** Carbonic anhydrase inhibitors such as dorzolamide (Trusopt) decrease aqueous humor production by approximately one half of baseline, thereby lowering intraocular pressure (IOP). Cholinergic agonists such as carbachol (Carboptic) cause pupil constriction, which does not affect aqueous humor production but increases its drainage. The glaucoma results from an increased production of aqueous humor, so increasing the production of aqueous humor would not resolve the problem. Increased outflow of aqueous humor is accomplished by a cholinergic agonist and nonselective sympathomimetics. **Cognitive Level:** Analyzing **Client Need:** Pharmacological and Parenteral Therapies **Integrated Process:** Teaching and Learning **Content Area:** Pharmacology **Strategy:** Recall that glaucoma is characterized by increased intraocular pressure (IOP). Associate the drug with the reversal of the disease process to make the correct selection. **Reference:** Deglin, J., & Vallerand, A. (2009). *Davis's drug guide for nurses* (11th ed.). Philadelphia, PA: F. A. Davis Company, pp. 1349–1355.

6 **Answer: 3 Rationale:** Because the drug is a cholinergic agent, it will reverse the effects of sympathomimetic drugs often used to treat asthma. Precipitation of an asthma attack is a systemic side effect of pilocarpine (Isopto Carpine). Other side effects include salivation, hypotension, diarrhea, nausea, and vomiting. Since the drug is a cholinergic agent, the client is more likely to have excessive salivation than dry mouth. This drug is more likely to cause hypotension rather than hypertension, and diarrhea rather than constipation. **Cognitive Level:** Applying **Client Need:** Pharmacological and Parenteral Therapies **Integrated Process:** Nursing Process: Assessment **Content Area:** Pharmacology **Strategy:** Associate the word *asthma* in the stem of the question with the word *wheezing* in the correct option. **Reference:** Deglin, J., & Vallerand, A. (2009). *Davis's drug guide for nurses* (11th ed.). Philadelphia, PA: F. A. Davis Company, pp. 1349–1355.

7 **Answer: 2, 5 Rationale:** In the adult client, the medication is most likely to flow into the canal if the pinna is pulled up and back before instilling otic solutions. The pinna is

pulled down in the child. Droppers should never be inserted into the ear canal, and the head should be tilted toward the unaffected side. **Cognitive Level:** Applying **Client Need:** Pharmacological and Parenteral Therapies **Integrated Process:** Nursing Process: Evaluation **Content Area:** Pharmacology **Strategy:** Select the option that is most likely to promote appropriate flow of the medication into the ear canal. **Reference:** Adams, M., Holland, L., & Bostwick, P. (2011). *Pharmacology for nurses: A pathophysiologic approach* (3rd ed.). Upper Saddle River, NJ: Pearson Education, pp. 25–26.

8 **Answer: 1 Rationale:** Ophthalmic beta blockers such as timolol (Timoptic) are administered to reduce intraocular pressure (IOP) by decreasing production of aqueous humor. The medication must be continued as lifelong therapy to maintain a stable IOP. Glaucoma already involves increased IOP so the medication is not given to raise it. Other drug groups may be utilized for the treatment of glaucoma as well as surgical intervention. **Cognitive Level:** Applying **Client Need:** Pharmacological and Parenteral Therapies **Integrated Process:** Nursing Process: Evaluation **Content Area:** Pharmacology **Strategy:** Recall first that timolol (Timoptic) is a beta-blocking agent since it ends in the suffix *olol.* Next recall the pathophysiology of glaucoma and select the option that correlates closest to the reversal of the disease process. **Reference:** Adams, M., Holland, L., & Bostwick, P. (2011). *Pharmacology for nurses: A pathophysiologic approach* (3rd ed.). Upper Saddle River, NJ: Pearson Education, pp. 769–770.

9 **Answer: 1 Rationale:** Because pupillary dilation pushes the iris over the area where aqueous humor normally drains, atropine (an anticholinergic agent) can precipitate an acute glaucoma crisis. Blurred vision, diplopia, photosensitivity, and dry eyes are the visual alterations associated with diphenhydramine (Benadryl). No visual alterations are associated with hydroxyzine (Vistaril). Contraindications associated with retelase recombinant (Retavase) include bleeding disorders, stroke, and severe uncontrolled hypertension. **Cognitive Level:** Applying **Client Need:** Pharmacological and Parenteral Therapies **Integrated Process:** Nursing Process: Implementation **Content Area:** Pharmacology **Strategy:** First recall the pathophysiology of glaucoma. Select the drug that represents a drug category that is most likely to cause structural changes that could increase intraocular pressure. Alternatively, recall that atropine dilates the pupil and associate this with blockage of the outflow of aqueous humor to make the correct selection. **Reference:** Adams, M., Holland, L., & Bostwick, P. (2011). *Pharmacology for nurses: A pathophysiologic approach* (3rd ed.). Upper Saddle River, NJ: Pearson Education, pp. 769–770.

10 **Answer: 2 Rationale:** If systemically absorbed, brinzolamide (Azopt) is eliminated via urinary elimination. In chronic renal failure with a urine output less than 30 mL/hr, the drug is retained. The drug is a systemic diuretic that could result in electrolyte imbalances. The drug has no known contraindications or side effects associated with the liver or the cardiovascular or skeletal systems. **Cognitive Level:** Applying **Client Need:** Pharmacological and Parenteral Therapies **Integrated Process:** Nursing Process: Implementation **Content Area:** Pharmacology **Strategy:** Correlate the drug category (carbonic anhydrase inhibitor) with the potential outcome of drug accumulation. **Reference:** Deglin, J., & Vallerand, A. (2009). *Davis's drug guide for nurses* (11th ed.). Philadelphia, PA: F. A. Davis Company, pp. 1349–1355.

Posttest

1 **Answer: 2** **Rationale:** Carteolol (Ocupress) is a beta-adrenergic blocker. If the client is monitored properly the beta-blocking agents will not mask symptoms of hypoglycemia. A serum glucose level significantly lower than normal can place the client at great risk more rapidly than an elevated blood pressure. Many clients live for long periods with hypertension without immediate risks to their health. Nonsteroidal anti-inflammatory drugs (NSAIDs) may reduce the antihypertensive effect of the drug so use is not helpful. Diarrhea needs to be controlled because of the potential fluid and electrolyte loss, but this is not the *first priority*. **Cognitive Level:** Applying **Client Need:** Pharmacological and Parenteral Therapies **Integrated Process:** Nursing Process: Evaluation **Content Area:** Pharmacology **Strategy:** Note that insulin is given for diabetes mellitus and that carteolol (Ocupress) is a beta-adrenergic blocker. Determine the relationship between these drugs to conclude that the carteolol could mask some signs of hypoglycemia. **Reference:** Wilson, B. A., Shannon, M. T., & Shields, K. M. (2012). *Pearson nurse's drug guide 2012.* Upper Saddle River, NJ: Pearson Education, pp. 1614–1618.

2 **Answer: 2** **Rationale:** Warming eardrops (if not contraindicated) makes administration of the medication more comfortable and prevents dizziness that can occur with the instillation of a cold solution. Microwaving the solution could result in hot spots that burn the tissue or could change the composition of the medication. The client is least likely to spend 5 minutes holding a bottle in the hands to warm it before each use. **Cognitive Level:** Analyzing **Client Need:** Pharmacological and Parenteral Therapies **Integrated Process:** Nursing Process: Evaluation **Content Area:** Pharmacology **Strategy:** Correlate the temperature of solution with common otic responses and use the process of elimination to make a selection. **Reference:** Adams, M., Holland, L., & Bostwick, P. (2011). *Pharmacology for nurses: A pathophysiologic approach* (3rd ed.). Upper Saddle River, NJ: Pearson Education, pp. 25–27.

3 **Answer: 4** **Rationale:** If systemic absorption occurs after the administration of betaxolol (Betoptic), the adverse effects such as increased airway resistance may override the effect of medications given to decrease airway resistance, which could result in dyspnea. The drug effects include vasodilation resulting in decreased cardiac output. The duration of betaxolol is 12 hours and

maintaining a therapeutic dose level would interfere continually with the respiratory drugs. **Cognitive Level:** Analyzing **Client Need:** Pharmacological and Parenteral Therapies **Integrated Process:** Teaching and Learning **Content Area:** Pharmacology **Strategy:** The core issue of the question is an understanding of the characteristics of the drug with the primary alterations associated with chronic obstructive pulmonary disease (COPD). **Reference:** Wilson, B. A., Shannon, M. T., & Shields, K. M. (2012). *Pearson nurse's drug guide 2012.* Upper Saddle River, NJ: Pearson Education, pp. 170–172.

4 **Answer: 1** **Rationale:** Because the tympanic membrane may be ruptured, the ear should be assessed before instilling medication. The old prescription may not be effective or may have deteriorated. Storage is an appropriate concern. In addition, the client should not risk inserting solution into a ruptured ear canal. Asking the client to diagnose and treat something that cannot be assessed directly by the nurse is inappropriate. There is no knowledge of how the drug has been stored. However, regardless of medication storage, the client must be assessed by a health care provider before starting a medication. **Cognitive Level:** Applying **Client Need:** Pharmacological and Parenteral Therapies **Integrated Process:** Communication and Documentation **Content Area:** Pharmacology **Strategy:** Associate the sudden change with increased pressure often occurring with an infection. With this in mind, conclude that this is a situation that warrants direct assessment and treatment by a health care provider. **Reference:** Adams, M., Holland, L., & Bostwick, P. (2011). *Pharmacology for nurses: A pathophysiologic approach* (3rd ed.). Upper Saddle River, NJ: Pearson Education, pp. 775–7756.

5 **Answer: 2** **Rationale:** Wiping from the inner canthus out prevents movement of microorganism-laden crusts from reaching the lacrimal duct. The client should avoid applying oil-based products on the eye. A washcloth is too coarse. To prevent irritation, the client should avoid using soap. If a cotton swab is used, sudden movement by the client could result in injury. **Cognitive Level:** Applying **Client Need:** Pharmacological and Parenteral Therapies **Integrated Process:** Nursing Process: Evaluation **Content Area:** Pharmacology **Strategy:** Utilize knowledge of the sterility of the mucous membranes of the eye in choosing the correct option. **Reference:** Adams, M., Holland, L., & Bostwick, P. (2011). *Pharmacology for nurses: A pathophysiologic approach* (3rd ed.). Upper Saddle River, NJ: Pearson Education, pp. 25–27.

6 **Answer: 2** **Rationale:** Otic gentamicin sulfate (Garamycin) is not approved for use in the United States. It is a safe and accepted practice for clinicians to prescribe ophthalmic gentamicin for otic use. The client should be informed of this practice. The pharmacist did not make an error in dispensing, and neither did the clinician. The client has questioned the appropriateness of the medication but has not provided evidence of lack of ability to correctly self-administer it. **Cognitive Level:** Analyzing

Client Need: Pharmacological and Parenteral Therapies **Integrated Process:** Teaching and Learning **Content Area:** Pharmacology **Strategy:** Compare and contrast ophthalmic medications with otic medications. Specific medication knowledge is needed to answer this question. **Reference:** Wilson, B. A., Shannon, M. T., & Shields, K. M. (2012). *Pearson nurse's drug guide 2012.* Upper Saddle River, NJ: Pearson Education, pp. 697–699.

7 **Answer: 3** **Rationale:** Acetazolamide (Diamox) inhibits carbonic anhydrase, which reduces the formation of aqueous humor. Because of the anticholinergic effects, atropine sulfate, glycopyrrolate (Robinul), and pralidoxime (Protopam) are contraindicated in clients with glaucoma. **Cognitive Level:** Analyzing **Client Need:** Pharmacological and Parenteral Therapies **Integrated Process:** Nursing Process: Implementation **Content Area:** Pharmacology **Strategy:** Correlate the drug's action with the primary problem associated with glaucoma. **Reference:** Wilson, B. A., Shannon, M. T., & Shields, K. M. (2012). *Pearson nurse's drug guide 2012.* Upper Saddle River, NJ: Pearson Education, pp. 11–14, 134–137, 709–710, 1243–1245.

8 **Answer: 4** **Rationale:** Ophthalmic anesthetic agents block the blink reflex. Because the eye is at risk for injury, an eye patch is applied for protection. Priority is given to protecting the cornea from irritants, debris, and rubbing. Since the medication is local, the airway is not compromised. Hypersensitivity reactions are not related directly to administration of ophthalmic anesthesia. The anesthesia would not change body temperature. **Cognitive Level:** Analyzing **Client Need:** Pharmacological and Parenteral Therapies **Integrated Process:** Nursing Process: Planning **Content Area:** Pharmacology **Strategy:** The primary concept is safety. Correlate the function of the eyelid movement with risks to the client. **Reference:** Burke, K. M., Mohn-Brohn, El, & Eby, L. (2011). *Medical-surgical nursing care* (3rd ed.). Upper Saddle River, NJ: Pearson Education, p. 1025.

9 **Answer: 1** **Rationale:** Atropine sulfate is commonly used preoperatively in outpatient procedures such as a colonoscopy.

The client needs to alert the staff about the diagnosis of glaucoma, since the use of atropine is contraindicated in narrow-angle glaucoma because it causes mydriasis, which results in reduced drainage of aqueous humor. Discontinuing medications could result in a significant increase in intraocular pressure (IOP). The health care provider cannot perform the procedure if the intestines are not thoroughly cleansed. The client should provide agencies and health care providers with the client's medical history in the event of a threat to their health. **Cognitive Level:** Applying **Client Need:** Pharmacological and Parenteral Therapies **Integrated Process:** Nursing Process: Evaluation **Content Area:** Pharmacology **Strategy:** Correlate the risks associated with preparation for general anesthesia and the client who needs to take medication to control the increased intraocular pressure (IOP) of glaucoma. **Reference:** Adams, M., Holland, L., & Bostwick, P. (2011). *Pharmacology for nurses: A pathophysiologic approach* (3rd ed.). Upper Saddle River, NJ: Pearson Education, pp. 769–774.

10 **Answer: 1** **Rationale:** Sudden severe pain accompanied by nausea may likely indicate a complication. This needs attention rather than masking the symptoms with medication. The nurse should not just accept the information provided by this level of staff, but instead should follow up with an assessment. Positioning the client with the affected eye up promotes gas absorption. Placement on the abdomen promotes floating of the gas against the retina, holding it in place. **Cognitive Level:** Analyzing **Client Need:** Pharmacological and Parenteral Therapies **Integrated Process:** Nursing Process: Assessment **Content Area:** Pharmacology **Strategy:** The critical word in the question is *contraindicated.* Consider the risks of administering medications aimed at symptoms without proper baseline assessment to make the correct selection. **Reference:** Ignatavicius, D., & Workman, L. (2006). *Medical-surgical nursing: Critical thinking for collaborative care* (5th ed.). Philadelphia, PA: W. B. Saunders, p. 1103.

References

Abrams, A., Pennington, S., Lammon, C., Goldsmith, T. (2009). *Clinical drug therapy: Rationales for nursing practice* (9th ed.). Philadelphia, PA: Lippincott Williams & Wilkins.

Adams, M., Holland, L., & Bostwick, P. (2011). *Pharmacology for nurses: A pathophysiologic approach* (3rd ed.). Upper Saddle River, NJ: Pearson Education.

Aschenbrenner, D., & Venable, S. (2012). *Drug therapy in nursing* (4th ed.). Philadelphia, PA: Lippincott Williams & Wilkins.

Deglin, J., Vallerand, A. (2010). *Davis's drug guide for nurses* (12th ed.). Philadelphia, PA: F.A. Davis Company.

Drug Facts & Comparisons® (Updated monthly). St. Louis, MO: A. Wolters Kluwer.

Karch, A. M. (2010). *Focus on nursing pharmacology* (5th ed.). Philadelphia, PA: Lippincott Williams & Wilkins.

Kee, J. (2009). *Laboratory and diagnostic tests and nursing implications* (8th ed.). Upper Saddle River, NJ: Pearson Education.

Lehne, R. (2010). *Pharmacology for nursing care* (7th ed.). St. Louis, MO: Mosby, Inc.

LeMone, P., Burke, K., & Bauldoff, G. (2011). *Medical-surgical nursing: Critical thinking in patient care* (5th ed.). Upper Saddle River, NJ: Pearson Education.

Skidmore-Roth, L. (2012). *Mosby's 2012 nursing drug reference* (25th ed.). St. Louis, MO: Mosby (an affiliate of Elsevier, Inc.).

Wilson, B. A., Shannon, M. T., & Shields, K. M. (2012). *Pearson nurse's drug guide 2012.* Upper Saddle River, NJ: Pearson Education.

ANSWERS & RATIONALES

Herbal Agents

16

Chapter Outline

Overview of Phytomedicines   Specific Phytomedicines   Nursing Management

Objectives

➤ Define the terms commonly associated with the use of herbs as supplements.
➤ Describe the general goals of therapy when administering specific herbal supplements.
➤ Describe the uses and dosages of various herbs used as supplements.
➤ Identify the cautions associated with the use of specific herbal supplements, including adverse effects, contraindications, and drug interactions.
➤ List the key client teaching points related to the use of herbs as supplements.

NCLEX-RN® Test Prep

Use the accompanying online resource, NursingReviewsandRationales, to test yourself with hundreds of NCLEX®-style practice questions.

Review at a Glance

bulk unpackaged, loose body of plant used for tea or decoction

decoction liquid form of herb brewed from seeds, bark, and root; herb is covered with boiling water, and covered, boiled, simmered and then strained with water added for consumption

extract a solution or preparation containing active ingredient of herb made by pressing herb and then soaking it in alcohol or water, which is allowed to evaporate; usually, it is put in a small amount of water for use

phytomedicine therapeutic agents or preparations made or derived from plants or plant parts

phytotherapy science of using plant-based medicines to treat illness

standardization act of conforming to a basis of comparison in size, weight, quality, strength, or the like

tea a liquid preparation using fresh or dried herb; boiling water is poured over the herb and allowed to steep for a period of time

tincture liquid extracts of herb most often alcohol-based, used internally or externally, taken in drops in small amount of juice or water; glycerin-based extracts are available when alcohol should be avoided

PRETEST

1 When the client asks the nurse about a magazine advertisement related to the therapeutic use of ginger, the nurse should focus on which of the following?

1. Client's ability to accurately assess reliability of information sources
2. Author of the article
3. Type of magazine in which the advertisement was found
4. Client's level of education

2 When a female client taking feverfew to prevent migraine headaches suspects she may be pregnant, the nurse should take which most appropriate action?

1. Instruct client to discontinue use of the feverfew.
2. Encourage client to have a pregnancy test performed.
3. Arrange for client to see her health care provider.
4. Suggest that client reduce the dosage of the feverfew.

3 The nurse interprets that a client is able to safely self-administer valerian root as a sleep aid after hearing the client state which information about valerian?

1. It is best to take the drug on an empty stomach.
2. It should not be taken with benzodiazepine derivatives.
3. It may be used safely in children over the age of 5.
4. It is not effective in the capsule form.

4 A client weighing 150 lbs wants to verify she is taking a safe dose of bilberry. Since doses of greater than 1.5 grams/kg/day could be fatal, the nurse informs the client to avoid exceeding which dose per day? Record your answer rounding to two decimal places.

_____ grams

5 After it is determined that the hot flashes and night sweats are not related to any underlying disease process, the nurse should support a 50-year-old client's use of which herbal phytomedicine?

1. Echinacea
2. Black cohosh
3. Bilberry
4. Valerian

6 The nurse interprets that which of the following statements best indicates that a client possesses sufficient knowledge of the potential therapeutic effectiveness of garlic?

1. "The effectiveness of garlic is based on scientific research."
2. "Garlic may be used safely with ginger."
3. "There are no remedies for bad breath caused by garlic."
4. "I can take garlic safely with over-the-counter medications."

7 The nurse includes a discussion about hawthorn in a seminar for clients interested in the use of herbal remedies. Which of the following statements by the nurse would be most accurate?

1. "You may use hawthorn for acute episodes of chest pain or angina."
2. "Hawthorn may increase your heart rate."
3. "You should not take hawthorn while taking captopril (Capoten)."
4. "Hawthorn is known to produce the same effects as verapamil (Calan)."

8 To increase mental concentration and physical stamina, a client has been ingesting nutritional bars containing ginseng for the past 2 weeks. The nurse should instruct the client to do which of the following?

1. Avoid operating machinery or driving a car while taking the nutrition bar.
2. Refuse to take this form of the herb, since it is known to increase adverse effects.
3. Avoid use of the nutrition bar with coffee, tea, or cola.
4. Continue use of the nutrition bar daily as desired.

9 Because a client is taking St. John's wort capsules to treat mild depression, the nurse should use which of the following statements to provide the client with appropriate information? Select all that apply.

1. "You may need to switch to another form of the herb."
2. "One dose of the drug may remain in the body for up to 24 hours."
3. "It may take several weeks for the therapy to become effective."
4. "You may find that the drug helps your arthritis as well."
5. "St. John's wort may not be effective for your type of depression."

10 Prior to supporting a client's decision to select evening primrose to manage a long history of insomnia, the nurse decides to perform which of the following assessments?

1. Ability to swallow
2. History of a seizure disorder
3. Where client learned about this function of the drug
4. Review medical record for red blood cell (RBC) count

➤ *See pages 527–528 for Answers and Rationales.*

I. OVERVIEW OF PHYTOMEDICINES

A. General information
1. The Food and Drug Administration (FDA) classification of herbs is as dietary supplements
2. Other than **phytomedicine** (therapeutic agents or preparations made or derived from plants or plant parts), names for herbal therapies also include botanicals, nutraceuticals, and dietary supplements
3. Herbal supplements are not substitutes for conventional medicine
4. The science of using plant-based medicines to treat illness is called **phytotherapy**
5. Doses of herbs are not yet standardized in many countries other than Germany; dosage of herbs is according to product literature, although in most cases a research-based safe dose is yet to be determined

6. Most herbs, except ginger, are contraindicated during pregnancy and lactation
7. The pharmacologically active chemicals in herbal products may come form one specific plant part or all parts, including the leaves, stems, flowers, rhizomes, or roots

B. Popularity
1. They are increasing in popularity in Western world
2. This may be partially a result of Western culture movement toward a "back-to-nature" approach to living

C. Frequency of use
1. More than 28 million Americans report taking one or more herbal supplements
2. Primary users tend to be college-educated women between the ages of 35 and 49
3. Many people use herbal products in addition to a conventional treatment, rather than a replacement

D. USP (United States Pharmacopoeia) Verification Program
1. Manufacturer submits products for examination of ingredients
2. If product meets stringent standards of USP it may carry USP label, which verifies that the product has been manufactured under acceptable standards of purity, has been tested for active ingredients stated on label, and is free of harmful contaminants
3. USP label is not a guarantee product is safe or effective

II. SPECIFIC PHYTOMEDICINES

A. Bilberry (*Vaccinium myrtillus*, European blueberry, huckleberry, whortleberry)
1. Description
   a. Relative of blueberry and cranberry

      b. Shrub with small, sweet black berries

      c. Active ingredients: anthocyanoside (antioxidant bioflavonoid), pectin (soluble fiber)

      d. Stabilizes collagen activity

       e. Prevents production and release of compounds that promote inflammation, such as histamine and prostaglandins

       f. Relaxes smooth muscle in vasculature

      g. Inhibits platelet aggregation

      h. Reduces permeability and strengthens capillary wall membrane

  2. Uses

       a. Most commonly used for treatment of simple diarrhea

      b. Prevention and treatment of eye disorders: diabetic retinopathy, night blindness, macular degeneration, glaucoma, cataracts

      c. Diabetes mellitus

      d. Antioxidant

      e. Possible treatment of varicose veins, hemorrhoids

      f. Lowers cholesterol

      g. Cardiovascular problems

  3. Dosage

      a. Dosage varies considerably

      b. **Standardization** (act of conforming to a basis of comparison in size, weight, quality, strength, or the like) should contain 25% anthocyanoside

      c. 240–480 mg bid or tid of standardized **extract** (a solution or preparation containing active ingredient of herb made by pressing herb and then soaking it in alcohol or water, which is allowed to evaporate; usually, it is put in a small amount of water for use)

      d. 20–60 grams of dried fruit daily

   4. Cautions

      a. May increase coagulation time

      b. May interfere with iron absorption when taken internally

      c. Use cautiously with acetylsalicylic acid (aspirin), anticoagulants, vitamin E, fish oils, feverfew, garlic, ginger, ginkgo

      d. Contraindicated in pregnancy and lactation

      e. Avoid long-term large doses, doses over 1.5 grams/kg/day may be fatal, doses over 480 mg/day may be dangerous

B. **Black cohosh** (*Cimicifuga racemosa,* black snakeroot, bugroot, rattleweed, rattleroot, squawroot, cimifuga)

  1. Description

      a. Active ingredients: triperpenoid glycosides, isoflavonones, aglycones

      b. Binds to estrogen receptors

      c. Inhibits luteinizing hormone

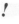   **d.** Apparent estrogen-like activity

  2. Uses

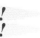   **a.** Primarily used to treat premenstrual syndrome (PMS) and postmenopausal symptoms

       b. Promotes labor of pregnancy

      c. Decreases blood pressure

      d. Treatment of snake bites

      e. Rheumatoid arthritis

      f. Recommended uses by herbalists: dysmenorrhea, antispasmodic, astringent, diuretic, expectorant, sedative

3. Dosage
   a. Research-based safe dosage yet to be determined
   b. 40 mg daily
   c. Possible stimulation of estrogen synthesis with 8 mg/day for 8 weeks
4. Cautions
   a. Contraindicated use with antihypertensives or hormone replacements
   b. May cause bradycardia, hypotension, joint pain
   c. Contraindicated in lactation
   d. Use in pregnancy only when birth is imminent to promote labor

C. **Chamomile** (*chamomilla recutita*)
   1. Description
      a. Derived from dried heads of German/Hungarian chamomile flower
      b. Flower heads and essential oil used
   2. Uses
      a. Commonly used as a mild sedative to aid in sleeping
      b. Antiflatulent and antispasmodic; often used to quiet GI spasms and upset
      c. Antimicrobial; may be useful for wound healing
      d. Anti-inflammatory
   3. Dosage
      a. Usually consumed in amounts of 1–4 cups daily as a **tea** (a liquid preparation using fresh or dried herb); boiling water is poured over the herb and allowed to steep for a period of time
      b. If taken by tablet, 400–1,600 mg daily
   4. Cautions
      a. Vomiting may occur with highly concentrated tea
      b. May increase bleeding if taken with antiplatelet agents, anticoagulants, NSAIDs
      c. **Tincture** (liquid extracts of herb most often alcohol-based, used internally or externally, taken in drops in small amount of juice or water) often contains valcohol; glycerin-based extracts are available when alcohol should be avoided
      d. Contraindicated in children, pregnancy, and lactation
      e. Do not use if allergic to asters, ragweed, or chrysanthemums; may cause severe allergic response

D. **Echinacea** (*Echinacea purpurea,* snake root, purple or American cone flower, sampson root, black sampson, hedgehog, survey root)
   1. Description
      a. Member of daisy family with 9 species
      b. Active ingredients: polysaccharides, alkylamides, flavonoids, caffeic acid derivatives (echinacosides), essential oils, and others
      c. Available in capsule, tablet, candle, glycerite, hydroalcoholic extract, fresh-pressed juice, lollipop, lozenge, tea, and tincture forms
      d. Activates T lymphocytes and intensifies phagocytosis of macrophages
      e. Stimulates tumor necrosis factor, interferon, and interleukin
      f. Nonspecific stimulation of immune system
      g. Stabilizes hyaluronic acid (a component of connective tissue) to protect cells and connective tissue from microorganism invasion and attack from free radicals
      h. Inhibits lipoxygenase to reduce inflammation
   2. Uses
      a. Most common: prevention or reduction of symptoms of cold or influenza
      b. Boost immune system and increase body's resistance to infection, particularly upper respiratory and urinary infection

    c. Treatment of herpes simplex and Candida infection

    d. Topically: improve wound healing, antioxidant protection from ultraviolet A and B light rays

  3. Dosage

    a. Standardized preparation should contain 3.5% echinacoside

    b. Available in capsule of powdered herb, expressed juice, tincture, water- or alcohol-based formula, fluid extract, solid extract, lozenge forms

    c. Dosage dependent on formula potency; varies according to source consulted

    d. Typically supplied in 380-mg capsules: 1–3 capsules tid at mealtime with water

    e. Regime should consist of 8 weeks on and 1 week off to reduce decreased effects with continued use

  4. Cautions

    a. Not to be used in presence of autoimmune disease (e.g., HIV/AIDS, collagen disease, multiple sclerosis (MS), tuberculosis), severe illness or allergy to sunflower or daisy family

    b. Not to be used with immunosuppressants (e.g., corticosteroids or cyclosporine)

    c. Prolonged use (longer than 8-week cycle) may cause hepatotoxicity and suppression of immune system

    d. Not to be used with other hepatotoxicants (e.g., anabolic steroids, amiodarone, methotrexate, antifungals such as ketoconazole)

    e. May influence fertility by spermatozoa enzyme interference

    f. Many tinctures contain large amounts of alcohol

    g. Contraindicated in alcoholism, children, pregnancy, and lactation

    h. Adverse effects: allergic reaction and anaphylaxis

  5. Herb-to-drug interactions

    a. Amiodarone

    b. Anabolic steroids

    c. Ketoconazole

    d. Methotrexate

E. Feverfew (*Tanacetum parthenium*, bachelor's button, febrifuge plant, feather few, feather foil)

  1. Description

    a. Short, bushy perennial; member of daisy family with yellow flowers and yellow-green leaves resembling chamomile

    b. Active ingredients: sesquiterpene lactones, especially parthenolide, essential oils

    c. Suppresses secretion of granules in platelets and neutrophils to inhibit platelet aggregation

    d. May suppress production of prostaglandins (thromboxane, leukotriene)

    e. Inhibits release of serotonin

  2. Uses

    a. Principle use: prevent recurrent migraine headaches, treat arthritis

    b. Relief of menstrual pain

    c. Asthma

    d. Dermatitis, psoriasis

    e. Antipyretic (promotes diaphoresis)

  3. Dosage

    a. Dosage varies according to source consulted

    b. Standardized preparation should contain 0.2% parthenolide

    c. Available in freeze-dried leaf, dried plant part, capsules, infusion

    d. Supplied in 380-mg capsules containing pure leaf and 250-mg capsules of leaf extract

    e. Most sources recommend anywhere from 50–125 mg of dried herb taken with or after meals to reduce GI colic

    f. Migraine: 0.25–0.5 mg to prevent attack; 1–2 grams to control attack

    g. May chew one fresh or frozen leaf/day to obtain dose, but may cause mouth sores or gastric distress

    h. Infusion: ½ to 1 tsp of herb in 1 cup boiling water, steep for 5–10 minutes, 2 cups daily

4. Cautions

    a. Long-term studies not done

    b. Contraindicated in pregnancy, lactation, and under age 2 years

    c. Cross allergy to ragweed

    d. Adverse effects: allergic reaction, lip and tongue swelling, mouth ulcers, abdominal colic, palpitations, increased menstrual flow

    e. Sudden withdrawal may cause post feverfew syndrome (muscles aches, pain, and stiffness); taper off to discontinue

    f. Other proven (conventional) remedies for relief of migraine should be used first

    g. May interfere with blood-clotting mechanism; not to be used with bilberry, garlic, ginger, ginkgo

    h. Discontinue use prior to surgery or dental extractions to reduce risk of bleeding

    i. Feverfew is known to cause rebound headaches

5. Herb-to-drug interactions that increase risk of bleeding: aspirin, heparin, nonsteroidal anti-inflammatory drugs (NSAIDs), warfarin, or other anticoagulants

F. Garlic (*Allium sativum*, stinking root or rose, nectar of the gods, camphor of the poor, poor man's treacle, rustic treacle)

1. Description

    a. Empirical support for effectiveness and use; most widely researched herb

    b. Active ingredients: (23 constituents), allicin (odorless, sulfur-containing amino acid), ajoene

    c. Should be crushed or bruised to effectively convert various enzymes, protein, lipids, amino acids, and other ingredients to active ingredient, allicin

    d. Allicin and ajoene are not found in dried garlic, but may be present if dried at low temperatures or taken in enteric-coated tablets

    e. Inhibits platelet aggregation

    f. Well-documented research shows that it inhibits metabolism of cholesterol, leading to reduction of cholesterol

    g. Increases bile acid secretion

2. Uses

    a. Principle use: reduce cholesterol (decreases triglycerides, low-density lipoproteins, increases high-density lipoproteins)

    b. Principle use: treatment of mild hypertension

    c. Reduce risk of stroke

    d. Antibacterial, antiviral, antifungal

    e. Anticancer properties

    f. Lower blood glucose

    g. Lay use: antihelminthic, antispasmodic, diuretic, carminative (relieves flatulence, digestant, expectorant, topical antibiotic)

3. Dosage

    a. Available in dried powder, fresh bulb, tablets (allicin total potential), tablets (garlic extract), antiseptic oil, fresh extract, freeze-dried garlic powder, garlic oil (essential oil)

    b. Commercial preparation not standardized; should deliver minimum of 10 mg daily or 5,000 mcg of total allicin potential

    c. A high dose of garlic can lead to GI problems

4. Cautions
   a. Avoid large amounts of garlic with other herbs affecting coagulation (bilberry, feverfew, ginger, ginkgo)
   b. May potentiate antidiabetic drugs
   c. Adverse effects: contact dermatitis, vertigo, garlic breath, hypothyroidism, GI irritation, nausea and vomiting with large doses
   d. Enteric-coated tablets containing powdered form may reduce bad breath, but are not as potent as raw garlic
   e. Contraindicated in pregnancy, GI (peptic ulcer disease and GERD), and bleeding disorders
   f. Chronic use may lower hemoglobin levels
   g. When used to decrease cholesterol levels, plan should be monitored by the health care provider
5. Herb-to-drug interactions
   a. Aspirin, NSAIDs, warfarin, or other anticoagulants (increased risk of bleeding)
   b. Insulin or oral antidiabetic agents (enhanced hypoglycemic effect)

Practice to Pass

Name 3 types of phytomedicines that are contraindicated in the client with a history of hemorrhagic stroke.

G. **Ginger** (*Zingiber officinal,* Jamaica ginger, African ginger, Cochin ginger, black ginger, race ginger)
   1. Description
      a. Green-purple flower resembling the orchid
      b. Active ingredient: sesquiterpenes, aromatic ketones (gingerols), and volatile oils
      c. Inhibits thromboxane production to enhance effects of anticoagulation
      d. Inhibits leukotrienes and prostaglandins to produce anti-inflammatory and analgesic effect
   2. Usage
      a. Principle use: antiemetic, improve appetite, treatment of motion sickness, vertigo
      b. Diuretic, digestion aid, dyspepsia
      c. Anti-inflammatory in treatment of rheumatoid arthritis and osteoarthritis
      d. Relief of muscle pain
      e. Antitumor, antioxidant, antimicrobial
   3. Dosage
      a. Dosage depends on use—consensus varies
      b. Available in capsules, liquid, powder extract, root, chewable tablets, tea, candied form
      c. Most commonly available in 500-mg capsules of powdered form
      d. Antiemetic: 500–1,000 mg in 4 divided doses/day of powdered ginger
      e. Dyspepsia, diuretic, vertigo: 2–4 grams/day in divided doses or 2 cups tea with 1 tsp fresh ginger root each or 15 tsp powdered ginger or two 1-inch squares of candied ginger that may be repeated every 4 hours as needed
      f. Antiemetic: 1–2 grams in 2 divided doses
      g. Motion sickness: 1 gram 30 minutes before traveling and 0.5–1 gram every 4 hours as needed during trip (most effective when regimen started several days before traveling)
   4. Cautions
      a. Adverse effects: headache, anxiety, insomnia, elevated blood pressure, tachycardia, asthma attack, postmenopausal bleeding
      b. Contraindicated in postoperative nausea caused by increased risk of bleeding
      c. Not to be used concomitantly with bilberry, feverfew, garlic, or ginkgo (increased risk of bleeding)
      d. Severe overdose: possible CNS depression and cardiac arrhythmias
      e. Dose in excess of 6 grams/day results in gastric irritation and ulcer formation

  f. Conflicting data related to safe use during pregnancy (relatively safe according to FDA); contraindicated in treatment of hyperemesis gravidarum

  g. Discontinue use 2 weeks before surgery or dental extractions

 5. Herb-to-drug interactions (increased risk of bleeding): aspirin, heparin, NSAIDs, warfarin, or other anticoagulants

H. Ginkgo (*Ginkgo biloba,* EGB 761, GBE, GBX, Tebonin, Tebofortan, Ginkogink)

 1. Description

  a. Active ingredients: flavone glycosides, flavonoids, terpene lactones (such as ginkgolides and bilobalide)

  b. Ginkgo biloba extract referred to as GBE

  c. Flavonoids act as antioxidants by destroying lipid layer of cell membrane

  d. Flavone glycosides produce mild platelet aggregation

  e. Ginkgolides antagonize platelet-activating factor to decrease coagulation

  f. Bilobalide increases cerebral circulation to improve tissue perfusion and increase memory

  g. Protects brain from effects of hypoxia

 2. Uses

  a. Cerebrovascular insufficiency and symptomatic relief of organic brain dysfunction to improve short-term memory loss

  b. Peripheral vascular disease (e.g., Raynaud disease, intermittent claudication), varicosities

  c. Senile macular degeneration

  d. Treatment of age-related mental decline related to short-term memory loss, poor concentration

  e. Treatment of depression-related cognitive disorders

  f. Treatment of depression in older adults particularly that are related to chronic cerebrovascular deficiency not responding to standard drug therapy

  g. Tinnitus, vertigo

  h. Improvement of symptoms of early-stage senility of Alzheimer's type

 3. Dosage

  a. Standardization should contain 24% flavonoids and 6% terpenes

  b. Available in capsule or tablet form containing 40 mg GBE, nutrition bars, sublingual sprays, tablets, concentrated alcohol extract of fresh leaf

  c. Treatment of vascular disorders, tinnitus or vertigo: 120–160 mg/day in 2 or 3 divided doses

  d. Treatment of dementia: 120–140 mg/day in 2 or 3 divided doses

 4. Cautions

  a. Effects may not be apparent for 4–8 weeks

  b. Not to be used concomitantly with bilberry, feverfew, garlic, ginger, or other anti-coagulants, such as ASA (aspirin) or warfarin (Coumadin)

  c. Avoid use of unprocessed ginkgo leaves that contain allergens related to urushiol, the chemical responsible for the itch in poison ivy

  d. Crude, dried leaf or tea may not contain sufficient active ingredients to be effective

  e. Large doses may cause restlessness, headache, nausea, vomiting, diarrhea

  f. Edible solid form sold in Asian shops should be kept out of reach of children as seeds may cause seizures

  g. Avoid use in pregnancy, lactation, children

 5. Herb-to-drug interactions

  a. Aspirin or NSAIDs

  b. Heparin, warfarin, or other anticoagulant

        c. Monoamine oxidase inhibitors (MAOIs)

        d. Tricyclic antidepressants (TCAs)

I. **Ginseng, Korean** (*Panax ginseng,* American ginseng)

   1. Description

      a. Active ingredients: triterpenoid saponin glycosides (ginsenosides, panaxosides)

      b. Possible effect on pituitary gland with action similar to corticosteroids

      c. Improves glycosylated hemoglobin (HbA1c) and amino terminal propeptide (PIIINP) concentrations

      d. Hypertensive effect with low doses, hypotensive effect with higher doses

      e. Improves serum cholesterol and triglyceride levels

   2. Uses

      a. Most common: counteract effects of physical and mental fatigue

      b. Improve stamina and concentration in healthy individuals

      c. Treatment of chronic hepatotoxicity related to alcohol and drug ingestion

      d. Improve body's ability to resist stress and disease, increase vitality

      e. Regulation of blood pressure

      f. Improve psychomotor performance (attention, auditory reaction time)

      g. Reduce serum cholesterol and triglyceride levels

      h. Regulation of blood glucose levels in type 2 diabetes mellitus

      i. Aphrodisiac

      j. Adjunct in cancer chemotherapy or radiation therapy

   3. Dosage

      a. Depends on species and strength

      b. Confirmation of standards varies according to source

      c. Available in capsule, extract, root powder, tea, cream, eye gel, nutrition bar, oil, **bulk** (unpackaged, loose body of plant used for tea or decoction); a **decoction** is a term referring to a liquid form of herb brewed from seeds, bark, and root; herb is covered with boiling water, and covered, boiled, simmered, and then strained with water added for consumption

      d. Little consensus on dosing with wide variations, but universal acceptance of ginseng-free period; dosing should be spaced at intervals (e.g., 2–3 weeks on, 12 weeks off)

      e. 0.5–1 gram in two divided doses for 2–3 weeks, 1–2 weeks off

      f. Best taken in morning, 2 hours before meal, not less than 2 hours after meal

   4. Cautions

      a. Most side effects reported related to excessive or inappropriate use

      b. Avoid concomitant use with stimulants (e.g., coffee, tea, cola)

      c. May potentiate MAOI actions

      d. Adverse effects: insomnia, palpitations, pruritus

   5. Herb-to-drug interactions

      a. CNS depressants

      b. Digoxin

      c. Diuretics

      d. Insulin or oral antidiabetic agents

      e. MAOIs

      f. Warfarin or other anticoagulants

J. **Ginseng, Siberian** (*Eleutherococcus senticosus,* five fingers, tartar root, Western ginseng, seng and sang, Asian ginseng, Jintsam)

   1. Description

      a. Active ingredients: eutherosides

      b. Pharmacologic actions not well understood

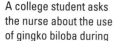

Practice to Pass

A college student asks the nurse about the use of gingko biloba during exam week to enhance performance on exams. What client education is necessary?

    c. Elevates lymphocyte count (T cells), boosts immune system

  2. Uses

    a. Enhance physical and mental performance under stress

    b. Improve athletic performance

    c. Increase oxygen metabolism, work capacity, and exhaustion time in variety of illnesses (e.g., atherosclerosis, diabetes, chronic bronchitis)

    d. Stimulate WBC production in clients undergoing antineoplastic therapy

  3. Dosage

    a. Little consensus on dosing with wide variations, but general consensus on ginseng-free period of 2–3 weeks every 4–8 weeks

    b. 0.6–3 grams daily

  4. Cautions

    a. Adverse reactions: hypertension, tachycardia, insomnia, and irritability

    b. Contraindicated in pregnancy, lactation, premenopausal women, hypertension, CNS stimulants, or antipsychotic medications

K. Glucosamine and chondroitin (glucosamine extracted from skeletons of crustaceans and other arthropods and synthetically; chondroitin extracted from shark or beef cartilage, bovine trachea, or synthetic)

  1. Description

    a. Compounds found in healthy cartilage and synovial fluid

    b. Ingredients may be taken separately but most often used jointly

    c. Helps slow cartilage degradation in osteoarthritis

    d. Improves pain and movement in osteoarthritis and temporomandibular joint (TMJ)

  2. Uses

    a. Osteoarthritis, TMJ

    b. Venous insufficiency, leg pain

    c. Inflammatory bowel disease, rheumatoid arthritis

    d. Chondroitin used to help with bladder control in interstitial cystitis, overactive bladder, and unstable bladder

  3. Dosage

    a. Glucosamine—1,000–1,500 mg/day

    b. Chondroitin—800–1,200 mg/day

  4. Cautions

    a. Avoid use in pregnancy and lactation

    b. Higher doses of glucosamine may be needed if taking diuretics

    c. Use with caution in kidney disease, diabetes, bleeding disorders, or if taking drugs that affect bleeding times

    d. Adverse effects: well tolerated; may cause GI upset, drowsiness, or insomnia

L. Hawthorn (*Crataegus oxyacantha*, Mayblossom, Maybush, whitehorn, LI 132)

  1. Description

    a. Small to medium tree of several species; leaves, flowers, berries (fruit) are used in standardized extracts

    b. Active ingredients: flavonoids, primarily procyanidins and proanthocyanidins

    c. Acts as antioxidant that decreases damage by free radicals to cardiovascular system by increasing levels of vitamin C intracellularly

    d. Increases coronary and myocardial circulation

    e. Decreases peripheral vascular resistance to decrease blood pressure

    f. Increases strength of myocardial contraction (positive inotropic effect) and decreases heart rate (negative chronotropic effect)

    g. Angiotensin-converting enzyme (ACE) activity that prevents conversion of angiotensin I to angiotensin II, a potent vasoconstrictor

       h. Decreases total plasma cholesterol and low-density lipoprotein (LDL) levels

       i. Improves cardiac function in clients with chronic angina and those with early congestive heart failure

2. Uses

       a. Treatment of mild hypertension

       b. Treatment of athero- and arteriosclerosis

       c. Treatment (prevention) of chronic angina: not intended for acute angina

       d. Treatment of early congestive heart failure

3. Dosage

       a. Standardized preparation should contain 18.75% oligomeric procyanidins and 2.2% flavonoids

       b. Available in extract, berry capsule, leaf capsule, extended-release capsule, dried fruit, tincture

       c. Dried fruit: 0.2–1 gram tid

       d. Liquid extract (1:1 in 25% alcohol): 0.5–1 mL tid

       e. Tincture (1:5 in 45% alcohol): 1–2 mL tid or 20–40 drops tid

4. Cautions

       a. Contraindicated with concomitant use of prescription antihypertensives or nitrates

       b. Supervision of health care provider necessary for those with existing cardiac disease

       c. May interfere with digoxin pharmacodynamics and monitoring

       d. Adverse effects: nausea, fatigue, perspiration and cutaneous eruption of the hands, increased CNS depression and sedation

       e. Contraindicated in pregnancy and lactation

5. Herb-to-drug interactions (drug effect)

       a. Digoxin additive

       b. ACE inhibitors

M. Milk thistle (*Silybum marianum,* Mary thistle, Marian thistle, Lady's thistle, Holy thistle, silymarin, the "liver herb")

1. Description

       a. Tall plant, prickly leaves, milky sap, member of daisy family

       b. Active ingredients: silymarin and its component silybinin to act as hepatoprotectant

       c. Promotes glutathione production, a powerful endogenous antioxidant

       d. Binds to hepatocyte membrane to block uptake of toxins into liver cell

       e. Stimulates nucleolar polymerase A activity to promote new liver cell growth

       f. Stimulates regeneration of liver by stimulating protein synthesis

       g. Inhibits action of leukotriene by Kupffer cells

       h. Binds to site on liver cell membrane, blocking availability for attack from phalloidin, the toxin in death cap mushroom

       i. Stabilizes liver cell membrane by decreasing turnover rate of phospholipids

2. Uses

       a. Reduces hepatotoxicity related to psychoactive drugs such as phenothiazines

       b. Adjunct therapy in liver inflammation related to cirrhosis, hepatitis, and fatty infiltrate related to alcohol or other toxins

       c. Treatment of overdose of death cap mushroom

3. Dosage

       a. Available in capsule, tablet, extract, and 200 mg concentrated seed extract equal to 140 mg silymarin

       b. 140 mg tid (dosage varies according to source)

       c. Standardization should contain at least 70–80% silymarin

 4. Cautions

   a. Insoluble in water, not to be taken in tea form

   b. Avoid alcohol-based extract in decompensated cirrhosis

 ! **c.** Cross allergy to ragweed

   d. Adverse effects: loose stools, diarrhea in high doses

   e. Contraindicated in pregnancy and lactation

   f. Close monitoring by health care provider in presence of active liver disease

N. Saw palmetto (*Serenoa repens,* sabal, American dwarf palm tree, LSESR)

 1. Description

   a. Shrublike palm tree with red–brown-black berries

   b. Active ingredients: saturated and unsaturated fatty acids and sterols from berries (liposterolic acid)

 ! **c.** Reduces action of 5-alpha-reductase enzyme that converts testosterone to dihydrotestosterone (DHT) in aging (effects similar to finasteride [Proscar] with fewer side effects)

 ! **d.** No effect on prostatic-specific antigen

   e. May reverse testicular and mammary gland atrophy

   f. May increase sperm production and increase sexual vigor

 2. Uses

   a. Symptomatic treatment of benign prostatic hyperplasia (BPH)

 ! **b.** Helps initiate urine stream, decreases urinary frequency, residual volumes, nocturia, dysuria; unclear whether actual prostatic size is reduced

   c. Lay uses: treatment of asthma, bronchitis, treatment of gynecomastia

 3. Dosage

   a. Standardized extract should contain 85–95% fatty acids and sterols

   b. Mild to moderate BPH: 160 mg standardized liposterolic acid twice/day with meals to decrease GI distress OR 1–2 grams fresh berry **decoction** OR 0.5–1 gram dried berry PO tid

 4. Cautions

   a. Long-term use with approximately 6 weeks for initial effects

   b. Insoluble in water, not to be taken in tea form

   c. Adverse effects: nausea, abdominal pain, hypertension, headache, diarrhea with large doses

 ! **d.** May interfere with iron absorption

 ! **e.** Supervision by health care provider necessary for diagnosed BPH

   f. Do not take with estrogen or hormone replacement

 5. Herb-to-drug information: finasteride (enhanced effect)

O. Red yeast rice (fermented rice, which obtains its color from cultivation with the mold *Monascus purpureus*)

 1. Description

   a. Inhibits action of HMG CoA reductase in liver

   b. Lowers total cholesterol, high-density lipid (HDL) cholesterol, and triglycerides

   c. Contains the substance monacolin K, the same substance contained in prescription drug lovastatin

 2. Uses

   a. Hyperlipidemia, elevated cholesterol and triglyceride levels

   b. Coronary heart disease, circulation

   c. Diabetes mellitus

 3. Dosage: 1,200 mg twice a day with food

 4. Cautions

   a. Do not take in conjunction with prescription cholesterol-lowering medications

   b. Contraindicated in liver disease

Practice to Pass

What phytomedicine is known as the liver herb? Why?

    c. Grapefruit juice may elevate drug levels

    d. Adverse effects: gastritis, abdominal pain, headache, muscle pain

    e. Increased risk of rhabdomyolysis if taken with cyclosporine, ranitidine, and some antibiotics

  5. Herb-to-drug interactions (drug effect)

    a. Additive effect may occur with benzodiazepines and barbiturates

    b. Altered drug levels can occur with thyroid medications, digoxin, St. John's wort, vitamin A, and coenzyme Q10

P. St. John's wort (*Hypericum perforatum,* amber, goat weed, touch-and-heal, St. John's wort, witch's herb, klamath weed, chasse-diable, devil's scourge)

  1. Description

    a. Yellow perennial flower with red pigmented leaves containing small black dots

    b. Active ingredient: hypericin from red pigment leaves, pseudohypericin and flavonoids, tannin, and others

    c. Inhibits reuptake of serotonin

    d. Low MAOI

    e. Actions not well determined or understood

    f. Effects comparable to imipramine (Tofranil)

    g. Produces fewer side effects than prescription antidepressants

  2. Uses

    a. Treatment of mild to moderate depression

    b. Not intended for treatment of suicidal ideation, psychotic behavior, or severe depression

    c. Possible antibacterial, antiviral, wound-healing properties

  3. Dosage

    a. Standardization should contain 0.14–0.3% hypericin

    b. Available in capsule, sublingual, dried plant, oil, tea, liquid tincture, topical cream

    c. Depression: capsules—300 mg tid; tincture—40–80 drops tid; tea—1–2 cups a.m. and p.m. with 1–2 heaping tsp dried herb per cup (steeped for 10 minutes); therapy should continue for 4–6 weeks

  4. Cautions

    a. Not to be used concomitantly with prescription antidepressants, especially selective serotonin reuptake inhibitors (SSRI) or MAOIs or foods containing tyramine (such as aged cheese, smoked meats, liver, figs, dried or cured fish, yeast, beer, Chianti wine)

    b. Not to be used concomitantly with opioids, amphetamines, OTC cold and flu preparations

    c. May inhibit absorption of iron

    d. Adverse effects (may continue for 2–4 weeks): GI distress, emotional vulnerability, fatigue, pruritus, weight gain, headache, dizziness, restlessness

    e. May cause photosensitivity; avoid sun exposure, especially if fair skinned

    f. May decrease digoxin levels

    g. Contraindicated in pregnancy, lactation, and children

  5. Herb-to-drug interactions

    a. CNS depressants or opioid analgesics

    b. Cyclosporine

    c. MAOIs

    d. Efavirenz or protease inhibitors (antivirals)

    e. Antidepressants: TCAs or SSRIs

    f. Reserpine

    g. Theophylline

    h. Warfarin or other anticoagulants

Practice to Pass

What are some other names used to identify St. John's wort?

Q. Valerian root (*valeriana officinalis,* wild valerian, garden heliotrope, setwall, capon's tail, all-heal, Amantilla, Baldrian wurzel, benedicta)

  1. Description
   a. Tall perennial with hollow stem, leaves, and white or red flowers
   b. Active ingredients: valepotriates and sesquiterpene derivatives, valeric acid, valeranone, and others
   c. Binds weakly to gamma aminobutyric acid (GABA) receptor sites to decrease CNS activity, causing sedation with decreased side effects
   d. Action similar to benzodiazepines, but nonaddicting, nondependence, no morning hangover
  2. Uses
   a. Sedative, reduction of anxiety
   b. Treatment of insomnia
   c. Adjunct therapy for benzodiazepine withdrawal
   d. Possible antispasmodic
  3. Dosage
   a. Standardization should contain minimum of 0.5–0.8 valerenic acid or 0.8% valeric acid; tincture should contain 2% essential oils
   b. Available in capsule, tablet tincture, tea
   c. Composition and purity vary widely
   d. Insomnia: 150–500 mg of root extract one-half hour before bedtime or as tea with 1 tsp dried root per cup; repeat dose 2 to 3 times if needed
   e. Anxiety: 200–300 mg each a.m.
  4. Cautions
   a. Valepotriate (which may be carcinogenic) should be removed from final product
   b. Not to be used concomitantly with other sedative/hypnotics, anxiolytics, or antidepressants
   c. May be used safely while operating machinery or car, although CNS effects should be monitored
   d. Sedation not increased with alcohol use, although caution should be exercised
   e. Adverse effects: headache, mild, temporary upset stomach
   f. Adverse effects with overdose or long-term use (overdose with 2.5 grams): excitability, insomnia, cardiac dysfunction, blurred vision, hepatotoxicity, severe headache, morning headache, nausea
   g. May cause hepatotoxicity; monitor liver function and avoid use in hepatic dysfunction
   h. Extract contains 40–60% alcohol; avoid use in those with alcoholism
   i. Contraindicated in pregnancy and lactation
  5. Herb-to-drug interactions (additive sedation): barbiturates, benzodiazepines, and CNS depressants

III. NURSING MANAGEMENT

A. General assessment
  1. Physical exam
   a. Vital signs, height, weight, lung sounds
   b. Depending on herb, liver, and kidney function status
  2. History
   a. Age
   b. Comorbid diseases
   c. Allergies, including food and others
   d. Use of prescription, over-the-counter medications, and phytomedicines, all to be entered into client's health record

    e. Cultural beliefs that may be related to race or ethnicity

    f. Pregnancy (or potential) and lactation

B. Principles of herbal administration

  1. General use

    a. Not intended for acute illness episodes or long-term therapy

    b. Appropriate as adjunct to conventional Western therapies

    c. Therapeutic effectiveness is slower than prescription medications; may take as long as several weeks, depending on herb

    d. Many herbs available in multiple forms, including teas, extracts, tinctures, capsules or tablets containing powdered or freeze-dried forms of herb

    e. Most herbs possess multiple uses, such as skin wash, gargle, compress, lotion, and eye bath

    f. They are not intended to replace healthy lifestyle

    g. Safe use in pregnancy and lactation is either contraindicated or unknown and may dry up breast milk during lactation

    h. Although they may be effective in children, phytomedicines should be avoided in acute, sudden onset illness

    i. Many interact with other herbs, food, and prescription medications

  2. Government regulation

    a. Dietary Supplement Health and Education Act (DSHEA) of 1994 defines herbs as dietary supplements

    b. Not defined as medicines, herbs cannot make therapeutic claims, only how they affect structure and function of human body

    c. Food and Drug Administration (FDA) does not regulate use of phytomedicines in United States but approves certain ones for their action on body (how they affect structure and function)

    d. FDA does not monitor herbs for their quality, composition, or preparation

    e. Formulations vary in their potency and recommended dosage with frequent lack of consensus on dosing

    f. The National Center for Complementary and Alternative Medicine (NCCAM), under National Institute of Health (NIH), is the main research component in the government on phytomedicine

  3. Safety, labeling, and purity

    a. Container labels must carry a disclaimer stating FDA does not evaluate product for treating, curing, or preventing disease

    b. Labels should contain specific directions for dosing and use

    c. Only the standardized extract, when available, should be used

    d. Not all phytomedicines have empirical support for their safety and efficacy

    e. Much of the research and standardization originates in Europe, where use of phytomedicine is popular, particularly in Germany

    f. Many herbs contain toxic substances (e.g., arnica, belladonna, hemlock, lily of the valley, and sassafras)

    g. Health care providers should report all adverse effects of phytomedicines to FDA

C. Client education

  1. Need for a complete history and physical before starting any therapy with herbs

  2. Phytomedicines are not effective for or to be used for acute illness or episodes

  3. Phytomedicines take longer to work than prescription medications, usually weeks

  4. Report use of all herbs to health care provider

  5. Start with one herb at a time, at lower than recommended doses, and closely monitor response

Practice to Pass

The client asks the nurse about safe use of phytomedicines. What should the nurse tell the client regarding what to look for on the container label?

6. Know particular use, dosing, and safe administration of each herb and take only as directed

!   7. Herbs may cause allergic reactions and adverse effects; if these occur, discontinue herb and report symptoms to health care provider

8. Become familiar with all herb–herb, herb–drug, and herb–food interactions

9. Purchase herbs from a reputable source and be aware of where and how herb was processed

10. Purchase standardized form of herbs, if possible

11. "Natural" or "all natural" does not equate with herb safety or efficacy

12. Become familiar with many various names by which particular herbs are identified

!   13. Avoid use of phytomedicines in pregnancy (potential for pregnancy), lactation, and in children

14. Accurately assess advertising claims; provide reputable sources of information, including referrals to the following resources on the internet: American Botanical Council, Herb Research Foundation, and National Center for Complementary and Alternative Therapy

Case Study

A 30-year-old female visits the health care provider's office with reports of migraine headaches. Vital signs reveal BP 118/76, pulse 82, respirations 18. She denies any allergies to medications. She states her neighbor takes feverfew with good results for relief of her headaches.

1. What other assessment data is necessary for the nurse to gather related to the possible use of the feverfew?

2. What client teaching should be done regarding the dosage of feverfew?

3. What are the pharmacologic actions of feverfew?

4. What client teaching is needed regarding discontinuation of the feverfew?

5. What over-the-counter (OTC) medications or herbs should the client be instructed to avoid?

For suggested responses, see page 546.

POSTTEST

1. Which nursing diagnosis is *most* significant when the nurse is assessing a client newly diagnosed with chronic renal failure (CRF) who is ingesting saw palmetto?

1. Risk for Injury
2. Disturbed Sleep Pattern
3. Impaired Skin Integrity
4. Risk for Imbalanced Nutrition: Less than Body Requirements

2. The nurse would interpret that glucosamine and chondroitin have met the intended therapeutic outcomes after assessing which of the following in a client?

1. Relief of signs and symptoms of osteoarthritis
2. Reduced severity of GI disturbances such as nausea, vomiting, and bloating
3. Reduction of hair loss and constipation
4. Decreased manifestations of anxiety disorder

POSTTEST

3 A client who uses fresh ginger for nausea does not like using kitchen spoons since they are not universal in size. The nurse provides the client with a medicine cup and instructs client to fill to which mL line for a single dose of ginger? Record your answer rounding to a single number.

_____ mL

4 Which appropriate information should be included in the home health nurse's notes in the health record of a client ingesting ginkgo biloba? Select all that apply.

1. Informed client to be alert for unexpected bleeding.
2. Informed client that ibuprofen decreases its effects.
3. Depression has improved since ingestion of ginkgo was initiated.
4. Instructed client to inform surgeon of long-term ingestion of the drug.
5. Informed client that drug is a potent enhancer of platelet activating factor.

5 The nurse would document which of the following predicted outcomes in a care plan for a client using St. John's wort?

1. "Client is aware of the need to cease bowling activities."
2. "Client demonstrated knowledge of the need to wear protective clothing and apply sunscreen."
3. "Client able to select foods high in tyramine from a list as preferred to foods low in tyramine."
4. "Client aware of the need to select a designated driver when ingesting alcoholic beverages with the drug."

6 Which of the following client behaviors is most indicative of a client's acceptance of the nurse's instructions before beginning the use of saw palmetto?

1. Requests that the assigned health care provider order liver function tests
2. Agrees to not ingest ibuprofen or aspirin concurrently
3. Agrees to not ingest laxatives or stool softeners concurrently
4. Requests that the assigned health care provider order a prostate-specific antigen (PSA)

7 Since a client is ingesting red yeast rice, the nurse should perform which follow-up activity?

1. Assess the client for heavy menstrual bleeding.
2. Make sure drug has been discontinued because of abortifacient properties.
3. Monitor the client for excessive bruising or bleeding.
4. Determine that the client is not taking any prescription cholesterol-lowering medications

8 The nurse instructs the client taking valerian root to avoid the use of which of the following medications?

1. Estrogen
2. Alprazolam (Xanax)
3. Digoxin (Lanoxin)
4. Aspirin

9 The nurse informs a client diagnosed with increased intraocular pressure (IOP) that use of which phytomedicine may decrease IOP?

1. Glucosamine chondroitin
2. Black cohosh
3. Aloe
4. Bilberry

10 Which of the following nursing diagnoses is most appropriate for the client ingesting chamomile?

1. Risk for Constipation
2. Disturbed Sleep Pattern
3. Ineffective Breathing Pattern
4. Impaired Gas Exchange

➤ *See pages 528–529 for Answers and Rationales.*

ANSWERS & RATIONALES

Pretest

1 **Answer: 1** **Rationale:** Because the herbal industry is not as highly regulated as traditional remedies, the focus should be on the client's ability to assess the reliability of the information source. Inability to use discretion could place the client at risk. The ability to make appropriate decisions about resources would include examining the author, the type of magazine, and the client's level of education. **Cognitive Level:** Analyzing **Client Need:** Pharmacological and Parenteral Therapies **Integrated Process:** Nursing Process: Assessment **Content Area:** Pharmacology **Strategy:** The wording of the question tells you that the correct option is likely to be one that is a broad statement rather than one that is narrow in focus. Evaluate each option, choosing the one that encompasses the other options within it. **Reference:** Adams, M. P., & Koch, R. W. (2010). *Pharmacology: Connections to nursing practice* (1st ed.). Upper Saddle River, NJ: Pearson Education, p. 1013.

2 **Answer: 1** **Rationale:** Regardless of the drug, avoiding the use of chemicals of any kind is a common underlying principle of management of the pregnant client. Reducing the dosage is insufficient. The client should not take any further doses of the herb unless it is determined that the client is not pregnant, but the pregnancy test itself is of lesser priority than immediately discontinuing the herb. **Cognitive Level:** Applying **Client Need:** Pharmacological and Parenteral Therapies **Integrated Process:** Nursing Process: Implementation **Content Area:** Pharmacology **Strategy:** The core issue of the question is knowledge that the use of the herb could be hazardous to the fetus during pregnancy. Consider that the primary concern is for the safety of the fetus to guide your selection. **Reference:** Lilley, L. L., Rainforth Collins, S., Harrington, S., & Snyder, J. (2011). *Pharmacology and the nursing practice* (6th ed.). St. Louis, MO: Mosby, Inc., p. 171.

3 **Answer: 2** **Rationale:** Since valerian root actions are similar to benzodiazepine and lorazepam is a benzodiazepine derivative, they should not be taken together. There is no evidence supporting the herb's safe use in children or of a relationship between the form of the herb and its effectiveness. **Cognitive Level:** Applying **Client Need:** Pharmacological and Parenteral Therapies **Integrated Process:** Nursing Process: Evaluation **Content Area:** Pharmacology

Strategy: Consider that medications and herbs should not be combined to eliminate one option. Next, eliminate a second option because the literature does not provide evidence of safe use of this herb in children. Apply knowledge of safe use of this herb to choose between the remaining options. **Reference:** Lilley, L. L., Rainforth Collins, S., Harrington, S., & Snyder, J. (2011). *Pharmacology and the nursing practice* (6th ed.). St. Louis, MO: Mosby, Inc., p. 199.

4 **Answer:** 1,020 **Rationale:** First convert the client's weight in pounds to kg by dividing 150 by 2.2 = 68 kg. Then multiply 68 by 1.5 grams to equal 1,020 grams. **Cognitive Level:** Applying **Client Need:** Pharmacological and Parenteral Therapies **Integrated Process:** Nursing Process: Planning **Content Area:** Pharmacology **Strategy:** First convert the client's weight to kg and then multiply it by the upper safe dose. **Reference:** Adams, M. P., & Koch, R. W. (2010). *Pharmacology: Connections to nursing practice* (1st ed.). Upper Saddle River, NJ: Pearson Education, pp. 173, 1347.

5 **Answer: 2** **Rationale:** One of the major uses of black cohosh is the treatment of postmenopausal symptoms, which include hot flashes and night sweats. Echinacea is commonly utilized to boost the immune response. Bilberry is commonly utilized to treat acute diarrhea. Valerian has been used to aid in sleep. **Cognitive Level:** Analyzing **Client Need:** Pharmacological and Parenteral Therapies **Integrated Process:** Nursing Process: Implementation **Content Area:** Pharmacology **Strategy:** Most menopausal signs and symptoms occur at night. Associate *black* with *night* to help make a connection between the client's symptoms and this herbal agent. **Reference:** Adams, M. P., & Koch, R. W. (2010). *Pharmacology: Connections to nursing practice* (1st ed.). Upper Saddle River, NJ: Pearson Education, pp. 173, 280, 522, 1201, 1347.

6 **Answer: 1** **Rationale:** The effectiveness of garlic is based on scientific evidence and clinical trials. Garlic has the ability to affect bleeding times and should not be taken with other herbs or over-the-counter medications, such as aspirin and ibuprofen, which also prolong bleeding times. Garlic is available in enteric-coated tablets, which is effective in reducing bad breath associated with the plant. **Cognitive Level:** Applying **Client Need:** Pharmacological and Parenteral Therapies **Integrated Process:** Nursing Process: Evaluation **Content Area:** Pharmacology **Strategy:** Specific knowledge is needed to answer the question. Apply information gleaned from current research regarding the herb to make a selection. **Reference:** Adams, M. P., & Koch, R. W. (2010). *Pharmacology: Connections to nursing practice* (1st ed.). Upper Saddle River, NJ: Pearson Education, pp. 173, 654.

7 **Answer: 3** **Rationale:** Hawthorn has an action that is similar to the action of angiotensin-converting enzyme (ACE) inhibitors, which reduce blood pressure by blocking the conversion of angiotensin I to angiotensin II, a potent vasoconstrictor. Its use should be restricted to chronic, self-limiting conditions and not for acute episodes of any nature. Hawthorn has a negative chronotropic effect resulting in a decreased heart rate rather than an increased one. Verapamil (Calan) is a calcium channel blocker that decreases blood pressure by blocking the influx of calcium ions across the cardiac and arterial muscle cell membrane. **Cognitive Level:** Analyzing **Client Need:** Pharmacological and Parenteral Therapies **Integrated Process:** Nursing Process: Planning **Content Area:** Pharmacology **Strategy:** Associate the drug with the angiotensins and the relationship to vasoconstriction and blood pressure. **Reference:** Adams, M. P., & Koch, R. W. (2010). *Pharmacology: Connections to nursing practice* (1st ed.). Upper Saddle River, NJ: Pearson Education, pp. 173, 540.

8 **Answer: 3** **Rationale:** Because ginseng is a stimulant, it should not be used in combination with coffee, tea, or colas. There is no evidence that the herb affects the ability to drive a car or operate machinery, or that it is related to increased incidence of adverse effects. A ginseng-free period is recommended, usually 2–3 weeks on and 1–2 weeks off. **Cognitive Level:** Applying **Client Need:** Pharmacological and Parenteral Therapies **Integrated Process:** Nursing Process: Implementation **Content Area:** Pharmacology **Strategy:** Associate the herb with stimulation. This will assist you to eliminate each incorrect option systematically. **Reference:** Adams, M. P., & Koch, R. W. (2010). *Pharmacology: Connections to nursing practice* (1st ed.). Upper Saddle River, NJ: Pearson Education, pp. 173, 590.

9 **Answer: 2, 3, 4** **Rationale:** The drug has a half-life of 24 hours so St. John's wort may take several weeks before the effects are evident. The effectiveness of almost all phytomedicines is slower than prescribed medications; however, many antidepressants have long onset time periods as well. The drug also has anti-inflammatory actions so it might be useful in managing arthritis. The time period does not correlate with the drug's characteristics. St. John's wort is appropriate for the treatment of mild to moderate depression. **Cognitive Level:** Applying **Client Need:** Pharmacological and Parenteral Therapies **Integrated Process:** Teaching and Learning **Content Area:** Pharmacology **Strategy:** Associate the herb with long onset and antidepressants and then use the process of elimination to make a selection. **Reference:** Adams, M. P., & Koch, R. W. (2010). *Pharmacology: Connections to nursing practice* (1st ed.). Upper Saddle River, NJ: Pearson Education, pp. 173, 313.

10 **Answer: 2** **Rationale:** Seizures are a side effect of this herb so assessing for a history of seizures would be of key importance. The ability to swallow is an appropriate assessment prior to drug administration but is not unique to this drug. Determining the credibility of resources is an appropriate assessment for planning client care but is not unique to this particular herb. Immunosuppression is a more likely side effect than altered red blood cell count. **Cognitive Level:** Applying **Client Need:** Pharmacological and Parenteral Therapies **Integrated Process:** Nursing Process: Assessment **Content Area:** Pharmacology **Strategy:** Associate the drug with epilepsy and match the herb with the critical word *seizure* in the correct option. **Reference:** Adams, M. P., & Koch, R. W. (2010). *Pharmacology: Connections to nursing practice* (1st ed.). Upper Saddle River, NJ: Pearson Education, p. 173.

Posttest

1 **Answer: 1** **Rationale:** The primary uses of saw palmetto include benign prostatic hyperplasia (BPH), male-pattern hair loss, prostate cancer, and prostatitis. Hypertension is a side effect of the drug and is also a common sign or symptom of chronic renal failure (CRF), putting the client at risk for hypertensive crisis or other adverse cardiovascular events. The herb does not deplete the client's nutritional stores. The drug is utilized to treat sleep disorders, but is not the most significant problem. **Cognitive Level:** Analyzing **Client Need:** Pharmacological and Parenteral Therapies **Integrated Process:** Nursing Process: Diagnosis **Content Area:** Pharmacology **Strategy:** Use knowledge of the combined risk of overlapping elements associated with the drug and the disease. Use the process of elimination and consider the option that represents the greatest harm to the client. **Reference:** Adams, M. P., & Koch, R. W. (2010). *Pharmacology: Connections to nursing practice* (1st ed.). Upper Saddle River, NJ: Pearson Education, pp. 173, 1232.

2 **Answer: 1** **Rationale:** The drug combination results in replacement of mucopolysaccharides, an element necessary for maintenance of the joints, tendons, and cartilages. GI disturbances, alopecia, and constipation are side effects of the drug. Anxiolytic properties are more commonly associated with kava kava. **Cognitive Level:** Analyzing **Client Need:** Pharmacological and Parenteral Therapies **Integrated Process:** Nursing Process: Planning **Content Area:** Pharmacology **Strategy:** Associate glucosamine and chondroitin with the musculoskeletal system. **Reference:** Fontaine, K. L. (2011). *Complementary and alternative therapies for nursing practice* (3rd ed.). Upper Saddle River, NJ: Pearson Education, pp. 133–134.

3 **Answer: 5** **Rationale:** The recommended dose of ginger is 1 teaspoon, which is equivalent to 5 mL. **Cognitive Level:** Applying **Client Need:** Pharmacological and Parenteral Therapies **Integrated Process:** Nursing Process: Planning **Content Area:** Pharmacology **Strategy:** Recall the recommended dose of ginger and then apply household to metric conversions to calculate correct answer **Reference:** Adams, M. P., & Koch, R. W. (2010). *Pharmacology: Connections to nursing practice* (1st ed.). Upper Saddle River, NJ: Pearson Education, pp. 173, 1013.

4 **Answer: 1, 4, 5** **Rationale:** Since ginkgo biloba can inhibit platelet activating factor, it can contribute to an increase in bleeding. Because of the risk of bleeding, the client should discontinue the drug until after any surgery. Nonsteroidal anti-inflammatory drugs (NSAIDs) such as ibuprofen are more likely to increase the risk of bleeding also. The drug is a potent inhibitor of the platelet activating factor. Gingko is not indicated for use in treating depression. **Cognitive Level:** Applying **Client Need:** Pharmacological and Parenteral Therapies **Integrated Process:** Communication and Documentation **Content Area:** Pharmacology **Strategy:** Evaluate the increased risk to clients with serious side effects associated with the drug. Specific knowledge of gingko biloba is needed to choose correctly. **Reference:** Adams, M. P., & Koch, R. W. (2010). *Pharmacology: Connections to nursing practice* (1st ed.). Upper Saddle River, NJ: Pearson Education, pp. 173, 360.

5 **Answer: 2** **Rationale:** One of the side effects of St. John's wort is photosensitivity requiring the client to avoid direct exposure to sunlight, especially if fair-skinned. Because it may increase the toxic effects of monoamine oxidase inhibitors (MAOIs), foods high in tyramine should be avoided. The drug's sedative effect is compounded by alcohol intake. The client should utilize a designated driver anytime ingesting alcoholic beverages. **Cognitive Level:** Applying **Client Need:** Pharmacological and Parenteral Therapies **Integrated Process:** Communication and Documentation **Content Area:** Pharmacology **Strategy:** Associate the side effects of the drug with risks to the client. **Reference:** Adams, M. P., & Koch, R. W. (2010). *Pharmacology: Connections to nursing practice* (1st ed.). Upper Saddle River, NJ: Pearson Education, pp. 173, 313.

6 **Answer: 4** **Rationale:** Saw palmetto is used primarily in the treatment of benign prostatic hyperplasia (BPH) and male-pattern hair loss. Additive bleeding risks associated with concurrent ingestion of nonsteroidal anti-inflammatory drugs (NSAIDs) is associated with use of ginger, gingko, and some other herbs, but not saw palmetto. Because the drug may cause a false positive prostate-specific antigen (PSA), the test should be done before starting the drug. **Cognitive Level:** Applying **Client Need:** Pharmacological and Parenteral Therapies **Integrated Process:** Nursing Process: Evaluation **Content Area:** Pharmacology **Strategy:** Apply knowledge of proper protocol associated with saw palmetto. **Reference:** Adams, M. P., & Koch, R. W. (2010). *Pharmacology: Connections to nursing practice* (1st ed.). Upper Saddle River, NJ: Pearson Education, pp. 173, 1232.

7 **Answer: 4** **Rationale:** Red yeast rice inhibits HMG CoA reductase, leading a decrease in total cholesterol, low-density lipoprotein, and triglyceride levels. Clients using this herbal supplement should avoid concurrent use of prescription drugs given to reduce these elements, since they can have a cumulative effect on liver function and increase the risk for impaired muscle metabolism and rhabdomyolysis. **Cognitive Level:** Applying **Client Need:** Pharmacological and Parenteral Therapies **Integrated Process:** Nursing Process: Implementation **Content Area:** Pharmacology **Strategy:** Associate the drug with reduced immunity. **Reference:** McCaffrey, R., & Younkgin, E. Q. (2010). *NP notes*. Philadelphia, PA: F. A. Davis Company, p. 214.

8 **Answer: 2** **Rationale:** Alprazolam (Xanax) is a short- to intermediate-acting benzodiazepine. Concomitant use of this drug with valerian root should be avoided since their actions are similar and the herb may potentiate the action of the alprazolam (Xanax). Valerian root may interact negatively with sedatives, narcotics, selective serotonin reuptake inhibitors (SSRIs), tranquilizers, and St. John's wort. Estrogen should be avoided with saw palmetto. Digoxin (Lanoxin) should be avoided with St. John's wort. Aspirin should be avoided with milk thistle. **Cognitive Level:** Applying **Client Need:** Pharmacological and Parenteral Therapies **Integrated Process:** Teaching and Learning **Content Area:** Pharmacology **Strategy:** Associate valerian root with Valium, a benzodiazepine that has diazepam as the generic name. **Reference:** Adams, M. P., & Koch, R. W. (2010). *Pharmacology: Connections to nursing practice* (1st ed.). Upper Saddle River, NJ: Pearson Education, pp. 173, 199.

9 **Answer: 4** **Rationale:** Increased intraocular pressure (IOP) is symptomatic of glaucoma. Bilberry is useful in the treatment of this and other eye disorders, such as diabetic retinopathy, night blindness, macular degeneration, and cataracts. Glucosamine chondroitin is used in the treatment of osteoarthritis. Black cohosh is used for the relief of postmenstrual symptoms, such as hot flashes and insomnia. Aloe is used for skin ulcerations and GI disturbances. **Cognitive Level:** Analyzing **Client Need:** Pharmacological and Parenteral Therapies **Integrated Process:** Nursing Process: Planning **Content Area:** Pharmacology **Strategy:** Associate bilberry with glaucoma. **Reference:** Adams, M. P., & Koch, R. W. (2010). *Pharmacology: Connections to nursing practice* (1st ed.). Upper Saddle River, NJ: Pearson Education, pp. 173, 1201, 1347.

10 **Answer: 1** **Rationale:** Chamomile has antispasmodic, anti-inflammatory, antimicrobial, antiflatulent, mild sedative, and calmative effects and is indicated for the treatment of GI spasms, insomnia or difficulty falling asleep, mouth ulcers, anxiety, and infant colic. **Cognitive Level:** Applying **Client Need:** Pharmacological and Parenteral Therapies **Integrated Process:** Nursing Process: Diagnosis **Content Area:** Pharmacology **Strategy:** Associate this drug with calming and sedative properties. **Reference:** Cox, H. C., et al. (2011). *Clinical applications of nursing diagnosis: Adult, child, women's psychiatric, gerontic and home health considerations*. Philadelphia, PA: F. A. Davis, p. 199. Fontaine, K. L. (2011). *Complementary and alternative therapies for nursing practice* (3rd ed.). Upper Saddle River, NJ: Pearson Education, p. 133.

ANSWERS & RATIONALES

References

Abrams, A. (2009). *Clinical drug therapy: Rationales for nursing practice* (9th ed.). Philadelphia, PA: Lippincott Williams & Wilkins.

Adams, M., Holland, L., & Bostwick, P. (2011). *Pharmacology for nurses: A pathophysiologic approach* (3rd ed.). Upper Saddle River, NJ: Pearson Education.

Adams. M. P., & Urban, C. (2013). *Pharmacology: Connections to nursing practice.* (2nd ed.). Upper Saddle River, NJ: Pearson Education.

Aschenbrenner, D., & Venable, S. (2012). *Drug therapy in nursing* (4th ed.). Philadelphia, PA: Lippincott Williams & Wilkins.

Drug Facts & Comparisons® (Updated monthly). St. Louis, MO: A. Wolters Kluwer.

Fontaine, K. L. (2011). *Complementary and alternative therapies for nursing practice* (3rd ed.). Upper Saddle River, NJ: Pearson Education.

Karch, A. M. (2010). *Focus on nursing pharmacology* (5th ed.). Philadelphia, PA: Lippincott Williams & Wilkins.

Kee, J. (2009). *Laboratory and diagnostic tests and nursing implications* (8th ed.). Upper Saddle River, NJ: Pearson Education.

Lehne, R. (2010). *Pharmacology for nursing care* (7th ed.). St. Louis, MO: Mosby, Inc.

LeMone, P., Burke, K., M., & Bauldoff, G. (2011). *Medical-surgical nursing: Critical thinking in patient care* (5th ed.). Upper Saddle River, NJ: Pearson Education.

Lilley, L. L., Collins, S. R., et al. (2011). *Pharmacology and the nursing practice* (6th ed.). St. Louis, MO: Mosby, Inc.

McCaffrey, R., & Younkgin, E. Q. (2010). *NP notes*. Philadelphia, PA: F. A. Davis Company.

Appendix A

➤ *Practice to Pass Suggested Answers*

Chapter 1

Page 6: *Suggested Answer*—The pregnant client is advised to avoid all medications during the pregnancy. Since she reports these discomforts occasional in frequency, the nurse may recommend some nonpharmacologic remedies for the headaches and backaches, such as taking a rest period or lying down during the day, or application of ice to the forehead or back.

Page 11: *Suggested Answer*—Most medications depend on a functioning renal system for excretion from the body. For a client with chronic renal failure, the priority considerations are related to appropriate dosing with the drug and to careful assessment of the client for toxic effects of the drug. The drug regimen for clients with chronic renal failure is often complex; the nurse will review with the client the prescribed drugs and the schedule for administration. If the client is being treated with hemodialysis for chronic renal failure, the nurse will review with the client what drugs are taken before and after the dialysis treatment.

Page 12: *Suggested Answer*—The correct volume to administer morphine sulfate 15 mg in this example is 0.6 mL. The problem can be set up this way: 25 mg: 1 mL = 15 mg: *x* mL.

$$25x = 15, x = 15 \div 25, x = 0.6 \text{ mL}$$

The nurse doing a drug calculation will review the answer and note that, if 25 mg is contained in 1 mL, then 15 mg will be contained in a volume less than 1 mL—in this case 0.6 mL. The nurse enhances client safety through accurate dosing by performing a "common sense" check at the end of each drug calculation.

Page 14: *Suggested Answer*—The intravenous (IV) route has no barriers to absorption of medication because it bypasses the gastrointestinal tract and does not need to be absorbed from muscle or subcutaneous tissue. Because it enters the bloodstream directly, it reaches the target tissues quickly and provides the most rapid action for analgesia or any other drug effect.

Page 15: *Suggested Answer*—There are several strategies the nurse can use in this situation:

- Do the teaching using short, simple sentences and provide a demonstration where possible.
- Use an interpreter or, if unavailable, ask a member of client's family to interpret.

- Search online or use other resources to find drug information materials in the client's language.
- Develop a diagram of the drug schedule that uses pictures and numbers.
- Observe the client for cues that signal lack of effective communication during the teaching session.

Chapter 2

Page 42: *Suggested Answer*—Assess number and characteristics of stools, abdominal cramping, if there is newly developed fever, and length of time on antibiotic therapy. If pseudomembranous colitis is suspected, arrange for a stool specimen for culture and sensitivity for *Clostridium difficile*. If specimen is positive for *C. difficile*, collaborate with the prescriber about discontinuing the antibiotic, initiating therapy with vancomycin PO or IV or with metronidazole (Flagyl) to treat the pseudomonas colitis, and about issues related to maintaining fluid and electrolyte balance. If the diarrhea is mild, the antibiotic may be continued. An absorbent antidiarrheal such as Kaolin and Pectin (Kao-tin) may be prescribed. Monitoring hydration status and potassium level will be important. Provide for good hygiene.

Page 48: *Suggested Answer*—Take tetracycline on an empty stomach with a full glass of water. Take 1 hour before and 2 hours after meals, and avoid ingestion of milk or milk products or antacids that would interfere with the efficacy of the drug. If the client is taking oral contraceptives, advise the client to use an alternative method of contraception during therapy and for one month after discontinuation of the tetracycline as the drug will interfere with effectiveness of oral contraceptives. Breakthrough bleeding may occur as well. Report severe side effects and clinical manifestations of Candida infection. Avoid direct sunlight and ultraviolet lights including tanning beds because of risk for photosensitivity. If in the sun, advise client to wear long sleeves, long-legged pants, hat, and sunglasses. Sunscreen and sunblocks may be used but may not prevent a photosensitivity reaction. Teach the client to store tetracycline in a tightly covered container protected from moisture and light—i.e., not in the medicine cabinet in the bathroom. Keep health care appointments for follow-up exams and tests.

Page 52: *Suggested Answer*—Peak and trough laboratory findings guide dosage and dosing schedule for certain drugs such as vancomycin (Vancocin). Changes will be prescribed based on these findings and the clinical manifestations of the client. Apparently the trough level was low and so the dosing schedule was increased from every 8 hours to every 6 hours. The dosage may also have been increased. If the trough is low, the therapeutic drug level is not being maintained, which could limit the drug's therapeutic effectiveness and allow microorganisms to replicate causing continuation or exacerbation of the infection. Explain the rationale for the change to the client. Ask for clarification of what the client means by "tied down," and facilitate the client's exploration of possible options to not being "tied down." Client compliance is necessary for effective outcomes.

Page 66: *Suggested Answer*—Explain to the client that taking the acyclovir (Zovirax) before symptoms occur better enables the antiviral drug to be effective in reducing the viral load and preventing complications. The drug's efficacy is best when the virus is residing in the body's cells and before the virus is released from the cell. The drug's effectiveness will diminish over time, but its effectiveness is optimized with early introduction as evidenced by persons with HIV not becoming symptomatic for longer periods. There are other antiviral agents available that are used in combination for future needs and to retard development of drug resistance. Offer to arrange for the client to discuss the treatment strategy with the prescriber if concerns persist.

Page 68: *Suggested Answer*—Xerostomia is dryness of the mouth. Amantadine (Symmetrel), an antiviral, is also an anticholinergic agent that can cause dryness of mucous membranes, such as in the mouth. Oral care is important for comfort and also to protect the integrity of the oral cavity that harbors pathogenic microorganisms. Frequent mouth rinses with water or warm saline solution can be refreshing and cleansing. Avoid hydrogen peroxide and commercial mouthwashes that contain alcohol because both can contribute further to dryness of the mouth. Sucking on hard candy may stimulate secretion of saliva, and there are artificial saliva products available. Keep the client hydrated.

Page 73: *Suggested Answer*—Determine first what the client means by *stuff* (the drug, the central line, or some other concern) and what is the client's understanding of "the bad things that can happen." As would be appropriate based on the information gleaned from the client, reaffirm the purpose of the therapy and explain what is done to minimize the risks or possible deleterious effects. For example, explain that premedication is provided to mitigate adverse reactions of the Amphotericin B (Fungizone), including antiemetic, antihistamine, and antipyretic agents. Analgesics are available if needed to maintain comfort as well. The client will also be hydrated before, during, and after the antifungal administration that will facilitate removal of toxins. Allow the client to verbalize concerns. Offer to arrange for the client to discuss concerns further with the prescriber if necessary. The client may prefer not to be alone, so arrange for someone (family, friend, pastoral care, volunteer) to be with the client during the drug

administration, if possible. Prudent nursing interventions can help this acutely ill client through a difficult time of treatment.

Chapter 3

Page 92: *Suggested Answer*—Three measures to prevent renal toxicity secondary to cisplatin administration include the following:

1. Assess of BUN and creatinine before administration and periodically during treatment.
2. Provide adequate intravenous or oral hydration (1,000 1,500 mL in 6–8 hours) before administration.
3. Administer mannitol (Osmitrol) or furosemide (Lasix) to promote diuresis.

Page 94: *Suggested Answer*—

1. Promote oral hygiene before meals and at bedtime with fluorinated toothpaste, a soft toothbrush, and dilute baking soda rinse.
2. Assess oral cavity daily and report any redness, irritation, or white patches observed (monilia).
3. Educate the client to report soreness at the first sign of irritation.

Page 98: *Suggested Answer*—

1. Ensure that IV site was not started more than 48 hours before administration.
2. Assess IV site for any redness or irritation, and restart if present.
3. Assess blood return and ensure that the vein is easily accessible and full.
4. Remove opaque or gauze dressing from the site to provide clear access during administration.
5. Ensure IV site is not positioned in the area of a joint (with underlying tendons and nerves nearby) or on the dorsal side of the hand.

Page 100: *Suggested Answer*—

1. Assess client's usual bowel history prior to administration.
2. Provide a high-fiber diet.
3. Obtain an order for stool softeners at least twice daily.
4. Auscultate abdomen Q shift for bowel sounds.
5. Assess bowel movements Q shift.
6. Obtain an order for laxatives if the client has not had a bowel movement after 48 hours of administration.

Page 106: *Suggested Answer*—

1. Take oral temperature at the same time every day and report to health care provider if greater than or equal to 101°F.
2. Maintain oral hygiene before meals and at bedtime.
3. Avoid eating raw fruits and vegetables.
4. Avoid proximity to fresh flowers or plants.
5. Refrain from emptying boxes filled with kitty litter, or fish tanks or aquariums.
6. Avoid large crowds and young children, and those with known infections.

Chapter 4

Page 128: *Suggested Answer*—A client who has been placed on anticoagulation therapy must understand that this treatment regimen will require close follow-up and long-term monitoring. The client must understand that the anticoagulant medication will make the client more susceptible to bleeding. Safety instructions must be given to the client to prevent bleeding episodes, such as using soft toothbrushes, electric razors, and avoiding trauma. The client must also be made aware of potential drug and food interactions. Compliance with the treatment regimen is an important process towards realizing the client's health goals. Both verbal and written instruction should be given to the client to enhance understanding and provide a reference post-discharge.

Page 131: *Suggested Answer*—Low-dose aspirin (ASA) therapy is used as a "blood thinner" for its antiplatelet effect. The dosage used is normally one baby ASA or 81 mg per day. If the client takes the normal adult dose of grains X or 650 mg q 4–6 hours, they will be taking medication to treat fever, aches, and pains. Taking too much ASA can lead to potential health consequences such as ASA toxicity. Gastrointestinal hemorrhage can occur with the prolonged use of ASA at high doses. The client can always be referred back to the prescriber for further clarification in writing of the required dosage.

Page 133: *Suggested Answer*—Nursing interventions aimed at preventing or reducing the likelihood of increased bleeding would include (1) minimizing the number of injections, (2) coordinating lab draws to avoid increased risk, (3) applying pressure after venipuncture and lab draws, (4) maintaining aseptic technique and limiting (if possible) the number of invasive procedures, (5) taking vital signs (using automatic blood pressure cuffs), and (6) continued assessment for possible bleeding sources (internal, retroperitoneal, intracranial, and gastrointestinal). The nurse must monitor the client closely and keep in close communication with the health care provider.

Page 137: *Suggested Answer*—It is important to know how long the topical agent has been in contact with the client's skin because there can be potential for skin damage upon removal of the agent. If the area is dry, then the nurse should irrigate the area gently with normal saline to minimize tissue irritation. Consult the health care provider or the pharmacist regarding removal and application procedures.

Page 146: *Suggested Answer*—Since anemia is a broad category and is sometimes a symptom of an illness as well as a disease entity, it is hard to make a general statement that medication by itself will restore adequate blood cell levels to correct anemia. Medication in conjunction with adequate dietary sources is a very effective treatment plan. However, if one is not sure of the underlying cause for the anemia, this may not be enough to restore blood levels. It would be important to verify the type of anemia that the client has in order to fully explore the answer. Clients who have vitamin B_{12}, folic acid, and iron-deficiency anemias can be treated successfully with combination diet and medication therapy in order to restore adequate blood cell levels.

Page 152: *Suggested Answer*—Cholesterol-lowering medications should be taken at night because the body normally performs the function of cholesterol synthesis at that time. If the body were normally undergoing that function, using the medication at that time would increase its biologic effect and efficiency.

Chapter 5

Page 163: *Suggested Answer*—OTC diet pills contain many unknown chemicals that might interact with Transderm-Nitro, an antianginal medication. This could put the client at risk for additional cardiac problems. The client should be praised for wanting to lose the weight, but advise her to contact the prescriber prior to taking OTC medications.

Page 167: *Suggested Answer*—Your client may be experiencing an adverse reaction to the beta-adrenergic blocking medication. The $beta_2$ receptors in the lungs are probably being affected. Evaluate the vital signs, check the pulse oximetry, and notify the prescriber. Be prepared to take further actions as ordered to relieve the client's symptoms and increase gas exchange.

Page 169: *Suggested Answer*—Assess the vital signs, including heart rate, BP, respiration, and mental status. Evaluate whether the client is experiencing any chest pain. The diltiazem (Cardizem) drip is a calcium channel blocker and may be causing a second-degree, Mobitz I (Wenckebach) heart block. Reduce the rate of the Cardizem drip by half and notify the prescriber. Do not leave the client alone.

Page 171: *Suggested Answer*—Turn off the infusion pump; remove the tubing but maintain a patent IV site with a saline lock or an NS infusion directly into the site. *Do not use the tubing containing the sodium nitroprusside (Nipride).* The client is experiencing profound hypotension with compensatory tachycardia from the Nipride drip. Notify the prescriber urgently. Assess the client's vital signs, including mental status, HR, and BP. Maintain an airway and the IV site, and monitor the client continuously.

Page 173: *Suggested Answer*—The client may be experiencing digitalis toxicity. Assess vital signs including mental status, heart rate, and blood pressure. Discuss the need to obtain a digoxin (Lanoxin) level and potassium with the prescriber. If necessary, draw the venous blood sample and send to the laboratory. Ask the client if he or she is taking other medications that might have interacted with digoxin.

Chapter 6

Page 195: *Suggested Answer*—Rhinitis or upper respiratory infection may decrease the effectiveness of this therapy. The information should be passed on to the prescribing health care provider. The client should be advised to contact the nurse again if there is any increase in urine output.

Page 196: *Suggested Answer* — The client should weigh herself daily. She is advised to notify the nurse if there is a weekly gain of more than 5 lbs since mineralocorticoids can alter fluid and electrolyte balance. Since this client has gained 5½ lbs in 2 days, the nurse should assess vital signs, edema, lung sounds, and skin to gather additional data related to fluid overload. Once the nurse has a comprehensive picture, the information should be reported to the prescriber.

Page 199: *Suggested Answer* — The nurse should encourage this action and should explain to the client the importance of wearing a MedicAlert identification. If the client should become ill or injured, the information about the client's health contained in this identification will have an impact on treatment. The most common side effects of glucocorticoid therapy are mental status changes, including affect, mood, behavior, aggression, and depression. Clients taking glucocorticoids should be advised to wear some sort of personal identification in the event that they become mentally incapacitated and cannot care for themselves temporarily.

Page 201: *Suggested Answer* — Increased effects of anticoagulant therapy can result when taken with thyroid medications. The nurse should monitor the client's prothrombin time (PT) or international normalized ratio (INR) to determine whether the warfarin (Coumadin) is being maintained in an appropriate dosage range.

Page 204: *Suggested Answer* — Digitalis toxicity and increased risk of dysrhythmias may result when these 2 drugs are taken together. Thus, the nurse should monitor serum digoxin levels and look for early signs of digoxin toxicity, such as anorexia and nausea. The nurse should also observe the cardiac monitor (if in use) for dysrhythmias, or look for an irregular pulse or change in pulse rate of a client who does not have a cardiac monitor in place.

Page 206: *Suggested Answer* — A musculoskeletal assessment needs to be performed, including inspection and gentle palpation of the vertebral column, particularly the lower thoracic and lumbar vertebrae. Back pain along with restriction of spinal movement and tenderness could be related to one or more compression fractures. Fractures in the distal end of the radius and the upper third of the femur may also occur.

Page 210: *Suggested Answer* — Insulin not in use should be refrigerated. Temperatures less than 36°F or greater than 86°F need to be avoided and all insulin should be kept away from direct heat and light. A slight loss of potency may occur if the bottle has been in use for more than 30 days, even when the expiration date has not been passed. Therefore, a spare bottle of insulin should always be available.

Page 211: *Suggested Answer* — The client's health care provider needs to be notified. Also, the blood glucose level needs to be monitored at least every 4 hours and the urine needs to be tested for ketones if the blood glucose level is greater than 240 mg/dL. Also, regularly prescribed insulin or oral hypoglycemics need to be taken and instructions must be given to drink 8–12 ounces of sugar-free liquids every hour.

Page 214: *Suggested Answer* — The nurse needs to assess the client's financial status and initiate an immediate social service referral to determine what resources may be available. The American Diabetes Association (ADA) has a toll-free phone number (800-232-3472 in the United States) and will refer a diabetic client to the appropriate agencies or resources. The American Association of Diabetes Educators (800-TEAM-UP-4) can also refer a diabetic client to a certified diabetes educator in the client's own area.

Chapter 7

Page 223: *Suggested Answer* — Cisapride (Propulsid) has been withheld by the Food and Drug Administration because of drug interactions that may lead to prolonged QT intervals and ventricular tachycardia.

Page 227: *Suggested Answer* — The client should contact a health care provider if diarrhea lasts longer than 2 days, which will allow the health care provider to rule out any infectious or colonic disorder.

Page 230: *Suggested Answer* — Activated charcoal should be given to counteract the effects of ipecac syrup. This may be administered orally as a flavored drink to disguise the taste, or it may be administered via a nasogastric tube.

Page 238: *Suggested Answer* — Misoprostol (Cytotec) can cause miscarriages. This information is vital for the pregnant client to be aware of so that the client can make informed decisions about whether or not to take this medication.

Page 240: *Suggested Answer* — The nurse should assess swallowing ability. Certain proton pump inhibitors must be swallowed whole while others may be opened and sprinkled on applesauce.

Chapter 8

Page 255: *Suggested Answer* — The nurse should assess the client for signs of hypersensitivity, which include any of the following: rash, urticaria, edema, and difficulty breathing. Hypersensitivity reaction is a medical emergency and must be assessed for and treated promptly.

Page 256: *Suggested Answer* — The nurse should assess the following three items:

1. Obtain a complete blood count (CBC) with differential and platelet count prior to the administration of colony-stimulating factors.
2. Assess CBC and platelet count following the administration of medication. Report a neutrophil count of 20,000/mm^3 to health care provider.
3. If CBC, particularly hematocrit, is rising rapidly (greater than 4% in 2 weeks), assess carefully for hypertension and seizure activity.

Page 260: *Suggested Answer*—The following items should be considered when determining learning objectives for a client who will be receiving immunosuppressant agents:

1. Educate regarding the prevention of infection (e.g., avoid overcrowded areas or people with known infections, take in adequate nutrition, maintain good hygiene practices).
2. Educate regarding all laboratory studies that should be conducted, such as CBC, platelet count, and renal and liver function.
3. Educate regarding supportive care for flulike symptoms.
4. Educate regarding action, side effects, and nursing implications of medications being administered.

Page 262: *Suggested Answer*—The following items should be incorporated into client teaching during an outbreak of hepatitis A:

1. Hepatitis A is transmitted by fecal–oral route.
2. Instruct on proper hygiene and sanitation.
3. Instruct on proper food preparation.
4. Hepatitis A transmission occurs from person-to-person contact and has been noted in areas with overcrowding, such as schools or day care centers.

Page 268: *Suggested Answer*—The following nursing interventions should be implemented to relieve flulike symptoms caused by medications used to treat multiple sclerosis:

1. Administer acetaminophen (Tylenol) for relief of pain or fever.
2. Provide adequate fluid intake to support fluid volume deficit.
3. Assess intake and output every 8 hours.
4. Provide adequate rest to promote healing.
5. Assess vital signs every 4 hours and administer antipyretic agents for temperatures over 101°F.

Chapter 9

Page 286: *Suggested Answer*—Assess the "diaper rash" before presenting a teaching plan. Take a history of the rash, the infant's usual foods, and the usual skin care the infant is now receiving. There can be several reasons for diaper rash—e.g., it might be caused by remaining in diaper too long, or by overingestion of a food to which the child is sensitive, or by some topical agent the mother is using. It also might be caused by a substance being used elsewhere, such as at a child care center. Sensitizers could be in soap, "baby wipes," topical powders, ointments, and even the diapers. Thus, the first step is to eliminate any food and any topical substance that are being used that seem likely to be sensitizers. The interventions aimed at restoring intact skin should be as simple as possible. There are skin protectants that might be helpful, such as A and D medicated diaper rash ointment or Balmex ointment. However, these are unlikely to be helpful if the culprit is a food. Directions for any topical preparation should be closely followed (e.g., "thicker is not better"). Exposure of the skin to air for 15 minutes four times a day can be helpful in drying out

a rash. If the steps are followed and there is no improvement after 7 days, a health care provider should be seen, since it could be a different problem, such as a fungal infection.

Page 288: *Suggested Answer*—The client might try Capsin, a topical analgesic lotion containing capsaicin in concentrations of 0.02% or 0.075%. The active ingredient is derived from capsicum oleoresin, which is found in a number of common chili pepper plant species. It can help manage minor pain associated with arthritis, sprains, strains, and simple backaches.

The precise mechanism of action is not fully known. However, capsaicin is believed to work by depleting the supply of the neurotransmitter substance P resulting in a reduction of pain perception. An initial burning sensation may occur after application, but generally will subside after continued use. It is applied to affected areas 3 to 4 times daily; if applied less often, optimum pain relief may not occur and the burning sensation may persist.

It is for external use only and contact with eyes, mucous membranes, and broken or irritated skin should be avoided. It should not be bandaged. If symptoms persist or worsen after 7 days of continued use, the health care provider should be consulted.

Page 289: *Suggested Answer*—Erythema (sunburn) is a familiar acute result of ultraviolet B overexposure, typically beginning 2–8 hours after irradiation and peaking at 24–36 hours. The lighter the complexion, the more severe the risk of sunburn. After severe overexposure, desquamation (peeling) occurs, reflecting changes in keratinocyte proliferation. There is a clear relationship in humans between the incidence of skin cancer and such variables as skin color, geographic latitude, and history of occupational and leisure-time exposure to sunlight.

The cousin needs advice on a photoprotection program. Sunscreens are a key ingredient in such a program and should be applied one half hour before exposure. Probably a strong sunscreen with a SPF of 15 or above would be prudent in this situation. Reapplication may be advisable after swimming or sweating. A broad-brimmed hat shields the face, neck, and ears. Planning to do outdoor activities early in the morning (before 10 a.m.) or late in the afternoon (after 3 p.m.) is a simple form of photoprotection.

Page 295: *Suggested Answer*—A typical client with head lice (pediculosis capitis) has few, if any, easily observable signs of infestation. The child may complain of itching around the ears and over the sides of the neck, but these changes occur so gradually that clients frequently give them little attention.

Nits represent eggs cemented to the side of hairs, and they cannot be removed easily. Lice are spread from human to human by direct physical contact and through fomites.

A shampoo with lindane 1% (Kwell), permethrin (Elimite cream, Nix liquid), or pyrethrin and piperonyl butoxide combination (Rid shampoo) would be used to treat pediculosis capitis. Kwell is the least desirable product for children because of risk of seizures. In this case, even if no nits are identified in the child's hair, it would not be wrong to use the shampoo as directed for the child. A nit comb is usually packaged with the shampoo and is used to contribute to the removal of nits from the hair.

All potentially contaminated articles of clothing, bedding, and personal hygiene products need to be disinfected. For head lice, the focus would be brushes, combs, hats, scarves, and coats. Items can be treated with rubbing alcohol or placed in home dishwasher. Towels, sheets, pillowcases, and bedding should be laundered in hot water. For items that are difficult to clean, freezing works well. It is not necessary to fumigate the house to rid the client of head lice.

Page 298: *Suggested Answer*—The client should use a topical product that contains salicylic acid to treat the wart. The product should be used as per its directions. General hygiene measures for the foot should also be discussed. This would include proper washing and drying of feet, wearing clean socks that are changed daily, and making sure to wear shoes (rather than go barefoot). If the wart does not heal within the time specified on the product directions, further treatment should be sought.

Chapter 10

Page 313: *Suggested Answer*—Discontinue the patient-controlled analgesia (PCA), call a physician stat, and be prepared to give an antihistamine or epinephrine for an allergic reaction.

Page 316: *Suggested Answer*—The client is probably experiencing acetaminophen toxicity because of taking acetaminophen (Tylenol) as well as cold medication with acetaminophen in it. Acetaminophen is toxic to the liver and should not be taken in doses exceeding 4 grams per 24 hours.

Page 323: *Suggested Answer*—The tube feeding usually needs to be turned off for 30 minutes to 1 hour prior to the medication administration and for 1–2 hours afterward. A nurse who has questions about the effects of a change in rate can also consult the agency pharmacist.

Page 329: *Suggested Answer*—Because of the multiple medication profile, medications such as antihypertensives and antidiabetic medications, including insulin, may need adjustment.

Page 333: *Suggested Answer*—Opioids, especially meperidine (Demerol), should not be administered because of possible fatal interaction between these medications.

Chapter 11

Page 356: *Suggested Answer*—Neuroleptic malignant syndrome (NMS) is a potentially fatal reaction to antipsychotic drugs. At one time it was thought to occur in about 1% of the clients taking antipsychotics with an accompanying mortality rate of up to 30%. Increased awareness and vigilance by nurses and others has significantly reduced both morbidity and mortality rates. It occurs most often when high-potency antipsychotic drugs are prescribed. Haloperidol (Haldol) is frequently cited as the causative neuroleptic. Onset is from 3 to 9 days after initiation of an antipsychotic. It is manifested by muscular rigidity, tremors, impaired ventilation, muteness, altered consciousness, and autonomic hyperactivity. The cardinal symptom is high body temperature. Temperatures as high as 108°F (42.2°C) have been reported. More likely, temperatures are 101° to 103°F. Dantrolene (Dantrium) and bromocriptine (Parlodel) are the drugs of choice for treating NMS and should be continued for 8–12 days after improvement. Antipsychotics should not be reinstituted for at least 2 weeks after complete resolution of NMS symptoms.

Page 363: *Suggested Answer*—Sexual dysfunction (e.g., anorgasmia, delayed ejaculation, decreased libido) is common, occurring in about 70% of men and women. Other common reactions include nausea (21%), headache (20%), and manifestations of CNS stimulation, including nervousness (15%), insomnia (14%), and anxiety (10%). Dizziness, fatigue, and anorexia associated with weight loss are also seen in clients taking fluoxetine (Prozac).

Page 368: *Suggested Answer*—The medication regime should include that lithium should be taken exactly as prescribed even if feeling "well." Other important points are:

- If a dose is missed, take as soon as remembered unless within 2 hours of next dose (6 hours if extended release).
- Medication may cause dizziness or drowsiness—do not drive or perform activities that require alertness or precision until response to medication is known.
- Low sodium levels may predispose client to toxicity; need to drink 2,000 to 3,000 mL of fluid each day and eat a diet with consistent and moderate sodium intake.
- Avoid excessive amounts of coffee, tea, and cola because of diuretic effect.
- Avoid activities that cause excess sodium loss—especially summer sun, hot weather, saunas, and exertion.
- Notify health care professional of fever, vomiting, and diarrhea.
- Advise client that weight gain may occur—review principles of low-calorie diet.
- Instruct client to discuss any OTC medication with health care professional before taking.
- Advise client to use contraception—notify health care professional if pregnancy suspected.
- Review side effects and symptoms of toxicity with client.
- Instruct client to stop medications and report signs of toxicity to health care professionals promptly.
- Explain to clients with cardiovascular disease or who are over 40 years of age about the need for electrocardiogram (ECG) evaluation before and periodically during therapy. Always report fainting, irregular pulse, or difficulty breathing immediately.

Page 375: *Suggested Answer*—Common side effects of lorazepam (Ativan) include daytime sedation, ataxia, dizziness, headache, blurred vision, hypotension, tremors, and slurred speech.

Page 383: *Suggested Answer*—The primary nursing priority for this client is maintaining physiological stability during the withdrawal phase. Other important priorities include to promote client safety, provide appropriate referral and follow-up, and to encourage client to participate in the intervention process and become familiar with self-help, rehabilitation, and aftercare.

Chapter 12

Page 394: *Suggested Answer*—Tinnitus, hearing impairment, deafness, vertigo or sense of fullness in the ears.

Page 401: *Suggested Answer*—Avoid potassium-containing agents or salts, anticholinergics, potassium-sparing diuretics, and angiotensin-converting enzyme (ACE) inhibitors.

Page 403: *Suggested Answer*—Modifiable factors for hypertension include increased sodium intake, obesity, excess alcohol consumption, decreased potassium intake, smoking, and sedentary lifestyle.

Page 403: *Suggested Answer*—Routine labs include BUN and creatinine, electrolytes, liver function tests, WBC, and differential.

Page 405: *Suggested Answer*—If the client is taking a medication with a potassium-sparing effect, salt substitutes, which are high in potassium, should be avoided. Otherwise, the client could develop hyperkalemia, which can cause cardiac dysrhythmias as well as other manifestations.

Chapter 13

Page 430: *Suggested Answer*—

1. Squeeze the prescribed amount of cream into the applicator and insert the cream deep into the vagina 1–3 times per week as directed.
2. Do not douche.
3. Remain recumbent for at least 30 minutes, and preferably use at bedtime to retain medication for a longer time.

Page 432: *Suggested Answer*—

1. Secondary sex characteristics such as pubic, axillary, chest, and facial hair; deepening voice; and enlargement of the testes and penis will begin to develop.
2. Testosterone can cause premature closure of the epiphyseal plates with subsequent loss of potential adult height; therefore, the health care provider may be ordering wrist x-rays every 6 months to monitor for this condition.
3. Acne may develop.
4. Libido may increase.

Page 433: *Suggested Answer*—

1. Liver function studies to determine whether or not hepatotoxicity has occurred.
2. HIV and hepatitis B and C panels because of needle sharing.

Page 436: *Suggested Answer*—Other medications can be used, such as papaverine with phentolamine (Cerespan) and alprostadil (Muse). However, sildenafil (Viagra) is the only oral medication. Viagra is also contraindicated with hypertension, recent myocardial infarction (MI) or cerebrovascular accident (CVA), and other cardiovascular diseases.

Page 439: *Suggested Answer*—

1. Has she ever had a deep vein thrombus (DVT), embolus, myocardial infarction (MI), or cerebrovascular accident (CVA)?
2. Is she taking any other medications, especially antibiotics and anticonvulsants?
3. When was her last monthly period? Could she be pregnant at this time?

Chapter 14

Page 460: *Suggested Answer*—This client appears to be suffering from bronchoconstriction as evidenced by wheezing and the dusky color. The pulse oximeter reading of 88% is too low. The client's color also indicates a low oxygen level. Appropriate actions by the nurse include administration of oxygen with continuous pulse oximetry to evaluate the effects of the oxygen. Since we do not know this client's history, starting oxygen at 2 L/min via nasal cannula is appropriate in case there is a history of chronic obstructive pulmonary disease. Further actions include obtaining an order for a bronchodilator and administration of the medication. Obtaining a nursing history and keeping the client on bed rest to conserve energy are also appropriate nursing interventions.

Page 461: *Suggested Answer*—This client has a theophylline level of 25 mg/dL, which is too high. More data are needed to determine the reason for the increased level. Dosage should be checked to be sure that the client is taking the medication as prescribed. Theophylline doses should be based on lean body weight as theophylline does not enter the adipose tissue; therefore, the proper dose should be calculated and adjusted accordingly. The reason for the elevated BUN and creatinine should be explored. Some theophylline is excreted via the kidneys—if there is renal disease, it could be part of the reason for the increased theophylline level. A liver profile will likely be ordered as theophylline is metabolized via the liver. The age of this client is not mentioned, but the nurse should consider the client's age and understand there is potential for increased sensitivity to theophylline in the elderly client and dosages may need to be decreased. The nurse should monitor the client for toxic effects of theophylline due to the elevated level. These include seizures, tachycardia, tremors, dizziness, hallucinations, restlessness, agitation, headaches, insomnia, nausea, vomiting, tachydysrhythmias, and chest pain. Adverse cardiac effects are not usually seen until the theophylline level exceeds 30 mg/dL. Seizure activity is not usually seen until levels exceed 40 mg/dL.

Page 464: *Suggested Answer*—The client needs to know the therapeutic action of theses medications. Albuterol (Proventil) is given to dilate the constricted airways. Proventil can be used for the prevention and the treatment of acute bronchoconstrictive attacks. Of the two medications listed, Proventil is the one that can be taken in the event of an acute attack, as beclomethasone dipropionate (Beclovent) is preventative. The difficulty with ventilation should improve with the administration of these agents; if it does not, the client should seek medical attention. Beclovent is an inhaled corticosteroid and is administered to decrease inflammation in the airways. Reassure the client that inhaled corticosteroids are not as likely to cause systemic side effects as corticosteroids that are administered orally. In addition to the action of the medications and the anticipated effects, the client should also be informed of potential side effects of the medications. Side effects of albuterol include hypotension, headaches, tremors, decreased potassium levels, increased blood glucose, nausea, vomiting, chest pain, irregular heart rhythm, restlessness, agitation, and insomnia. Side effects of beclomethasone include pharyngeal irritation, coughing, dry mouth, oral fungal infections, sore throat, and sinusitis. The client may also experience diarrhea, nausea, and vomiting. The nurse should utilize wording that the client understands and not give too much information in the first session. This client is newly diagnosed and may not hear all that is said due to the anxiety caused by a new diagnosis. Remember each client should be treated as an individual and some clients need and can assimilate more information than others. The basic information that is needed in this case is the way the medications work, how they are to be administered, signs that the medications are working properly or not working properly, and the potential side effects of the medications. Additional information can be given at a later date or as indicated by the individualized needs of the client.

Page 471: *Suggested Answer*—Fexofenadine (Allegra) is an antihistamine. The action of the medication is to block the action of histamine by competing with histamine for receptor sites and therefore decreasing the response of the client to histamine. This medication should ease breathing and decrease allergic secretions. The medication is used prophylactically to decrease allergic reactions and should be taken regularly, not during an acute allergic attack. Fexofenadine (Allegra) is a nonsedating antihistamine that has a rapid onset after oral administration. This medication is to treat the symptoms, but the cause of the allergic reaction should be avoided when possible. Fexofenadine (Allegra) may be tolerated better if taken with meals. Some of the side effects can include drowsiness, dry mouth, visual changes, constipation, and difficulty with urination. The client may also experience nausea, vomiting, diarrhea, dizziness, syncope, muscular weakness, unsteady gait, restlessness, and nervousness. Fluid intake should be increased to decrease the potential dry mouth effect and also to thin respiratory secretions and therefore ease expectoration. The medication should be taken exactly as prescribed. The prescriber should be contacted prior to taking any over-the-counter (OTC) medications. Alcohol and other central nervous system depressants should be avoided while on this medication. Hard, sugarless candy may help if the client has a problem with dry mouth. Prolonged exposure to the sun can cause sunburn.

Page 476: *Suggested Answer*—Dimetane-DC is an opioid antitussive medication. There is a potential for respiratory depression with these medications. The client is 80, which makes her more at risk because of potential for the effects of medications to intensify in older adults. She may have decreased renal function and not be able to excrete the medication as readily. The client is definitely in respiratory difficulty as evidenced by a respiratory rate of 5 per minute and cyanosis. The client is also lethargic, which may be because of the narcotic but also could be related to decreased oxygenation and increased CO_2 levels. The client should be started on oxygen, and oxygen saturation should be measured continuously. Respiratory effort should be monitored. Arterial blood gases should be drawn, and a work-up should be done to determine the cause of the cough. No more antitussive agents should be administered. The client will likely have an chest x-ray and be admitted to the hospital for possible intubation and mechanical ventilation. Education of the daughter and the client (when she is more responsive) should be initiated to discuss the adverse effects of opioid antitussive medications. Assessment of the underlying reason for the cough (such as respiratory disease) is important. Two weeks is an excessive period for the administration of antitussive medications. Teaching is indicated to correct this as well. The client should be assessed for liver, renal, thyroid, and adrenal diseases as any of these can intensify the effects of opioid antitussive medications. The nurse should also obtain a history as to the concurrent use of central nervous system depressants such as alcohol and antianxiety agents, as these can intensify the effects of opioid antitussive medications.

Chapter 15

Page 494: *Suggested Answer*—Oral acetazolamide (Diamox) may cause gastrointestinal (GI) side effects such as anorexia, nausea, vomiting, and weight loss. To reduce risk of GI side effects, the client should take the medication with food or milk. Since acetazolamide also causes diuresis, instruct the client to take medication early in the day to avoid nocturia. Acetazolamide may also exacerbate renal stones. Unless contraindicated, the client should be instructed to consume at least 2,000 mL of fluid per day and a diet high in potassium and low in sodium. The client should also maintain follow-up visits to monitor for fluid and electrolyte imbalances.

Page 495: *Suggested Answer*—Instruct the client to administer pilocarpine one hour after the administration of latanoprost (Xalatan). Inform client of side effects such as blurred vision, photophobia, burning, stinging, and itching. Latanoprost may also cause an increase in iris pigmentation. The client should remove contact lenses before use, and for 15 minutes after instillation of the medication.

Page 498: *Suggested Answer*—The eye is cleansed of crust and drainage before the administration of ophthalmic medications. To properly clean the eye, use a cotton ball moistened with sterile normal saline or other prescribed solution. Wipe the eye from the inner canthus towards the outer canthus.

To avoid contamination of the other eye, use a separate cotton ball for each eye. The eyelid and eyelashes are cleansed.

Page 500: *Suggested Answer*—Proparacaine hydrochloride (Ophthaine) temporarily causes a loss of the blink reflex due to the effects of anesthesia. To protect the cornea, an eye patch is applied until the blink reflex returns. Instruct the client to avoid touching or rubbing the eye until the anesthesia has worn off. Because the client had a foreign body removed, instructions also include reporting drainage, severe irritation, delayed healing, or any other symptoms that may indicate an infection.

Page 503: *Suggested Answer*—Initially, an examination of the client's ear canal is done to determine the presence of cerumen or edema, which would prevent the flow of medication into the canal. If cerumen is present, it is removed by the clinician. If edema is present, a wick may be inserted to allow absorption of the medication. If the ear canal is clear, evaluate the client's administration technique. Instruct the client to pull the pinna up and back, tilt head toward the unaffected side or lie on the side with the affected ear up. After the medication is instilled, allow time for the medication to flow into the ear canal by remaining in the position for 2–3 minutes.

Chapter 16

Page 516: *Suggested Answer*—Three types of phytomedicines that are contraindicated in the client with a history of hemorrhagic stroke are bilberry, feverfew, and garlic (also ginkgo and ginger). Since a hemorrhagic stroke is caused by a bleed, any medication or herb (such as these) that prolongs coagulation time should be avoided.

Page 518: *Suggested Answer*—Ginkgo is recommended for age-related mental decline. By increasing cerebral circulation, it is believed to improve short-term memory and concentration. New evidence suggests effective use in the treatment of Alzheimer's disease and dementia. The appropriate phytotherapy for this client would be American ginseng, which will help the client (student) improve concentration and stamina, and increase the body's ability to resist stress.

Page 521: *Suggested Answer*—Milk thistle is known as the liver herb. It has been shown to protect hepatocytes from toxins and enhance regeneration of the liver cells. It has also been shown to be effective in reducing hepatotoxicity with concomitant use of psychoactive drugs such as phenothiazines and in treating overdose of the death cap mushroom.

Page 522: *Suggested Answer*—Some other names used to identify St. John's wort are amber goatweed, Johnswort, klamanthweed, God's wonder plant, touch-and-heal, witch's herb, chassediable, and devil's scourge. Since many of the herbs are identified by several names, including the English common, brand name, or foreign translation, it is important to be familiar with these names to help the client identify them appropriately.

Page 524: *Suggested Answer*—The ability to assess labeling of the container is necessary for safe and effective use of phytotherapy. Read the label for the specific, intended use. Also, the client should read the label for dosage, placing more trust in phytomedicines that contain a standardized form of the herb. The dosage should be clear and include length of therapy required for expected results. The client should also read the label to determine where the herb was manufactured. Although some European herbs are highly regulated and standardized, caution should be taken with those herbs manufactured or purchased outside of the United States, because the herbs may be contaminated. The letters *USP* (United States Pharmacopoeia) demonstrate standards were followed in the herb's manufacture and that the herb has an approved use by the FDA. If use of the herb has not been approved by the FDA, the label should read "NF" (National Formulary), meaning that the manufacturer has at least followed the same standards of quality and purity.

➤ *Case Study Suggested Answers*

Chapter 1

1. The nurse will assess this client's ability to read the medication labels accurately since the client has diminished vision; the nurse is also concerned with client's ability to accurately draw up the prescribed dose of Humulin since the insulin syringe calibrations are small. Assessment of the client's short-term memory in relation to the medication regimen is also indicated. The client may forget to take ordered medications or may take the medication and then forget and take the dose again. The nurse plans ahead to make these assessments in a way that is sensitive to the older client's feelings about age-related changes.

2. During this home visit, the nurse will gather data on the client's current blood pressure, blood glucose level, and the client's report of pain in knees. These data will provide information on the effects of the drug regimen.

3. Based on the nurse's assessment of the client's ability to be accurate and to comply with the drug regimen, the nurse may suggest measures to assist the client with medication management:
   - Use of a drug dosing box that can be prepared weekly and serves to remind client of time of dose for each day
   - One week's doses of insulin can be prepared and placed in refrigerator with labels for each day's use
   - Prepare a large-print label for the medication supply
   - A family member can be enlisted to assist the client with this activity, keeping track of the number of pills in the supply as a way of evaluating the client's use of the drug

4. The client's report of feeling dizzy should be carefully assessed in this client. Client safety during these episodes is of high priority. The nurse will listen to the client's description for information on the timing and circumstances of feeling "dizzy"; the drug lisinopril (Zestril) has

a side effect of orthostatic hypotension, which may cause the symptom of dizziness when the client changes position, especially from sitting to standing. The nurse will measure the client's blood pressure when the client is lying down and again when standing to note if there is significant difference in these values. The symptom of dizziness, especially associated with weakness and sweating, may occur if the client experiences hypoglycemia that may result from inadequate food intake and the dose of Humulin; the effects of Humulin last for 24 hours after injection and its peak effects occur at 4–12 hours after injection. The nurse will instruct the client to move positions slowly and to have an available source of sugar at hand to deal with onset of this symptom; the nurse may make a judgment to contact the physician to discuss this situation.

5. The nurse will plan to use printed educational materials for this client based on the following:
   * The client's interest in reading about the prescribed drug therapy
   * The client's reading level as compared to the reading level of the prepared materials
   * The print size of the prepared materials
   * The client's primary language

The nurse will introduce the materials one at a time and spend time reviewing them with the client to prevent sensory and information overload.

Chapter 2

1. Assess allergies to previous penicillin therapy and to cephalosporins because there is cross-sensitivity between the two classes of antibiotics; occurrence of mild erythematous, maculopapular rash is not a hypersensitivity reaction but needs to be reported to the health care provider. Gastrointestinal side effects do not preclude the client from taking amoxicillin (Amoxil).

   Assess vital signs, especially temperature, to establish baseline febrile status, to assess the immunologic response, to determine if interventions are indicated for client's comfort, and to determine baseline for future evaluation of drug therapy effectiveness.

   Determine if the client is pregnant. Safe use during pregnancy has not been established although antibiotic therapy will probably be implemented. The risks for rheumatic heart disease and acute glomerulonephritis as sequelae to a "strep throat" infection are significant.

   Assess renal function since the drug is usually excreted through the kidneys; periodic assessment of BUN and creatinine would be indicated for prolonged therapy.

   If complete blood count (CBC) results are available, leukocytosis with elevated neutrophils, bands, and stabs would be expected with this diagnosis of an acute bacterial infection.

   Assess concurrent medications that may interact, such as tetracycline, which may interfere with the

anti-infective property of the amoxicillin; and probenecid (Benemid), which delays excretion of the antibiotic and prolongs its effect.

2. Assess for improvement of clinical manifestations including fever, dysphagia, malaise, and inflamed, erythematous posterior oropharynx and tongue with white pustules. Improvement of signs and symptoms should be observed within 48–72 hours of antibiotic therapy. Identify negative results on re-culture of oropharynx and resolution of leukocytosis if respective laboratory findings are available. No or minimal side effects occur.

3. Assess number and characteristics of stools. Pseudomembranous colitis is characterized by at least 4 to 6 watery stools a day with blood and/or mucus, a newly developed fever, and abdominal cramping. If pseudomembranous colitis is suspected, arrange for culture and sensitivity on a stool specimen. If positive, collaborate with the prescriber regarding discontinuation of the antibiotic and initiation of vancomycin (Vancocin) or metronidazole (Flagyl) to treat the colitis.

   If the diarrhea is mild, yogurt or buttermilk can be added to the diet to counter eradication of the normal intestinal flora. An absorbent antidiarrheal agent as kaolin and pectin (Kao-tin) may be prescribed. In either case, ensure hydration and assess for hypokalemia, which often demonstrates nonspecific symptoms such as muscle weakness, fatigue, anorexia, nausea, irritability, and depressed T wave.

4. The full course of antibiotic therapy must be completed in order to better ensure eradication of the pathogenic organisms, to prevent regrowth of organisms that can occur with premature discontinuation of the antibiotic, and to decrease the risk for drug resistance to develop.

   The antibiotic should be continued for at least 48–72 hours after clinical manifestations of the infection are resolved. Further, this client with a hemolytic streptococcal infection needs at least 10 days of antibiotic therapy to prevent complications such as acute glomerulonephritis and acute rheumatic fever.

   If the drug is not used and is kept available for future self-administration, the client may not be taking the correct type of anti-infective and/or the drug potency may be less.

   The 2 infectious sequelae that could occur are acute rheumatic fever and acute glomerulonephritis.

5. If the client is taking oral contraceptives, advise client that the antibiotic may interfere with the effectiveness of the oral contraceptive and an alternate method of contraception will need to be used during therapy with amoxicillin and for one month after treatment has been discontinued. Breakthrough bleeding may occur.

   Take medication around the clock at evenly spaced intervals without interrupting sleep, as possible. This schedule better ensures sustaining a therapeutic drug level.

   If a dose is missed, take as soon as remembered, but do not double-dose at the next administration time.

Report side effects such as rash, urticaria, wheezing, and GI adverse effects that are severe such as nausea, vomiting, and diarrhea. May take dose with food to minimize gastrointestinal distress. Practice good hygiene including washing hands frequently, disposing of tissues properly, and not sharing eating utensils. Encourage fluid intake of at least 8 glasses a day. Explain rationale for completing full course of treatment and for follow-up.

Chapter 3

1. The most important nursing diagnoses include the following:
   - Risk for Infection related to intravenous administration of antineoplastic agents and resulting myelosuppression.
   - Risk for Decreased Cardiac Output related to administration of a cardiotoxic chemotherapeutic agent.
   - Risk for Injury: Hemorrhage related to intravenous administration of antineoplastic agents and resulting myelosuppression.
   - Risk for Imbalanced Nutrition: Less than Body Requirements related to intravenous administration of antineoplastic agents, which cause excessive nausea and vomiting.
   - Deficient Knowledge related to the side effects of chemotherapy.
   - Risk for Impaired Oral Mucous Membranes related to intravenous administration of antineoplastic agents.
   - Risk for Impaired Tissue Integrity related to the administration of an intravenous vesicant chemotherapeutic agent.

   The nursing diagnoses are listed in priority from the most life threatening to the least. Since the development of infection is the most life threatening, it is listed first. Doxorubicin (Adriamycin) can cause cardiomyopathy and is therefore listed second. All of the agents can cause myelosuppression; therefore, the risk for development of thrombocytopenia needs to be assessed. Excessive nausea and vomiting can cause nutritional alteration. Although deficient knowledge is an actual problem, the potential problems that precede it are more life threatening, should they occur. Methotrexate (Folex) and 5-FU commonly cause impaired mucous membranes, which can also promote nutritional alterations. While extravasation of a vesicant is a potential problem, it is listed last since it is rare.

2. The following are important diagnostic or assessment values that need to be obtained before initiating the chemotherapy:
   - Ejection fraction from the multi-gated acquisition (MUGA) scan. If less than 50%, the prescriber should be notified before administration of Adriamycin.
   - Liver function studies (LFS) and complete blood count (CBC). If LFS are elevated, the prescriber should be notified for potential dosage reduction. The WBC and differential should be assessed to ensure the absolute granulocyte count (AGC) is greater than or equal to 1,500/mm³.
   - Obtain ultrasound of the liver and ensure no abnormality is found.
   - Client's vital signs, including weight, height, temperature, blood pressure, and pulse.

3. A pretreatment teaching plan for this client could include the following outlined elements:
   - Discuss chemotherapy agents prescribed.
   - Discuss potential side effects and mechanisms of preventing
     - Nausea and vomiting.
     - Stomatitis.
     - Extravasation.
     - Hemorrhagic cystitis.
     - Sterility.
   - Teach client to report burning or sting of chemotherapy upon administration.
   - Teach client mechanisms to prevent infection.
   - Teach oral care and demonstrate mixing of solutions.
   - Discuss contraceptive methods if appropriate.

4. The orders that need further clarification with the prescriber are as follows:
   - Loading dosage of ondansetron (Zofran) exceeds the recommended dose of 20 mg.
   - The dose of 5-FU seems to be too low. Is it a transcription error?
   - Since this is the client's first dose of chemotherapy and he does not have a central venous line (CVC), does the health care provider intend on placing a temporary CVC such as a peripherally inserted central catheter (PICC) or triple-lumen catheter (TLC) for this treatment?

5. The following should be done to prepare the client for discharge from the hospital:
   - Reinforce continuation of oral hygiene after discharge.
   - Reinforce mechanisms to prevent infection.
   - Identify primary caregiver and/or financial resources to obtain one temporarily.
   - Teach anticipated nadir period, and signs and symptoms to report to the health care provider.

Chapter 4

1. A weight-based heparin therapy protocol is being used as it is the most effective method for achieving a therapeutic anticoagulation level in a short amount of time. Weight-based therapy helps individualize the dosage, client response, and therapeutic level. It takes into account individual requirements because the drug dosage is based on the client's weight. Many times, in adult clients, the dosage will be the same for all clients regardless of size and weight (e.g., antibiotic therapy). However, in most acute-care settings, it is important to go back to weight-based dosing to achieve a safe and therapeutic effect.

2. Activated partial thromboplastin time (APTT) would help to establish therapeutic blood levels of heparin

administration. It would be important to obtain baseline complete blood count (CBC) with differential, serum chemistry, and coagulation studies. In addition, labs should be done per protocol and the results trended to establish therapeutic levels. A Doppler/vascular study may be necessary to evaluate the client's deep vein thrombus (DVT).

3. The nurse can help to decrease client's anxiety by explaining why lab tests are necessary. It is important to offer the client information and emotional support to make the client feel a part of the health care team. It is important to spend time with the client and determine whether or not this anxiety is related to "frequent blood tests" or if there are any other underlying reasons that could be causing the client to be anxious.

4. It is important to give both verbal and written instructions for warfarin (Coumadin) therapy to the client before discharge. Referral to a dietitian and continued follow-up will help to have the client feel that a health care team is available to supply necessary information and support. It would be important to include family members in the client teaching so that the client can meet therapeutic goals in a safe environment. It may be helpful to share with the client that many people are on this medication on a long-term basis and live well within the guidelines without adverse effects.

Chapter 5

1. You would need several pieces of information before addressing discharge medications.
   - What type of myocardial infarction (MI) did the client have?
   - Has the client been taking any medications?
   - Does the client have the financial resources to comply with treatment?
   - Is the client interested in complying with treatment?

2. Assess vital signs including HR, BP, and respiration to become familiar with client's baseline. Assess the client's baseline knowledge of the MI and long-term consequences so teaching can proceed from the level of understanding that the client currently has. Assess baseline knowledge of the role of each medication for the same reason. Ask the client about daily habits (getting up, eating, bedtime) as these will affect the teaching plan.

3. Teach the client as you assess the importance of each measurement. Instruct the client how to measure pulse and blood pressure. Discuss where the client could purchase a BP cuff. Discuss the importance of following the cardiac rehabilitation program if needed. Inform the client about available resources. Start teaching at least 24 hours before discharge. Do not wait until the client is dressed and ready to leave! After your initial assessment of the client's knowledge, use many resources to provide medication instructions. Use a written chart with specific names and doses of medications. Decide the best times of day for the client to take medication. When completed,

make several copies. Attach one to the client's teaching record and give the remaining copies to the client.

4. Tell the client not to stop the medications because the client may experience worsening symptoms, including sudden hypertension (be certain to use language appropriate to the knowledge level of your client). This could lead to another MI or even stroke (cerebrovascular accident, or CVA). Instruct the client to obtain enough medication before vacation because sometimes (depending on the location) a person might not be able to obtain the correct medication if a refill is needed.

5. Before discharge, sit down with the client and ask the client to tell you about the medications. Allow the client to look at the chart you have constructed together. This should not be a threatening time for the client. Encourage the client by reinforcing correct information, and fill in any missing information. Encourage the client to ask questions and to call prescriber with any questions.

Chapter 6

1. It is important to inform the client that type 1 diabetes mellitus (DM) can occur at any age but is most likely to occur in childhood and adolescence. In type 1 DM, the beta cells of the pancreas are destroyed, which yields an absence of insulin. Type 1 DM is an autoimmune disease in which the immune system kills the insulin-producing cells, which causes the client's need for insulin injections. It is important to inform the client of the genetic predisposition to diabetes mellitus. Approximately 1 in 20 children of a parent with diabetes will become diabetic.

2. The clinical manifestations of DM are caused by glucose molecules, which accumulate in the blood causing hyperglycemia. This leads to increased blood volume because of increased osmolality and increased renal flow with osmotic diuresis (polyuria). Glucose is then excreted in the urine, which is known as glucosuria. Since these factors cause dehydration, the client experiences polydipsia (increased thirst). The client will then become lethargic and experience excessive hunger. The excessive hunger is called polyphagia. Thus, polyuria, polydipsia, and polyphagia are the cardinal signs of diabetes mellitus.

3. Hyperglycemia is a glucose level above 110–120 mg/dL. The normal blood glucose (BG) is 70–110 or 80–120 depending on the laboratory. It is important that the client understand that a sudden BG decrease to 45–60 mg/dL is considered hypoglycemia and should be treated with a quick-acting sugar. Severe hypoglycemia can cause coma and ultimately death. An increase in blood glucose can result from overconsumption of food, lack of exercise, decrease in insulin administration, or onset of illness or infection. Manifestations of diabetic ketoacidosis are a blood glucose level of 250 mg/dL or higher and a plasma pH less than 7.3. The client's bicarbonate level will be less than 15 mEq/L. The client will present with glycosuria and ketonuria, which could also lead to coma or death if untreated.

4. It is important that the client understand that she should consume breakfast and supper approximately one half hour after taking her regular insulin. The peak of the regular insulin and the onset of action of the NPH insulin will occur at the time her breakfast or dinner are being metabolized, thus raising the blood glucose. Her lunch will be affected by the peak of her NPH insulin. Also the midafternoon snack will provide the body with energy to counteract the remaining NPH insulin. It is important that the evening meal be consumed approximately one half hour after the evening insulin dose. The peak of the regular insulin will occur at the time the supper meal is being digested and metabolized. The evening snack will maintain the proper BG through the night to prevent an insulin reaction.

Chapter 7

1. The symptoms the client is describing are related to gastroesophageal reflux disease, which is the backward flow of gastric acid into the esophagus from the stomach. This explains why he is experiencing heartburn and cough, particularly at night.
2. In regards to the client's diet, alcohol consumption increases the gastric acid leading to reflux. It is important that the client understand that he should not consume food or fluids prior to retiring. It is important that he understands that lying recumbent will increase the chance of gastric acid reflux. Also, the foods he is consuming prior to bedtime will contribute to acid reflux such as coffee, mint, and dairy products.
3. In the event of *H. pylori,* omeprazole (Prilosec) can be combined with clarithromycin (Prevpak) to eradicate the infection.
4. Antacids and proton pump inhibitors reduce gastric secretions and promote healing of erosive esophagitis. These medications will also relieve the symptoms of heartburn. The client should be instructed to maintain his medication schedule in order that complications of gastroesophageal reflux disease such as Barrett's esophagus will not develop. Barrett's esophagus is caused by a change in cells lining the esophagus and increases the risk of esophageal cancer development.

Chapter 8

1. The priority nursing diagnoses preoperatively include the following:
   - Risk for Injury related to impaired clotting
   - Activity Intolerance related to illness state and fatigue
   - Impaired Tissue Integrity related to edema
   - Ineffective Family Coping related to fear of the unknown
   - Acute Pain related to liver enlargement
   - Deficient Knowledge related to surgical experience
   - Excess Fluid Volume related to diminished liver function

The most important nursing diagnoses postoperatively include the following:
   - Ineffective Airway Clearance related to pain and surgical incision
   - Acute Pain related to surgical procedure
   - Fear related to life-threatening surgery
   - Disturbed Body Image related to extensive scarring
   - Deficient Knowledge related to postoperative care, medication administration, and infection-related side effects of immunosuppressant medications.
2. It is important for the following laboratory studies to be assessed prior to and during the administration of the medications:
   - Aspartate aminotransferase (AST)/alanine aminotransferase (ALT)
   - Blood glucose
   - Blood urea nitrogen (BUN) and creatinine
   - Electrolytes: sodium, potassium, calcium, magnesium, and phosphorus
   - Complete blood count (CBC) and platelet count
   - Uric acid
3. The teaching plan for the client and family should include the following elements:
   - Discuss medications that have been prescribed by the physician.
   - Discuss potential side effects of medications.
   - Instruct the client and family on prevention of infection, since the goal of immunosuppressant therapy is to decrease the immune response and prevent rejection of the transplanted liver.
   - Instruct about pain relief measures.
   - Instruct on coping mechanisms to assist in preventing anxiety and depression.
4. Nursing interventions that should be implemented prior to discharge after portal vein repair include the following:
   - Instruct on signs and symptoms of bleeding, and report any sign of bleeding to the health care provider.
   - Instruct on care of the incision site.
   - Instruct on prevention of infections.
   - Instruct on proper nutrition.
   - Assess for signs and symptoms of liver failure.
   - Assess AST/ALT periodically as available.
   - Assess vital signs frequently.
   - Instruct the client on turning, coughing, and deep breathing to prevent atelectasis.
   - Provide pain relief measures.
5. Methylprednisolone (SoluMedrol) is administered following the portal vein repair to decrease the inflammation within the liver and diminish the likelihood of organ rejection.

Chapter 9

1. Benzaclin is a combination of Benzoyl peroxide and clindamycin. Benzaclin provides an antibacterial and keratolytic activity. It should be applied twice daily after

cleansing of the affected areas. The client should be assessed for reaction to the medication. The client should be assessed for hypersensitivity reactions.

2. Isotretinoin is Accutane, which is a retinoic acid derivative. It is used for severe recalcitrant nodular acne that is unresponsive to conventional therapy. It should only be administered for 15–20 weeks. The dosage can increase from 0.5–1 mg/kg/day in divided doses to 2–4 mg/kg/day. It is contraindicated in clients who are sensitive to parabens. Parabens are used as preservatives. The action of the medication is that it normalizes keratinization and decreases the size of the sebaceous glands. It is important that the young client be assessed for any psychiatric disorders, asthma, liver disease, anorexia, and diabetes. Although this is not particular to this case, any sexually active woman of child-bearing age should be taking oral or topical contraceptives.

3. This is the proper dose for this client but it could be raised to 2–4 mg/kg/day in divided doses.

4. The client should protect his skin from the sun due to the photosensitive nature of both medications. The client should apply sunscreen when exposed to the sun. He should avoid using vitamin A products. He should not use Tetracycline due to increase potential for the development of pseudotumor cerebri. He should be aware that food taken with medication increases absorption, thus it should be taken with food. Instruct him that alcohol use may increase hypertriglyceridemia. The client should report any visual disturbances, joint pain, or muscle pain.

Chapter 10

1. Questions to ask the family upon arrival should include the following:
   - When did the client have his last seizure?
   - When did the client last take his seizure medication?
   - What other medications is the client taking, both prescription and nonprescription?
   - Is the client currently experiencing an unusual amount of stress?

2. Initial assessments should include level of consciousness (LOC), mental status, and vital signs. These provide a baseline measurement of the client's neurologic, cardiac, and respiratory status.

3. The priorities of care for the client while he is in the emergency department include to keep him seizure-free and explore why the client experienced the seizure.

4. The client education points that are of highest priority prior to discharge home include the following:
   - Medication regimen including dose, schedule, side effects, and adverse effects
   - When to call health care provider
   - The importance of always taking prescribed medication
   - Health care follow-up needed to ensure therapeutic dosage levels

5. Medications or foods that could interfere with the client's seizure medication include the following:
   - Phenytoin: alcohol, antacids, antineoplastics, and antihistamines (note: the only foods that interfere with phenytoin are tube feedings, which do not apply to this client).
   - Phenobarbital: theophylline, corticosteroids, and doxycycline

Chapter 11

1. Disulfiram (Antabuse) is taken by clients with alcoholism to help them refrain from drinking alcohol. This drug discourages drinking by causing severe adverse effects if alcohol is ingested. Disulfiram has no applications outside the treatment for alcoholism. It works in the following way:
   - Disulfiram disrupts alcohol metabolism by causing irreversible inhibition of aldehyde dehydrogenase (the enzyme that converts acetaldehyde to acetic acid).
   - Then, if alcohol is ingested, acetaldehyde will accumulate to toxic levels, producing unpleasant and potentially harmful effects.

2. Clients must be thoroughly informed about the potential hazards of treatment:
   - Teach clients that consumption of any alcohol can cause potentially hazardous or fatal effects.
   - Teach clients orally and in writing to avoid all forms of alcohol, including alcohol in sauces, cough syrups, and vanilla extract.
   - Inform client that disulfiram effects will persist for about 2 weeks after the last dose is taken—alcohol must not be taken during those 2 weeks.
   - Encourage client to carry identification indicating this status.

3. The purpose for use of disulfiram is to help individuals avoid alcohol use until their recovery program is established and they are better able to avoid alcohol without the use of disulfiram.

4. Other treatment options available include 12-step recovery program meetings (Alcoholics Anonymous or other self-help programs), group therapy, aftercare groups, individual counseling if necessary, and group therapy if indicated.

5. Therapy may last for months or even years but should be used only with individuals who are healthy and motivated toward abstinence from alcohol.

Chapter 12

1. When administering lisinopril (Prinivil, Zestril), the client should be informed to report any signs or symptoms of angioedema such as laryngeal edema or facial edema. The client should report any fever, infection, or sore throat. The medication should be taken daily.

2. The client should adhere to a low-sodium diet. The client should not use salt substitutes due to the increased risk of hyperkalemia.

3. The medications can cause an increase in liver enzymes, so liver function and kidney function tests should be evaluated at intervals throughout administration. The client should be instructed of the following adverse effects: dizziness, headache, fatigue, orthostatic hypotension, muscle cramps, hyperkalemia, diarrhea, nasal congestion, impotence, dyspepsia, nonproductive cough, and angioedema.

4. The action of lisinopril may result from suppression of the renin–angiotensin–aldosterone system, thus lowering blood pressure.

Chapter 13

1. Dinoprostone (Prepidil, Cervidil) is FDA-approved for cervical ripening prior to the induction of labor. Prepidil intracervical gel contains 0.5 mg of dinoprostone and is inserted into the cervix after direct visualization via speculum. Cervidil vaginal insert contains 10-mg dinoprostone, and one insert is placed into the posterior cul-de-sac, with the string protruding out of the vagina. The client should remain recumbent after administration.

2. Labor induction is accomplished by starting a peripheral IV, using either Y-tubing or piggy-backing into the main line, and infusing the oxytocin (Pitocin) solution via infusion pump. The oxytocin (Pitocin) solution is most commonly diluted as 10 units in 1 liter of IV fluid (although some practitioners will order 20 units in 1 liter.) The Pitocin is begun at 1 or 2 milliunits, and increased every 20–30 minutes until adequate contractions occur.

3. Because of the hypertension of preeclampsia, the oxytocin (Pitocin) solution infusion rate would be increased. If this did not control the hemorrhage, carboprost tromethamine (Hemabate) would be utilized, as it produces less increase in blood pressure than do either methylergonovine (Methergine) or ergonovine (Ergotrate).

4. Magnesium sulfate is most commonly used for the seizures of eclampsia. A 4- to 6-gram loading dose is given over 20 minutes, and then 1–2 grams per hour is usually given via IV infusion.

5. Breastfeeding women can use progestin-only preparations for contraception. This includes medroxyprogesterone acetate (Depo-Provera) IM, levonorgestrel intradermal implants (Norplant), or oral norethindrone (Micronor or Nor-QD).

Chapter 14

1. Albuterol (Proventil) is a beta-adrenergic agent that is given orally or by inhalation and is used to treat and prevent bronchoconstriction. Albuterol will dilate constricted airways to ease breathing, and should be taken exactly as ordered. Beta$_2$-specific actions may be diminished at larger than prescribed doses. Therefore, the client may experience cardiac symptoms such as increased heart rate, and at larger doses, she may also experience nausea, anxiety, and tremors. The effects of this medication can be intensified by decongestants and some antihistamines. The prescriber should be notified prior to taking any OTC medications. Some clients experience hypotension and vascular headaches with albuterol. The client should have blood pressure and heart rate monitored regularly to ensure there are no cardiac side effects. She should be taught the proper use of an inhaler. The client should note the color, amount, and character of sputum. Oral doses of this medication should be taken with meals to decrease gastric upset. She should keep a record of when medications are taken and whether or not symptoms subside to determine the effectiveness of the medication. Inhalations of different medications should be taken at least one minute apart or longer depending on product literature. The client should avoid eye contact with the spray of an inhaled medication. Wheezing and dyspnea should decrease with the administration of this medication. If this does not occur, the prescriber should be notified. She should take the inhaler to school with her so that it can be taken as needed in the event of an acute asthmatic attack. She should begin to note which allergens cause her difficulty and attempt to avoid them. Also, increased fluid intake will help liquefy any secretions and ease expectoration.

2. Beclomethasone (Beclovent) is an inhaled corticosteroid that is thought to decrease the release of bronchoconstricting substances. Swelling in the airways is thought to diminish. This medication is to be used preventatively and not for an acute attack. She should take the medication whether or not symptoms are present. Inhaled corticosteroids are not as likely to cause the typical systemic effects of corticosteroids because of the route of administration. Symptoms of a cold or the flu should be reported to the physician immediately due to the potential for suppression of the immune system. This is less likely with inhaled corticosteroids than with oral corticosteroids. Allergens should be identified and avoided. She should be aware of symptoms and notice any increase or decrease. Difficulty should be reported to the health care provider. She should be taught to note the amount, color, and character of sputum. Increased fluid intake helps thin secretions and ease removal. Hard candy decreases difficulty with mouth dryness. She should wear a bracelet that identifies her as one who takes corticosteroids. The medication should be taken exactly as prescribed and not overused. The medication should not be stopped abruptly. The correct use of the inhaler should be taught as well as the need to rinse the mouth after inhalation of medication.

3. It is important for the nurse to understand the teenage client. Acceptance by the peer group as well as being similar to the peer group is very important to the 14-year-old. Exploration of ways the client can administer the needed

medications without making her appear different from her peers would be beneficial. Another aspect to consider is that teenagers are normally healthy. Sickness in a teenager makes the young person different from the norm. Attempting to help the client incorporate the illness into her self-concept will aid in acceptance as well as compliance. The nurse should respond with compassionate understanding of the real issues faced by the client even if it seems insignificant to the health care worker. Assisting her to determine ways that she can participate in the normal activities of a 14-year-old in spite of her illness will help with acceptance and compliance.

4. The anticipated effect of albuterol is to dilate the airway and ease breathing. With proper use of the medication, she should experience less wheezing and dyspnea. Some of the side effects of albuterol are listed in the answer to question 1. Additional side effects include tremors, hypokalemia, hyperglycemia, nausea, vomiting, chest pain, dysrhythmias, paradoxical bronchospasms, and urinary retention. The anticipated effect of beclomethasone is to decrease inflammation of the airway and therefore ease breathing. She should notice a decrease in the symptoms of dyspnea and wheezing. Potential side effects include pharyngeal irritation, coughing, dry mouth, oral fungal infections, sore throat, and sinusitis. Some clients experience diarrhea, nausea, vomiting, and stomach upset. Menstrual disturbances are possible and should be reported to the prescriber.

5. The nurse should assess respiratory function. She should talk to the client about the disease and assess her acceptance of the disease and the treatment. The nurse should determine whether or not medications are taken regularly and properly. It would be helpful to observe the client with self-administration of the inhaled medications to be sure her technique is appropriate. Determine whether or not the client is experiencing any side effects. Explore her thoughts and feelings about the disease and its treatment, about the medications and whether or not the symptoms are controlled. Determine whether or not she can participate in the activities that are important to her. Talk to her about whether or not she feels accepted by her friends and if she has any feelings about being different from her friends. This will give the nurse information about her acceptance of the disease and her tolerance not only of the disease, but of the treatment for the disease as well. Acceptance of the disease and its treatment will aid in compliance.

Chapter 15

1. Glaucoma is a disease of the eye characterized by elevated intraocular pressure. The increase in intraocular pressure results from excessive production of aqueous humor or a decrease in the outflow of aqueous humor. Persistent high intraocular pressures may lead to blindness. The medication prescribed, betaxolol (Betoptic), is a beta-adrenergic blocking agent that decreases the production of aqueous humor, thereby reducing intraocular pressure.

2. Because of its ß selectivity, Betoptic is the drug of choice for clients with pulmonary disease. However, beta-blocking agents are used cautiously in clients with pulmonary disease (risk of bronchospasm). The client should be monitored for cardiopulmonary complications.

3. Local side effects include burning, stinging, and eye irritation. Systemic absorption may lead to bradycardia, congestive heart failure, cardiac dysrhythmias, bronchospasm, insomnia, dizziness, vertigo, and gastrointestinal disturbances. The client should report these symptoms to the health care provider.

4. Photophobia may result from use of Betoptic. The client should wear dark sunglasses and avoid bright lights.

5. Instruct the client to wash hands, look up toward the ceiling, pull down the lower eyelid to form a sac, and then instill the medication into the sac. Instruct the client to avoid touching the eye, and to avoid touching the eyedropper to the eye or any other object. Instruct the client to use nasolacrimal occlusion (press on the tear duct) to minimize systemic absorption.

Chapter 16

1. The nurse should assess the client for cross allergy to ragweed, pregnancy (or potential for) or lactation. The client history and physical should be performed to assess for contraindications to the use of feverfew, such as bleeding disorders and the use of any anticoagulants or herbs that increase bleeding time, such as bilberry, ginger, garlic, and ginkgo.

2. There is not consensus on the dosage of feverfew. Most sources recommend anywhere from 50–125 mg of the dried herb, which should be taken with or after meals to reduce GI colic. An accepted dose to prevent a migraine attack is 0.25–0.5 mg and 1–2 grams to control a migraine attack.

3. Feverfew is effective in the prevention and treatment of recurrent migraine headaches by inhibiting the release of serotonin. It is believed that the activation of cerebral neurons containing serotonin (as well as norepinephrine) are responsible for the precipitation of a migraine headache.

4. Feverfew may cause post–feverfew syndrome (muscle and joint pain, aching, and stiffness) when discontinued abruptly. To reduce the risk of these symptoms, the client should taper off the feverfew.

5. The client should be instructed to avoid any medications that have an anticoagulant effect, such as ASA (aspirin) and ibuprofen (Motrin). It is important to include education regarding accurate assessment of labels on other OTC medications, such as cold and influenza preparations that may contain these medications. Any other herbs that may play a role in blood clotting should be avoided, including bilberry, garlic, ginger, and gingko.

Appendix B
Reference Tables

Appendix B-1	Common Abbreviations in Pharmacology		
ac	before meals	mg	milligram
ACE	angiotensin-converting enzyme	ml, mL	milliliter
ARB	angiotensin II receptor blocker	NSAID	nonsteroidal anti-inflammatory drug
ASA	acetylsalicylic acid (aspirin)	OTC	over-the-counter
bid	2 times a day	OU	both eyes
cc	cubic centimeter	pc	after meals
COX	cyclooxygenase	PO	oral, by mouth
DMARD	disease modifying antirheumatic drug	PPD	purified protein derivative
DPI	dry powder inhaler	PR	per rectum
gm	gram	PRN	as needed
h, hr	hour	q	every
HRT	hormone replacement therapy	qid	4 times a day
IM	intramuscular(ly)	qod	every other day
IV	intravenous(ly)	SubQ/SQ	subcutaneous(ly)
kg	kilogram	sl	sublingual
KVO	keep vein open	stat	immediately
l, L	liter	tid	3 times a day
MAOI	monoamine oxidase inhibitor		
MDI	metered dose inhaler		

| Appendix B-2 | Therapeutic Drug Levels |

Generic (Trade) Names	Level in Conventional Units	Level in SI Units
acetaminophen (Tylenol)	0.2–0.6 mg/dL; toxic: greater than 5 mg/dL	13–40 micromoles/L
carbamazepine (Tegretol)	4–12 mcg/mL	375–900 nmol/L
digoxin (Lanoxin)	0.5–2 ng/mL	1–2.6 nmol/L
lidocaine (Xylocaine HCl)	1.5–6 mcg/mL	6–21 micromoles/L
lithium (Eskalith)	0.5–1.5 mEq/L	0.5–1.5 mmol/L
phenytoin (Dilantin)	10–20 mcg/mL	40–80 mcg/mL
procainamide (Pronestyl)	4–8 mcg/mL	17–40 micromoles/L
quinidine (Quinalgute)	2–6 mcg/mL	4.6–9.2 micromoles/L
salicylate (acetylsalicylic acid; Aspirin)	100–200 mg/L; toxic: greater than 200 mg/L	724–1448 micromoles/L; toxic: greater than 1450 micromoles/L
theophylline (Theo-Dur)	10–20 mcg/mL	55–110 micromoles/L
valproic acid (Depakene)	50–100 mcg/mL	350–700 micromoles/L
vancomycin (Vancocin)	30–40 mg/mL (peak); 5–10 mg/mL (trough)	20–40 mg/dL (peak); 5–10 (trough)

dL, deciliter; L, liter; mcg, microgram; mEq, milliequivalent; mg, milligram; mL, milliliter; ng, nanogram; nmol, nanomole

| Appendix B-3 | Selected Medication/Poison Toxicities and Antidotes |

Substance at Toxic/Poisonous Level	Antidote
Acetaminophen (Tylenol)	acetylcysteine (Mucomyst)
Anticholinergics	physostigmine (Antilirium)
Benzodiazepines	flumazenil (Romazicon)
Calcium channel blockers	calcium chloride, calcium gluconate
Copper	penicillamine (Cuprimine)
Cyanide or nitrate	methylene blue (Urolene blue)
Digoxin (Lanoxin)	digoxin immune fab (Digibind)
Doxorubicin	dexrazoxane (Zinecard)
Heparin	protamine sulfate
Insulin	glucagon
Iron	deferoxamine (Desferal)
Isoniazid	pyridoxine (Nestrex)
Lead	succimer (Chemet)
Methotrexate	leucovorin calcium (Wellcovorin)
Nondepolarizing neuromuscular blockers	neostigmine (Prostigmin)
Opioids	naloxone (Narcan); nalfemene (Revex)
Warfarin sodium (Coumadin)	vitamin K (Aquamephyton)

Appendix B-4   Common Equivalents in Weights and Measures

Volume Equivalents		Mass Equivalents	
1 milliliter	= 0.034 fluid ounce	1 milligram	= 0.0154 grain (apothecary)
			= 1000 micrograms
1 liter	= 1000 milliliters	1 gram	= 15.4 grains (apothecary)
	= 33.8 fluid ounces		
	= 2.11 pints		
	= 1.06 quarts		
1 cubic centimeter	= 1 milliliter	1 grain (apothecary)	= 64.8 milligrams
1 fluid ounce	= 29.6 milliliters	1 ounce (apothecary)	
	= 2 tablespoons		
1 teaspoon	= 5 milliliters	1 ounce (avoirdupois)	= 28.4 grams
1 tablespoon	= 15 milliliters	1 pound (avoirdupois)	= 454 grams
	= 3 teaspoons		= 0.454 kilogram
			= 16 ounces
1 cup	= 237 milliliters	1 kilogram	= 2.2 pounds (avoirdupois)
	= 8 fluid ounces		
1 pint	= 473 milliliters		
	= 16 fluid ounces		
	= 2 cups		
1 quart	= 946 milliliters		
	= 32 fluid ounces		
	= 2 pints		
1 gallon	= 3785 milliliters	**Temperature Conversion**	
	= 128 fluid ounces	(Celsius degrees × 9/5) + 32 = Fahrenheit degrees	
	= 4 quarts	(Fahrenheit degrees −32) × 5/9 = Celsius degrees	

Index

Page numbers followed by b indicate box; those followed by f indicate figure; those followed by t indicate table.